THE
PHYSICAL FITNESS
ENCYCLOPEDIA

Prepared and Edited

by

CHARLES T. KUNTZLEMAN

PAUL F. EYANSON, *Assistant Editor*
ARNE L. OLSON, *Consulting Editor*

RODALE BOOKS, INC.
Emmaus, Pennsylvania 18049

Standard Book Number 87596-046-4
Library of Congress Catalog Number 76-116512
Copyright MCMLXX by Rodale Press, Inc.
ALL RIGHTS RESERVED
PRINTED IN THE UNITED STATES
Second Printing—July, 1971

G-742

To—

Mr. and Mrs. John F. Emhardt
Rev. and Mrs. Walter A. Kuntzleman

Grandparents of Deborah, John and Thomas

Acknowledgments

Grateful acknowledgment is made to the following for permission to use material in this book:

Dr. P. O. Astrand for the chart on the energy cost of activities from the *Canadian Medical Journal*, 1967, XCVI, 907.

Dr. Kenneth H. Cooper for the chart on running activity taken from *Aerobics*, c. 1968, by Kenneth H. Cooper and Kevin Brown and published by M. Evans and Company of New York.

Dr. Thomas K. Cureton for the Progressive Balance Beam Test and the 18 Item Motor Efficiency Test from Physical Fitness Workbook, 1947, C. V. Mosby Company, St. Louis, Missouri.

Dr. M. F. Graham for the charts on determining body surface area and on the obesity cycle, from *Prescription for Life*, c. 1966, New York. Reprinted by permission David McKay Company, Inc.

Harper and Row, Publishers for the graphs on pulse rate from *Science and Medicine in Exercise and Sports*, 1960, Harper and Row, New York.

Dr. Edmund Jacobson for the material on the relaxation techniques of the arm for *Self Operations Control*, c. 1964, J. P. Lippincott Company, Philadelphia.

Dr. Ernest Jokl for the charts on age and athletic performance from *Physiology of Exercise*, 1964, Charles C. Thomas, Springfield, Illinois.

Dr. H. C. Lehman for the charts on age and athletic performance from "Chronological Age vs. Proficiency in Physical Skills, *American Journal of Psychology*, 1957, LXIV, 161.

Donald K. Mathews for the material on the RSP program from *Beginning Conditioning*, c. 1965, by Wadsworth Publishing Company, Inc., Belmont, California. Reprinted by permission.

Dr. Jean Mayer for the chart on body weight from the *American Journal of Clinical Nutrition*, 1956, IV, 169.

Dr. Laurence E. Morehouse for material on training from *Sports Medicine for Trainers*, 1964, W. B. Saunders Company, Philadelphia, Pennsylvania.

H. Pollack, C. F. Consolazio and G. J. Isaac for the chart comparing energy costs of activities from "Metabolic Demands as a Factor in Weight Control," *Journal of the American Medical Association*, 1958, CLXVII, 216.

Nathan W. Shock for the chart on aging from "The Physiology of Aging," c. 1962, by Scientific American, Inc. All rights reserved.

This Week magazine and Crown copyright for material from the 5BX

Acknowledgments

and XBX programs in *Royal Canadian Exercise Plans for Physical Fitness,* 1962, Queen's Printer, Ottawa, Canada.

KATHERINE F. WELLS for the material on the range of motion in selected joint movements, from *Kinesiology,* c. 1960, W. B. Saunders Company, Philadelphia, Pennsylvania.

Foreword

The Physical Fitness Encyclopedia is an appropriate contribution to the national interest in physical fitness. Government leaders, physicians, educators, recreators, fitness experts are continually urging the American public to be more active and resist the narcotic of easy living.

To increase our incentive to exercise, researchers are continually discovering new health benefits related to regular exercise, and fitness experts are developing new conditioning techniques. The volume of new and reliable information is so great that categorizing it all into one easy-to-get-to file is difficult for experts, unpractical for the general public.

Congratulations and thanks are due to Charles Kuntzleman for his Herculean achievement in drawing the most pertinent of that information into a single volume. A "thank you" is also due for all the time he has saved those of us who have the continued need for a quick reference to physical fitness information. The fitness-seeking American will find this work invaluable in clarifying his questions about physical fitness.

GLENN SWENGROS
Formerly Director of Program Development for the President's Council on Physical Fitness and Kansas State Director of Health and Physical Fitness

Preface

Perhaps no book is more timely than *The Physical Fitness Encyclopedia*. One of the most pressing reasons for its completion is the fact that most Americans are suffering from "health myopia." They are beset with physiological and psychological ills and do not have the clearness of vision to prevent them. They eat incorrectly, smoke and drink excessively and rest sporadically. And most importantly, they think of exercise as a chore that is to be tolerated mildly and avoided if possible.

This book is an effort to clear the air of the misinformation that clouds the public's understanding of proper health habits. It gives primary emphasis to healthful exercise, although it was written with the knowledge that exercise and fitness are not panaceas for all our maladies. We believe it is most important for each person to be made aware of the direction toward better health indicated by the latest research.

Exercise is pivotal in the real achievement of physical fitness, for it has a salutary effect on all of the body's systems. Yet our mechanized society forces man into inaction, and today, despite his potential, he is much less the vigorous physical creation he was centuries ago. The result? New ailments that once were of trivial importance today cut him down, and he is powerless to resist. Although science has been able to make his life easier, it has not been able to make it longer or more vigorous.

When a caged animal is first captured and placed in a zoo, it is robust, muscular and full of life. But inactivity soon reaps its toll, and it becomes sluggish, fat, irritable and aloof. Modern man is like that caged animal. Whereas he once had to depend on his physical stamina for his existence, today he is actually prevented from accepting any physical challenge. But his body, the same basic organism that served man 6,000 years ago, has become incompatible to the new environment of man's creation.

I am hopeful that this book will not only underline the need for exercise but also provide many avenues for its achievement. If you want to exercise because you feel the need to become more fit, you will benefit from this book. If you've neglected to exercise because you have been unable to find a program that is enjoyable, practicable and adaptable, you will also benefit. To allow for individual needs, I have included programs for fitness through many sports and activities. Use them as stepping stones to better health.

You won't find entries for the traditional sports like football, basketball, baseball and soccer because it's hard for the normal person to get 20 people together 3 or 4 times a week who are interested in those activities as a route to fitness. Should you be interested in those or other sports that have no entries, refer to the sections on CARRY-OVER SPORTS and SPORTS.

Before you read any section of this book, it might be advisable to read the following sections in this order: (1.) PHYSICAL FITNESS; (2.) METABOLISM; (3.) ENERGY COST OF ACTIVITIES; and (4.) INTENSITY OF EXERCISE. Those articles present the concept of physical fitness used in this book, together with information on how the exercise programs were established and how to go about setting up your own program.

There is an endless list of people to whom I am indebted for assistance in making this book a reality, and it is impossible to thank them all. A special thanks goes to Robert Rodale for conceiving the idea of the Encyclopedia and giving me the opportunity to act as editor. It was a tremendous challenge and a rewarding educational experience. Mr. Rodale's concept of health and fitness is dynamic and exciting, for he brings an immediacy to bear on his innovative philosophy that makes fitness a working part of every day.

A special thanks is also extended to John Haberern, editor, and Glenn Johns, managing editor, of FITNESS FOR LIVING magazine for their guidance. Both men gave considerable advice that bettered the book. Mr. Johns had the huge task of special project director. The entire staff at Rodale Press is to be congratulated for their cooperation and helpful suggestions.

I want to thank my wife Carol for her understanding during the five years it took to complete this book. Her personal sacrifices were many. She also read the manuscript and made valuable suggestions.

Finally, a special thanks to the many people involved in physical fitness work whose research and findings form the core of this book.

May 11, 1970   CTK

Contributors and Consultants

AEHNLICH, PAUL C., M.S., Instructor, Department of Physical Education, United States Air Force Academy, Colorado 80840. (Water Polo)

ANDERSON, J. L., Secretary, the Federated Mountain Clubs of New Zealand, Inc., P. O. Box 1604, Wellington, New Zealand. (Tramping)

ARNOLD, JAY, Ed.D., Department of Health, Physical Education and Recreation, Philadelphia, Pennsylvania 19122. (Schools)

BANASZEWSKI, WILLIAM A., M.Ed., Instructor, Department of Health, Physical Education and Recreation, State University of New York at Buffalo, Buffalo, New York 14214. (Obesity)

BENDER, JAY A., Ph.D., Deceased, Formerly Professor of Physiology, Southern Illinois University, Carbondale, Illinois 62901. (Isometrics)

BERENSON, L. STANLEY, President and General Manager, Miami Jai-Alai, Inc., Miami, Florida 33101.

BOSLOOPER, THOMAS, Ph.D., The Reformed Church of Closter, High and West Streets, Closter, New Jersey 07624. (Femininity)

BOYD, ELLSWORTH, 5405 Morello Road, Baltimore, Maryland 21214. (Skin Diving)

BRUESS, CLINT E., Ed.D., Associate Professor, Department of Health Education and Physical Education, West Chester State College, West Chester, Pennsylvania 19380. (Benefits of Exercise, Heart Disease, Tennis)

CASADY, DONALD R., Ph.D., Associate Professor, Department of Physical Education for Men, University of Iowa, Iowa City, Iowa 52240. (Mental Health)

CERUTTY, PERCY W., Director, International Athletes Camp at Portsea, Victoria, Australia. (Aging, Fartlek, Interval Training, Staleness)

CHAMBERLAIN, SHELDON A., JR., M.Ed., Instructor, Department of Health and Physical Education, Montgomery County Community College, Conshohocken, Pennsylvania 19428. (Longevity)

DAVEY, COLIN P., M.Ed., Lecturer, Department of Physical Education, University of Melbourne, Victoria, Australia. (Squash)

DAYTON, O. W., Head Trainer, Yale University, New Haven, Connecticut 06515. (Injuries)

DICKEY, GARLAND M., E.D.D., Professor and Head of Department of Physical Education; Director of Athletic Activities, Berry College, Mount Berry, Georgia 30149. (Community Fitness)

DRAEGER, DONN, Kodokan, Tokyo, Japan. (Judo, Karate)

DUNCAN, W. RAYMOND, M.D., Simon Fraser University, Burnaby, British Columbia, Canada. (Pulse Rate)

EYANSON, PAUL F., M.S., Department of Health and Physical Education, Seton Hall Preparatory School, South Orange, New Jersey 07079.

FRANZ, MAURICE, Managing Editor, Organic Gardening and Farming, Emmaus, Pennsylvania 18049. (Gardening)

FULTON, GERE B., Ph.D., Associate Professor and Coordinator of Health

Education, Department of Health and Physical Education, Trenton State College, Trenton, New Jersey 08685. (Weight Training, Weight Lifting)

GOOD, LARRY, Ed.D., Associate Professor, Department of Physical Education, University of Southern Illinois, Carbondale, Illinois 62901. (Scuba Diving, Skin Diving)

GRABER, RALPH, Ph.D., Professor, Department of English, Muhlenberg College, Allentown, Pennsylvania 18104.

GRAHAM, M. F., M.D., Director of Research and Medical Education, Doctors Hospital, Dallas, Texas 75246. (Ischemic Heart Disease)

HABERERN, JOHN, B.S., Editor, *Fitness For Living*, Emmaus, Pennsylvania 18049. (Community, Low Back Pain, Yoga)

HASKILL, WESTON B., JR., A.B., President, Sport House (SCIA, Inc.), Concord, Massachusetts 01742. (Cross Country Skiing)

HECHT, JEAN A., M.S., Assistant Professor, Department of Physical Education, Muhlenberg College, Allentown, Pennsylvania 18104. (Camping, Hunting, Skiing)

HETTINGER, T., M.D., Privatdozent fur Arbertsmedizen, Sozialhygiene Mediznische Fabultat der TH Aacheu Werksarzt der Rheinstahl Hutteniverke AG, Mulheim (Ruhr), Friedrich-Ebert-Str. 171. (Strength)

HILL, LEE L., Assistant Professor, Department of Physical Education, Fairleigh Dickinson, University of Madison, Madison, New Jersey 07940. (Cholesterol)

HORSTMAN, ROBERT, President, Rodale Manufacturing Co., Emmaus, Pennsylvania 18049. (Surfing)

HOSPODAR, HELENE H., M.A., Assistant Professor, Department of Physical Education, Muhlenberg College, Allentown, Pennsylvania 18104.

JOHNS, GLENN F., M.A., Managing Editor, *Fitness For Living*, Emmaus, Pennsylvania 18049. (Equipment)

JOHNSON, ALEX J., M.A., Research Assistant, Department of Physiology, Southern Illinois University, Carbondale, Illinois 62901. (Isometrics)

KAPLAN, HAROLD M., Ph.D., Professor of Physiology, Southern Illinois University, Carbondale, Illinois 62901. (Isometrics)

KENDALL, BRUCE, M.D., 1416 Cedar Swamp Road, Brookville, New York 11545. (Relaxation)

KINDIG, LOUISE E., Ed.D., Assistant Professor, Department of Health, Physical Education and Recreation, Temple University, Philadelphia, Pennsylvania 19122. (Women)

KING, DOUGLAS W., Ph.D., Assistant Professor, Department of Physical Education for Men, Washington State University, Pullman, Washington 99163. (Jogging)

KRUGER, D. A., T.E.D., Principal, Salvokop Primary School; Secretary, South African Jukskei Board, Pretoria, South Africa.

KUNTZLEMAN, CHARLES T., M.Ed., Assistant Professor, Department of Health and Physical Education, Lehigh County Community College, Schnecksville, Pennsylvania 18078.

LEPHART, S. A., M.S., Lecturer, Department of Physical Education, University of Melbourne, Victoria, Australia. (Canoeing)

LEWIS, A. S., B.A., Department of Physical Education, Olympic Trainer, University of Canterbury, Christchurch, New Zealand. (Body Type, Rowing, Target Training)

LOVINGOOD, BILL W., Ph.D., Associate Professor, Department of Physical

Education, University of North Carolina, Chapel Hill, North Carolina 27514. (Body Composition Determination, Drugs)

MALINA, ROBERT, Ph.D., Assistant Professor, Department of Anthropology, University of Texas, Austin, Texas 78712. (Body Composition, Growth, Races)

MAPES, DONALD F., Ph.D., Associate Professor, Department of Health, Physical Education and Recreation, Western Illinois University, Macomb, Illinois 61455. (Waist)

MARSH, RICHARD L., M.S., Assistant Professor, Department of Health, Physical Education and Recreation, State University of New York College at Buffalo, Buffalo, New York 14222.

MACKEY, RICHARD T., Ed.D., Professor, Department of Health and Physical Education, Miami University, Oxford, Ohio 45056. (Swimming)

McDERMOTT, LAWRENCE, Ed.D., Department of Health, Physical Education and Recreation, Temple University, Philadelphia, Pennsylvania 19122. (Schools)

McHARGUE, PATRICK H., M.A., Executive Office, Department of Physical Education, United States Air Force Academy, Colorado 80840. (Reconditioning)

McPHERSON, BARRY D., M.A., Department of Physical Education, University of Wisconsin, Madison, Wisconsin 53706. (Personality, Psychological Values)

MERRIFIELD, H. H., Ph.D., Associate Professor, Department of Physical Therapy, Ithaca College, Ithaca, New York 14850; Visiting Associate Professor, University of California, Berkeley, when articles were written. (Kinesthesia, Rehabilitation)

MEYERS, CARLTON R., Ed.D., Professor and Acting Chairman of Department of Instruction, Faculty of Educational Studies, State University of New York at Buffalo, Buffalo, New York 14214. (Intelligence, Waterskiing)

MITCHELL, CURTIS, Writer, member National YMCA Committee on Health and Physical Fitness, 5 West Parish Road, Westport, Connecticut 06880. (Altitude, Jogging)

NELSON, JACK K., Ed.D., Associate Professor of Health, Physical Education, and Recreation, Louisiana State University, Baton Rouge, Louisiana 70803. (Altitude)

NELSON, RAY, Public Relations Assistant, American Bowling Congress, Milwaukee, Wisconsin 53201. (Bowling)

NETTLETON, BRUCE, B.A., Lecturer, Department of Physical Education, University of Melbourne, Victoria, Australia. (Hiking and Camping)

NOBLE, BRUCE, Ph.D., Associate Professor, Department of Health and Physical Education, Director, Human Energy Research Laboratory, University of Pittsburgh, Pittsburgh, Pennsylvania 15213. (Work)

OLSON, ARNE L., Ph.D., Professor and Chairman, Department of Health and Physical Education, East Stroudsburg State College, East Stroudsburg, Pennsylvania 18301.

OSNESS, WAYNE H., Ph.D., Assistant Professor, Department of Physical Education and Recreation, University of Kansas, Lawrence, Kansas 66044. (Diet)

OXENDINE, JOSEPH B., Ed.D., Professor and Chairman, Department of Health, Physical Education and Recreation, Temple University, Philadelphia, Pennsylvania 19122. (Motor Learning, Reaction Time)

PATTERSON, CARL, Ed.M., *Deceased,* Assistant Professor and Gymnastics Coach, Department of Health, Physical Education and Recreation, Temple University, Philadelphia, Pennsylvania 19122. (Sailing)

PATTERSON, THOMAS C., B.S., North American Senior Moth Champion, 1965. Department of Health, Physical Education and Recreation, Temple University, Philadelphia, Pennsylvania 19122. (Sailing)

PENCE, ROBERT G., Executive Secretary, National Horseshoe Pitchers' Association, 341 Polk Street, Gary, Indiana 46402.

POWELL, JOHN T., Ph.D., Professor and Director, School of Physical Education, University of Guelph, Ontario, Canada. (Calisthenics)

PUSCHOCK, THOMAS A., A.B., Managing Editor, *Health Bulletin,* Rodale Press, Emmaus, Pennsylvania 18049. (Feats of Fitness)

REES, CARL D., M.A., Assistant Professor, Department of Health, Physical Education and Recreation, University of Pittsburgh, Pittsburgh, Pennsylvania 15213.

RODALE, ROBERT, Publisher, *Fitness For Living,* Emmaus, Pennsylvania 18049. (Bones, Indian Clubs, Motivation, Shooting, Work, Government)

ROSS, WILLIAM D., Ph.D., Assistant Professor, Physical Development Center, Simon Fraser University, Burnaby, British Columbia, Canada. (Pulse Rate)

ROWE, JOANNE, M.S., Assistant Professor, Department of Health and Physical Education, Berry College, Mount Berry, Georgia 30149. (Community Fitness)

RYAN, ALLAN J., M.D., Associate Professor, Department of Physical Education, Clinical Associate Professor, Department of Surgery, Athletic Teams Physicians, University of Wisconsin, Madison, Wisconsin. (Salt Tablets)

SAGE, JOHN N., Ed.D., Assistant Professor, Department of Physical Education, University of California at Riverside, Riverside, California 92507. (Social Context)

SANDSTROM, E. R., M.S., Lecturer, Department of Physical Education, University of Melbourne, Victoria, Australia. (Flexibility, Motor Fitness, Skill)

SCAGNETTI, JACK, 22611 Crespi Drive, Woodland Hills, California 91364. (Jogging)

SHAWN, TED, Honorary M.P.E. (Springfield College) Founder-Director of the Jacob's Pillow Dance Festival and "The University of the Dance." Cor 287, Lee, Massachusetts 01238. (Dance)

SHEEHAN, GEORGE, M.D., Cardiologist, 79 West Front Street, Red Bank, New Jersey 07701. (Running)

SHEETS, NORMAN L., Ed.D., Dean, School of Health, Physical Education, West Chester State College, West Chester, Pennsylvania 19380. (Handball)

SLOCAIN, SEAN, O., General Secretary, Gaelic Athletic Association, Croke Park, Dublin 3, Ireland.

SMITH, ROBERT W., M.A., Economist, United States Government, Author of five books and hundreds of articles on boxing, wrestling and Asian combatives, Graded 3-Dan in Judo. (Karate, Judo)

STOCKHOLM, ALAN J., M.A., Assistant Professor, Department of Men's Physical Education, State University College, Cortland, New York 13045. (Stress)

SWARD, SIDNEY B., Ph.D., Professor, Department of Physical Education, Norfolk State College, Norfolk, Virginia 23504. (Myths)

SWEENEY, ROBERT T., M.Ed., Associate Professor, Coordinator of Elementary Health and Physical Education, Department of Health, Physical Education and Recreation, East Stroudsburg State College, East Stroudsburg, Pennsylvania 18301. (Childhood Fitness)

TEUFEL, ROBERT J., B.A., Vice President, Rodale Press, Emmaus, Pennsylvania 18049. (Fencing)

VINCENT, MURRAY L., Ed.D., Assistant Professor, Department of Health and Physical Education, University of South Carolina, Columbia, South Carolina 29208. (Ergogenic Aids)

WALTERS, MARSHALL L., Professor and Chairman, Department of Health, Physical Education and Recreation, Appalachian State University, Boone, North Carolina 28607. Editor, USVBA Volleyball Guide and Rule Book. (Volleyball)

WHITE, PAUL DUDLEY, M.D., Eminent Heart Specialist, 264 Beacon Street, Boston, Massachusetts 02116. (Health)

WILLEE, ALBERT W., Ph.D., V.R.D., Director of Physical Education, University of Melbourne, Victoria, Australia. (Fads and Fitness)

WILMORE, JACK H., Ph.D., Assistant Professor, Department of Physical Education, University of California at Berkeley, Berkeley, California 94720. (Oxygen Debt, Oxygen Intake)

WISE, ANTHONY, M.B.A., Promoter of Lumberjack World Championship, Hayward, Wisconsin 54843.

YOUMANS, JOHN G., Ph.D., Recreation Chairman, Department of Health, Physical Education and Recreation, Temple University, Philadelphia, Pennsylvania 19122. (Dance)

YOUNG, GLORIA, M.S., Teaching Assistant, Department of Health, Physical Education and Recreation, Temple University, Philadelphia, Pennsylvania 19122. (Horsemanship)

ZIMMERLI, WILLIAM H., M.Ed., Instructor, Department of Health, Physical Education, Recreation, State University of New York at Buffalo, Buffalo, New York 14214. (Golf)

ABDUCTION

The 600+ muscles of the body work in close harmony with one another to provide smooth efficient movement of the body. To cause movement, however, the muscles must contract; and because of their attachments and insertion to bones, they cause a limb or part of the body to move. One muscle, for example, may allow you to raise your arm upward, while a second muscle, a partner, causes you to reverse that movement.

Abductor muscles are those muscles that allow you to move a part of the body, usually a limb, away from the midline of the body. Once started, the movement is called abduction despite the fact that the limb may be coming back toward the center of the body. In other words, if you are in a standing position and raise your arm at your side, you are abducting the arm at the shoulder joint. But if you continue to raise the arm, you will notice that the arm moves past the shoulder and starts to turn back toward the midline of the body. The arm is still being abducted.

Abduction is usually considered in terms of the entire leg or arm; there is no abduction of the elbow or knee joint. A few of the better known abductors are the *deltoids* which abduct the arm and the *gluteus medius* and *gluteus minimus* which abduct the leg.

The muscles that reverse the movement of the abductors are the adductors. See ADDUCTION. For a related discussion, see EXTENSION, FLEXION, and MUSCLES, SKELETAL.

ACTIVITY DRUNKARDS

The term "activity drunkard" was coined by Ellis H. Champlin, former director of physical education at Springfield College. It is used to describe an overtrained, overactive, overstimulated, overanxious and overdeveloped person. He may be extremely nervous and unable to relax or sleep and usually has very high physical fitness index scores. See PHYSICAL FITNESS INDEX.

ADAPTATION

Adaptation refers to one of the physiological principles of training; if the body is subject to physical stress as in the training techniques required by running and lifting, it will usually adapt to that stress. If the body is made to work harder, it will soon be able to work harder. Generally, adaptation is measured by improvement in performance, a principle which is important in establishing an exercise program. It implies that the program selected should be gradual in its application.

As an example of adaptation, suppose you are currently engaged in an exercise program that involves running two miles in 30 minutes. At first, the schedule may be quite demanding and

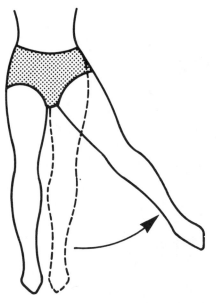

Abduction is the movement of a limb away from the body's midline.

leave you virtually exhausted. After a period of time, however, you will find that the run becomes easier and less fatiguing. When the adjustment occurs, your body has *adapted* to the stress imposed upon it. Adaptation occurs in any form of activity: exercise, work, etc. See TRAINING.

ADDUCTION

Adductor muscles are those muscles that enable you to move a part of the body, usually a limb, toward the midline of the body.

Adduction is usually considered in terms of the entire leg or arm; there is no adduction of the elbow or knee. A few of the better known adductors are the *pectoralis major* and *latissimus dorsi* which adduct the arm and the adductor group of the thigh which adduct the leg.

The muscles that reverse the movement of the adductors are the abductors, see ABDUCTION. For a related discussion see EXTENSION, FLEXION, and MUSCLES, SKELETAL.

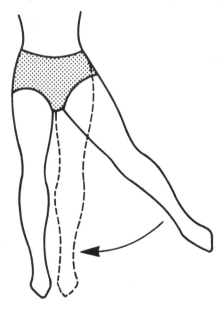

Movement of a limb toward the midline of the body is called adduction.

AEROBIC EXERCISE

Aerobic exercises refer to those exercises or activities that place a reasonable amount of stress on the circulorespiratory system. Aerobic exercises are concerned with performances with oxygen but not to the extent where the body craves oxygen. (See OXYGEN DEBT for a discussion of what happens to the body when it does not receive sufficient oxygen for the task at hand.) Those exercises tax the circulo-respiratory and biochemical systems that are involved with oxygen usage and transport throughout the body.

Aerobic exercises produce a positive training effect upon the body, such as a more efficient heart, better breathing during exercises, better blood supply to the muscles, and other circulatory and respiratory improvements. In reality, your body increases its capacity to bring in oxygen and transport it around the body, especially to the vital tissues. As a result, your endurance increases. See CIRCULO-RESPIRATORY ENDURANCE and MUSCLE ENDURANCE. Aerobic exercises are important because of their positive influence on the circulatory, respiratory, endocrine and muscle systems.

In general, however, the exercises should not be so intense that the body is unable to receive sufficient oxygen for the performance. An exercise such as sprinting is so demanding that the body cannot possibly be supplied with sufficient oxygen and it goes into oxygen debt. See ANAEROBIC EXERCISES.

AGE AND ATHLETIC PERFORMANCE

Such outstanding performances of teenage athletes have caused people to wonder about the best age for performance in various sports. Youngsters

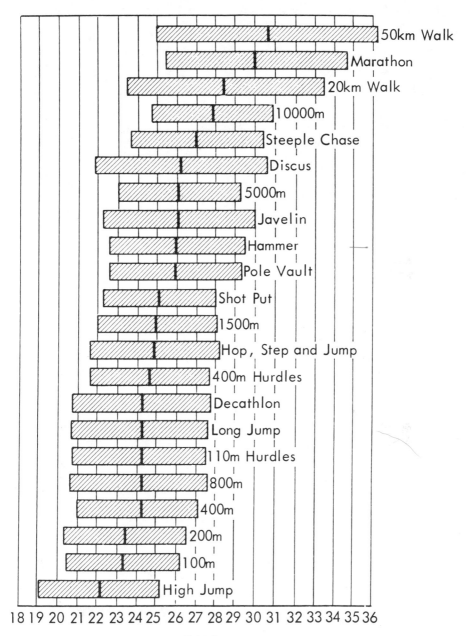

18 19 20 21 22 23 24 25 26 27 28 29 30 31 32 33 34 35 36

YEARS

This unique bar graph shows the age distribution of track and field athletes at the 1960 Olympic Games in Rome. The thick vertical lines indicate average ages, while the length of each horizontal column shows the standard deviations of ages.

in their teens have contributed significantly to world class performances. Robert Mathias, age 17, won a gold medal in the grueling decathlon. At the age of 16, Jim Ryun ran the mile in 4:08.2; at 17, he became the first high school boy to break 4 minutes in that event, and at 19, he set a new world mile record of 3:51.3 and a half mile record of 1:44.9. The 1960, 1964 and 1968 Olympic games further dramatized the age factor when teenagers, some as young as 13, made smashing victories and significant contributions for their teams in the swimming events.

At the other end of the continuum, there have been performances by those considered up in their years for athletic participation. In the 1952 Helsinki Olympics, for example, the oldest competitor was 66—the sport was clay bird shooting. Many other participants in the 1952 Olympics were well over 45 years of age.

Endlessly you read or hear accounts of individuals in their 60's or 70's who perform athletic or physical skills that astound the world, such as cross-country walking, marathon runs and distance cycling.

Several investigations and reviews of age and athletic performance have tried to establish which are man's best years in various sports. One of the earliest was conducted by Harvey C. Lehman, who listed the best age and performance of United States Olympic contestants through the years 1920 to 1936.

Lehman also presented the age of best performance in other sports.

The charts represent averages. In a few instances, the age groups would be different if the social environment had been different. For example, the age of best performance for professional football players might be lower if it were not for the fact that most professional football players do not begin to play until they are 21 or 22

years of age because of their college career.

Amateurs appear to achieve their best performance earlier than professionals, probably because amateurs discontinue participation at an earlier age. Professionals, on the other hand, frequently continue to participate as long as possible for the financial rewards. Generally, indications are that the age of maximum performance in athletes is between 20 and 33 years of age. That generalization may be further refined to state that activities requiring speed, power and explosiveness are indicative of lower age groups, while those activities requiring endurance and finer motor skills are excelled in by somewhat older people.

Track and field activities offer one method of illustrating the terms speed, power, explosiveness and endurance. The shorter races require speed, while the longer races are dependent upon endurance. The field activities such as the various jumps require power and explosiveness. The average age for championship performance in track and field events is from 22 to 29.

The capacity for moderate work does not need to decline with age. Instead, the decline is more evident when the requirement includes hard, explosive work.

Older people, however, who are accustomed to physical activity are able to perform at a rather high level of performance. Dr. Peter V. Karpovich describes that fact very graphically, by reporting a study in which "13 Bulgarians, 55 to 80 years of age (average 63) hiked across mountainous terrain at altitudes between 4,900 and 8,900 feet for 30 days, covering 435 miles. After the hike, they were in good health."

The United States excels in those activities that are primarily classified as speed, power and explosive events, especially in those sports associated with the Olympics. Many reasons have

AGE OF BEST PERFORMANCE

Activity	Age	Activity	Age
Baseball (Professional)		Professional Football	23-27
Non-Pitchers	27-29	Automobile Racing	27-30
Pitchers	26-28	Corn Husking	27-31
Professional Boxing	21-25	Bowling—Amateur	30-34
Golf		Duckpin Bowling	
Prof. & Amateur	25-34	Men	30-34
Tennis		Women	25-29
Prof. & Amateur	25-29	Rifle and Pistol	25-34
Roller Skating (Amateur)	14-18	Billiards	30-34
Ice Hockey	24-28		

U.S.A. OLYMPIC CONTESTANTS
1920-1936

Event	Most Common Ages of Performance
Swimming (women only)	17-21
Swimming (men only)	20-24
Boxing	19-22
Lacrosse	20-25
Cycling	19-22
Baseball	20-24
Handball	20-23
Hurdles, jumps, pole vaults, hop-skip-and-jump	21-25
Rowing	20-24
Races up to and including the 5000 meter race	21-24
Discus, shot put, hammer throw, and javelin throw	21-25
Wrestling	21-25
Field Hockey	26-28
Weight lifting	24-28
Steeple chase 3000 meters	21-25
Gymnastic events	22-26
Ice Hockey	24-28
Speed Skating	22-26
Basketball	23-27
Soccer	26-29
Figure Skating	23-27
Yachting	19-23
Fencing	23-27
Skiing	26-29
10,000 meter race and the marathon	26-30
Bob Sledding	30-34
Equestrian events	32-36

been given for that phenomenon. One of the most plausible is that the speed and explosive sports are those in which the younger age group excels. Most of the participants train in college or high school. Once their educational careers are ended, only a handful continue to train, reducing the number of active participants. Also, many of the athletes become involved in occupations that use up their time and do not permit adequate training. The establishment and support of more athletic and fitness clubs would help rectify that situation.

AGILITY

Agility is the ability to change direction quickly and correctly while moving at full speed. It requires nimbleness of movement without expending a great deal of force. This particular component of motor ability is extremely important in many activities, i.e., ballet and basketball. A reasonable degree of agility is also desirable for some daily activities like walking across a busy street. For the most part, however, the average individual does not need to develop agility to a great extent.

Determine for yourself what level of agility is necessary for your life and participation in recreational activities. The most popular tests are zigzag and

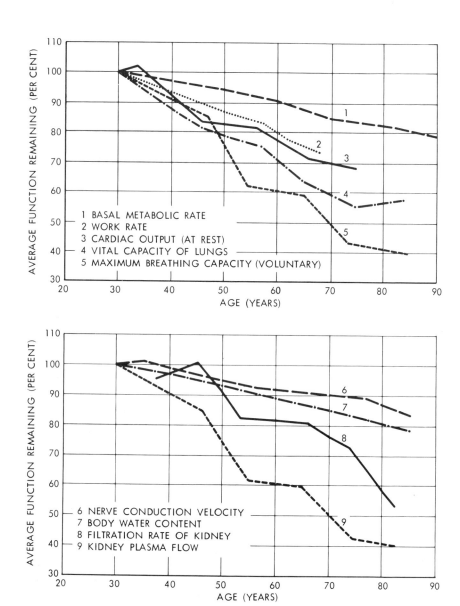

Percentage changes with age for different physiological functions are shown in these diagrams. The average value for each function at age 30 is taken as 100 per cent. Small drop in basal metabolism (1) is probably due simply to a loss of cells.

shuttle runs. See PHYSICAL FITNESS and TESTS.

AGING

Benjamin Franklin, who lived to be 84, went swimming for 80 of those years. A retired insurance man named Jesse F. Hyde celebrated his 75th birthday with a 24-hour, 75-mile hike. Those and many other instances of active oldsters, plus the near-miraculous extension of the human life expectancy in recent years, have led to a popular interest in the science of the aging process (gerontology).

"Aging" may begin during early middle age, but the typical signs—decreased vigor; increased weight; less joint flexibility, strength and mental flexibility; changed bowel and bladder habits; a change in sight and hearing; and the adjustments associated with the "Change of Life"—usually do not occur until 45 to 50 years of age.

The reason for their occurrence is not known; but Dr. Nathan Shock advances an interesting theory that aging is the result of changes that take place in cells and tissues, causing the organism's continuing decline and eventual death.

While aging is inevitable, it is important to note that, at least during the middle years, the changes are probably the result of disuse rather than "the aging process." It is apparent, therefore, that you need not age as fast as expected. Exercise and diet can slow down the process by making the various organs and their tissues more efficient.

Many geriatric authorities believe that regular exercise can postpone the effects of aging, to the extent that a person can retain 50 per cent of the

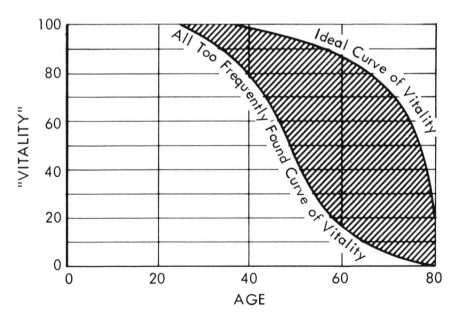

Regular exercise and proper hygiene will retard the aging process. This graph by Dr. C. McCloy shows that 50 per cent of our youthful vitality may remain at age 75.

vitality he had in his prime, even up to age 75. Without regular exercise, an individual may drop to the 50 per cent at age 50, as demonstrated by Dr. C. McCloy. People who exercise little and practice poor hygiene have less than the desired level of vitality. The effects of exercise and proper hygiene reveal that the decline does not need to begin until the late thirties or early forties.

Of course, it is not always true that conditioning exercises will lengthen your life, but that is a strong possibility, according to the latest findings in cardiovascular research and obesity. Certainly there will be an increase in the productivity of life because regular exercise can postpone many of the typical indications of aging. The committee on Aging of the American Medical Association in its book, *The Health Aspects of Aging,* says: Exercise helps maintain muscle tone, including that of the heart itself; promotes a milking action of the muscles on the veins, thereby assisting in the venous return of the blood; promotes an improved digestion, mainly through relief of tension; helps to control obesity; and causes deeper respiration, thereby improving the gaseous exchange and the state of the lung tissue. And the best part of all—those benefits will come to all who exercise, regardless of age.

Although there is a need for more exercise on the complex subject of exercise and aging, enough is now known to state definitely this undeniable fact: Exercise retards the aging process.

The kind of exercise that an older person should do is largely an individual matter. Dr. Paul D. White, the late President Eisenhower's physician, feels that the type is not important, except that it should suit the person's strength, ability and interest. In fact, vigorous exercise may be enjoyed by people well into their 80's. Percy W. Cerutty, director of the International Athletes' Camp at Portsea, Victoria, Australia, gives this specially prepared account of how he regained fitness after 40:

"When I was 48 years old, I resumed an athletic career in long distance running after a 25-year absence from competitive sport.

"That is all the more interesting when you realize that, at 43, I had regressed into a physical condition that hindered proper digestion of many common foods; and I boasted a body weight of 112 pounds instead of my normal 130 pounds.

"This debilitation was corrected by adopting a diet of almost entirely uncooked foods in their natural state and the near-total exclusion of animal fats in any form from the diet.

"The struggle for life had alerted the instinct for survival. I decided to exercise. In the beginning, that meant a return to walking, swimming, and later, running. I was unable to swim more than 25 yards, had difficulty in walking more than a mile or two, and was unable to run more than 100 yards or so, at the slowest pace.

"However, after seriously taking up athletics at 48 years of age, I ran almost 8,000 miles in the ensuing 5 years; and after 3 years of consistent training, I achieved a State Marathon (26 miles 385 yards) Championship and Record, as well as accomplishing record runs up to 60 miles. I ran, in a little over 8 hours, a trek along a country road with a light pack on back, completing 100 miles in 23½ hours.

"What can be learned from my experiences?

"In a normally fit person, there is no risk of strain or physical harm from strenuous exercises or sporting pursuits, providing the cardiovascular system, according to a medical authority has not suffered any organic changes. The limiting factors are a hardening of the arteries and a consequent above normal blood pressure.

"However, you need to maintain certain intelligent attitudes. In the old, as the young, the undue calling up of the will to perform some feat of strength, or endurance, can always be considered foolhardy. Grave risks are engendered when pride, conceit or ambition override common sense and intelligence.

"Certain symptoms are applicable to all. Heat exhaustion is the most dangerous. Its symptoms are an intense feeling of heat in the head and dizziness.

"Another risk is from attempting feats of strength; repeated efforts, such as repetitive lifts of an unduly heavy barbell, or overcompetition with younger men in such sports as rowing, are dangerous.

"Other than those reasonable precautions, no harm is likely to result from even the most prolonged physical efforts at almost any age, providing that the heart and arteries are in condition to sustain the imposed loads. In general, the heart is efficient when the resting pulse rate is around the low sixties, and the blood pressure is not higher than 90mm Hg. during diastole and 130mm Hg. during systole.

"As long as the cardiovascular system can sustain the level of effort, there is no age at which athletic performance is deleterious or even dangerous. But the age of efficiency, or desirability, will differ greatly with each individual. From middle age onwards it is wise to avoid undue enthusiasm for exhaustive competitive efforts."—*Percy W. Cerutty*. See AGE AND ATHLETIC PERFORMANCE, LONGEVITY, MIDDLE AGE.

ALBUMINURIA

Albumin and other protein substances are not generally found in the urine of healthy persons, but occur in injured kidneys. Yet, many times when a urinalysis is performed on healthy individuals after they have engaged in strenuous exercise, albumin is found in the urine. The albumin found is temporary; the condition is called exercise albuminuria. It is not serious, but merely a response to exercise that occurs because the blood is temporarily diverted from the kidneys to the skin and exercising muscles. Large amounts of lactic acid, furthermore, appear in the blood, and the acid condition makes kidney tubules more porous to albumin. After extended exercise, circulation is sluggish; and the kidneys do not get sufficient oxygen. These occurrences cause the membranes to allow the albumin to pass from the blood to the kidneys.

Apparently, repeated exercise does not cause permanent damage to the kidney tissues. See EXCRETORY SYSTEM.

ALCOHOL

Mix alcohol and exercise, and what do you get? Not much in the way of performance, most coaches and researchers agree. Although personal opinions and half-truths often obscure the reasons for athletes abstaining from alcoholic beverages, the general agreement is that drinking inhibits maximum physical accomplishment.

The alcohol found in beverages is a variable solution of ethyl and grain alcohols, with organic extracts added for flavor. Wine, for example, is made from fermented grapes or fruit; beer from barley; rum from molasses, etc.

The resulting product is not a stimulant but a narcotic. The apparent "stimulation" that some persons feel while drinking is really a result of depression in the higher nerve centers. The prime nerve center affected is that of inhibition.

Alcohol is absorbed directly into the blood. Its ultimate effect on the body is to produce heat and some energy. Like sugar, however, it contains no vitamins, minerals, or proteins. At one time, beer and wine were a good source of the B-complex vitamins; but because of modern techniques of manufacturing, that is no longer true.

Alcohol may be called a fuel food; but it is not a desirable one, since it has little nutritive value and has a narcotic effect on the body.

Although alcohol cannot be stored in the body, drinking it may lead to an overweight condition when other food fuels are stored instead of burned. Even an 8 ounce glass of beer can unbalance the average diet because it contains 105 calories. (1½ ounces of Bourbon equal 120 calories; 1½ ounces of gin produce about 105 calories.)

Since it is a depressant, alcohol consumed before exercise will lower your efficiency. If you're engaging in a skill-type activity such as hitting a baseball, shooting a clay pigeon or swinging at a golf ball, you'll find that alcohol will affect your performance because it has altered the reaction time and the precision of movement.

Here's a final reason to abstain from alcohol: It prevents some hemoglobin in the blood from releasing oxygen at the tissue level. At that level, oxygen leaves the hemoglobin and gets into the cells by enzyme action. But alcohol immobilizes some of those enzymes for up to 12 hours, and the oxygen is not released in sufficient quantity. The result is premature fatigue and a limiting of endurance.

ALL-OR-NONE LAW

A muscle fiber is the individual unit of skeletal muscle. Billions of fibers are required to make up the more than 600 skeletal muscles of the body. Each fiber is separate from the others. That is, they may touch one another, but physiologically they are single fibers. Fifty to 100 of the fibers are bound together in groups, called a motor unit.

A unit has five basic parts: the nerve cell, the motor nerve fiber, the muscle fibers, the motor end plate and the endomysium, or connective tissue. When a motor nerve stimulates several muscle fibers, fiber contracts completely—not partially. That maximal contraction is known as the "All-or-none" law. If the stimulus is sufficient to stimulate the fiber, it is a threshold stimulus and causes the fiber to contract with all its strength. If, on the other hand, the stimulus is not sufficient, or a sub-threshold stimulus, the fiber makes no movement.

The contraction of a muscle, therefore, is dependent upon the number of fibers stimulated. If many receive a threshold stimulus, the contraction will be strong; if only a few are stimulated, the contraction will be weak. Experience tells you how much strength is needed in order to perform a certain task. If maximum effort is needed to lift a weight, most of the fibers of the muscle are stimulated. But if you lift a pencil, only a few fibers are stimulated.

An interesting phenomenon that you have probably experienced is when you attempt to lift an object you think is very heavy. Upon lifting the object, you find it much lighter than you initially thought. Many muscle fibers were stimulated to lift the supposedly heavy object. That type of action naturally is extremely inefficient. The reverse also is true, for when you attempt to lift a 50 pound object that

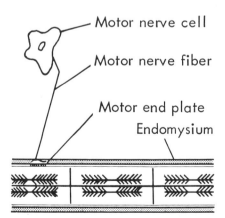

Motor nerve cell

Motor nerve fiber

Motor end plate

Endomysium

The muscle fiber is a necessary muscle component. The average muscle contains hundreds of thousands of muscle fibers.

you think is only 5 pounds, no movement takes place because not enough fibers have been stimulated.

The all-or-none law applies only to the muscle fibers and not to the whole muscle. If it involved the entire muscle, your movement would be extremely inefficient. See MUSCLES, SKELETAL.

ALTITUDE

See ENVIRONMENT.

ANAEROBIC EXERCISE

Anaerobics are very demanding on the circulo-respiratory system because as the word implies, they are done "without oxygen." They include short bursts of maximum effort, such as running or swimming as far and as fast as you can. There are two types of anaerobic activities. (1.) Those that require a fairly high degree of oxygen and are cut short voluntarily, usually as a result of lack of motivation or because you are forced to breathe harder than you wish. (2.) Those that are exceptionally demanding on the intake of oxygen and are cut short involuntarily because they are just too hard. Activities of that nature last about 20 to 30 seconds.

In anaerobic exercise, the exercise is so intense that your body is just not able to supply it with sufficient oxygen. As a result, you start to breathe heavily to supply the body with the life giving, energy producing oxygen. You have created what is called an oxygen debt; see OXYGEN DEBT. If the exercise is truly anaerobic, your body cannot be supplied with adequate amounts of oxygen. The oxygen must be repaid quickly. To do that, you must stop or slow down considerably so that the oxygen can be supplied.

Anaerobic exercises are necessary for athletic training but are of lesser value in a personal physical fitness program. In fact, if you have been sedentary or if the heart is damaged, the exercises can be quite harmful. You should concentrate on the aerobic exercise (see AEROBIC EXERCISE) if you want to improve circulo-respiratory endurance. Once you have surpassed the sedentary level and as your circulo-respiratory endurance improves, you will find that some anaerobic exercises will be necessary for further conditioning.

ANGINA

Angina pectoris is a symptom that the heart muscle is not getting enough blood and oxygen for the work it is doing. In short, it is an indication that the blood supply to the heart is reduced. There is no actual injury, however, as there is in a heart attack, where the blood supply is stopped and there is resulting muscle injury.

Many names have been used to describe the symptoms of angina pectoris; the most common are heart pain, coronary pain, anginal pain and angina. It actually means "strangling in the chest."

A person with angina will generally complain of a slight feeling of tightness in his chest, right behind the breast bone. It is a feeling of pressure, rather than pain. Occasionally, some individuals may feel a slight tingling along the inner side of the left upper arm.

Generally, the pressure is absent during rest, and occurs during physical exertion or under emotional stress. At times, minimal exertion after a heavy meal may cause that feeling of pressure.

The heart, like other muscles of the body needs to receive food and oxygen; and the demand for them increases as heart rate increases. The food and oxygen are carried to the heart muscle by the coronary arteries. If the arteries are narrowed by atherosclerosis, a portion of the heart does not get enough blood. The result may be anginal pain, varying from very mild to quite severe.

To control angina, a physician will generally prescribe nitroglycerin or some form of nitrate that will dilate the coronary arteries when the heart muscle demands more blood and oxygen. He will probably tell the patient to notice which activities cause the feeling of pressure, and to avoid or reduce them.

Of paramount importance is that the patient understand his condition and that he prevent anginal discomfort. That can be done by following the guidelines listed above, plus avoiding emotional stress situations.

If coronary arteries are narrowed by atherosclerosis, the nearby arteries will often get wider and open up tiny new branches to deliver blood to the area not receiving adequate blood supply. That is called collateral, compensatory, or substitute circulation. If the collateral circulation develops adequately, the patient may be able to increase his physical activity.

For some, collateral circulation matches the onset of atherosclerosis, hence they feel no anginal pain and do not suffer heart attacks. On the other hand, if the atherosclerosis de-

velops fast and collateral circulation does not, heart disease develops.

The peak age for angina in the United States, according to Dr. E. G. Dimond, is 42. In other countries, it is around 52. There are four reasons for this difference, says Dr. Dimond: 1. The stress of life in the United States; 2. the highly competitive society; 3. the lack of exercise; and 4. the rich diet. Only one other nation approaches the United States in a similar pattern —West Germany. Coronary disease is increasing there, too.

What can be done about angina? Follow the advice of a physician, who will undoubtedly tell a patient to take off excess weight, to reduce the animal and dairy fats in his diet, and to substitute vegetable fats such as corn oil, soybean oil, cottonseed oil and fish oils. He will also explain to the patient the cause-and-effect relationship between cigarette smoking and coronary atherosclerosis.

The possibility of developing angina can be lessened in light of the four reasons cited by Dr. Dimond. Although there is little you can do to reduce the stress and the competitiveness of society, you can teach yourself how to relax and to avoid or reduce

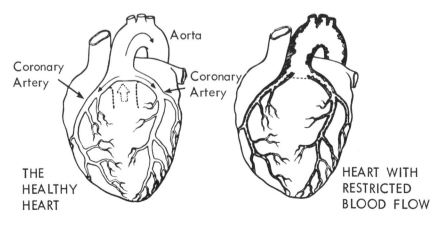

A heart kept healthy with exercise and diet maintains clear coronary arteries. When arteries become narrowed, the blood supply is reduced, and angina pain may occur.

stressful situations. You can gradually increase daily exercise level by following the guidelines set forth in this book —that is, continuous, rhythmical exercise. Restricting the fat content in your diet will aid also in reducing the possibility of angina. The percentage of fat caloric intake should be reduced from the traditional 40-45% to 25-30% of the total daily diet.

The American Heart Association has outlined the following six point program for protecting the heart:

1. Reduce if overweight.
2. Decrease saturated fats in the diet.
3. Stop smoking cigarettes.
4. Control high blood pressure.
5. Exercise regularly.
6. Shun needless tensions.

See ARTERIOSCLEROSIS, BLOOD PRESSURE, DEGENERATIVE CARDIOVASCULAR DISEASE, HEART DISEASE, LOAFER'S HEART, and ISCHEMIC HEART DISEASE.

ANTIGRAVITY MUSCLES

Erect posture is maintained by the constant pull of certain muscles on the bones. Those muscles are called postural or antigravity muscles. The constant pull on them is called *muscle tone* or *tonus*. Muscle tone varies for a number of reasons some of which are discussed under MUSCLE TONE. The antigravity muscles include those of the neck that hold the head upright, the erector muscles of the spine, the gluteals, the quadriceps on the front of the thigh, the gastrocnemius of the lower leg and the abdominals. With the exception of the abdominals, all of those muscles are extensors. That is, they straighten joints, thereby extending the body against the pull of gravity.

ANTHROPOMETRY

Anthropometry is the branch of anthropology that is concerned with measurements of the human body.

Measurements include height, weight, linear and circumferential measurements. Linear measurements include length and width of various body parts. The most common sites of circumferential measurements are the neck, chest, waist, thigh, calf, arm and forearm.

Linear and circumferential measurements are easy to obtain and are valuable in revealing changes related to growth, activity and inactivity.

A third type of anthropometric

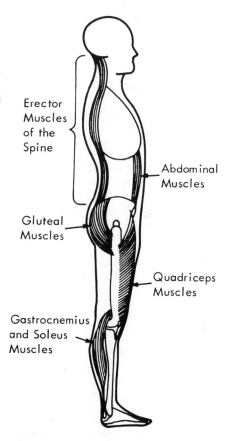

Erector Muscles of the Spine

Abdominal Muscles

Gluteal Muscles

Quadriceps Muscles

Gastrocnemius and Soleus Muscles

This sketch shows the location of the antigravity muscles. Because they help maintain a satisfactory upright position, they are often also called postural muscles.

measurement is the fat or skinfold measurement. It is taken with a device known as a fat caliper, by measuring the thickness of a fold of skin. Such measurements are useful in determining the specific density of the body as well as the amount and locations of adipose tissue (fat) on the body. Skinfold measurements are also useful in relating the amount of body fat to physical performance.

Presently anthropometric measurements are used to:

1. Classify individuals as to body type. See BODY TYPE.
2. Relate body types to degree of success in various athletic activities.
3. Make comparisons between populations.
4. Make studies of particular populations.
5. Relate body structure to physiological and psychological functioning.
6. Analyze posture.

Anthropometry is a relatively young study, and its usefulness will undoubtedly increase as the means of taking measurements and analyzing data improve. One recent and valuable advance in the field is photogrammetry, the use of photographs to take measurements and judge posture. That procedure helps to reduce the likelihood of human error in taking measurements.

APPARATUS

See EQUIPMENT.

APPETITE

Almost every day, you hear statements about the effects of exercise on appetite. The most prevalent adage is that an increase in exercise level and intensity will increase your appetite. It is generally concluded, then, that because exercise makes you want to eat more, it is ineffective in weight control.

Some people carry this to further extremes and state that exercise makes them gain weight because they must consume more calories than the exercise causes them to use.

But they're wrong, according to researchers. Dr. Jean Mayer, for instance, notes that it is a misconception to think that an increase in physical activity *always* causes an increase in appetite and food intake, which equals or is greater in energy value than that of the energy cost of the exercise. He reveals that under sedentary conditions there is a voluntary increase in food intake. That leads to an increase in weight and an accumulation of fat. With normal daily exercise, calorie intake appears to be proportional to the caloric output and weight remains constant. With exhausting physical exercise, it appears that there is a reduction in food intake and a subsequent weight loss.

A study by Dr. Mayer and two associates demonstrated the relationship of food intake, body weight and exercise. It can be seen, then, that appetite is *not* adversely affected by exercise. That is, moderate or intense exercise will not cause an increase in appetite that will negate the energy expenditure. Rather, a sedentary disposition has a tendency to increase caloric consumption and is a sure means of increasing weight. See CALORIES.

ARCHERY

Archery developed in the very earliest times and has taken many forms. The popular variations are target, and field shooting, including the actual hunting of small and large game.

Target Archery

The target archer shoots at a target that has four rings around the bull's-eye. He receives from 1 point for an arrow in the white outside circle up to 9 points for an arrow in the gold bull's-eye. In tournaments, he shoots a pre-

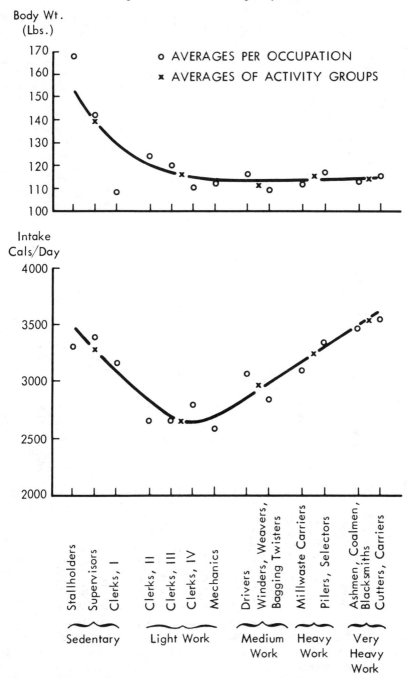

These graphs show how body weight is dependent upon caloric intake and exercise in adult men. Often the amount of exercise involved in a person's occupation will play a major role in his total body weight.

scribed number of arrows from various distances, trying for the highest possible number of points.

Equipment

The typical bow ranges from 5 to 6 feet in length and varies greatly in finish. Some cost $200 or more. Select a bow that can be pulled back to the point of the arrow and held steadily while aiming at a target. Bows vary according to their "weight"—the number of pounds of pull it takes to draw the arrow its full length. Bows are made of red cedarwood, lemonwood, fiberglass or aluminum. Arrows are usually 24 to 32 inches long, the length determined by the height and reach of the archer. They are most often made of aluminum or cedar.

You may find it helpful to purchase a leather cuff to protect the forearm from scraping by the string as it snaps forward. A three fingered glove for the shooting hand will help protect the finger tips from being cut or injured by the string.

Archery can develop a high degree of arm and shoulder strength, depending upon the weight of the bow you select. It will also aid in developing a moderate amount of abdominal strength. You'll find that when you draw the bow back, the abdominal muscles contract, thereby placing stress on those muscles.

Conditioning Programs

Since archery is a highly skilled activity requiring hand-eye coordination, the best method of training is to practice at varying distances.

General exercises for the shoulder, upper and lower arm, and abdominal muscles will aid the prospective archer. See EXERCISES. You can undertake more specific exercises for the muscles used in archery after consulting the WEIGHT TRAINING and ISO-METRICS sections.

Anyone may participate in archery, provided that he selects a proper

length and weight bow and a proper arrow length. A normal beginning adult (male or female) will find a 20-25 pound bow best. Although some people may feel that weight bow too light, most people will find it more important to learn the proper technique and experience some success before progressing to a heavier bow.

Associations:

National Archery Association of the United States (NAA), 23 East Jackson Boulevard, Chicago, Illinois 60604.

National Field Archery Association (NFAA), Route 2, Box 514, Redlands, California 92373.

ARM

The muscles of the arm are relatively easy to develop through concentrated exercise. At the top of the arm is the *coracobrachialis*. That small muscle draws the arm forward and toward the center of the body. Here's an exercise that will help to develop the muscle and several other muscles nearby. Sit on the floor between two chairs, and rest your arms on them. Now force the elbows down toward the seat pads for ten seconds.

The exercise also affects the *pectoral* muscles of the chest, and the *rhomboids, latissimus dorsi* and the *teres major* of the back.

The *biceps brachii* is perhaps the most popular muscle of the body. The muscle is located in the front of the arm and is the muscle children refer to when they say "make a muscle." It flexes the arm and rotates the forearm outward.

An isometric exercise to strengthen the biceps is to grasp a bar and exert a pull for ten seconds.

An alternate form of the exercise is to grasp your desk and exert a pull for ten seconds.

The *brachialis* assists the biceps in flexing the arm at the elbow. The *triceps brachii* is located on the back of the arm, is an antagonist of the *biceps brachii*, and extends the forearm.

To strengthen the triceps, do push-ups. Be certain, however, that when performing the exercise the hands are directly under the shoulders and the back is kept straight.

A modification of the push-up is to perform the push-up with the knees bent.

The muscles of the forearm are numerous. For the sake of clarity, the muscles shall be grouped according to action, that is, flexors, extensors, supinators and pronators.

The flexors (front side of the arm) are the *flexor carpi radialis*, the *pal-maris longus*, the *flexor carpi ulnaris*, *flexor digitorium sublimis*, and the *brachioradialis*. Their function is to flex the wrists, fingers and elbow joint.

To develop the flexors of the hand, hold a dumbell or a book in your hand and rest your forearm on a support. Your palms should be facing upward. Extend the hand fully and then curl the hand upward to maximum height.

The extensor muscles (the posterior side of the arm) include the *extensor carpi radialis longus*, the *extensor carpi radialis brevis*, *extensor digitorum*, *extensor digiti minimi* and *extensor carpi ulnaris*. They extend the wrist and fingers.

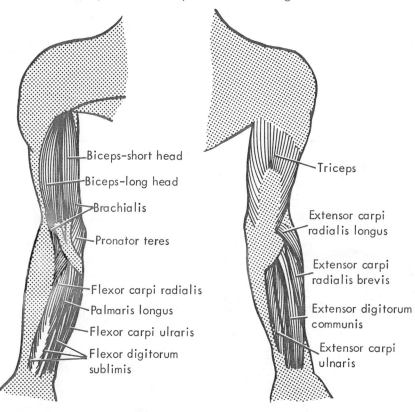

Biceps-short head
Biceps-long head
Brachialis
Pronator teres
Flexor carpi radialis
Palmaris longus
Flexor carpi ulraris
Flexor digitorum sublimis

Triceps
Extensor carpi radialis longus
Extensor carpi radialis brevis
Extensor digitorum communis
Extensor carpi ulnaris

FRONT VIEW   BACK VIEW

To develop those muscles, rest your hand on a support with your palm facing down. Again a dumbell or book is held. Then extend the hand to a maximum height and return.

The *supinator* is a muscle that acts in supination (turning out) of the wrist. Its antagonist is the *pronator teres*. The muscle, as the name implies, rotates the arm inward (pronates).

To develop the pronators and supinators of the forearm hold a book or single bell in a handshake position. Lower the book or bell inward until it is horizontal and return, to tax the pronators. Then lower the book or bell outward until it is horizontal and return, placing stress on the supinators. Also see: EXERCISES, ISOMETRICS, WEIGHT TRAINING.

ARMED FORCES

In the 20th century the armed forces have been vitally concerned about the physical fitness of the people of the United States, particularly its youth. That concern, naturally, is an outgrowth of the need to have physically qualified men in the armed services. Individuals with faulty posture, poor muscle strength, poor muscle endurance and low cardio-respiratory endurance are an extreme liability there.

The status of our youth was dramatically illustrated by the fact that in 1913, 35 per cent of the men called to the military service were rejected. During World War II, four million men were rejected, of which 700,000 had remediable defects. During President Eisenhower's administration, 40 per cent of the young men were turned down for purely physical reasons.

Historically, the armed forces' emphasis on physical fitness has been called physical training, or "P.T." When the United States entered World War I in April 1917, the military leaders stated that the development of a military fitness program was of paramount importance. Since there was no specified program of physical fitness, two basic programs evolved. First authorities established formal conditioning exercises such as combatives (wrestling, judo, hand-to-hand combat), marching, drill and calisthenics. Second, they developed a recreational program of games and sports. Eventually, those two programs merged into a physical fitness or physical training program.

As a result of that wartime program, calisthenics or the "daily dozen" played a vital role in the military and school programs. From the military interest in fitness a concern for the handicapped also developed. Shouldn't those people, too, be given an opportunity to improve their physical condition?

The second World War brought the nation out of the doldrums economically. It also woke the American public up to the fact that its youth were not physically fit. Both the armed forces and several physical education leaders demanded a new emphasis on fitness.

The military experimented extensively with fitness programs in an effort to derive optimum fitness benefits. The most notable were the Navy

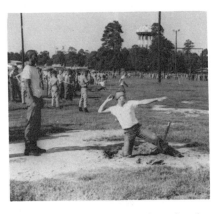

Historically, the military has placed a heavy emphasis on physical conditioning. Here a Marine combines coordination and strength to throw a grenade.

V-5 and Navy V-12 programs. The Army, likewise, in conjunction with large universities, trained specialized personnel for various military positions.

Those programs stimulated interest in research, tests and measurements in physical fitness. Soon, there were a number of changes in the nation's high schools. More time was devoted to physical education; and more schools, counties and states made it compulsory. A great deal of the revision was a result of a booklet put out by a joint committee of physical educators and representatives of the armed forces, entitled *Physical Fitness Through Physical Education for the High School Victory Corps*. Since women were actively engaged in the service, there resulted an increase in interest in physical fitness for the distaff set.

A few years after the war, however, interest in physical fitness again began to wane. Emphasis was placed on a variety of sports, particularly carry-over sports.

With the Korean conflict, interest in physical fitness renewed. The Kraus-Weber tests dramatized the low level of fitness of the American youth.

This time, however, President Eisenhower added his interest to the on-again, off-again problem of physical fitness. The subsequent result was a President's Council on Youth Fitness, which eventually evolved into the President's Council on Physical Fitness and still later the President's Council on Physical Fitness and Sports. Since the time of the First Conference meeting of the council in 1957, the interest in physical fitness has increased considerably, spurred on by research that demonstrated the benefits of exercise and their role in retarding the degenerative decrease of modern man.

Since that time, the interest has not been confined to the military and physical educators, and many people now show a genuine concern. The armed forces still demonstrate a great deal of interest in the area of physical fitness.

For example, the vigorous training for men at the various service academies, the concern of pilots and astronauts to maintain their flying status, and the hard training encountered at boot camp. At Parris Island, North Carolina, a Marine basic training camp, physical training sessions may last 4 hours. Caloric intake of the overweight is restricted and dietary supplements for underweight are added. A recruit may lose a pound or more a day. The Corps, furthermore, has a Marine Corps Physical Fitness Test that is given to many high school students. It holds regional contests in an effort to dramatize physical fitness and encourage physical fitness among the youth.

In 1968, the Marine Corps Physical Fitness Academy was established at Quantico, Virginia. Its primary purpose is to improve the combat readiness of the Marine by improving his physical condition. To accomplish that objective, that academy educates physical training instructors and specialists who have the responsibility of establishing and conducting the physical training and combat survival programs for the Corps. The potential teachers get comprehensive instruction in anatomy, physiology, kinesiology and principles of training. Instruction is also given in vigorous sports and conditioning programs. See PROGRAMS.

Today, physical fitness is the concern of many individuals and groups; and some organizations are making a profound effect in alerting people to improve their level of fitness. We owe a great deal to the armed forces for their continued interest in physical fitness throughout this century, during times that few people could clearly see that need.

ARTERIOSCLEROSIS

Arteriosclerosis is a chronic degenerative disorder of the blood vessels,

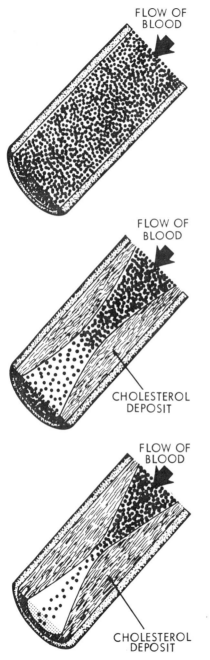

FLOW OF BLOOD

FLOW OF BLOOD

CHOLESTEROL DEPOSIT

FLOW OF BLOOD

CHOLESTEROL DEPOSIT

As cholesterol progressively limits the flow of blood, the tissues supplied by the blood receive less nutrients. When those tissues are in the heart, kidneys and brain, severe complications may occur.

affecting the walls of the arteries. A common cause of high blood pressure and heart attacks, the disease may take several forms. One is *hardening of the arteries;* a second is *atherosclerosis.*

Hardening of the arteries is due to the deposit of calcium in the arterial wall, causing the arteries to become inelastic. Because the heart has to pump the blood into rigid vessels, it has to work harder; and the blood pressure is increased. That condition increases the possibility of a break in the arterial walls. A break of a vessel in the area of the brain produces apoplexy or "stroke." Likewise, poor circulation in the heart or kidneys can cause serious problems in those organs.

Hardening of the arteries appears to be caused by emotional stress, heredity, infection and metabolic disturbances (such as deficiencies in estrogen, insulin, thyroxin and adrenalin which may contribute to hypercholesterolemia).

Atherosclerosis is characterized by deposits of fat—rich in cholesterol—occurring on the inner linings of the arteries. The deposits may extend into the middle layer of the arterial wall and affect the blood-carrying capacity of the vessels. They also may produce a blood clot (thrombosis), which may break off and lodge in another part of the body. That occurrence is called an embolism.

Like hardening of the arteries, atherosclerosis may affect the heart, brain and kidneys.

The heart can be temporarily or permanently damaged if one of its arteries is narrowed or blocked. The formation of a large clot within an artery of the heart will cause a "heart attack," properly called *coronary thrombosis.* If the heart muscle is injured because of the blocked artery, the result is *myocardial infarction.*

A reduced blood flow to the kidneys, due to a hardening or narrowing of the kidney vessels, will lower the kidneys' efficiency in removing waste. If the damage is severe, *uremia* (poisons in the blood stream) may result.

In the brain, a rupture or a clotted vessel will result in a stroke, or oxygen starvation of a portion of the brain—which probably will result in irreparable damage. In severe cases, that brain damage may lead to partial or total paralysis of certain portions of the body or even in death.

Hypertension (high blood pressure) is a sign that a person has arteriosclerosis. High blood pressure is characterized by a narrowing of the arterioles, which increases the pressure needed to force the blood through. The heart, therefore, must work harder.

What can be done about arteriosclerosis depends upon the individual and the condition of his vascular system. Although there is no best treatment prescribed for arteriosclerosis, drugs, surgery, psychotherapy, special diets and prescribed exercise have been helpful. See also DEGENERATIVE CARDIOVASCULAR DISEASE, HEART DISEASE and ISCHEMIC HEART DISEASE.

ARTHRITIS

Arthritis, the disease of inflammation of the joints, is often used synonymously and erroneously with rheumatism. Rheumatism refers to a broad group of diseases affecting body tissues that have to do with moving about, such as the muscles, tendons, ligaments and joints. Arthritis, on the other hand, is only one aspect of what doctors call the rheumatoid diseases. Here's a typical classification of diseases under rheumatism:

A. Arthritis
1. Arthritis due to specific infection agents
2. Arthritis due to direct trauma
3. Rheumatic fever
4. Rheumatoid Arthritis
5. Osteoarthritis
6. Gout
7. Less common diseases of joints
B. Nonarticular rheumatism
1. Bursitis
2. Tenosynovitis and tendinitis
3. Fasciitis
4. Myositis and mylagia
5. Fibrositis
6. Disorders of fatty tissues
7. Reflex sympathetic dystrophies
8. Psychogenic rheumatism
C. Other

The most common forms of arthritis are rheumatoid arthritis, osteoarthritis and gout.

Rheumatoid Arthritis

Rheumatoid arthritis is 3 times more prevalent in women than in men. The reason is not clear, however. Generally that form of arthritis may appear after an infection or a wound. Occasionally, emotional shock may cause an attack. Whatever the cause, there are several signs that are easily recognized. The hands feel numb, and the skin is cold and clammy. You may feel "under the weather" with digestive upset and emotional depression.

Although the entire body suffers, the joints cause the most discomfort. Usually the smaller joints, i.e., fingers, are affected first. Later, the larger joints (hips and knees) may be affected. Occasionally, the first sign of rheumatoid arthritis may occur in the larger joints. Regardless of where the pain occurs it may come slowly and with sharp twinges. Swelling also appears.

The pain may come and go for years. If a joint on the left side is affected, the same joint on the right may demonstrate a similar affliction. When a person allows his condition to go untreated, each attack will become more severe and the swelling will increase until movement is greatly restricted. Proper treatment, however, can avoid that incapacitating situation.

Continuous medical supervision is

very important. Although there is no complete cure, prompt medical attention and the patient's cooperation will go a long way in limiting the malady. The most commonly prescribed medication is aspirin. Hormones, carefully prescribed, may also be used, however, treatment consists of much more than a few aspirin tablets. The doctor will set up a well balanced diet for the patient; undoubtedly nutrients (vitamins, minerals, etc.) will be added. It is important that overweight patients lose weight and that the underweight gain.

Exercise will play a role in the treatment of rheumatoid arthritis once the condition of the patient improves. The exercise is initiated by experienced people (physical therapists) and conducted under medical supervision. It entails limited exercise of the joints; either active (on one's own) or passive (someone else moves the joint). After sufficient progress has been made, a member of the family under the guidance of a physical therapist, may take over the exercises. The exercises are to be gradual and progressive. Care is taken that the patient does not experience pain or, at least, has a minimum of pain.

An effort is made to reestablish the full range of motion of the joint which may take several weeks and months. It is also imperative that the muscles be developed and maintained, for if they are weakened, additional stress or pressure may be put on the afflicted joints.

Osteoarthritis

Osteoarthritis, sometimes called degenerative joint disease involves a breakdown of the cartilage and other tissues which make the joint move properly. It is often called the wear-and-tear disease, and over 97% of people over 60 show signs of it.

Osteoarthritis is most common in the hips, knees, spine and base of big toe and thumb. The cause is not clear although heredity may be a factor. A joint that has received particular stress may also be a cause.

A person with osteoarthritis may not even know that he is suffering from the disease. But when there is trouble, the most prevalent symptom is pain. Generally, it is only a mild ache or soreness on movements; in other cases, the pain may be constant, even at rest. Another symptom is loss of movement. Although that is usually not severe, it inhibits the ability to perform easy, comfortable movements of the joints.

There are two basic kinds of osteoarthritis—primary and secondary. The primary kind starts by itself, but secondary is a result of a stress or strain.

Although osteoarthritis cannot be cured, the symptoms can be alleviated and the joint function improved. Drugs have been used successfully, but the physician must be careful in prescribing because of reactions to various medication. Heat and surgery have also been successful. Sometimes splints, crutches and/or braces are used to rest the joints and relieve pressure. Rest is particularly helpful in relieving strain on the affected joints. Too much rest, however, is not good. If the patient is immobilized too long, he may lose use of his joints and muscles. A special diet may be prescribed to maintain good health or correct a specific deficiency.

Physical therapy and exercise have been used successfully, along with the previously mentioned techniques, in treating osteoarthritis patients. It may be the most valuable treatment. Muscle weakness and loss of normal joint motion are serious end results of the disease, thereby disabling the patient. The main objective of physical therapy is keeping joints flexible, maintaining strength of the muscles so that the joints retain their stability, and protecting the joints from further injury.

Physical therapy treatment must be carried on continuously, since the disease is progressive. For that reason, a member of the family should learn from the therapist what exercises should be done.

The key idea in the exercise is to see that the joints are moved through the entire range of motion, several times daily. It is extremely important, because if one joint has restricted movement, another part of the body may be affected. For example, if one hip joint is stiff, the patient may favor that side, thereby weakening the muscles of the affected side and over-developing the muscles of the other side. Posture is affected and abnormal stresses are placed on various parts of the body, increasing the possibility of developing osteoarthritis in joints experiencing the stress.

The exercises selected are gentle rather than vigorous. Some of them are active, done alone by the patient; other exercises are passive, in which he is assisted. The active exercises primarily develop the musculature, while the passive ones are directed more toward the range of motion.

A person may feel that his daily activities will be sufficient to develop his musculature and maintain or increase his range of motion. But, too often, daily activities do not place the joint through the entire range of motion progressively. Some daily activities, furthermore, may be violent and sharp, thereby placing strain on the osteoarthritic joints. The doctor may prescribe some daily activities, that he feels will not cause pain but will add to the muscle development and the range of motion.

ASTHMA

Asthma, a noncontagious disease of the lungs, subjects the asthma sufferer to periodic attacks of difficult breathing, ranging from mild to very severe. Asthma may start in childhood or may appear at almost any age.

An asthmatic does not have symptoms all the time; but his attacks may last for minutes, hours, or days. Since he cannot get enough air into or out of his lungs, a person suffering from an attack feels that he is choking. His labored breathing is very loud.

In normal respiration the air breathed in through the nose and mouth enters the windpipe (trachea). The windpipe then divides into two smaller tubes called the bronchi. The bronchi divide again into smaller tubes called bronchioles which become so small that they are no larger than a fine piece of thread. At the end of each bronchiole, there is a tiny cluster of air sacs called alveoli. In those sacs, oxygen from the air is picked up by the blood to be carried throughout the body. At the same time the blood is absorbing oxygen, it is releasing the waste product carbon dioxide which is then exhaled. The process is repeated about 16 times every minute.

When a person suffers an asthmatic attack, the small bronchial tubes are narrowed, making breathing very difficult. The narrowing usually is the result of a swelling of the membrane which lines the tubes or of mucus blocking the tubes. Therefore, the person cannot breathe in or out satisfactorily. If the attack is severe, he feels as though he is choking. The choking feeling increases the patient's anxiety, causing further restriction and more labored breathing. The patient may turn bluish, perspire and experience heavy breathing.

Generally, most attacks of asthma are mild, but they are very disturbing to the person experiencing them.

The most common cause? Allergic reaction. Substances that cause the asthma may be food; some property in the air such as pollen, or air pollution; bacterial reactions, especially those that involve the sinuses, throat and nose.

An asthmatic should be tested to determine the cause.

It is important that you do not diagnose yourself or child as having asthma. Let a doctor decide. He has the sophisticated techniques to determine what the affliction is. You may be suffering from some other ailment. For instance, see EMPHYSEMA.

If your child is suffering from asthma, do not assume that he will outgrow it. It is far better to have it treated. Doctors have noted that it is much more likely that untreated childhood asthma will grow worse rather than go away.

Included in the treatments the doctor may give are injections such as adrenal steriods; to relieve the stress of an attack; medications; and various tests. The asthmatic can follow many procedures to help relieve or reduce the incidence of the attack. Some of those will be recommended by the family physician. Here are some basic recommendations.

Diet—Diet must be adequate in both quality and quantity. Extremes of under- or over-weight are not good. Your doctor will recommend what to eat. Avoid gas-forming foods because they may interfere with the movement of the diaphragm. Ice cold drinks are also out.

Temperature—Avoid sudden temperature or humidity changes. Extreme heat or cold will be distressing, as will high humidity or very warm dry air. The most comfortable temperature is slightly warmed air.

Colds—Avoid persons with colds and stay away from crowds during cold or flu seasons.

Fatigue—Avoid overwork or inadequate sleep. Emotional stress will also lead to fatigue. Don't allow it.

Emotions—A relaxed mental state is very important. Healthy emotions are necessary in preventing attacks and in shortening any attacks that may develop. Worry will certainly never help asthma.

Respiratory Irritants—Be on the look out for respiratory irritants. These include smoking, dust, allergic substances, alcoholic beverages (espe-

cially if you are allergic to particular cereal grains), drugs and sedatives unless they are prescribed by your doctor.

Other—Stay away from quack cures that claim overnight results. Your doctor is the one to see for treatment of asthma.

See EMPHYSEMA for several types of breathing exercises to benefit the asthmatic. Consult a physician before you attempt those exercises, as they may be completely unnecessary if the condition is under control.

Asthma patients for years have been restricted from such normal activities as baseball, running, gymnastics and dancing. Physicians used to insist on long periods of rest for asthmatics. More recently, however, that trend has been dropped. Doctors are learning about the value of exercise in helping the asthmatic toward a more enjoyable and productive life.

The National Jewish Hospital, in Denver, Colorado, with a grant from the U.S. Vocational Rehabilitation Administration, conducted a study on exercise and asthma. They discovered that 60 minutes of calisthenics such as sit-ups, push-ups, pedaling a stationary bicycle, and weight lifting allowed two out of three patients to improve in physical endurance, and three out of four to better their heart-lung efficiency. Improvement, once obtained, persisted for three months. The study indicated that controlled physical activity does not harm an asthmatic's bronchial tubes, and that physical conditioning can help the asthmatic lead a more useful life. Martin Nacman, director of rehabilitation at the hospital, and Dr. Irving H. Itkin, who conducted the study, both emphasized that asthmatic children cannot be sent out to playgrounds every day to play with other children or to participate in games. In a school situation, the school doctor or nurse can help them determine when to play and when to abstain. Otherwise, the asthmatic children must decide when they are able to participate.

Mr. Nacman noted that there is some indication that games with intermittent running are better for asthmatics than sports which require steady running. One of the most encouraging results of the study, the researchers noted, was that increased physical condition of the children gave them greater self-confidence.

A report in the 1965 *Medical Tribune* demonstrated the value of physical conditioning to asthmatics. Dr. Thomas R. McElhenny, of the University of Texas, related a 3-year pilot program of asthmatic boys, aged 8 to 13. The actual conditioning program, under the direction of Dr. Kay H. Peterson at the University, had the young boys report to the gymnasium for 2 or 3 hourly sessions each week for a year. Each child had instruction in breathing exercises and basic body skills, which included running, throwing and catching. At the outset of the program, the boys demonstrated a low fitness level and poor coordination. After the training program, they increased their vital capacities by 20 per cent, improved their performances in the standing broad jump, sit-ups, agility run, grip strength, and 50-yard dash. Ninety per cent of their teachers noted that the boys' emotional stability improved. It was also noted that there was a 40 per cent decrease in both duration and severity of asthmatic attacks.

The 1958 *Journal of the American Medical Association* contained a report by Dr. Merle S. Scherr and Lawrence Frankel. Those men conducted an experiment at the YMCA in Charleston, W. Va. Twenty-five children who were being treated for bronchial asthma were involved in the study. The program was divided into four broad phases. They were basic breathing techniques, postural exercises, gymnastics and adaptation conditioning (combatives). Each child was encour-

aged to compete with his own record rather than another child. For many children, it was their first real experience with physical exercise. The investigators reported that the majority of the children demonstrated an improvement by increasing their amount of time involved in church, school and home activities. The frequency and severity of the attacks were reduced. Pulmonary function tests also demonstrated an improvement, and the children showed a better emotional state.

It is becoming increasingly apparent that exercise is being recognized as an important adjunct for asthmatic treatment. It is not a panacea, but it should not be neglected by those people working with asthmatics, for it has both psychological and physiological values. *The Rehabilitation Record, Journal of the Vocational Rehabilitation Administration,* has noted in summary of the National Jewish Hospital Study: "The beneficial results of exercise for asthmatic patients have implications for the psychological and vocational adjustment of these individuals. These results suggest that, from a physical standpoint most asthmatic individuals, even those who are severely ill need not be restricted in physical activity as heretofore thought."

ATHLETE'S HEART

Strenuous, endurance exercise may give you a larger and stronger heart than that of an inactive person of the same physical type. That increase in size (hypertrophy) of cardiac muscle is gradual and is a beneficial adjustment to exercise. It is not the same as pathologically "enlarged" heart that occurs in some kinds of heart disease.

The term "athlete's heart," then, refers to a physiological enlargement of the cardiac muscle and does not indicate any deleterious effect. The increase in size, instead, may indicate a more efficient heart.

The athlete's heart is superior to the normal heart in several ways. With each beat, the trained heart can pump up to twice as much blood as the normal or untrained heart, therefore pumping more oxygen and nutrients with fewer beats.

Experiments with animals have shown the effect of training on the heart. Most studies involved splitting a number of animals into two groups. When one group was trained and the other group led a sedentary life, postmortem investigation revealed that those which led an active life had larger, stronger hearts than their sedentary counterparts.

Exercises of speed or strength produce little change, if any, in the size of the heart. During exercise, the healthy heart will decrease in size,

never increase. Afterward, it will return to its former size. An increase in size during exercise is usually an indication that there is an impairment in the heart, such as leaking aortic valves. In some instances, the hypertrophy of the muscle is difficult to assess, for the heart is a hollow organ and the walls may thicken inward as well as outward, thereby making X-ray evaluation difficult. In healthy hearts, physical training cannot cause injury. See LOAFER'S HEART.

ATHLETIC FITNESS VERSUS PHYSICAL FITNESS

Many people believe that athletic fitness and physical fitness are synonymous. Because of that belief, some shy away from trying to achieve physical fitness. You must realize that the basic elements of fitness are strength, mus-

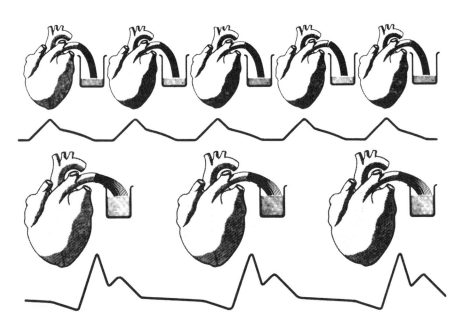

Physical conditioning will help the heart work better. In the above illustration each drawing represents a single heartbeat, and the beakers hold the blood pumped per beat. The loafer's heart (top) emits a weak, rapid beat. The beat of the trained heart at the bottom is strong and powerful.

cle endurance, flexibility and circulo-respiratory endurance. They are extremely important even if you never intend to participate in sports, because they are health factors. See STRENGTH; MUSCLE ENDURANCE; FLEXIBILITY, and CIRCULO-RESPIRATORY ENDURANCE for a discussion of those terms.

If you plan to participate in sports, other fitness components come into play—power, reaction time, movement time, speed, kinethesis and coordination. They are components which help you improve in your sport but are not that important from a health viewpoint. Athletic fitness might appropriately be called motor ability. See that listing. See also PHYSICAL FITNESS.

ATHLETIC PARTICIPATION FOR YOUNGSTERS

A good deal of controversy has been centered around allowing children and adolescents to participate in athletic contests. There has been a tendency to lower the age at which children are permitted to participate in interscholastic and interclub competition, and a lot of pressure has been placed on schools and communities to develop competitive activities for children. The argument supporting the activities goes: "Children will compete anyway, so why not make the competition safer by providing supervised team activity?" But is it safer?

The argument is also advanced that some children mature faster and are ready for competition at an earlier age and that their bodies can stand a great deal of stress with no apparent ill effects. But can they?

The Division of Men's Athletics of the American Association of Health, Physical Education and Recreation has divided athletic competition into three categories—elementary school, junior high school and senior high school. Its elementary school athletics are limited to informal games between teams from two or more schools on occasional sport days. Spectators are discouraged from attending, and emphasis is placed on competition for all children. The most important comment the division makes, however, is that "high-pressure programs of interscholastic athletics, in which varsity teams compete in regularly scheduled contests that are attended by partisan spectators, should not be allowed under any circumstances."

In junior high schools, the physical and emotional immaturity of the children must be controlled. The primary emphasis is on the participants rather than on winning teams.

In senior high school, the interscholastic athletic program should include sports in accordance with the school enrollment, facilities and budget. All should be encouraged to participate.

The basis for those guidelines established by the Division of Men's Athletics is based upon sound research and should not be taken lightly. Dr. Jiri Kral has made recommendations concerning training and competition among young children and adolescents. Although many people consider his findings too conservative, he has evidence that caution must be exercised in allowing young children to vigorously engage in competitive athletics.

Dr. Kral, a noted cardiologist and sports physician, feels that every male or female, regardless of age, must be given an extensive medical examination annually prior to the training for competition.

The most significant aspect of the three charts is not the age of competition, but rather the age at which training begins. Most training begins two years before the start of competition; and even then, the competition is generally modified.

This "go-slow" policy in competitive athletics is based on sound physiological and psychological principles.

The human body is not developed

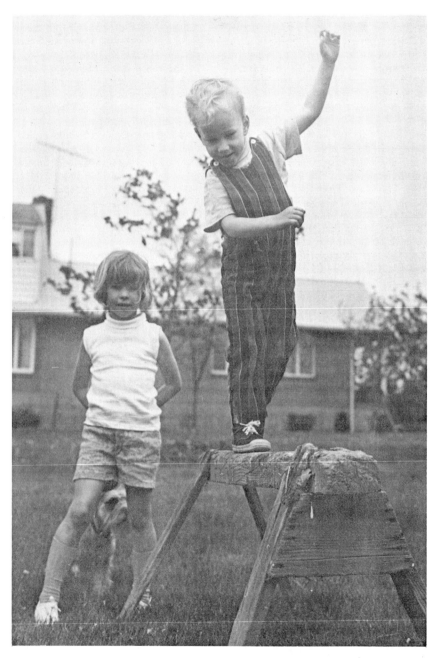

Organized competitive sports are fine for grown up boys and girls, but younger children like their play unrestricted and free. By substituting that kind of activity for team sports, your children may bypass highly pressurized activity at an early age.

TRAINING AND COMPETITION CHART FOR CHILDREN
AND ADOLESCENTS IN ATHLETIC CONTESTS

ACTIVITY	BOYS		GIRLS	
	Earliest Age to Begin Training	Earliest Age to Begin Competition	Earliest Age to Begin Training	Earliest Age to Begin Competition
Archery	9	11	11	13
Basketball	14	16	14	16
Boating				
Canoe	13	16	Only Recreation	
Kayak	13	16	13	16
Rowing	11	17	11	17
Sailing	13	16	13	16
Boxing	13	16	NO	
Cycling	11	16	16	18
Fencing				
Foil	11	11	13	16
Saber	14	16	NO	
Epee	16	18	NO	
Field Events				
Discus	13	13	16	16
High Jump	11	11	11	13
Javelin	13	13	16	16
Long Jump	11	11	11	13
Pole Vault	13	16	NO	
Triple Jump	16	18	NO	
Field Hockey	13	16	13	16
Golf	11	13	11	13
Handball	13	16	13	16
Horse Riding	11	16	13	18
Ice Hockey	10	16	NO	
Jiu Jitsu	13	14	14	16
Mountain Climbing	16	18	18	18
Rugby	13	16	NO	
Soccer	13	16	NO	
Table Tennis	13	16	13	16
Tennis	11	16	11	16
Volleyball	13	16	13	16
Water Polo	13	16	NO	
Wrestling	13	14	NO	

completely until late adolescence or young adulthood. The lack of development is especially at the joints, important where development is often delayed until the 19th to 21st year. Because of the tendon attachments, a severe strain from excessive training and competition may result in a bone growth disturbance or deformity.

"Little League Elbow" is such an injury, occurring as a result of strain and stress placed on a joint. It's a catch—all description of at least two common ailments, *epiphysitis* and *osteochondritis*. Epiphysitis is an inflammation of the still growing ends (epiphyses) of the bones. Osteochondritis is inflammation and fragmentation of cartilage. Both of the conditions result from an exaggerated throwing action in baseball. Little League Elbow has occurred in boys 10 to 13

TRAINING AND COMPETITION CHART FOR CHILDREN AND
ADOLESCENTS IN RUNNING AND SWIMMING CONTESTS

ACTIVITY	BOYS		GIRLS	
	Earliest Age to Begin Training	*Earliest Age to Begin Competition*	*Earliest Age to Begin Training*	*Earliest Age to Begin Competition*
Running				
25 yards	6		6	
50 yards	8	11	8	
75 yards		14		13
100 yards		16		16
150 yards		16		18
220 yards		16		20
440 yards		18		
880 yards		13		After 19
1000 yards		16		
1 Mile		18		
Long Distance				
1 Minute	Up to 9			
2 Minutes	9-11			
2-4 Minutes	11-13			
4-7 Minutes	13-16			
7-15 Minutes	16-18			
3 Miles		18		
6 Miles		21		
Marathon		23		
Cross Country	Same as Long Distance Training			
X-Country				
1 Mile		14		17
2 Miles		16		18
3+ Miles		18		
Hurdles				
50	11		13	
75		13		13
100		16		16
100-440		18		
Swimming				
Natural Form	6		6	
Strokes	11		11	
50 Yards		11		11-13
100 Yards		13		16
200 Yards		16		16-18
All		18		18
Diving				
1 Meter	11	13	11	13
3 Meters		16		16
10 Meters		18		

years of age. If untreated, either condition may lead to growth disturbances or deformity.

The psychological problems associated with sports are greater and perhaps more damaging than the physiological aspects. Some children are forced into competition by their well-meaning parents, who feel that "Johnny needs the exercise" or that he

TRAINING AND COMPETITION CHART FOR CHILDREN AND ADOLESCENTS IN WINTER SPORTS EVENTS

ACTIVITY	BOYS		GIRLS	
	Earliest Age to Begin Training	*Earliest Age to Begin Competition*	*Earliest Age to Begin Training*	*Earliest Age to Begin Competition*
SKATING				
A. Figure				
3 hr. week	8		8	
6 hr. week	11		11	
Modified competition		11-16		11-16
Normal competition		16		16
B. Speed	From 6 on in the form of free sport			
500	15	16	16	16
Mile		16		18
Long Distance		18		18
C. Ice Hockey			NO	
Techniques	10			
Training	15			
Competition		16		
SKIING				
Cross Country Training				
Natural form	6		6	
Moderate slopes	11		11	
Racing Style	13		13	
Competition				
1 Mile		11		14
3 Miles		13		16
5 Miles		16		18
10 Miles		20		
Above		23		
Descents				
No Obstacles	11		11	
Normal Competition		18		18
Ski Jumping				
30 Meters	13			
50 Meters	16			
Normal Competition		18		
Slalom				
Training Competition	11		11	
150 yards (20° slope)		11		13
500 yards (25° slope)		16		16
Normal Competition		18		18

must be as athletic as other neighborhood boys.

Many times, children are pressured into feats they are incapable of performing. For example, an adult finds it difficult to hit a ball that is pitched to him 60 feet 6 inches away. Yet a little leaguer must attempt to dupli-cate that feat, from a distance of 40 feet.

The child reacts with frustration. He is unable to do the things expected of him; yet he feels he must, or he will suffer humiliation from his peers and parents.

Another problem is that many elementary children are not ready for highly organized play. Look at any reputable elementary physical education program, and you will see the emphasis placed on free play, rhythmic, explorative activities. Any games played usually lack formal organization.

The pressures exerted on children in organized sports like Little League is unbelievable. Here are a few situations encountered by a Little League Football coach:

"The mothers thought it would be nice to have cheerleaders for the games. So they made uniforms for the young girls, some five years of age, and had them lead the crowd in cheers during the game.

"The size limit for the boys was 112 pounds. One boy, at the beginning of the year, weighed 125 pounds. He was encouraged to sweat down to 112 pounds to make him eligible to play. (He was only weighed once during the season.) He competed against boys who ranged from 70 pounds to 112 pounds.

"Parents and friends were encouraged to attend; a collection was taken. They offered such encouraging remarks to their boys age 8 to 12, as: 'Get that bum out of there,' and 'That kid stinks,' or 'No, don't put them in there.' "

Another serious problem encountered in Little League competition is that many times, well-meaning people, without the necessary knowledge of exercise and the sport, direct a little league program. All too often, they are former high school athletes who coach essentially the way they were taught 20 years before. As a result, they may have the boys using improper exercises or techniques that are outdated and considered dangerous to the participant.

A parent should not believe that because his child is engaging in sports he is achieving fitness. To achieve fitness, a well rounded selection of sports and exercise must be made.

Today, children are forced into competitive activities before they are ready physiologically and psychologically. The tendency to start too soon has caused considerable heartbreak and cut many an athlete's career short. The important thing to remember is that a child should be given a diversity of activities from his early childhood. The activities selected should be diverse enough so that all body areas are affected and should include tumbling, hanging, jumping, running, skipping, rough and tumble play and many lead-up ball activities. As a child gets older, lead-up games and the various sports should be included. The activities must last several hours a day.

When a child is introduced to an activity, it ought to be in free form. Let him experiment on his own in the form of lead-up games. As he begins to develop, the games and activities may become more structured, until he is ready for training and competition.

A parent must be aware of what contributions various activities make to physical fitness. Sport programs are advantageous for child fitness, but early competition and training are dangerous.

Dr. Thomas K. Cureton and Dr. Allan Barry have demonstrated at the Sport-Fitness School of the University of Illinois that the combining of exercise with sport activities is necessary to achieve fitness in youth. They state that elementary school children should experience 30 minutes of continuous rhythmical exercises daily prior to participating in sports, games, dances, swimming and outdoor living. Strength activities and exercises must become progressively harder and longer so that the cardiovascular system is developed. They also feel that such activities as interval training, circuit training and steeplechase must be used. As you will note, all those activities are quite vigorous and demanding.

The primary emphasis is on the attainment of physical fitness, and sports play a vital role in the achieving of fitness. A child does not develop his fitness potential, however, by participating in only one or two sports. Diversification is necessary, making a child compete in organized athletics at too early an age will restrict his physical fitness development. See CIRCUIT TRAINING, INTERVAL TRAINING, GROWTH, INJURIES, SPORTS and TRAINING.

ATHLETIC SICKNESS

After a short but exhausting exercise bout, you may experience extreme weakness, heavy perspiration, throbbing head, nausea, vomiting, blurred vision, or a feeling of light-headedness. The phenomenon is known as *athletic sickness*. It is a result of sugar being withdrawn from the blood to the exercising muscles at such a rapid rate that the liver is unable to replenish the sugar immediately, and *hypoglycemia* occurs. After a brief period of rest, the condition usually disappears. See BLOOD.

BACK

The back muscles are more often thought of as a source of discomfort than as a building stone toward physical fitness. Given a moderate amount of attention and exercise, however, back muscles can be developed to a degree that will help avert most of the common back ailments.

Individual Muscles

The *splenius capitis* muscle is located at the back of the neck and draws the head backward and to the side. It also acts with other muscles in supporting the head in an erect position.

An excellent exercise to strengthen that muscle and other neck muscles is to place your hands in back of your head and press with your head back into your hands. Then place your hands on the forehead and push your head into your hands. Be certain the pressure is exerted by the head or neck and not by the hands.

The *sacrospinalis* is a deep, large muscle that starts in the hip region and travels all the way to the neck. The muscle, itself, splits into three columns which are called the *iliocostalis*, the *longissimus* and the *spinalis*. Those muscles aid in holding up the spine and connect the column to the ribs. The muscles also aid in bending the back backward.

To strengthen the *sacrospinalis* muscles lie flat with your chest on the floor and your hands along the sides of your body. Then lift your upper body from the floor; be certain that your rib cage is completely off the floor.

To stretch the muscles, lie with your back on the floor; and the arms at a 45° angle. Bring your legs over the head, together, and touch the toes to the floor. Keep your legs straight.

The *trapezius* is a large flat triangle shaped muscle that covers the upper back and the upper and back part of the shoulders and neck. It aids in lifting the arms or in carrying a load on the shoulders. It also plays a part in shrugging the shoulders, extending the head from side to side.

Here's an isometric exercise to strengthen the trapezius. Stand in a doorway and turn your palms out pushing against the door jam. Keep the elbows as straight as possible. Exert a maximum force for 10 seconds.

The *latissimus dorsi* muscle is a triangular cover of the lower middle part of the back and the back part of the rib cage. Part of the muscle is attached to the humerus (arm bone). Because of that attachment, the muscle helps in moving the arm backward, rotating the arm inward, and bringing the arm toward the body. It is used considerably in swimming and rowing. To increase the strength of the muscle, place both hands between a doorway. The hands should be above the head with the palms turned out. Press the hands outward against the door jams and keep the elbows straight; hold for 10 seconds.

The *rhomboid* muscles, located in the upper portion of the back near the neck, act with other muscles to steady the shoulder bone (scapula) when the arm is moved. They also retract and depress the shoulder.

Exercises can be used to increase the strength of the rhomboid muscle. See: EXERCISES, ISOMETRICS, WEIGHT TRAINING. See especially LOW BACK PAIN.

BACK PACKING

See HIKING.

BACKYARD FITNESS

"I wish my children would exercise more, but the 'Y' is too far away." The solution to that dilemma is as close as your backyard. Use it as your family's path to fitness.

Swing Set

Swing sets are popular in America's backyards; but often, when Dad puts up a set, he neglects the extras, like rings, chinning bar and rope. Perhaps he had to struggle to get the main part of the swing up, and forgot the extra items; or perhaps Mom was afraid the children would get hurt climbing around like monkeys.

Whatever the reason, it is unfortunate; for the extra equipment is excellent for developing arm and shoulder

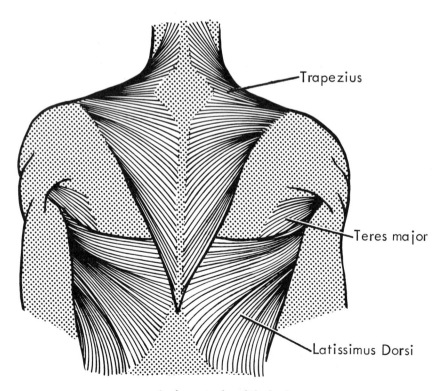

Surface muscles of the back.

muscles—areas which are greatly underdeveloped in American youth.

The rings and the chinning bar are used for pull-up and skin-the-cat exercises. As the child develops, he can add gymnastic activities, like half-lever exercises, belly grinds and birds' nests.

Rope

Don't forget the rope. At first children will merely swing on it, tarzan style. Later, they will climb to the top, with or without their feet. Some will even try climbing upside down.

From a sturdy tree limb, hang a knotted rope, ¾ inch in diameter. Tie the first knot about 4 feet from the ground, spacing the rest every 12 to 18 inches apart. The knots make excellent hand-holds for children. When a child is first learning, he should not exceed three knot lengths. As he becomes more proficient, he can gradually increase his height until he reaches 15 to 20 feet above the ground. For safety, line a bed, around the base of the rope, with sand, pine needles, sawdust or shavings. If the bed is long enough, it may be used for a high jump or broad jump pit.

For additional challenge to rope climbing, hang two ropes about 2½ feet apart and have the children climb the ropes at the same time.

Give the children other ropes, about ¼ inch in diameter; they will find a hundred uses for them, from rope skipping to rope high jumping.

Tires

Old tires are a fitness challenge to children. If tires are not available, substitute logs. Have the children run through the tires by stepping in the holes. They can alternate legs or jump with both legs from one tire to another. Add a competitive element by having the children run through the tires as rapidly as possible. They can also roll the tire on the ground with a stick.

A tire tied to a rope hanging from a tree is a unending source of physical entertainment. Children will swing on it, jump through it, or throw a ball or other object through it.

House Ladder

A ladder is an excellent device to challenge your child to be more active physically. Lean the ladder against the house, being certain that is is securely anchored. In that position, it is a substitute chinning bar. Pull-ups, knees to the chest, and half lever positions are a few possible ladder gymnastics.

Or place the ladder horizontally between two trees or some other sturdy base. Then the children can jump up and grasp a rung with both hands and advance forward, monkey-style.

All those exercises are particularly good for developing the upper arm and shoulder muscles.

Chinning Bar

Put up chinning bars throughout the yard. They should be of varying heights for different sized children.

A pipe 1¾ inches in diameter makes an excellent bar. For beginners, put the bar at chest height. The children can hang from the bar, curling their legs up behind them and attempting to pull themselves up. See EXERCISES.

Other

There are many other techniques that can be used in backyard fitness.

Provide balls of all sizes and shapes and watch the children improvise. Select a playing site for badminton, volleyball or deck tennis. If you have a concrete or smooth macadam driveway, hopscotch and shuffleboard are naturals.

Are you handy with tools? You can easily build some of the equipment, for example, chinning bars or a sawhorse for balancing stunts.

Children will also get a big kick out of jumping off objects of various heights. The pile of dirt that you just don't know what to do with, the sawhorses, a pile of railroad ties—anything of reasonable height can be used.

If you have a swimming pool or some other elaborate recreational facility, your fitness program has a head start already.

At first, TV might have an iron hold on your family, creating an anti-exercise feeling. So make them follow your lead. Soon they will pick up the idea and start to tell you what to do or what can be done.

Do not be surprised if you get interested in many of the activities the children are doing and attempt to duplicate their feats. Participating along with the children will do you a world of good. Remember, children are great imitators. If you dump yourself in front of the television every minute and allow yourself to become overweight, they will too. If you are active, your children will be active. What you are, they will become.

A recent study by W. A. Ruffer in the *Research Quarterly* revealed that active high school students had active parents who encouraged their children to be active. Inactive students had inactive parents who did not encourage physical activity among their children.

See: CALISTHENICS, DAILY ACTIVITIES, DUAL RESISTANCE EXERCISE, FAMILY PHYSICAL FITNESS, ISOMETRICS, MEDICINE BALL ACTIVITIES, PROGRAMS, ROPE SKIPPING, SPORTS, TRAINING and WEIGHT TRAINING.

BADMINTON

Badminton is a high-energy activity that will make a big contribution to fitness if played vigorously (not as it is practiced in most backyards).

Depending upon the vigor and length of play, a regular player can expect to achieve a high level of circulo-respiratory fitness, leg muscle endurance, abdominal muscle strength, and increased endurance and flexibility in the dominant arm and shoulder.

You can find useful exercises for the sport by consulting the diagrams in the WEIGHT TRAINING and ISOMETRICS sections. Additional help can be obtained from volleying a pee-gee ball against a wall and swinging the racket around, fast enough to make a swishing sound.

The game is played indoors or outdoors on a flat surface. The players

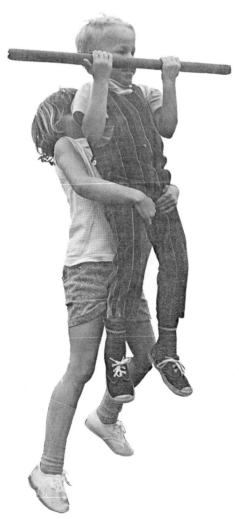

When the facilities are handy and the encouragement is substantial, youngsters can have fun while they build healthier bodies right in their own backyard.

(two for singles, four for doubles) use rackets weighing about five ounces to hit the shuttlecock, or bird, over a net in mid-court, tennis fashion. The shuttlecock is a ball, usually of cork, with a skirt of feathers or plastic to slow its speed of flight.

Only the serving player can score. If a player loses the rally, which he put in play with the serve, he loses the serve to his opponent. In doubles, before a team loses its opportunity to serve, both players on the team have an opportunity to serve. The game is usually played to 15 points by men, and 11 points by women.

On the initial serve of the game, in both singles and doubles play, opponents serve and receive from their respective right hand courts. With each serve, they alternate right- and left-hand courts. At the time of the serve, both feet must be in contact with the floor.

Physical Qualities Needed

Age is no barrier to badminton playing. So long as a person has been fairly active and has maintained a good physical condition, he can enjoy playing well after age 60.

Playing requires good hand-eye coordination; and to experience any kind of success, practice is essential—both in hitting the shuttle on the serve and on the volley. Practicing hitting a pee-gee ball will help develop hand-eye coordination.

A reasonable degree of circulo-respiratory endurance must be developed to prevent excessive fatigue during play. Lacking that type of endurance, play will deteriorate rapidly because of the great amount of running and movement involved. Also needed are a moderate degree of arm strength, adequate abdominal strength and low back flexibility to make the many difficult plays, and leg muscle endurance.

Association:

American Badminton Association, (ABA), 1330 Alexander Drive, San Diego, California 92107.

Since badminton is a high energy cost activity, it may be used to help improve your fitness level, especially your circulo-respiratory and muscle endurance. Below is a badminton program that takes into account the important principles of training.

If you desire to improve your strength and power for the activity, see WEIGHT TRAINING and ISOMETRICS. The weight training and isometrics exercises may also be used to prepare your body for athletic competition.

* BADMINTON PROGRAM
(Vigorous) **

Chart 1	Chart 2
1. 10 minutes	1. 38 minutes
2. 15 minutes	2. 40 minutes
3. 18 minutes	3. 43 minutes
4. 20 minutes	4. 45 minutes
5. 23 minutes	5. 50 minutes
6. 25 minutes	6. 53 minutes
7. 30 minutes	7. 55 minutes
8. 33 minutes	8. 58 minutes
9. 35 minutes	9. 60 minutes

* See ENDURANCE and ENERGY COST OF ACTIVITIES for an explanation of the charts.
** Doesn't include rest periods, time outs, etc.

Fitness 1

If you achieved a score of poor or low average on the *Harvard Step Test* or a score of very poor or poor on the *12 Minute Run*, start on Chart 1-Level 1 and spend 1 week at each level until Chart 2-Level 9 is reached. It is recommended that you participate 4 to 5 days a week. When Chart 2-Level 9 is reached, 4 days a week is sufficient.

Fitness 2

If you achieved a score of high average on the *Harvard Step Test* or fair on the *12 Minute Run*, start on Chart

1-Level 2. Spend one week on Chart 1-Levels 2, 4, 6, 7, 9, and Chart 2-Levels 2, 4, 5, 7, and 9. It is recommended that you participate 4 to 5 days a week. When Chart 2-Level 9 is reached, 4 days a week is sufficient.

Fitness 3

If you achieved a score of good or excellent on either the *Harvard Step Test* or *12 Minute Run*, continue your current program or select Chart 2-Level 9 as your level of participation. Four days a week is sufficient.

BALANCE

Balance, a component of motor ability, involves reflexes, vision, the inner ear, the cerebellum and the skeletal-muscular system. It is closely related to the kinesthetic sense. According to Dr. Edwin Fleishman, there are three types of balance: static, dynamic and balancing of objects. Static balance is the ability to hold the body in some natural or unnatural position for a length of time. It is usually measured while a person is standing on one foot or doing a hand balance. Dynamic bal-

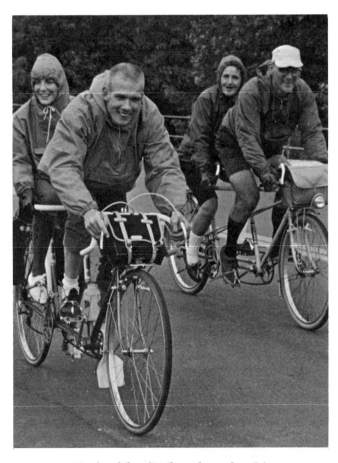

Tandem bikes distribute the work and fun.

ance is the ability to maintain your equilibrium while performing some other task (like rail walking or balancing yourself on a large ball).

The ability to balance an object is also an aspect of fitness and is usually measured by having a person balance a yardstick on the end of a finger or a ball on the back of a hand.

Persons with good balance normally excel in diving and/or trampolining. To improve your balance, simply make repeated attempts at the desired feat.

See COORDINATION, KINESTHESIA, PHYSICAL FITNESS and TESTS.

BICYCLING

Bicycling or cycling has four aspects —recreation, transportation, racing and fitness.

In some areas, the bicycle is a weekend plaything; while in European and Asian nations, it is often a person's daily transportation. Recent endorsements of the bicycle by medical au-

thorities like Dr. Paul Dudley White, the noted heart specialist, have increased the popularity of bike riding for exercise in the United States.

Dr. Irvine H. Page, president of the American Heart Association, said recently, "We ought to replace automobiles with bicycles. . . . It would be better for our coronaries, our dispositions and certainly our finances."

People vary in their use of a bicycle. Some may use it only on weekends; others make it a daily habit. Some pedal leisurely; others enjoy vigorous pedaling.

Generally, the casual rider will use a one-or-three-speed bicycle; they're usually best for short jaunts. He will sit almost straight up and pedal sedately. A person who uses a bicycle over longer stretches will undoubtedly use a 5, 10 or 15 speed model. Here the rider leans forward and pedals vigorously.

Racing cyclists have many distances and forms of races from which to

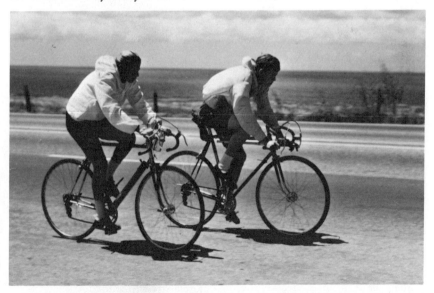

Two ways to ride a 10-speed bicycle. Cyclist on the left puts hands on the top of the handlebars for normal driving, while the cyclist on the right demonstrates the use of the dropped handlebars for speed racing or for extra leverage on hills.

choose, varying from short sprints, middle and long distance races, up to road races that take several days. Some races occur on special cycling tracks, some on improvised facilities (unused air fields, motor speedways, auto drag strips, stadium tracks, parking lots, etc.), and still others on highways. The bicycle will vary according to the type of race, as well as to the rules and preference of the individual.

Often, to supplement or spice up the traditional short and long distance races special races are held. Those include:

The Slow Race: The last rider across the finish line wins. The rider must stay within a prescribed lane and cannot allow his feet to touch the ground.

The Unknown Distance Race: The race is performed best on a stadium or cycle track. All riders start together with the sound of a gun. While the cyclists are moving around the track, the starter randomly selects a lap number. The starter then fires the gun to signal the rider that only two laps remain. The first to cross the finish line wins.

The Laggard: The race is performed on a stadium or cycle track. The last rider after each lap is disqualified. The race is run until only one rider remains.

Naturally, all cyclists do not want to race. Touring or vigorous pleasure riding will develop fitness, too. Here are some guidelines for enjoying bicycle touring from cycling authorities.

The reason many people are sore after extensive trips is that they choose any old bike and start riding. They never take the trouble to make the preliminary adjustments. The saddle is too low, the frame too heavy or too whippy, the tires too big or too small. A person can no more pick up the first bicycle he sees and be comfortable on it than he can in somebody else's shoes. Therefore, get a bike to fit you! Do not ride a borrowed bicycle. Buy one.

Once you bring your bike home, observe these points for the most pleasure and beneficial exercise:

Pedal with the ball of the foot, not the heel or arch. Don't use too "high" a gear during your first rides; "down-shifting" avoids strain and fatigue.

Avoid the pitfall of setting the seat too low. Ideally, the seat should be high enough so that when a leg is extended fully, the heel rests on the bottom pedal. That creates a slight bend in the leg when the ball of the foot is placed properly on the pedal.

The "up in the air" feeling you get, after first adjusting the seat properly, will soon disappear. You'll learn to mount the bike by stepping up on the top pedal, and to get off by stepping from the bottom pedal as you come to a stop.

Keep to quiet streets or parks while learning to ride. In large American cities, there has been a movement in recent years to designate special bicycle routes along streets where auto traffic is low. Some cities go so far as to designate "bicycle only" routes during certain weekend hours.

Contribution to Fitness

Age is no barrier to bicycling. As a rule, a bike ride can be enjoyed by anyone who can walk. Furthermore, cycling can make a significant contribution toward physical fitness. The degree of fitness, naturally, depends upon the vigor with which you participate.

If you ride at 12 miles an hour or more (on the level) for at least 30 minutes, four or five days a week, you can expect to develop excellent leg muscle strength and endurance. There will also be an improvement in hip, knee and ankle flexibility. Vigorous cycling (racing) will improve arm, abdomen, chest, shoulder, back and neck muscle strength and endurance.

The biggest and most important contribution of cycling, however, is circulo-respiratory fitness. Since that

*CYCLING PROGRAM (BALLOON TIRE–COASTER BRAKE)

Chart 1	Chart 2
1. 1¼-1½ miles in 7 minutes	1. 3¾-4 miles in 20 minutes
2. 1½-1¾ miles in 8 minutes	2. 4-4¼ miles in 20 minutes
3. 1¾-2 miles in 10 minutes	3. 4¼-4½ miles in 22 minutes
4. 2-2¼ miles in 11 minutes	4. 4½-4¾ miles in 22 minutes
5. 2¼-2½ miles in 12 minutes	5. 4¾-5 miles in 25 minutes
6. 2½-2¾ miles in 13 minutes	6. 5-5½ miles in 25 minutes
7. 2¾-3 miles in 14 minutes	7. 5¼-5½ miles in 27 minutes
8. 3-3½ miles in 16 minutes	8. 5½-6 miles in 30 minutes
9. 3½-3¾ miles in 18 minutes	9. 6½ miles in 30 minutes

* See ENDURANCE and ENERGY COST OF ACTIVITIES for an explanation of the charts.

Fitness 1

If you achieved a score of poor or low average on the *Harvard Step Test* or a score of very poor or poor on the *12 Minute Run*, start on Chart 1-Level 1 and spend 1 week at each level until Chart 2-Level 9 is reached. It is recommended that you participate 4 to 5 days a week. When Chart 2-Level 9 is reached, 4 days a week is sufficient.

Fitness 2

If you achieved a score of high average on the *Harvard Step Test* or fair on the *12 Minute Run*, start on Chart 1-Level 4. Spend one week on Chart 1-Levels 2, 4, 6, 7, and 9, and Chart 2-Levels 2, 4, 5, 7, 8, and 9. It is recommended that you participate 4 to 5 days a week. When Chart 2-Level 9 is reached, 4 days a week is sufficient.

Fitness 3

If you achieved a score of good or excellent on either the *Harvard Step Test* or *12 Minute Run*, continue your current program or select Chart 2-Level 9 as your level of participation. Four days a week is sufficient.

---

is extremely effective in reducing the incidence of degenerative cardiovascular disease, it is important to include in your program a continuous, rhythmical activity that will make such a contribution to circulo-respiratory fitness.

Many noted health and medical authorities have given testimonials to cycling for fitness. A poll among 14,000 doctors during a Bicycle Health Week campaign in England attested to the value of the bicycle and its effect upon every group in the population.

The best training for bicycling is simply riding a bicycle. However, those interested in a complete regimen should consult the TRAINING section and the diagrams in the WEIGHT TRAINING and ISOMETRICS sections.

Associations:

Amateur Bicycle League of America (ABLA), 6411 Orchard, Dearborn, Michigan 48126.

American Cycling Union (ACU), c/o Harvey C. Black, 192 Alexander Street, Newark, New Jersey 07106.

Bicycle Institute of America, 122 East 42nd Street, New York, New York 10017.

League of American Wheelmen, Inc. (LAW), 5118 Foster Avenue, Chicago, Illinois 60630.

Since bicycling is a high energy cost activity, it may be used to help improve your fitness level, especially your circulo-respiratory and muscle endurance. Below are two cycling training programs that take into account the important principles of training.

*CYCLING PROGRAM (RACING BICYCLE)

Chart 1	Chart 2
1. 2 miles in 7½ minutes	1. 5 miles in 18½ minutes
2. 2 miles in 7 minutes	2. 6 miles in 23 minutes
3. 3 miles in 12 minutes	3. 6 miles in 22½ minutes
4. 3 miles in 11½ minutes	4. 6 miles in 22 minutes
5. 4 miles in 15½ minutes	5. 7 miles in 27 minutes
6. 4 miles in 15 minutes	6. 7 miles in 26½ minutes
7. 4 miles in 14½ minutes	7. 7 miles in 26 minutes
8. 5 miles in 19½ minutes	8. 8 miles in 31 minutes
9. 5 miles in 19 minutes	9. 8 miles in 29-30 minutes

* See ENDURANCE and ENERGY COST OF ACTIVITIES for an explanation of the charts.

Fitness 1

Same as balloon tire cycling program.

Fitness 2

If you achieved a score of high average on the *Harvard Step Test* or fair on the *12 Minute Run,* start on Chart 1-Level 2. Spend one week on Chart 1-Levels 2, 3, 6, 8, and 9, and Chart 2-Levels 2, 4, 6, 7, 8, and 9. It is recommended that you participate 4 to 5 days a week. When Chart 2-Level 9 is reached, 4 days a week is sufficient.

Fitness 3

Same as balloon tire cycling program.

BLOOD

If the network of blood vessels were likened to a subway system, the blood would be the train within that system. The capillaries would be the stations and terminals where passengers enter and exit. The passengers would be oxygen, carbon dioxide, nutrients and other substances which are carried in the blood to and from the cells and tissues.

Despite its appearance, blood is not entirely liquid. It is a fluid tissue made up of various cells and a liquid called *plasma.* Those cells are actually solid microscopic particles which are carried throughout the body in the liquid plasma. The average adult circulatory system contains 10 pints of blood.

Arterial blood is bright red on its way to the tissues. After it leaves the tissues as venous blood, it is a darker purplish color. The oxygen in arterial blood gives it the red color. The color change accompanies the release of oxygen from the blood to the tissues. At the same time, the carbon dioxide content of the blood increases, as a result of cell activity. The blood retains the purplish color until it reaches the lungs, where carbon dioxide is expelled and the oxygen supply is renewed. During that process of external respiration, the blood once again assumes a bright red color. See CIRCULATORY SYSTEM and RESPIRATION.

Blood Volume

Blood volume falls at the outset of training and increases as training progresses, persisting several weeks after training. The rise may be as much as 25 per cent. During prolonged bed rest, the opposite occurs—the blood volume decreases during the immobilization and increases when the patient is reconditioned. Therefore, exercise plays a critical role in blood volume.

The values of increased blood volume are: It aids in heat dissipation during severe exercise. See ENVIRONMENT. The muscle tissues, during exercise, need more blood. The increased volume will allow a more adequate venous return to the heart, which is critical during severe or heavy exercise.

Red Corpuscles

Even short exercise periods will increase the number of red cells, dependent upon the intensity of exercise. The normal count is around 5 million per cubic millimeter. Vigorous exercise may increase that level by as much as 25 per cent. Whether the increase is a result of stored cells being released, or the manufacture of more cells is not clear. However, the increase is of short duration and will gradually diminish a few minutes after exercise. Within a half to two hours, it will return to the pre-exercise level. The increase is due to a compensatory adjustment of the body so that the tissues exercised are more adequately supplied with blood and oxygen.

Whether or not training produces an increase in red cell count per cubic millimeter of blood has been the subject of many investigations. Evidence is conflicting. Logically, you may infer that since there is an increase in blood volume there is also an increase in red blood cell count, but not necessarily the number per cubic millimeter of blood.

Some investigators note that even if, during training, there is an increase in red blood cells, a researcher might not be able to find that increase while the subject is at rest. It is possible that the cells are diverted from circulation and stored somewhere in the body until needed. The telltale sign that convinces most investigators that training produces an increase in red blood cells is that the bone marrow, under training, becomes much redder, indicating an increase in red blood cell production.

With an increase in red cells, the oxygen carrying capacity of the blood is increased. Because of the increased

oxygen supply to the muscles, endurance increases.

White Blood Cells

Exercise of any type increases the leukocyte count. If the exercise is exhausting, the white blood cell count may rise from the normal 5,000 to 9,000 count to 30,000—the greater the stress, the greater the increase. Less fit individuals show a greater rise in white cells after exercise.

Most exercise physiologists agree that the reason for the rapid increase is that there is a literal "washing out" of the white corpuscles from such places as the spleen, liver, lungs and bone marrow.

Training appears to have very little effect on the number and percentage of white blood cells. The only apparent change is that the number of younger white cells increases.

Immediately after exercise, the number of platelets (small colorless corpuscles) decreases rapidly by 15 to 30 per cent. The period of decline is followed by a rapid increase and overproduction of those cells. The platelet count may exceed the normal count by 20 per cent. Several hours after exercise the platelet count stabilizes itself.

A number of research studies have demonstrated that vigorous exercise has an effect on reducing the plasma level of some typical blood fats (triglycerides).

Furthermore, many studies indicate that cholesterol levels are reduced as a result of endurance training. Low fat diets and a reduction of stress also contribute to reducing the cholesterol level. See CHOLESTEROL.

There are two popular theories on the cause of atherosclerosis and arteriosclerotic heart disease. One maintains that a fatty substance is deposited in the arterial walls, and reduces the diameter of the blood vessel—the *lipid deposit theory*. See ARTERIOSCLEROSIS. A second, the fibrin deposit theory, advocates that fibrin is deposited in the arterial wall, causing a thrombus to be formed. The thrombus also decreases the diameter of the vessel.

Regardless of the theory accepted, it is evident that blood clots do block important vessels and cause heart attacks and strokes. The research findings indicate that exercise and training increase the clotting time of the blood and speed the clot's lysis (dissolving) time. That conclusion indicates that exercise may prevent the formation of a thrombus or aid in dissolving one.

Blood sugar may increase during and after vigorous exercise. If exercise is prolonged for several hours, blood sugar may drop. How far it drops, and whether it will drop below normal, depends primarily upon the amount of carbohydrate stored in the body.

After a certain exertion, the phosphate content of the blood will drop; but it will not drop as low in the trained man as in an untrained man.

Should you exercise after donating blood? The answer generally is that you may exercise 24 hours later. Be certain the workout is not exhausting, and try not to do more than the previous day's workout. Giving blood is not harmful to the body; but performance, especially endurance, will be affected for several days after the blood loss. In some instances, performance has been affected for as much as 18 days.

BLOOD PRESSURE

Circulation of blood begins with the heart, the pump of the circulatory system. The arteries carry the blood from the heart to various parts of the body. After each contraction, the heart relaxes temporarily. When it does, the aortic valve closes; and the blood flows through the aorta to the other arteries. As the blood passes through the arteries, they expand to adjust to the increased volume. The expansion can be felt as a pulse. To continue circulation, the blood must be pumped under pressure, which is provided by the heart as it contracts. When it relaxes, there is virtually no pressure in the valves of the heart, but the aortic valve keeps pressure within the arteries.

Blood flows out of the heart into the aorta when the heart contracts, creating pressure within the heart. Since the pressure is greater in the aorta, the blood flows into the subsequent smaller arteries. It leaves the arteries for the capillaries, the capillaries for the veins, and the veins for the right auricle. The process is simple; blood always flows from a region of higher pressure to a region of lower pressure.

Age and Blood Pressure

The normal arterial blood pressure of an individual varies considerably with age. At birth, systolic pressure may be as low as 20 to 60 mm Hg; but by the first month, the average pressure rises to 70 to 80 mm Hg. There is a gradual increase in blood pressure until old age. At 20 years of age, or so, a typical blood pressure is: systolic blood pressure—120, diastolic blood pressure—80, recorded as 120/80.

There are indications that, although the gradual increase after 40 years of age is typical, it is not necessary. The increase is attributed to a gradual decrease in the elasticity of the arterial walls. In many instances, if that elasticity is maintained, the blood pressure

INFLUENCE OF AGE ON BLOOD PRESSURE

Age	Systolic Pressure	Diastolic Pressure
6 mo. male	89	60
6 mo. female	93	62
10 yr. male	103	70
20 yr. male	120	80
30 yr. male	123	82
40 yr. male	126	84
50 yr. male	130	86
60 yr. male	135	89

will not continue to rise. There are many individuals over 60 years of age who have systolic pressure of 120 and diastolic pressure of 70 or 80, a commendable reading for any adult.

The normal resting systolic blood pressure for men is from 110 to 135 mm Hg., while the normal diastolic pressure is 60 to 99 mm Hg. Those ranges may vary and still be normal for a particular individual.

Sex

The normal resting blood pressure of women is about 10 mm Hg. lower than the normal resting blood pressure for men.

Emotions

Emotions, such as excitement, fear and anxiety may cause an increase in blood pressure. Therefore, the emotional state of the individual should be considered when taking a reading. A person who is subject to a life of anxiety or stress will have above normal pressures.

Body Position

Blood pressure is affected by the position of the body. For example, when a person stands up from a reclining position, there is usually a momentary reduction in the blood pressure. The decline is a result of a slower blood return to the heart via the veins. The body attempts to adjust for the momentary drop; and in doing so, it usually overadjusts. The overadjustment causes the blood pressure to jump up to 10 to 15 mm Hg. higher than it was in the reclining position.

In a few instances, a feeling of dizziness or faintness may result after rising. That sensation sometimes comes from the failure of the body to adjust the blood pressure with the change in posture. The blood pressure, instead of rising to adjust, falls and insufficient pressure causes the feeling of dizziness. The condition is not usually serious.

The blood pressure change from the reclining to the standing position is often used as a general measure of physical fitness. However, there is not enough evidence to substantiate that relationship for everyone.

Exercise

Since excitement will cause a rise in blood pressure, athletes often experience an anticipatory rise in blood pressure prior to competition. The rise may occur days, hours, or minutes before competition. It is dependent upon the gravity of the contest, mental preparation, and various individual factors, such as the amount of leisure time (time to think about performance) and the nature of the contest.

During exercise, there is a greater demand for oxygen. To meet the demand, the amount of blood passing through the lungs and muscles must be increased. The pressure around the arteries is greater during muscular effort, and the blood pressure must be increased to overcome that greater pressure. Also there is an increased stroke volume (amount of blood pumped per beat) of the heart which results in an increased pressure on the walls of the aorta and the arteries.

Mild exercise, such as slow walking, affects systolic blood pressure very little. In fact, after a leisurely walk, the systolic pressure of some persons drops slightly.

As exercise becomes more intensive, systolic pressure rises. During vigorous exercise, the pressure rises quickly at the beginning, then levels off, and may drop slightly. Continued exercise, however, may produce a gradual second increase. The reason for the rapid rise, leveling off, and subsequent second rise may be a result of the adjustments the body is making to the exercise stress.

Immediately after exercise, the systolic pressure may fall; but shortly after, there is a dramatic increase, reaching a maximum level sometime within the next minute. The reason for the decline and the sudden increase after exercise is not clear, although it may be a result of a slowing down of the return of the blood to the heart through the veins. That phenomenon is somewhat similar to the dizzy feeling experienced by some people after lying down for some time and then standing quickly.

An abnormal systolic response to exercise will reveal an increase similar to that described above. However, after maintaining a plateau for a short time, the blood pressure will fall rapidly to the original level and lower. The drop is attributed to fatigue of the heart that has not adapted to the physical stress.

Although there is a considerable degree of controversy concerning the response of diastolic blood pressure to exercise, it appears that among people in good condition the pressure falls during exercise; while among those in poor condition or with hardened arteries, diastolic pressure will rise. The reason given for the difference is that the decrease in diastolic pressure is the result of the arterioles and capillaries opening up for better circulation. The opening causes a decrease in their resistance; thereby causing better efficiency. The tissues receive more oxygen and the body becomes better cooled. During mild exercise, the diastolic blood pressure of a person in good condition will remain almost unchanged.

Type of Exercise

The type of exercise affects blood pressure. In strength exercises, such as weight training, there is a sudden rise in blood pressure, without a great change in pulse rate. After exercise, however, the pressure drops very quickly. Exercises that are continuous and rhythmical, on the other hand, produce a gradual increase during the exercise of both heart rate and blood pressure, and a slow gradual drop to normal afterward.

The blood pressure response to exercise has several implications for prescribing exercise for individuals who may have cardiovascular diseases or weaknesses. Exercises involving heavy lifting may place a dangerous stress on blood vessels and, therefore, on the cardiovascular system, due to the sudden increase and decrease of blood pressure.

Speed exercises, such as sprinting, cause an increase similar to weight lifting. Although the pressure does not usually go as high, there is a rapid increase during the event and a rapid decrease after the event.

During endurance-type exercises the pressure rises above that of sprinting but not to the level reached in weight lifting. In severe endurance events, such as a 10,000 meter race, the blood pressure may drop below normal 10 to 15 minutes after cessation of the race. That decrease may continue for several hours before the pressure starts an upward swing.

Generally, the greatest blood pressure response is generated through strength exercises, followed by endurance exercises. Finally, the least response comes with rhythmical exercises.

Training

Although training has little effect on *normal* resting systolic blood pressure, there is considerable evidence accumulating to indicate that above normal systolic blood pressure levels may be reduced through endurance type exercises. These endurance exercises also apparently reduce elevated diastolic blood pressures. It is also important to note that the general increase in systolic blood pressure due to aging is much less rapid in the person who remains active throughout life.

Disorders in Blood Pressure

Several disorders may affect blood pressure. Perhaps the most common is high blood pressure or *hypertension,* where pressure is permanently as high or higher than that of a normal person who is exercising. The systolic blood pressure may be 300 mm Hg. or more, while the diastolic pressure may rise to 180 mm Hg.

High blood pressure is attributed to an increase in peripheral resistance (a narrowing or constriction of the arterioles throughout the body). Why there is an increase in that peripheral resistance is not definitely established, although body chemistry, heredity, and emotions probably play critical roles. Because of the abnormal narrowing of the arterioles, greater pressure is required in the arteries to force the blood through. The heart works harder, though not necessarily faster, to accomplish that; and the blood pressure rises.

See ANGINA, ARTERIOSCLEROSIS, CIRCULATORY SYSTEM, DEGENERATIVE CARDIOVASCULAR DISEASE, HEART DISEASE, and ISCHEMIC HEART DISEASE.

BODY COMPOSITION

Physical activity has long been recognized as a potent factor in the regulation and maintenance of body weight. Body weight, however, is a gross measure and it is doubtful whether it measures anything of significance. For example, what is the significance of body weight in two individuals weighing 200 pounds, one a 21-year old athlete, the other a 21-year old sedentary office worker? At first glance, such information indicates very little, for we need to know also the varying contributions of different tissues to the person's total weight and build. The study of body composition in recent years has led to a more complete understanding of body mass, the dynamics of its composition, and its relationship to physical activity.

Weight is a complex of vertical, transverse, and sagittal dimensions. It is a composite of independently varying tissue components—primarily bone, muscle, fat and viscera—of which body fat is the most labile. Thus, body weight is not a completely adequate measure of growth, nutritional status, or physical fitness, the capacity for sustained physical activity without undue fatigue. It is relatively variable and is affected by a number of factors, two of which are most significant—nutrition and physical exercise. The study of body composition attempts to ascertain the components of the mass and has taken a variety of approaches seeking to explain the relationships and significance among its various parameters.

Biochemists see the overall composition of the body in terms of a four component system—water, protein, minerals and fat. For all practical purposes, however, the two component system of A. R. Behnke is perhaps the most efficient and effective approach for analyzing growth patterns in body composition as well as the relationships of the body's composition to physical activity. Behnke divides the body mass into two compartments, the lean body mass and fat. The former refers to the fat-free protoplasmic portion of the body plus the skeletal structures, whereas the latter refers to the highly variable and labile nonlean tissue, fat.

In recent years, researchers have given increased importance to understanding the composition of the human body. As a result, a variety of procedures have evolved, including many highly refined anthropometric, densitometric, radiographic, physiologic, and radioactive techniques. All are essentially aimed at determining one thing: the quantity of lean versus fatty tissue in the body. The use of radiography and skinfold thicknesses provide a direct regional estimate of body fat, from which researchers predicate total body fat. The former utilizes an X-ray of selected body regions, most frequently the upper arm and lower leg, while the latter utilizes a caliper to measure the thickness of a double fold of skin plus subcutaneous tissue (superficial fat). The two most frequently studied sites are the triceps (back of the upper arm) and subscapular (just below the shoulder blade) areas.

Growth in the lean and fat tissues generally parallels the pattern for height and weight to adolescence. During the preadolescent years, sex differences in composition are minor. Boys generally have more lean tissue than girls, while the reverse is true for fatty tissues. During adolescent years, there is a sharp acceleration in the rate of growth, so that sex differences in body composition become marked. The adolescent spurt in growth is rather abrupt, particularly in males. They show a marked increase in lean tissue, especially muscle and a decrease in body fat. Females, on the other hand, show a slight spurt in the lean body mass and a slight increase in fat. There is a sex difference in the timing and the nature of the adolescent growth spurt; it occurs earlier and is less intense in females than in males. Also, adult values are reached earlier in females—approximately 15-16 years—as opposed to 18-20 years in males. The impact of the adolescent spurt in growth is so marked that in early adulthood females have approximately twice the amount of body fat as do males. C. M. Young in a study of college women found her sample to have 28.7% of body weight as fat, where as males of a comparable age in studies by J. Brozek and Keys and L. R. Pascale *et al.* showed 10.92% and 11.17% body fat respectively. That sex difference persists into the later adult years with both sexes showing a gradual, slight increment in the percentage of body weight as fat.

Physical Activity

Obviously, physical activity implies a training program—a systematic regimen of organized exercises and activities, as opposed to the relatively infrequent, irregular activity bouts of the American "weekend athlete." With

training, there is an increase in the lean body mass and a decrease in body fat. According to J. Parizkova, that is true for both sexes during the growing years and throughout the adult years. And it's especially true for athletes. L. P. Novak, for example, noted striking differences in body composition between high school football and basketball players and a random control group. The athletes were taller and heavier, with the overall size difference being reflected in a greater lean body mass and less fat. The athletes had approximately one-half the amount of fat of the non-athlete controls (7.2% compared to 14.9% of body weight as fat). G. B. Forbes reported similar results for college football players. The observed weight difference between a group of players and non-playing controls, equated on the basis of age and stature, were entirely due to a greater lean body mass in the athletes, as is evident in the data presented below:

Age	Players	Controls
Age	19.9 yrs.	19.9 yrs.
Height	5.7 ft.	5.8 ft.
Weight	168.5 lb.	156.6 lb.
Lean body		
mass	152.5 lb.	135.5 lb.
Fat	16 lb.	20.9 lb.

It is evident, therefore, that training exerts a beneficial effect on the overall leanness/fatness ratio comprising body weight. We can also see that an increase in body weight is not necessarily identical with obesity and, thus, emphasizes the relative futility in evaluating body weight changes alone without any estimate of which components in this complex mass are changing.

Continued Activity

Data based upon adults, suggests that continued activity is essential to maintain the favorable effects brought about by chronic physical activity. Tanner, for example, in a study of weight training, noted increases in muscle and slight decreases in fat. However, measurements taken on the subjects four months after the prescribed training program had ceased, showed that almost all measurements had reverted to the pre-training values. Such results illustrate the favorable effects of exercise on body composition; but more important, clearly indicate the need for continued activity in maintaining the exercise induced alterations. Hence, the favorable changes in the ratio of fat to lean tissue produced by systematic exercise programs are dependent upon continued activity for their maintenance.

Physiologically, a great percentage of the body weight as lean tissue is significantly related to maximum oxygen consumption, which in turn is one of the best indicators of physical or organic fitness. Parizkova has shown the close relationship of the percentage of lean body mass and maximum oxygen consumption in both children and adults respectively, the greater the percentage of lean tissue, the greater the maximum oxygen consumption.

The significance of body composition relative to growth, strength and motor performance has been recently reviewed by Malina and Johnston. Strength is a composite expression dependent upon anatomical, mechanical, physiological and psychological factors. It is related to motor performance in that a degree of strength is essential to move the body in the performance of gross motor tasks. Rarick and Thompson, for example, reported significant relationships between calf muscle size and ankle extensor strength in 7 year old boys and girls. Although boys were only 5% larger than girls in muscle size, they were 13% stronger, suggesting a greater strength per unit of muscle area in males. Similar results were also reported by Dempsey concerning muscle size and strength in the upper arm. Boys were 5% larger than girls in upper arm muscle size and 11%

stronger in elbow flexor strength.

In a study of performance and body composition in preadolescent boys, Ismail, *et al.*, reported a body fitness factor, which had its highest statistical loading on the percentage of lean body mass. A closer look at the data indicates a positive relationship between performance in selected events, namely, the vertical jump, standing broad jump, and 50-yard dash, and the lean body mass, emphasizing the importance of the amount of lean tissue in performance. Leedy, *et al.*, reported similar results in adult males and concluded that the percentage of lean body mass is of greater importance in activities where the whole body is involved rather than the absolute amount of lean tissue. It is apparent, therefore, that body composition and gross motor performance are related, with the percentage of lean tissue being the critical factor; and excess fat exerting deleterious effects on performance.

In summary, the available evidence suggests that body composition is intimately and dynamically related to the level of physical activity characteristic of an individual. With training, there is an increase in lean tissue at the expense of the fatty tissues. The converse is true when physical activity ceases or sedentary habits are resumed. The leanness/fatness ratio is related to maximum oxygen consumption, strength and gross motor performance in both children and adults. Individuals with a greater percentage of lean body mass demonstrate greater functional efficiency in terms of the criteria described. Those observations are true during both the growing years and adulthood. Nevertheless, the relative value of such training programs during the growing years in inducing permanent changes which persist into adulthood remains inconclusive and requires further inquiry.—*Robert M. Malina*

Body Composition Determination

The human body is never stable and static in form and composition; its metabolic processes are in a continual state of change, both on the molecular level and in terms of overall composition, or the ratio of lean body mass to fat. J. Parizkova relates that the continual process of change, a fundamental characteristic of living matter, is brought about by a multitude of factors associated with growth and development, and aging and senescence, upon which are superposed further influences—e.g., the intensity of energy intake and output, chiefly reflecting nutrition and physical activity.

Measurements of human body density, or "specific gravity," have been undertaken since the middle of the 18th century. Practically all the earlier experiments were influenced by the unknown quantities of gases in the body, especially in the lungs.

From the earlier measurement efforts, a lone conclusion may be drawn "that obesity tends to decrease specific gravity."

In recent years both the medical and physical education professions have become interested in the topics of fat and physical fitness. An inverse relationship seems to exist between the two factors. The attention given obesity by the medical profession, and efforts to control it by physical educators, may play a key role in determining whether the future of America will be fatness or fitness.—*Bill W. Lovingood*

BODY MECHANICS

Many people go through life without paying any attention to proper or efficient body movements; and many of the same people wonder why they have low back pain, become rapidly fatigued, or are awkward in performing a physical skill.

Proper body mechanics can prevent injuries, retard fatigue and improve the aesthetic quality of a movement. Naturally, body mechanics not only apply to athletic or recreational skills but also are extremely important in daily tasks such as walking, standing, sitting, carrying and lifting.

The vertebral column, a central consideration in body mechanics, is not perfectly straight. It has several gentle curves that aid in absorbing shock. The column is supported by muscles and connective tissue; and in turn, along with the muscle and tissue, the column supports a great deal of the body weight. Therefore, erect posture in sitting, standing, or walking is extremely important. Good posture places little strain on the muscles and ligaments that hold the various vertebrae together.

Sitting

To correctly sit down in a chair stand with your back to the chair and move one foot back comfortably. Bend both knees, allowing the hips to be lowered under control. As the body is lowered, lean the trunk forward slightly. If the seat is longer, it may be necessary to slide back after sitting.

While sitting, allow your body to follow the contour of the chair. By doing so the hips should be well back in the chair. That type of sitting allows the back muscles to relax because weight is taken off the spinal column.

When rising, follow the reverse of the sitting down mechanics. If the seat is deep, you may have to slide forward before rising.

Generally, the same procedure should be followed for all chairs. If the chair has arms, they may offer some assistance when sitting down or arising. The arms, however, should not do the majority of the work. One specific sitting position need not be held for a long period, for it is desirable to shift position frequently to avoid muscle fatigue and poor blood circulation.

When sitting at a desk or table, be sure it is high enough so that you are not forced to bend over to any great extent. The trunk may be brought forward slightly. Continued bending may cause fatigue of the back or neck, with resulting pains.

Standing

In standing, maintain a posture that places the body weight on the vertebral column rather than the supporting muscles. For the body to be in balance, the center of gravity must be over the feet. That is best achieved by having the feet relaxed, the pelvis level, the shoulders directly above the hips, the head in position above the shoulders, and the chin level.

If the head is allowed to droop, there is a tendency for the upper back and lower back curves to increase.

An increased lower back curve can cause low back pain by placing undue strain on the vertebral column, compressing the articular processes. To correct such faulty posture, hold the head high and the shoulders back, the abdomen in and the pelvis level. The posture should not be military, but relaxed and aligned.

Another point to remember is that if the abdominal muscles are weak, the pelvis cannot be held properly; it will droop forward. The dropping of the pelvis is a rotation which causes the sacral area of the spinal column to turn or rotate inward. That rotation causes the lumbar vertebra to dip forward; increasing the lumbar, or low back, curve. The condition is called a "sway back." The accentuated curve causes a squeezing of the articular processes of the vertebra creating a pressure on the nerves and producing pain.

Walking

The general body position in walking is the same as for standing, except that inertia must be overcome by moving the center of gravity forward. That is done by bringing one foot forward to be a "supporting foot" and then swinging the other leg up to that foot and beyond, so that the swinging leg becomes the supporting leg. The supporting foot is also the pushing foot as the swinging leg moves forward.

Point the toes of the feet forward, with the inner borders of the feet falling along a line. The arms should swing easily and alternate the action of the leg movement. That easy swing and arm action aids in reducing trunk rotation and in moving the upper body forward.

Throughout the day, many tasks require proper body mechanics. The correct application of basic principles are essential for aesthetic, efficient, and injury-free movement.

Pushing and Pulling

Many pushing and pulling tasks are, for the most part, relatively light in nature; but some involve the application of considerable force, such as moving furniture, pushing a baby carriage, or pushing a stalled automobile. When an object to be moved is on wheels, the friction is reduced. Every effort, therefore, should be made to place the object on wheels or on some type of tarp if it is too heavy to be carried.

A long rope should be used to pull a cumbersome object. Attach it to a point in line with, or below, the center or gravity of the object. Stand facing the direction of movement with the feet in a walking position and point the toes straight ahead, with the trunk leaning forward. Bend the knees so that the powerful leg muscles do the most work. The degree to which the knees are bent depends upon the force necessary to move the object. At times, to start moving a heavy load, you may have to stand facing the load in a sitting-backward position. Be sure to avoid falling backward when it moves by spreading your feet to maintain balance. Moreover, be ready to turn quickly once the object starts to move.

If you desire to push an object, place the hands near a point opposite

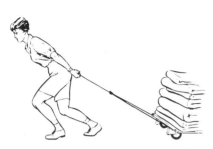

To pull unwieldy objects attach a long rope to the center of gravity. Face the direction of movement with feet in a walking position.

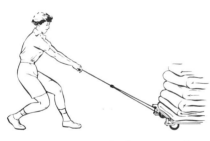

To move a heavy load you may have to stand facing it. Keep your feet spread to reduce the tendency to fall when the object starts to move.

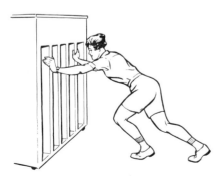

Place hands at the center of gravity to push heavy objects. Bend the knees but keep the back straight, thereby forcing strong leg muscles to do the work.

the object's center of gravity, and bend the knees with a minimum bending of the waist. That position forces the leg muscles to do the majority of the work, thereby again avoiding excessive strain on the small of the back. Stand away from the object so your center of gravity is ahead of the pushing foot and take care that the hands are spread apart for better control.

Those principles can also be applied to pushing an object upward or pulling it downward. The upward or downward movement can be made safely if the body weight is placed as near as possible to the object.

Holding and Carrying

When you hold an object, remember that the weight becomes a part of your total body weight. That shifts your center of gravity in the direction of the weight; and you must make a compensating adjustment so that the center of gravity is over the feet. Make that adjustment from the ankles rather than from the waist. Thus, the entire body is used to balance the newly-acquired weight. To keep the adjustment at a minimum, make every effort to keep the object as close to the body as possible.

Other adjustments also can be made; for example: carrying an object at one side of the body shifts the center of gravity to the side, slightly over the base of support. Raising the opposite arm sideways usually counterbalances the newly acquired weight. Many times people incorrectly lean the body to counterbalance the weight. The improper lean usually places a strain on the lower back.

Stooping and Lifting

Many people attempt to pick up an object, by bending from the waist with the knees kept almost straight. Picking up a heavy object in that manner places a strain on the back muscles, the end result being a possible severe lower back injury.

When you must lift an object, assume a stooping rather than a bending motion. By stooping, you utilize the stronger leg muscles and keep the object close to the body's line of gravity.

There are two common techniques for stooping. If the object to be lifted is located in front of the body, assume a wide stride. The knees should be bent and the hips lowered. When you return to a standing position, hold the object close to the body, straighten the knees and the back. That technique can be rather awkward for a woman, especially if she is dressed in a skirt. Here's a second technique. Place the object close to the body, as before;
but place the feet in a walking position and locate the object along side of the body. That walking position provides greater balance. As in the first method, let the legs do the lifting, not the back.

Remember, immediately, stop any attempt to lift an object if you cannot keep the hips under the upper body as the legs are extended. In such a case, additional help is needed to do the lifting.

Physical Fitness and Body Mechanics

A high level of fitness aids in the development of good body mechanics. If the muscles of the body are in good tone and have adequate strength, the body is better able to withstand fatigue and to provide the strength for performing tasks. The presence of fat in certain portions of the body may affect the center of gravity, especially if the fat is centered around the abdomen.

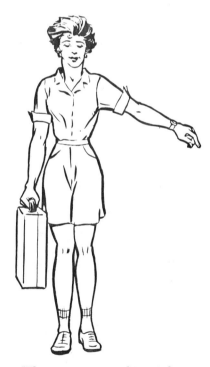

When you carry an object, it becomes part of your total body weight and your center of gravity shifts toward it. Raising the opposite arm can counterbalance the newly acquired weight to maintain an erect posture.

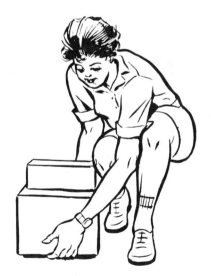

Stoop, don't bend, to lift a heavy object. That will enable you to utilize the strong leg muscles and keep the object close to your center of gravity, thereby reducing the chance of injury to the lower back.

When there are heavy fat deposits in the abdomen, the spinal column cannot support a great deal of the weight and the muscles of the back must work harder to support the body.

Weak abdominal muscles can cause low back pain, since the weakened muscles cannot provide adequate support of the pelvic area, and the lumbar curve is accentuated. See LOW BACK PAIN.

Good body mechanics contribute to physical fitness because good posture can be a preventive or curative agent for certain injuries. Many aches, pains, and symptoms of fatigue can also be eliminated by correct body mechanics. See POSTURE.

BODY TYPE

People come in different shapes and sizes. Some are very fat, others very muscular, and still others very thin. Those differences are determined by many factors. Bone structure, the number of muscle fibers per muscle, and the length of the intestine are determined before birth and play a major role in the basic body type. Over the years, man has attempted to classify the many varieties of the human physique into three basic types: fat, muscular and thin.

Somatotyping

Somatotyping is a method of classifying the human body into those three basic types by estimating the dominance of fat, muscle, or bone. There are many differences in the physical structure of people. Some individuals have a short stocky build, others a tall lean build; and there are many variations and graduations between physical types.

The differences are largely a result of inherited characteristics, such as bone structure, number of muscle fibers and the length of the intestines. Dr. W. H. Sheldon has done extensive work in this area and has recognized

that there are three distinct types of body structures.

In his classification system, Dr. Sheldon utilizes the three embryonic layers; endoderm (the inner layer), the mesoderm (the middle layer), and the ectoderm (the outer layer). The digestive organs are derived from the endoderm, the muscles and bones from the mesoderm and the skin from the ectoderm. Those words developed into terms, describe his classification system. For instance, a person with considerable bone and muscle development would be classified as a mesomorph, a person with high visceral development is an endomorph, and one with significant development in skin and nerve tissue is an ectomorph.

Endomorphy

The endomorph possesses a roundness or a softness to his body. Normally, he has little muscle development and small bones. His weight is centered in the front of the body around the abdomen. The arms and legs are comparatively small with very little muscle development. The breasts of men are feminine in appearance. There are heavy pads of fat around the backs of the hips, abdomen, buttocks, thighs and arms. Other common characteristics include a round face and a short neck with a double or triple chin. He is usually extremely poor in athletic events requiring support of body weight, speed, agility, endurance or jumping, although he may be adept at such activities as golf, archery and swimming.

Mesomorphy

The mesomorph is muscular and big-boned. Noted for hardness and ruggedness, he normally is of moderate height, longnecked and, broad shouldered, with a large chest, relatively slender waist and broad hips. His arms and legs are well developed and he is strong enough to lift or carry heavy objects. The mesomorph usually

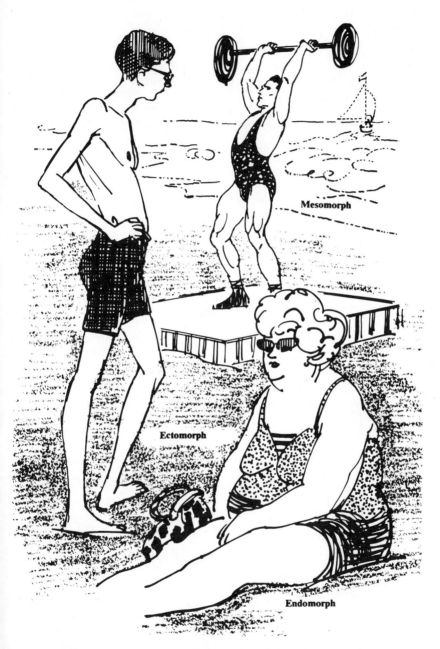

It is easy to distinguish between the three basic body types—endomorph, meso-morph and ectomorph. The challenge in body-typing is to distinguish between the variations of those three physical types. A pure ectomorph, mesomorph or even endomorph is extremely rare. Most people fall somewhere between the extremes.

enjoys vigorous and exciting activities.

Collectively, mesomorphs usually excel in activities that require strength, power, agility and endurance; such activities as wrestling, football, lacrosse and baseball. People with that body build or type usually have a tendency to put on weight upon cessation of regular exercise.

Ectomorphy

The ectomorph is thin muscled and thin boned. His body looks fragile and delicate. His trunk is short while his neck, arms and legs are long. The shoulders are usually rounded. Weak upper arms and thighs are typical of the extreme ectomorph. There is very little fat on his body. Generally, his posture is rather poor because he lacks the muscular strength to hold himself up properly. He usually excels in athletic events that require little body contact since he is susceptible to bodily injury. Activities such as badminton, tennis and endurance running are his best ventures.

Classification

Sheldon's technique of classification hinges on the premise that each person possesses qualities of endomorphy, mesomorphy and ectomorphy in varying degrees. Each component is rated on a seven-point scale, the highest being seven and the lowest, one. Three digits are combined into a number that indicates the degree to which each component exists in a person. Very few people possess a single extreme somatotype although they do exist. But no one has a 111 or 777 classification, for no one can be extremely low or high in all three categories.

The great majority of individuals fall somewhere between the extremes, generally with one component higher than the others. For example, you might be basically muscular but have many soft characteristics (an endomorphic mesomorph) and be classified as a 461. That means you're relatively

high (4) in fat, high in muscle development (6) and low in thinness (1). A muscular thin person (mesomorphic ectomorph) might possibly have a somatotype of 254 or 154.

Anyone can roughly estimate into what somatotype grouping he falls. That method would be rather subjective, but it can serve as a rough guide. It may also be fun to have your spouse or a friend rate you.

Selection of Activities

Body type influences the type of athletic activities in which a person will be most successful. A heavily muscled person excels in contact sports such as wrestling and football, while ectomorphs do well in activities like distance running and tennis.

Dr. Frank Sills and P. W. Everett note that these differences exist in the physical performance of *extreme* somatotypes:

Mesomorphs are stronger than endomorphs and ectomorphs.

Endomorphs are stronger than ectomorphs (though not in strength per pound of body weight).

Ectomorphs are superior to endomorphs in speed, agility and endurance.

Mesomorphs are superior to both endomorphs and ectomorphs in agility, speed and endurance.

Excess weight is a handicap to endomorphs, and insufficient strength is a handicap to ectomorphs in the performance of physical tests.

Dr. Thomas K. Cureton extended Dr. Sheldon's analysis and applied it to champion athletes, illustrating the relationship between performance and body build. Figure contains some of his evaluations.

That doesn't mean that a somatotype of 252 will make you a champion wrestler. The body type merely sets limits. Speed, training, motivation, coordination and motor abilities influence the degree to which your somatotype potential can be attained.

SOMATOTYPE RATING SCALE

A. Scale for rating fat status (endomorphy)

1 2	3 4	5 6 7
Extremely low in adipose tissue and relatively small anteroposterior dimensions of the lower trunk.	Average tissue and physical build of lower trunk.	Extremely obese with large quantities of adipose tissue and unproportionately thick abdominal region.

B. Scale for rating muscular status (mesomorphy)

1 2	3 4	5 6 7
Extremely underdeveloped and poorly conditioned muscles squeezed or pushed in the contracted status (biceps, abdominals, thighs, calves).	Average in skeletal muscular development and condition.	Extremely developed with large and hard muscles in the contracted state; firm under forceful squeezing.

C. Scale for rating skeletal status (ectomorphy)

1 2	3 4	5 6 7
Extremely thick and heavy bones, short and ponderous skeleton with relatively great cross-section at ankle, knee and elbow joints.	Average size bones and joints in cross-section and length.	Extremely thin frail bones; tall linear skeleton with relatively small cross-section of ankle, knee and elbow joints.

Note: After one rating is selected from each of A, B and C, the digits are combined into one rating, for example, 2-5-4. The sum of the three digits should equal 11.

(From Cureton, T. K. *Physical Fitness Appraisal and Guidance.* St. Louis: The C. V. Mosby Co., 1947. With permission of the publishers.)

BODY TYPES OF CHAMPION ATHLETES

Somato- type	Activity
171 } 271 }	Weight Lifting
372	Fullback, Football
252	Wrestling, Gymnastics, Diving
154	Tennis, Distance Running
162	Jockeying
453	Distance Swimming
354	Baseball Pitching

Sports and Body Type

Body-typing alone, however, cannot provide a reliable means of determining either athletic ability or suitability of a sport for a person. It is concerned with shape only and takes little account of size and no account of the size of body segments. Measurement or *anthropometry* is, therefore, a necessary accompaniment of body typing since it supplies information not only on gross size but also on the type of limb levers. Anthropometry is a much older science than somatotyping but standardization of methods and improvements in instruments in recent years have made its application more widespread and reliable. See ANTHROPOMETRY.

The importance of physique as a determining factor in athletic achievement can be seen by examining briefly the main factors contributing to success. These are:

(1) Physique somatotype—the way a person is built, his size, body proportions, bone and muscle structure.

(2) Physiological factors—heart rate, oxygen carrying capacity of the blood,

utilization of body fuel, exchange of gases in the lungs, tolerance of oxygen debt and many associated body functions concerned with exercise.

(3) Psychological factors—motivation, determination, aggressiveness and mental preparation for competition.

(4) Skill—the ability to perform efficiently and economically all the movements associated with a particular sport.

The physiological, psychological and skill factors can all be influenced and, to a large measure, controlled. Training, for instance, can bring about substantial physiological changes to produce what is generally termed "fitness." Psychological conditioning can similarly take place to produce what might be termed "mental fitness" for the particular sport. Specific skills can be taught by a good teacher or coach who makes use of up-to-date technological knowledge. Of the four factors, physique is the only one that cannot be significantly changed. No amount of training or playing of sport is likely to alter substantially the way an individual is built. There can be no joy for the lightly built boy who is forced to participate in rugged contact sports; and there can be nothing but frustration for the boy who aspires to be a high jumper but is too heavy in the bone to win the fight against gravity. Such obvious observations reinforce the findings of recent investigations which show that certain types

BODY TYPE AND ACTIVITY PARTICIPATION

	Physical Qualities that are Typical of Certain Body Types					Activities in Which You Can Expect to Experience Most Success													
	Strength	Endurance	Power	Agility	Body Support	Archery	Badminton	Basketball	Bowling	Cycling	Golf	Handball	Hiking	Jogging	Skiing	Swimming	Tennis	Running	Wt. Training
Endomorphy																			
Meso-Endomorphy																			
Mesomorphy																			
Meso-Ectomorphy																			
Ectomorphy																			

of physiques are attracted to certain sports; and in those sports, certain physical characteristics mark the successful athlete. In the search for prospective champions, therefore, coaches should select persons with the physique suited to the sport before setting about serious conditioning and training.

There have been few body types studies of games players, but such evidence as exists indicates that psysiques cluster around a distinctive mean type. There is a strong tendency for the better class of players to be more mesomorphic. That is particularly true of contact sports such as Rugby football and American football. The solid bulk of the players exhibits a strong combination of endomorphy (F) with the mesomorphic component. J. E. Carter has shown that College football Lettermen have a mean somatotype of 4¾ 5½ 2 with some slight differences according to position as well as to level of competition. Knowledge of those differences could greatly facilitate selection. Dr. Sheldon once observed that a coach who cannot distinguish between a 5½ and a 6 mesomorphy might not win many football games.

Studies of Olympic athletes by J. M. Tanner have shown marked differences according to the event. The throwing event athletes have somatotypes close to 362 with the shot putters being the most ponderous. Jumping event athletes are low in endomorphy (F) with mesomorphic (M) and ectomorphic (L) components fairly evenly balanced within the medial range. Among runners, all classes are low (between 2 and 3) in endomorphy (F). Sprinters are highest in mesomorphy (M = 5-6); but among other runners, there is a slight decrement in mesomorphy (M) accompanied by a slight increment in ectomorphy (L) with distance of race or need for endurance. Those facts demonstrate that

the "dead weight" of the endomorphic body build is a handicap to that type of performance. There is a relationship between mesomorphy and the output of power.

Additional measurements of body proportions give further information on appearance. Middle distance runners are long in the leg. Sprinters and long distance runners have shorter legs, but the former have much larger muscle girths. High jumpers are tall with long legs relative to trunk length, thus giving a high center of gravity. Hurdlers look like sprinters but have longer legs. Throwers are taller and heavier than either jumpers or runners, and discus throwers have very long arms.

Objective measurements will never supplant the trained eye of a successful coach or selector. Body typing and anthropometry, however, may become valuable aids both in the school and on the sports field. It is clear that certain physiques are more suited to one kind of sport than another, and it is valuable to know their characteristics. It is also possible that size and body proportions may give valuable clues of potential ability, particularly if enough factors are considered. An apparent deficiency may be compensated for by excellence of other qualities. The study of appearance or shape must, therefore, be made as objective as possible. Information gained can then effectively help sports administrators, not only in guiding young people into a satisfying sport, but also in the selection and development of successful athletes and sports teams. See BODY COMPOSITION—*A. S. Lewis*

BONES

Because the bones of the skeletal system are composed of living tissue with many vessels, vigorous exercise has an immediate effect on the bones of the body. Most people don't realize that exercise builds bone just as it builds muscle. Professional athletes not only have bigger and stronger muscles than nonathletes, but they have thicker and stronger bones as well. The pull and tug of muscle against bone that occurs when you exercise stimulates the vital life processes which go on in healthy bones, and causes them to grow in size to meet that challenge. The health and strength of your whole body increases as a result. To the contrary, when a person does not exercise, bones become weaker. That has been proven beyond doubt by several experiments with healthy young people who volunteered to lie in bed with their bodies encased in plaster casts. Within a few days they began to excrete much larger than normal amounts of calcium in their urine, proving that the stores of calcium in their bones were being depleted by lack of exercise. If bed rest or extreme sedentariness is continued for long periods, bones can become seriously weakened.

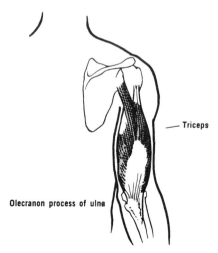

Olecranon process of ulna

— Triceps

Although most muscles are attached to the bone by tendons, some muscle fibers are connected directly to the bone structure. The pull and tug of muscle against bone stimulates bone growth.

Exercise for Your Bones

Your bones will benefit from almost any type of exercise that you do to increase muscular strength or cardiovascular fitness. The lower legs and arms are among the regions of the body most vulnerable to fractures—although we all know that you can break almost any bone if the shock is great enough. Hips are vulnerable in people with osteoporosis. Walking is often recommended as the ideal exercise and there is good reason to believe that it is the best movement prescription for older people vulnerable to bone weakness. It will exercise both the legs and the hips. For a variety of reasons, including bone-building, every mature person who doesn't do other rhythmic exercise should walk an hour a day, regardless of the weather. Jogging is also very good for people who don't have physical limitations that preclude that activity.

Exercising the arms is more of a challenge. Swinging Indian clubs is one activity that can be highly recommended, because it increases joint flexibility as well as providing the muscular resistance needed to stimulate bone growth.

People who have advanced stages of osteoporosis, as diagnosed clinically, should follow the exercise prescriptions of their physician. (Low back pain and back stiffness are early signs of the disease.) But if you are healthy just step up all your exercise activities to build better bones.—*Robert Rodale*

BOWLING

Bowling is a mild exercise that is quite popular in the United States. It appeals to young and old, men and women, the strong and the handicapped. Wheelchair bowling is widespread, and there have even been classes in the sport for the blind.

Bowling requires comparatively few skills. Neither strength nor endurance is necessary, but rhythm, relaxation and coordination are useful. As a result, bowling does little to improve physical fitness other than contribute to relaxation, recreation and social interaction.

The casual, or once a week, league bowler does little conditioning for the sport. Some will go out for a few warm-up sessions, mostly to polish their timing and approach. The professional bowler, on the other hand, will practice and work at the game all year, so there are actually no pre-season drills.

Bowling has been recommended for heart patients, even after attacks, as a means of relaxation. That, of course, precludes any strenuous tournaments or competition.

Injuries are rare because of the nature of the sport. Obviously, if a bowler plays too much, he can develop blisters and callouses on the thumb and fingers, but the casual participant rarely has any such problems.

The most popular type of bowling in the United States is *tenpins*, but there are many variations, such as *lawn, duckpins, barrel pins* and *candle pins*. They all involve the use of small pins and small balls. The fundamentals of all the games are essentially the same.

Bocce is an Italian form of bowling, played outdoors. The participants roll balls toward a smaller ball that has been rolled previously. The one who rolls closest to the small ball wins.— *Ray Nelson*

Associations

American Bowling Congress (ABC), 1572 E. Capitol Drive, Milwaukee, Wisconsin 53211. (Also American Junior Bowling Congress (AJBC) at same address).

American High School Bowling Congress, 8142 Indiana Avenue, Chicago, Illinois 60619.

American Lawn Bowls Association (ALBA), 1525 Ridge Court, Wauwatosa 53213.

National Bowling Associations (NBA), 1324 Dorr Street, Toledo, Ohio 43607.

National Bowling Council (NBC), 1414 Eye Street, N.W., Washington, D.C. 20005.

National Duck Pin Bowling Congress (NDPBC), 1420 New York Avenue, N.W., Washington, D. C. 20005.

Woman's International Bowling Congress (WIBC), 1225 Dublin Road, Columbus, Ohio 43212.

BUSINESS

Today's executive is a man on the go. Appointments, deadlines, engagements, trips, pressures, commitments jam his day. That kind of life is a dangerous one, for he often neglects his health and lets his physical condition deteriorate.

Except for an occasional round of golf (which often ends at the 19th hole), the executive of today gets very little exercise. A recent study by the Life Extension Institute found that 12 per cent of corporate executives take daily exercise; 35 per cent exercise merely on weekends, and 52 per cent do not exercise at all.

With a life pattern like that many executives are headed for trouble. Rich diets may raise their weight, waistline and cholesterol, increasing the chance of degenerative diseases. See DEGENERATIVE CARDIOVASCULAR DISEASE.

Dr. Hans Selye, director of the Institute of Experimental Medicine and Surgery at the University of Montreal, has noted that stress of long duration may cause a stress syndrome that can, in turn, cause high blood pressure, colitis, diarrhea, gastric ulcers and even death. The apparent solution is the avoidance of the stress; but in the competitive business world, that is impossible. Some relief is possible through progressive relaxation, tension release exercises performed at the office or home, wholesome recreation, developing and maintaining circulo-respiratory fitness, and learning to live more active lives.

Proper Relaxation

To help fight tension, rest is essential. The ability to sleep at night is a real help, and a "cat nap" for about 5 minutes once or twice a day is a good release mechanism.

Allied with and often necessary for sleep, is relaxation. The critical point in the relaxation process is being able to recognize stress and tension, then doing something about it. The progressive relaxation technique developed by Dr. Edmund Jacobson is an excellent means of relieving tension. The idea is to recognize the tension, reduce it with muscular contractions, and then release the muscles. For a description of his concept and technique, see RE-LAXATION.

Tension Release Exercises

Tension release exercises are relatively easy and can be performed in the office, often without anyone else really knowing.

Shoulder Shrug

Sitting at the desk, draw your shoulders toward your ears as far as possible. Pull up hard. Then press the shoulders down hard, stretching to make a long neck. The downward motion is very important for releasing the tension. Do several times.

Round the back by pressing your arms and shoulders forward and dropping your head. That action stretches the upper back muscles. Now press both shoulders back as far as possible. Tilt the head slightly upward and lift the chest. Do several times.

The Reach

Raise your arms high above the body and touch the ceiling without leaving the floor. Then relax. Repeat several times.

Feet on Desk

Put your feet on the desk. Cross one leg over the other, raise both legs into the air and hold for 5 seconds. Then place the other leg on the bottom, so it gets its share of work.

Chair Press-Up

Several times a day, place both feet on the floor and your hands on the arms of the chair. Do a push-up while keeping your body in the sitting position. Then lower yourself and relax. Be careful the chair doesn't tip over.

Neck Roll

Sit in the chair and let your head fall forward. Let it hang for 5 seconds. Roll the head to the right side; then move it back and forth. After 10 seconds, roll the head to the other side and repeat. Do several times a day.

Foot Rotation

Place the feet about 10 inches apart and rotate them inward, bringing the toes together. Then rotate them outward as far as possible. Do about 10 times.

Heel Lift

Place the feet flat on the floor. Keeping the toes and ball of the right foot on the floor, raise the heel as high as possible, then lower and relax. Repeat with the left leg. Do about 10 times.

Waist Twist

Stand with your feet about 2 feet apart. Twist the upper body to the right as far as possible and return. Repeat to the left. Do 8 times.

Desk Curl

Sit with your hands under a heavy desk. Try to lift the desk. Hold for 5 seconds and relax completely. Do 3 times.

Waste Basket Press

Hold a waste paper basket at arms' length in front of the body. Press hard as though you were trying to make your hands meet.

Charles Atlas

Hold your left fist in the palm of your right hand. Press down with the left and up with the right. Hold 5 seconds, then relax completely. Do 3 times, then change hands.

Knee Press

Sit back on a chair, hold your legs straight out, and place the palms of your hands above your knees. Press down with your hands and up with your legs. Hold 5 seconds and relax. Do 3 times.

Telephone Squeeze

Grasp the telephone and squeeze it as hard as possible. Hold 5 seconds and relax. Repeat with the other hand. Do each time you use the phone.

Wholesome Recreation

A percentage of the day should be set aside for recreation, providing it's stimulating and satisfying. (One man's recreation may be another man's work.) It is important to experience some degree of success with the activity, or you will soon want to drop it. The recreation need not be a sport or exercise; it may involve a musical instrument, playing cards, stamp and coin collecting, etc. See also CARRY-OVER SPORTS, and MENTAL HEALTH. See CIRCULO-RESPIRATORY ENDURANCE, CONTINUOUS RHYTHMICAL EXERCISE, DEGENERATIVE CARDIOVASCULAR DISEASE, PROGRAMS and SPECIFIC SPORT ENTRIES.

Learning to live with Fitness Built in

Learning to be more active is extremely important in today's society. Techniques that can be employed to help improve fitness levels include getting off a train a few blocks from your place of work and walking the remaining distance, walking behind the lawn mower rather than riding one, and so on. See DAILY ACTIVITIES.

Industry's Responsibility

Industry is constantly seeking ways to get the best returns on its investment in executive talent. On the job training programs, educational courses and self-improvement programs are a few methods used to stimulate executive thinking. In recent years, programs have been designed to improve the physical fitness of top management. More and more heads of industries are realizing that a physically fit management team will contribute more than executives who pay little attention to their health. Research has shown that the fit are more alert, less prone to absenteeism, and have a longer productive tenure.

A recent Metropolitan Life Insurance Company survey of business and professional men, listed in the 1950-51 edition of *Who's Who in America*, showed that they "have lived on the average distinctly longer than men in the general population." When those men were compared with men in similar occupations who had not reached prominence, the men in *Who's Who* had a 40 per cent lower death rate. Metropolitan Life concluded that the longer life span among prominent businessmen "is believed to reflect in large measure their *physical and emotional fitness* for positions of responsibility."

Some ideas being adopted by industries are:

Exercise breaks should take the place of coffee breaks. Several industries in Russia have adopted that procedure. In the United States, the coffee break is so ingrained that it may be difficult to change completely. But an additional ten minute exercise period in both the morning and the afternoon would be a solution.

Industries in Russia, Austria, West Germany and Sweden provide extensive recreational facilities for the families of the employed in the evenings. American industries are doing so on a less elaborate level.

Such recreational facilities might be carried one step further if they were opened to the employees during the day. Fitness, Inc. located in Cambridge, Mass. has developed a plan in which it offers exercise programs to industries, as has Fitness Finders Inc. located in Emmaus, Pennsylvania.

Fitness training centers or clinics might be set up for executives, first giving the executives a thorough physical examination and battery of tests, then a tailored exercise education program on fitness.

Industry should also support development of sports facilities and programs throughout the respective communities, counties or states. One such program is the Life Time Sports Foundation established by the Brunswick Company and the AMF (American Machine and Foundry Company). See LIFETIME SPORTS.

BUST

See CHEST.

CALF

See LEGS.

CALISTHENICS

No wonder calisthenics are in disfavor. Exercises appear to be an unpleasant start to any session of activity —the sooner over with, the better. If there is no fun, if the exercises have no purpose, if they are just "part of the show" or just a prelude to the real content of the lesson, they do not fulfill their need. What, then, are the purposes of exercises?

(a) So that *EVERYONE* will be basically exercised in a pattern of systemized movements, thoroughly obeying all the elements of motor fitness! i.e., Balance - Power - Speed - Strength - Flexibility - *ENDURANCE*.

(b) To be effective, exercises should be continuously performed—to a pattern, for exercises are a part of training, and training can be *specific* or *general.*

General Exercises

(a) They have a pattern for their aim, which is to exercise a man, or a woman, bi-laterally, yet all over. They find weaknesses and help to correct them, and they do not pander to a person's strengths.

(b) Effectiveness depends upon the manner and the spirit in which they are performed.

(c) In themselves exercises will do nothing. It is how they are taught and where the stress is placed that makes exercise effective.

(d) For them to be efficacious, they should be varied and should not be duplicated. Usually, exercises giving the same effect should *not* follow one another—that does not mean that the same body area should not be exercised successively.

(e) With general exercise, a specific order of exercises is not necessary. However, all areas should be covered: lateral, abdominal, dorsal, leg, arm, shoulder, trunk, thigh, knee, ankle, wrist, neck, etc.

Some exercises should be rhythmic, some even static, some for speed, some for balance, some *with* power, some for mobility, but *all* with variety, contributing to endurance, and for fun.

Specific Exercises

(a) They are performed as a part of training towards an end and are devised so that a *specific* end may be realized. For example, calisthenics for fencing might utilize different types of exercises for legs (power, agility, and endurance) and for upper body (speed and range of movement). Calisthenics for sprinting might include speed of reaction and coordinative movements of arms, shoulders and trunk, with specifics for ankle, knee, hips, calf, thigh (power and rhythmic-range work).

(b) Exercises are stressed differently. Sometimes they are repeated, sometimes increased in intensity by repetition, by increasing the load, changing the tempo, increasing the leverage. Or an area is exercised repeatedly by change of exercise, *but* the stress is kept in the same area. However, progression is ever-important.

(c) Exercise should never be boring. Tough, hard, demanding full range, energetic—yes! A person in training has, occasionally, to know punishment.

(d) If done conscientiously, exercises have their part in the preparation of one for the task set.

Calisthenics allow you to be fit *to play* without *having* to play. In that way they permit you to be able to apply the techniques of the game or sport: See EXERCISES for specific exercises.—*John T. Powell*

CALORIES

A calorie is a heat unit used to measure the energy requirements of the body and the energy supplied by various foods. Specifically, it is the amount of heat energy needed to raise the temperature of approximately 4 pounds of water 1 degree Fahrenheit. When used in diet and health measurements, it is called the "large calorie." A "small calorie," used in physics, is the amount of energy that will raise the temperature of 1 gram of water 1 degree Centigrade.

The body needs calories to supply energy to sustain the life processes (heart beat, respiration, blood pressure, muscle tone, and so on), to main-

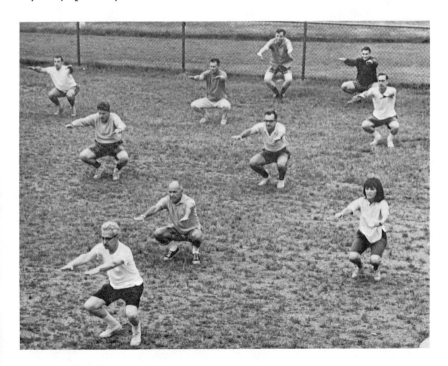

When they begin a fitness program, many people find calisthenics boring. The trick is to select exercises that are energetic but do not duplicate themselves.

tain body temperature, and to carry on physical activities. Carbohydrates and fats are the main source of calories. Proteins will also supply energy, but their principal function is to maintain, repair and build tissues. In a healthy body, enough calories are furnished by fats and carbohydrates so that proteins need not be consumed.

Man is dependent upon food for his source of energy. The quantity of energy used normally is reflected either by a gain in body weight (stored energy) or by a loss in body weight (utilized energy).

Nutritionists normally use the term *calorie* for measuring the energy needs and expenditures of a person and the energy value of food. Speaking in terms of body health, a calorie is a quantity of food capable of producing a certain amount of energy when it is burned by the body. Obviously, if the food you eat contains too many calo-

CALORIES OF COMMON FOODS

Food	Calories	Food	Calories
Angel Food Cake 2 in. sec.	110	Lettuce, headed 2 leaves	7
Apples, raw 1 med.	87	Lima Beans 1 cup	152
Apple Juice 1 cup	124	Liver, beef 2 oz.	118
Applesauce 1 cup	85	Lobster, raw ½ average	88
Asparagus 1 cup	36	Marshmallows 5	98
Banana 1 med.	132	Molasses, cane 1 tbsp.	50
Beets, red 1 cup	56	Muffins 1	135
Bran flakes 1 cup	117	Noodles 1 cup	107
Bread, rye 1½ slices	57	Olives, green 10	72
Bread, white 1½ slices	63	Onions, raw 1 2½ inch	50
Broccoli 1 cup	25	Oyster Stew 1 cup	244
Brussels Sprouts 1 cup	60	Pancakes, wheat 1 4 inch	60
Butter 1 tbsp.	100	Peaches, raw 1 cup	175
Cabbage, raw 1 cup	24	Peanut Brittle 1 ½x¼ piece	66
Cashews, roasted 1 cup	810	Peanut Butter 1 tbsp.	92
Cauliflower 1 cup	30	Pears, raw 2½	80
Celery, raw 1 cup	18	Peas 1 cup	111
Clams, raw 4 oz.	92	Popcorn 1 cup	57
Cocoa 2 tsp.	15	Porterhouse 3 oz.	293
Corn, sweet 1 ear	92	Potato, baked 1 med.	97
Corn flakes 1 cup	96	Potato, sweet 1	185
Cottage Cheese 1 oz.	21	Pretzels 5 small sticks	18
Crackers, graham 2 med.	55	Puffed rice 1 cup	55
Crackers, saltines 2 med.	34	Rice flakes 1 cup	117
Cucumbers 1 cup	140	Roast Beef 3 oz.	189
Custard, baked 1 cup	283	Sardines 3 oz.	182
Doughnuts 1	136	Sauerkraut 1 cup	32
Flounder 4 oz.	78	Scallops 4 oz.	90
Frankfurter 1	124	Sherbet ½ cup	118
Fruit Cocktail 1 cup	180	Shrimp 3 oz.	110
Grapefruit, raw 1 cup	77	Soybeans, dry 1 cup	695
Grapes, 1 cup	84	Spinach 1 cup	46
Ham 3 oz.	340	Sponge Cake 2 in. sec.	117
Hamburger 3 oz.	316	Squash 1 cup	97
Hard Candy 3 pieces	31	Sugar, brown 1 tbsp.	51
Honey 1 tbsp.	62	Swiss Cheese 1 oz.	101
Ice Cream 1 slice	167	Tomato Ketchup 1 tbsp.	17
Kale, raw 1¾ cup	70	Watermelon ½ slice	97
Leg Roast 3 oz.	314	Whipped Cream ½ cup	280

AMOUNT OF ACTIVITY NEEDED TO CONSUME VARIOUS FOODS

Activity (In Minutes)

Food (calories)	Lying Quietly	Driving A Car	Golf	Walking	Table Tennis	Vig. Walking	Water Skiing	Skiing Downhill	Hand-ball	Bicycling	Swimming Crawl	Running
Tomatoes 1 med. (30)	23	13	7	6	5	4	4	3	3	3	3	2
Puffed Wheat 1 cup (43)	32	18	12	8	7	6	5	4	4	4	3	3
Carrots, raw 1 cup (45)	34	19	11	9	8	7	6	5	5	4	4	4
Jellies 1 tbsp. (50)	38	22	12	10	8	7	6	5	5	4	4	4
Whole Wheat Bread 1½ slices (55)	41	24	14	11	9	7	6	6	6	5	5	4
Salad Dressing 1 tbsp. (60)	45	26	15	12	9	8	7	6	6	5	5	5
Oranges 1 med. (70)	53	30	17	13	10	9	8	7	6	6	6	6
Egg 1 med. (77)	58	33	19	15	12	10	9	8	7	6	6	6
Strawberries 3 oz. (80)	62	35	19	16	13	11	10	8	8	7	7	6
Cola 6 oz. (33)	62	35	20	16	14	12	10	8	8	7	7	6
Milk, Nonfat 1 cup (87)	67	37	21	17	14	13	11	9	8	8	7	7
Mayonnaise 1 tbsp. (92)	69	39	22	17	15	13	12	9	9	8	8	7
Bacon, fried 2 slices (97)	73	42	23	18	16	14	12	10	10	9	8	8
Margarine 1 tbsp. (100)	75	43	25	19	17	14	12	10	10	9	8	8
Potato Chips 10 Med. (103)	81	46	26	21	18	15	14	11	11	9	9	8
Cereal 1 cup (120)	83	47	27	23	18	16	14	11	11	10	9	9
Grape Juice 1 cup (120)	90	52	30	23	21	18	15	12	12	11	11	9
Beer 12 oz. (125)	93	53	30	23	21	18	15	12	12	11	11	10
Oatmeal 1 cup (150)	113	65	40	27	25	22	19	15	15	15	13	12
Milk, Whole 1 cup (165)	125	71	41	32	28	24	21	17	17	15	14	14
Tuna Fish 3 oz. (170)	120	73	45	32	28	24	21	17	17	15	14	14
Veal Cutlet 3 oz. (184)	138	79	45	35	30	26	23	18	18	17	16	15
Round Roast 3 oz. (197)	148	84	48	38	33	28	24	20	20	18	17	16
Spaghetti, cooked 1 cup (220)	165	95	54	42	37	31	28	23	22	20	19	18
Chuck Roast 3 oz. (265)	199	113	65	50	44	38	33	27	27	23	23	22
Pumpkin Pie 1 slice (275)	208	118	67	52	46	39	34	28	28	25	24	23
Candy Bar 1 average (300)	226	129	73	57	50	43	38	30	30	27	26	25
Turkey 4 oz. (305)	231	130	74	58	51	43	38	31	30	28	26	25
Apple Pie 4 inch. sec. (330)	256	142	81	63	55	47	42	33	33	30	29	28
Duck 4 oz. (370)	277	159	90	71	62	53	46	38	37	34	32	31
Raisins, dry 1 cup (430)	323	184	105	82	72	61	54	43	43	39	37	36
Macaroni & Cheese 1 cup (464)	348	199	113	88	77	66	58	47	46	42	40	39
Rib Chop 4 oz. (480)	361	206	117	91	80	69	69	48	48	47	42	40
Mince Pie 1 piece (515)	387	221	126	99	86	74	64	52	52	47	45	43

ries and the calories are not expended day after day, the remainder is stored in the body as fat.

Calorie Balance

To maintain your weight, you must balance your *caloric* intake (food eaten) with your *caloric outgo* (activity). To lose weight, your body must burn more calories than it absorbs in food. If the caloric outgo is greater than the caloric intake, you will lose weight, simply because the body needs energy to exist, even when you are at complete rest. When enough calories are not taken on by the body and energy is needed, the body will begin to metabolize (burn up) the fat of the body.

There are many available charts that indicate the number of calories in various portions of food and the energy expenditure of various activities. The latter are approximations, however. Energy expenditure is affected greatly by body weight, age, sex, musculature and present physical condition. Most of the lists were compiled for a man weighing 154 pounds and a female weighing 120 pounds. The charts, however, may be used rather effectively to help you determine the intensity of the activity.

Naturally, the most popular way to burn up extra calories quickly is through some form of exercise. The following tables demonstrate how long it takes to burn up a given amount of calories and the number of calories in the typical American foods.

See WEIGHT CONTROL for further information and specific caloric charts. See also METABOLISM.

CAMPING

More and more people are heading toward campgrounds equipped with tents, car-top sleeping accommodations, tent trailers, or other types of trailers. The modern conveniences you carry depend entirely upon choice.

Camping is becoming more modern and is a far cry from "roughing" it in the woods when you slept under the open sky and made meals over an open fire. Families are finding that camping is an inexpensive way to spend vacation time together and still have all members enjoy themselves. Although the initial cost you invest in equipment may run high, careful planning of essentials will eliminate foolish buying.

There is fun and enjoyment awaiting you when you set out to discover a new way of life. It can be relaxing when you leave the fast pace of life behind. You experience the feeling of aliveness and an awakening of the senses as new sounds are heard, new sights discovered and new smells experienced.

Each type of living quarters has both advantages and disadvantages. There is a wide selection of tents available in different materials, sizes, shapes and prices—the A-wall, umbrella, car-tent, miner, Baker, pop, open or campfire style, the common pup tent, the cottage tent, the mountain tent, and the Plains Indian tepee, just to name a few. In the small models, the tents are easy to pack and carry. With a larger tent, it is wise to set it up in the yard a few times to familiarize yourselves with the procedure. Some tents have screened windows, sewed-in floors, awnings for windows and doors, aluminum poles, metal fittings, strong zippers and vents. There is also a tent made that encloses the rear of a station wagon.

Car-top sleeping quarters may include a platform of wood on which air mattresses and sleeping bags are placed. A folding metal frame supports a tent cover for use when sleeping. Another type is a box construction which contains an innerspring mattress. A frame supports a tent cover during use and folds flat when traveling. You reach the sleeping quarters by use of a short metal ladder.

The camping trailer is a compact unit with one or two wheels, attached to the rear bumper and pulled by a car. Most models have a metal or wooden body and a canvas top which opens into living quarters when set up in camp. Some trailers have an aluminum frame over which canvas tops are stretched. Others have a frame which is cranked up to position or a push-button method which operates from a battery. Extra features include additional rooms to one side of trailer body, kitchen cabinets, stoves, sinks, iceboxes, closets for clothing, heaters and storage cabinets.

The pickup coaches and house trailers are compact but have more luxurious living quarters. They can be hooked up to electricity, water and drainage when parking in a trailer camp. A pickup coach is fitted onto a half-ton or larger pickup truck. They come in various sizes, although most experienced sportsmen prefer a house trailer from 15 to 19 feet long and about 7 feet wide. Both trailers and pickup coaches may have such luxuries as a gas stove and oven, gas refrigerator, shower, flush toilet, separate bedroom and living room, a pressure or electric water system, a heater and plenty of storage space.

Another type of camping vehicle is the compact van, manufactured by different car companies. Although it features many conveniences, some campers prefer not to have to take their living quarters with them whenever they leave camp to sightsee or do errands.

First-hand information from owners will give you the pros and cons of the various techniques so that you can purchase the best type of camping equipment.

Activities in Camping

Camping offers a variety of activities, some requiring severe physical endurance and others that are quite relaxing. Usually there is much to see

within walking distance of the camping area. Some areas have designated hiking trails with posted information or a guide to inform you of the historic and scenic information. The pace set in hiking ranges from a leisurely stroll to a vigorous stride. It's best to condition the body beforehand if you expect to do a lot of hiking in rough terrain. A high degree of cardio-respiratory endurance is demanded for long and difficult hikes. See HIKING.

Swimming is another activity which many campers enjoy. Many times campers will sunbathe on the beach and take only occasional dips in the water. Such activity is very relaxing but certainly not conducive to fitness.

Many campers desire to see the countryside on horseback. You can ride for an hour or two, take a day trip, or an overnight trip. You will feel stiff the next day if you do not condition your body to horseback riding. The best conditioning is to ride frequently before you decide to explore the surroundings when you are camping. Muscles have to be toned into shape.

Water sports can be great fun when there is a lake or river nearby. Water skiing is popular on large lakes where motor boats of all sizes are permitted. Other water sports are canoeing and rowing.

Fishing can be a refreshing activity, especially in the early morning or the sunset hours, when nature is seen at its finest. Wild animals can be seen around the lakes. Knowledge of how to cast, what type of lure or bait to use, and the habits of fish makes the sport so much more enjoyable. See FISHING for conditioning requirements and benefits.

Conditioning

Most camping activities can be performed without any prior conditioning. However, often a satisfactory physical condition will mean the difference between enjoying the activity to the fullest and suffering with aches, pains and blisters. A conditioned body will not become fatigued as easily, nor develop muscle soreness as quickly.

Common Injuries

The most common injuries are blisters of the hands and feet, cuts and wounds of hands and feet, leg cramps when hiking too much, and sprains of the ankles.—*Jean A. Hecht*

Associations:

National Campers and Hikers Association (NCHA), 7172 Transit Road, Buffalo, New York 14221.

American Camping Association (ACA), Bradford Woods, Martinsville, Indiana 46151.

Family Camping Federation (FCF) (at the same address).

CANOEING

The art of handling a canoe is a telltale mark of a true woodsman. Commonly associated with the Indians of Northeastern America, canoeing originated as a mode of travel in the area surrounding the Great Lakes and the St. Lawrence River. Although it is generally thought of as a quiet, restful activity often involving tent camping and touring by waterway, canoes are raced in the Olympic Games.

In Olympic competition, two types of canoes are used: The Canadian canoe is an extreme modification of the standard canoe, paddled by a single-blade paddle. Either one or two men compete. The Kayak class is a variation of the familiar Eskimo craft, with a rudder to keep it on course. Double-blade paddles are used.

Contribution to Fitness

Since canoeing can be enjoyed at any level of physical exertion, its contribution to physical fitness is entirely dependent upon the effort made in paddling. As an Olympic event, it requires an extraordinary amount of circulo-respiratory fitness as well as muscle endurance and strength in the arms, shoulders and trunk. At lower levels of participation, however, the most noticeable requirement is endurance in the arms and shoulders.

Aside from general good health, there is no specific physical fitness level required to begin canoeing. No particular skill is required, but it's a good idea to know how. Canoe tripping for any distance, however, may require a knowledge of map reading, camp-crafts and first aid. As a canoeist progresses, it is advisable to build up the arm, shoulder and trunk muscles. That can be accomplished by canoeing itself or by any exercise program which simulates paddling movements, such as a continual raking or sweeping movement.

Although there are no particular physical prerequisites for the beginning canoeist, there are certain factors which should be kept in mind while planning the beginning program. For instance, the choice of a place to canoe is very important in that excessive wind and/or water turbulence make handling very difficult. Similarly, cold weather, rain, fog or other unpleasant conditions make canoeing uncomfortable and should be avoided until he has attained some degree of skill and confidence. Ideal conditions consist of a rather small lake or large but slow moving river, with warm sunshine and little or no wind.

Injuries

Injuries are rare although muscular soreness and joint stiffness are fairly common. Use of the sitting position can lead to soreness in the abdominal and lower back muscles. Capsizing in fast water can cause lacerations, bruises, fractures, or even drowning. A life jacket and crash helmet are advised for "shooting the rapids."— *S. A. Lephart*

*CANOEING PROGRAM

Chart 1	Chart 2
1. 1-1.2 miles in 15 min.	1. 4.6-5.0 miles in 70 min.
2. 1.3-1.6 miles in 20 min.	2. 5.1-5.3 miles in 75 min.
3. 1.7-2.1 miles in 25 min.	3. 5.4-5.8 miles in 80 min.
4. 2.2-2.5 miles in 30 min.	4. 5.9-6.3 miles in 90 min.
5. 2.6-2.9 miles in 35 min.	5. 6.4-6.9 miles in 100 min.
6. 2.9-3.1 miles in 40 min.	6. 7.0-7.3 miles in 105 min.
7. 3.2-3.5 miles in 45 min.	7. 7.4-7.7 miles in 110 min.
8. 3.6-4.2 miles in 50 min.	8. 7.8-8.2 miles in 115 min.
9. 4.3-4.5 miles in 60 min.	9. 8.3+ miles in 120 min.

* See ENDURANCE and ENERGY COST OF ACTIVITIES for an explanation of the charts.

Fitness 1

If you achieved a score of poor or low average on the *Harvard Step Test* or a score of very poor or poor on the *12 Minute Run*, start on Chart 1-Level 1 and spend 1 week at each level until Chart 2-Level 9 is reached. It is recommended that you participate 4 to 5 days a week. When Chart 2-Level 9 is reached, 4 days a week is sufficient.

Fitness 2

If you achieved a score of high average on the *Harvard Step Test* or fair on the *12 Minute Run* start on Chart 1-Level 1. Spend one week on Chart 1-Levels 1, 2, 4, 6, 8 and 9, and Chart 2-Levels 1, 3, 4, 5, 7 and 9. It is recommended that you participate 4 to 5 days a week. When Chart 2-Level 9 is reached, 4 days a week is sufficient.

Fitness 3

If you achieved a score of good or excellent on either the *Harvard Step Test* or *12 Minute Run*, continue your current program or select Chart 2-Level 9 as your level of participation. Four days a week is sufficient.

Association:

American Canoe Association (ACA), Office of the Secretary, 400 Eastern Street, New Haven, Connecticut 06513.

Since canoeing is a moderate-energy cost activity, it may be used to help improve your fitness level, especially your circulo-respiratory and muscle endurance. Below is a canoeing training program that takes into account the important principles of training.

If you desire to improve your strength and power for that activity, see WEIGHT TRAINING and ISOMETRICS. The weight training and isometrics exercises may also be used to prepare your body for athletic competition.

CARDIO-RESPIRATORY ENDURANCE

See CIRCULO-RESPIRATORY ENDURANCE.

CARDIO-RESPIRATORY SYSTEM

See CIRCULO-RESPIRATORY SYSTEM.

CARDIOVASCULAR ENDURANCE

Cardiovascular endurance refers to the fitness and efficiency of the heart and the blood vessels. Many times it is incorrectly interchanged with circulo-respiratory endurance, which involves the respiratory and circulatory system. Although cardiovascular refers only to the circulatory system, it is difficult to separate it from the respiratory system, for they work in very close harmony.

A person with good cardiovascular endurance will have a low heart rate (at rest and during exercise), high stroke volume, and low blood pressure during exercise.

See CIRCULO-RESPIRATORY ENDURANCE.

CARDIOVASCULAR SYSTEM

The cardiovascular system includes the heart and the blood vessels of the human body. Many times the cardiovascular system is used interchangeably with the circulo-respiratory system, largely because they work so closely together. The cardiovascular system, however, refers to the circulatory system.

See CIRCULATORY SYSTEM AND CIRCULO-RESPIRATORY SYSTEM.

CARRY-OVER SPORTS

Carry-over sports are those activities engaged in after high school and college when organized athletics cease. They can be enjoyed individually or with one partner, often for an entire lifetime.

Carry-over sports may be used for relaxation, fitness, recreation, and/or the joy of competition.

Sport Selection

The selection of the carry-over activities or sports will depend a great deal upon a person's interests, needs and capacities.

There are several important aspects of the human body to consider in the

CARRY-OVER SPORTS

Strenuous	Moderate	Mild
Bicycling	Archery	Boating
Cross Country Running*	Badminton*	Billiards
Diving*	Bobsledding*	Canoeing (Recreational)
	Calisthenics	Croquet
	Camping	Curling
	Dancing	Fishing
Gymnastics*	Deck Tennis	Horseshoe Pitching
Handball*	Fencing*	Quoits
Hiking	Gardening	Rowing (Recreational)
	Golf	Shuffleboard
	Hunting	Walking (Leisure)
	Horseback Riding	
Mountaineering*	Indian Clubs	
Oriental Martial Arts*	Ice Skating	
Orienteering*	Jogging	
	Netball	
Rowing*	Rollerskating	
Running	Rope Jumping	
Scuba Diving*	Sailing	
Skiing*	Shooting	
Skin Diving*	Surfing*	
Squash*	Table Tennis	
Swimming	Tobogganing	
Tennis*	Walking (Vigorous)	
	Water Skiing*	
Wrestling*	Weight Lifting*	
	Yachting	
	Yoga	

selection of a carry-over activity. During early maturity (24 to 30 years of age), physical development is completed. Skill capacity is at its highest so that vigorous skill type of activities are popular. During this period, an occupation is usually selected. If the job is sedentary, then it is desirable to pick an activity that will retard physical degeneration.

At maturity (30 to 50), the capacity for endurance is at its highest. Skill and speed have leveled off and may have started to decline, and job pressures may be restricting activity.

Late maturity (ages 50 and above) reveals a maintenance or decline in endurance and skill, depending upon previous activity, and in speed and strength. It is also an age when bone fractures are common. At this age carry-over sports should not involve short bursts of effort unless preparatory work is done (warm-up). More moderate activities rhythmical in nature, should be continued.

Chronological age is not the best means of determining the age for participating in an activity. A more valid age, yet one that is difficult and sometimes impossible to measure, is fitness age. Some men at 70 or 80 who have kept themselves in good condition through life are able to participate in vigorous activities and out-perform a man of 35 who repeatedly refuses exercise and is able to engage only in the mildest form of activity. See LIFE-TIME SPORTS.

The basic advantages of carry-over sports are (1) they encourage participation until at least 50 years of age, and (2) may be performed on an individual or partner basis. For a more complete discussion see the listing under the individual activities.

Carry-over sports range from strenuous to mild. Some activities may defy classification, depending on the vigor with which they are performed. In the list on p. 72 an asterisk (*) next to an activity indicates it may be too strenuous for people over 30-35 years of age. However, if you have remained truly active all your life and make moderate or strenuous exercise a part of your daily program, you will find that the age limit of 30-35 is meaningless.

CHEST

Chest development appeals to both men and women for appearance's sake, but the health benefits of improved posture are even better reasons for exercising the three main chest muscles.

The *pectoralis major* is the thick muscle located in the upper part of the chest, which helps rotate the arm inward and pull the arm toward the body.

The *pectoralis minor* is smaller, has about the same functions, and lies underneath the pectoralis major. Both pectorals, if developed, can aid in giving a pleasing appearance to the feminine bustline.

The *serratus anterior* muscle lies on the side of the chest. It's the one that causes a rippled, "washboard" effect when well-developed. It functions in pushing and punching movements. Push-ups help develop the serratus muscle if care is taken to keep the body straight and the hands under the shoulders.

Building the Bust

Serious physicians long ago concluded that the bust line of almost any normal female can be enhanced through the right type of exercises. A build-up of the pectoral muscles which lie under the breasts and an increase in overall chest expansion will improve the appearance automatically. Added to those are the important benefits to be derived from postural reeducation. Exercise will make the fibers of the pectoral muscles become broader and open new capillaries to feed the muscle. The increased blood supply carries the energy and tissue-building materials to the working muscles. Protein will be carried and utilized for new tissue growth; and fats, also carried in the blood stream, may be deposited between the muscle fibers as well as under the skin and over the muscle. In this way, a new natural form takes shape without disturbing or irritating these delicate glands.

Exercises

The following exercises will firm up the muscles beneath the mammary glands, increase the size of the muscle fibers, and provide a new natural shape.

Hold a book in each hand while lying on your back. Extend your arms toward the knees. Then raise the books over your head, reaching as far back as possible. Repeat 10 times, using books heavy enough so that 10 repetitions feels like all you can do.

Lie on your back with the arms at right angles to the body and a book in each hand. Raise the arms so that they point straight up, pulling in your abdomen at the same time. Ten daily repetitions of the routine are enough for increasing the bustline. More would serve to increase muscle endurance.

Finally, clasp hands at various heights above the body while standing or sitting. Hold each position 10 seconds, while tensing the arms.

Men can benefit from the same exercises, in terms of chest development.

See EXERCISES, ISOMETRICS and WEIGHT TRAINING.

CHILDHOOD FITNESS

At present, in the American society, great emphasis is placed upon learning. Education is now one of our

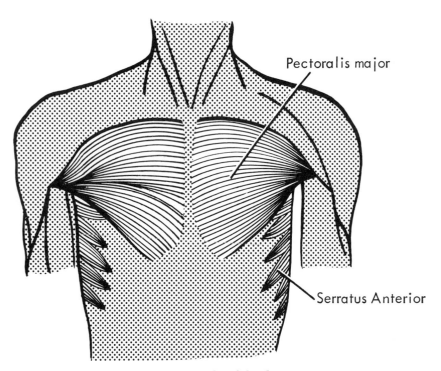

Main muscles of the chest.

Pectoralis major

Serratus Anterior

nation's largest businesses. Within education, there is a noticeable trend toward learning during the first 6 years of life. That trend, because of the age group of the subject, is of concern for parents and educators alike. The quantity and quality of nursery or preschool programs are increasing with the availability of finances and the importance attached to early learning. Federal, state, district, and agency programs provide early learning experiences for all upper, middle and lower classes.

For this discussion, the term preschool child includes children from 2 years 6 months, to 6 years 11 months inclusive. Physical capacities refer to the measureable physiological responses during or after exercise and scores collected from physical and motor fitness test items. The collected data is descriptive in nature. Materials collected in the realm of exercise physiology (responses), were prepared by P. O. Astrand, A. S. Robinson and Elda Robb. Data in the physical or motor fitness areas was researched by Rachel E. Metheny and J. Keogh.

Energy Requirements

Robb conducted a study of energy requirements necessary for maintenance, commonly referred to as basal metabolism, and the energy requirement necessary for quiet activity of 3- and 4-year-old children. She used the basal metabolism part of her study as the basis for the energy cost of the quiet activity section. She used a respiration chamber, an absorption system, and a gas analysis apparatus as her instrument. Her subjects were four girls and three boys. From her results, she concluded: "The energy expanded during quiet play has been found to range from 3.20 to 4.25 calories per kilogram per hour for the girls and from 3.80 to 4.20 for the boys, averaging 3.62 for the girls and 3.98 for the boys. The percentage increase over the average basal value has been

found to range from 40 to 101 per cent for the girls and from 61 to 79 per cent for the boys, averaging 66 to 69 per cent respectively." Drawing implications for child development she states, "Thus the cost of similar activity appears to be approximately twice as great for preschool children as for adults, furnishing another explanation for the comparatively high energy requirement of children."

Pulse Rates

Astrand provides information regarding pulse rate. Being nondefinitive of specific age, he states, "Robinson registered 190-200 as the highest average pulse rate for those in the age range of 6 to 30 years." His own research reveals, "Pulse rate values during maximal physical work for subjects 4 to 30 years old averaged about 200." "Maximal pulmonary ventilation for 4-to-6-year-old boys was 40 l/min. The ventilation per liter absorbed oxygen is greater for children and aged people than for persons 20 to 30 years old at maximal. The vital capacity is relatively lower in children than in

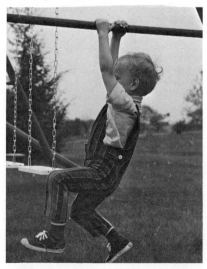

Physical activity for young people is gaining strong support from the physical education and medical communities.

adults. Thus, 7- to 9-year-old children reached 16 ml./cm. body height, the 12- to 13-year-old subjects 21 ml., and the adults 32 ml./cm. Maximal tidal air during work averaged, for the youngest subjects (ages) 4 to 30, one or two per cent below 50 per cent and for the adults 54 per cent of the vital capacity. According to Nielsen a tidal air of 50 per cent of the vital capacity should be most economical as far as effective pulmonary ventilation and cost of respiratory work is concerned. Blood lactic acid concentration levels for one to 6 minutes after maximal muscular work during 4 to 6 minutes were increasingly higher for older age groups: 56 mg. per cent for the 4- to 6-year-olds and 112 mg. per cent for the adults."

Breathing Capacity and Grip Strength

Metheny, in 1940, collected data on breathing capacity and grip strength of preschool children. Her extensive review of literature including studies done from 1894 to 1940, shows a con-

sistent increase in mean scores for each age group and between age groups from the first to the last study. The steady increase in scores could be attributed to improved testing procedures or physically larger, healthier children. Averaging the reported mean scores, the scores for breathing capacity reported in cubic inches are as follows:

Metheny presented her study data on breathing capacity in similar fashion but provided the range of scores.

By averaging the mean scores of her related literature on grip strength, she computed the following averages and ranges of scores. Note the year in which the study was conducted. The low range scores were reported in the earlier studies, the high scores in the later studies.

Metheny reports higher scores for her population. The scores of her lower range equal the average of mean scores of her related literature. She reports the following data:

Using analysis of covariance or grip strength scores, Metheny concluded,

GRIP STRENGTH

	No.	Boys	No.	Girls
4 year old	77	46.5	66	45.6
5 year old	418	55.8	327	49.0
6 year old		65.1		57.6

BOYS' BREATHING CAPACITY IN CUBIC INCHES

Age in Years	Number	Mean Scores	Range
2.6-3.5	18	42.05	26 to 57
3.6-4.5	31	51.24	42 to 70
4.6-5.5	44	69.32	47 to 91
5.6-6.5	22	74.32	50 to 100

GIRLS' BREATHING CAPACITY IN CUBIC INCHES

Age in Years	Number	Mean Scores	Range
2.6-3.5	22	33.86	23 to 44
3.6-4.5	23	46.64	26 to 61
4.6-5.5	28	56.62	36 to 81
5.6-6.5	18	68.84	46 to 84

AVERAGE OF MEANS OF GRIP STRENGTH (KILOGRAMS)

Age	Number	Mean Scores	Range-Year
BOYS: Studies from 1900 to 1940			
3 yr. old	41 (one study)	5.1	5.1 (1935)
4 yr. old	166 (five studies)	5.9	5.0 (1900)- 7.6 (1935)
5 yr. old	497 (six studies)	7.1	4.9 (1902)-10.2 (1935)
6 yr. old	(ten studies)	8.3	6.1 (?) -11.4 (1935)
GIRLS:			
3 yr. old	30 (one study)	4.3	4.3 (1940)
4 yr. old	112 (three studies)	5.3	4.0 (1900)-6.4 (1940)
5 yr. old	391 (four studies)	6.8	4.7 (1902)-8.4 (1940)
6 yr. old	(six studies)	7.1	5.1 (?) -9.2 (1940)

MEAN GRIP STRENGTH OF STRONGER HAND IN KILOGRAMS

Age	Number	Mean Scores	Range
BOYS:			
2.6-3.5	21	7.92	5.1 to 9.7
3.6-4.5	27	9.52	6.0 to 13.6
4.6-5.5	42	11.72	7.0 to 16.5
5.6-6.5	26	18.10	9.3 to 17.0
GIRLS:			
2.6-3.5	19	6.83	4.3 to 10.0
3.6-4.5	20	8.91	6.5 to 11.1
4.6-5.5	26	10.09	7.0 to 12.6
5.6-6.5	19	11.25	9.5 to 13.6

"These analyses produce the interesting findings that at 3 and 4 years old the differences in mean grip strength for boys and girls when adjusted for height are not great enough to be statistically significant. At 5 years of age, it is highly probably that boys have a greater grip strength than girls for their height and at 6 years, it may be stated with considerable assurance that the girls of this preschool group are the weaker sex."

Motor Performance

Keogh studied motor performance using many test items found in physical fitness, motor fitness, or motor capacity test batteries. He used 1,171 subjects in grades kindergarten through sixth in Santa Monica, California. The scores of the 5- and 6-year-old subjects were selected.

Keogh's test items and their results follow:

Keogh summarized, "The data obtained in the Santa Monica test program are similar to data for other California children, indicating that the Santa Monica children consistently scored well on all tests in comparison with other reports, and it appears to be true for California normative information for 10, and 11, year, olds."

These studies present sparse data in the areas of energy cost, maximal pulse rate, maximal pulmonary ventilation, vital capacity, maximal tidal air and blood lactic acid. However, they do present more extensive but still inadequate information in the areas of breathing capacity and grip strength. The latest data collected in the physical and motor fitness areas completed

		AGE 5		AGE 6	
Test		*Girl*	*Boy*	*Girl*	*Boy*
30-yard Run	N.	33	40	41	58
(seconds)	M.	7.67	7.47	6.69	6.78
	S.D.	0.71	0.64	0.50	0.60
Standing Broad Jump	N.	36	44	41	58
(inches)	M.	33.1	35.9	41.2	42.9
	S.D.	6.1	6.7	5.0	7.2
50-ft. Hop	N.	37	45	33	32
(seconds)	M.	10.2	10.6	7.3	7.4
Balance Beam	N.	34	44	31	29
(seconds)	M.	22.1	23.2	33.7	30.1
	S.D.	9.5	10.1	10.2	10.8
Beam Walk	N.	34	44	31	29
(steps)	M.	15.7	15.7	20.6	17.8
	S.D.	5.7	5.7	5.9	6.6

N = Number, M = Mean, S.D. = Standard Deviation.

Scores reported for 6-year-old subjects alone are the following:

Test		*Girl*	*Boy*
Side Step	N.	41	58
(points)	M.	8.2	8.8
	S.D.	2.2	2.6
Cable Jump	N.	41	58
(jumps)	M.	3.5	1.8
	S.D.	2.7	2.3
Shuttle Run	N.	41	58
(seconds)	M.	13.83	13.83
	S.D.	1.02	1.13
Ball Throw	N.	41	58
(feet)	M.	19.0	34.1
	S.D.	7.4	11.9
Accuracy Throw	N.	41	58
(points)	M.	12.4	9.1
	S.D.	5.1	6.2
Mat Hop	N.	41	58
(points)	M.	24.6	18.9
	S.D.	10.9	9.0

by Keogh covers a more extensive number of test items.

The quantity of available information concerning the physical capacities of preschool children, as stated previously, is negligible. The quality of research of the earlier studies can also be questioned because of research tools and methods used then and now.

The preschool age group is a relatively unresearched population. Implications for study are prevalent. The future of physical education in the nursery school is gaining impetus. The time is right to establish the position and determine its effect upon further development of the preschool child.—*Robert T. Sweeney*

CHOLESTEROL

Cholesterol is a fat-like solid alcohol that is soluble in organic solvents but almost insoluble in water. Cholesterol belongs to the group of compounds called sterols, is known to be of considerable physiological importance, but has an obscure biochemistry. It is found abundantly in the digestive bile and in all animal fats, such as butter, cream, egg yolk, and the fat in meat. Some gallstones are composed of it.

Cholesterol has been closely related to atherosclerosis, the cause of most heart attacks and strokes, and, therefore, elevated cholesterol levels has become a problem of national interest. From the experiments conducted by doctors and other professional people, it has been found that cholesterol and other fats are deposited on the internal lining of arteries making the surface rough and, in extreme cases, ulcer-like. The condition progressively becomes more acute as additional deposits are made. When it reaches a point where there is restriction of the blood supply to the heart, the result may be fatal.

You should be careful in selecting a diet and keep the intake of cholesterol small. In general, land animals yield hard or saturated fats, while fish and marine animals contain unsaturated fats, as do some vegetable oils. A high fat diet tends to be associated with high incidence of heart disease. Low fat diets tend to have a very low blood cholesterol level and a low death rate from heart disease. Since the liver produces cholesterol in the body, the amount present should be controlled through diet and extended exercise.

Exercise and Cholesterol

Research studies have been conducted on animals and humans to determine the effects of exercise on blood cholesterol levels. The trend of the studies is that regular, vigorous exercise and the eating of low-saturated-fat food will reduce blood cholesterol formation. The type of exercise, however, is very important. The exercise must place sufficient stress on the circulo-respiratory system or the reduction will not occur. Running,

cycling, vigorous walking and swimming are examples of the type of strenuous activities that are beneficial in reducing blood cholesterol levels. Weight training exercises and isometrics are illustrations of exercises that do not affect cholesterol levels. Blood cholesterol levels that are high are most affected by vigorous exercise.

Moreover, body type has a great deal to do with blood cholesterol levels. Mesomorphs (people with muscular builds) tend to build up cholesterol easily if they fail to exercise regularly and eat high-saturated-fat food. Proper exercise appears to play a major role in reducing the mesomorph's cholesterol level.—*Lee H. Hill*

See ANGINA, ARTERIOSCLEROSIS, BLOOD, DEGENERATIVE CARDIOVASCULAR DISEASE, DIET and BLOOD.

CIRCUIT TRAINING

In 1957, R. E. Morgan and G. T. Adamson introduced a fitness training program of "timed exercises," called circuit training, at the University of Leeds, England. Basically, circuit training is an organized course of exercises, and its object is to complete a prescribed number of exercises in a shorter period of time each day.

A series of exercise stations are placed around a room or gymnasium. The performer does a certain number of repetitions of the exercises at each station. When he completes the repetitions at a station, he immediately moves to the next station. Each task is to be completed correctly, but as rapidly as possible. The performer moves from one station to another quickly, without a pause, trying to complete three laps around the circuit. A typical series of exercise stations follows:

Station #1	push-ups
Station #2	squat thrusts
Station #3	sit-ups
Station #4	bar-dips
Station #5	barbell ½ squats

SAMPLE CIRCUIT PROGRAM

Station No.	Exercise*	Circuit Level		
		Beginning	Intermediate	Advanced
1	Push-ups	10	20	30
2	Squat Thrusts	10	14	18
3	Sit-Ups	12	20	24
4	Bar-Dips	3	7	11
5	Barbell ½ Squats	120 lbs. @ 6	130 lbs. @ 6	145 lbs. @ 6
6	Toe Raise	120 lbs. @ 10	130 lbs. @ 10	145 lbs. @ 10
7	Rope Climb	15'–2 times	15'–4 times	15'–7 times
8	Pull-ups	3	6	10
9	Barbell Curls	30 lbs. @ 6	40 lbs. @ 6	50 lbs. @ 6
10	Side Leaning Leg Raiser	7 (each side)	12	18

Note: Remain at the beginning level until your target time is reached. At that point, retest yourself and advance to the intermediate level.

* The various exercises may be found at EXERCISES, ISOMETRICS and WEIGHT TRAINING.

Station #6   dumbbell jumps
Station #7   rope climb
Station #8   pull-ups
Station #9   barbell curls and
Station #10   side sit-ups.

Method

On the first day, make sure you understand the correct techniques for performing the exercises. Then complete the three laps of a beginning program. Do not hurry through the exercises, but concentrate on correct performance. On the second and third day, continue at your own rate of speed for correct execution.

On the fourth day, test yourself at each station. On exercises such as the bar-dips and pull-ups, record the total number of times you can perform the movement. On other exercises such as the sit-ups and squat thrusts, place a time limit on the test, i.e., number of sit-ups performed in ½ minute (minimum) or 1 minute (maximum). When taking the test, stay in the circuit order, and between tests, take one-minute rests.

From the test data, you can determine the suitable number of repetitions for each exercise station. Generally, halving the test score produces the repetition number.

On the fifth day, you are ready for a time trial. Do three laps around the circuit as quickly as possible. (The number of repetitions that you perform at each station has been determined by the test results of the previous day.) When you complete the three laps, record your time. On the basis of that time, set a "target time" which you must achieve before you may be tested again. When you reach the target time, give a retest. From those test results, you may add to the *beginning* or *initial* circuit and establish an *intermediate* circuit. Set a new target time. When that goal is reached, give yourself a third retest, and start a third, or *advanced*, circuit.

(See Sample Circuit Program for an explanation of beginning, intermediate and advanced circuits.)

The target should be high enough that it will take three weeks or more to achieve it. For an unfit person, a big reduction in time—around one-third—is reasonable. A person in generally good condition cannot be expected to drop his time that much.

Main Characteristics

Circuit training has three main characteristics: it enables you to develop the physical fitness components of muscular and circulo-respiratory endurance, it utilizes the principle of progressive (gradual) overloading (placing of additional stress), and it allows a large number to train at one time.

Circuit training is not a fitness test but rather a physical training program. It may be used effectively in training athletes, students, businessmen, or anyone else interested in establishing a vigorous fitness program.

Guidelines for Establishing a Circuit

The following points are essential in establishing a suitable circuit program:

1. Select exercises that include the major muscle groups of the body. The circuit may be designed, however, to include only certain muscles for specific development.

2. Choose rather vigorous exercises.

3. Warm-up prior to engaging in the circuit.

4. Design the number of stations according to the nature of the exercises (if easy, more; if difficult, less) and the equipment and space available.

5. Set a circuit time limit between 10 and 30 minutes.

6. Make comparisons on *your* performance, not on another.

Alternate Method

Persons in a classroom, Y program, or lunch-hour break, may use a time limit adaptation of circuit training. Using the same physical setup of stations, try to complete the circuit as often as possible in the time allotted for exercise. For example, if 20 minutes is available and you attempt the beginning circuit on the chart, you may find that you are able to go around the circuit two complete times plus station #1 on the third trip.

According to that performance, you have gone through the circuit 2.1 times. Therefore, set your target or goal by increasing the test result of 2.1 by ⅓ to produce a goal of 2.8. When you achieve that goal, retest yourself, set a new goal, and start a new assault. All other principles apply as in the regular circuit training.

Poor Man's Circuit

Individuals who have no equipment available may devise a "poor man's circuit" by selecting push-ups, sit-ups, squat thrusts, leg hops, knee bends, V-seats, side sit-ups, body arches, running-in-place, etc., as alternate exercises for the circuit. This type of circuit can be set up in the basement, garage, or backyard.

Adaptability

Circuit training is infinitely adaptable and can be tailored for developing or maintaining any fitness level, depending on your physical condition, ability and motivation.

CIRCULATORY SYSTEM

The human body is made up of billions of microscopic structures called cells. In order for the cells to carry on their life functions, they must be supplied with various substances, especially oxygen and nutrients. Also, certain waste products must be removed. Those functions of supply and removal are performed by the circulatory system, or the cardiovascular system.

The components of the circulatory system are the heart, the blood vessels and the blood. The heart is the pump for the system; the blood vessels are the intricate set of tubes through which the heart pumps the blood to all parts of the body and the blood is the means by which the oxygen, nutritive substances and wastes are transported through the system.

The Heart

The function of the heart is to pump blood throughout the system in sufficient amounts to satisfy the needs of all the cells. The heart is extremely efficient and adjusts automatically to changing body needs. In twenty-four hours, it pumps about 5,000-6,000

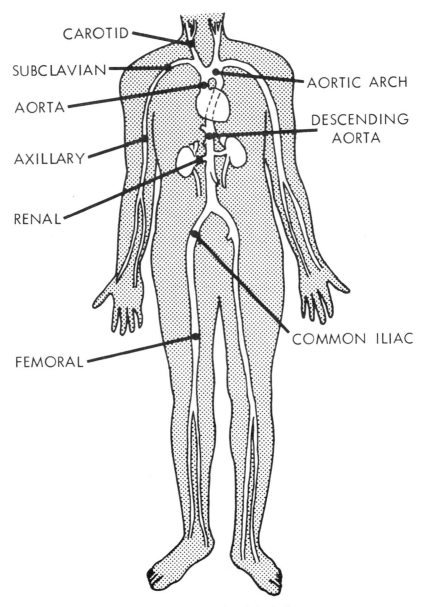

The main arteries of the body.

quarts of blood through the vascular system, a system of blood vessels. The body's entire blood supply, approximately 10 pints in the average adult, makes a complete circuit through the vascular system in less than one minute. In the average lifetime, the heart beats some 2½ billion times, with its only rest coming between beats. Its rich blood supply makes heart muscles almost untiring.

The heart is a four-chambered muscular organ about the size of a man's fist. It lies just above the diaphragm with two-thirds of its mass to the left of the midline of the body. It is enclosed in a protective loose-fitting covering called the *pericardium*. The same kind of membrane covers the outer surface of the heart. The slight space between the two membranes contains a lubricating fluid called *pericardial fluid*, which affords the heart protection from friction. The heart wall consists primarily of special muscle tissue called cardiac muscle, or myocardium. Lining the interior of the myocardial wall is a delicate tissue known as the endocardium.

The heart is divided into a right and left side by a leak proof wall called the septum and each side has two chambers. The smaller upper chamber is called an atrium or auricle, while the lower chamber is called a ventricle. The ventricles are larger and have thicker muscular walls than the atria because their pumping responsibility is bigger.

Circulatory System and Exercise

Below is a summary of the effects of exercise (training) on the circulatory system:

An increase in the number of capillaries, which results in improved endurance.

An increase in the use of latent capillaries, which also results in better endurance.

A decrease in the resting heart rate

and an increase in stroke volume. That means the heart gets more rest each minute, yet the same amount of blood is pumped throughout the body.

A decrease in the recovery time of the heart rate after exercise, indicating that the body adjusts more quickly to stress.

An increase in blood volume and in red blood cell count, which permits greater work performance because more oxygen is getting to the muscle tissue.

A larger cardiac output, enabling a greater amount of blood and oxygen to be carried to the tissues every minute.

Because of the increase in capillaries, there is an increase in the amount of oxygen that is picked up by the blood in the lungs and an increase in the amount of oxygen fed to the muscle tissue.

The removal of lactic acid is more efficient as a result of the increased capillaries and blood. Since lactic acid is removed more efficiently, fatigue is reduced or delayed.

Exercise and the Heart

Despite substantial evidence, the notion still persists that strenuous exercise leads to a heart attack, particularly in older people. Cardiologists state, however, that normal hearts cannot be injured by physical training. Proper exercise does not cause heart disease, but rather various heart diseases often develop from a lack of exercise.

The human heart is an extremely capable, fascinating, and fantastic machine, for it pumps 5,500 quarts of blood per day. In order that the heart can continue that effort, it must supply its muscular tissue with sufficient blood. The heart is supplied through two coronary arteries and their branches which surround the heart. If the heart is healthy, the linings of the arteries and smaller vessels are smooth and clear. If the heart is unhealthy, however, the walls are thickened and rough. The unhealthy conditions are caused, for the most part, by a slow deposit of a wax (fatty in nature) called cholesterol. The cholesterol is like rust in a pipe and retards the flow of blood to the heart tissue. See CHOLESTEROL.

Lack of exercise, smoking, emotional stress, obesity, fat-rich foods, and other factors (heredity and age) contribute to the narrowing of the arteries. Because the arteries are narrowed, the blood flow is restricted, and insufficient oxygen reaches the heart. An increased demand for oxygen can cause a heart attack because the necessary blood cannot get through the rusting arteries. That inability to obtain sufficient blood causes a heart attack. When the narrowed artery is blocked by a clot, it is called a thrombosis.

Although the reason for the rusting cannot be specifically pinned down to one condition, it appears that physical exercise retards and even reduces the condition.

Epidemiological research supports that theory. An article in a 1958 issue of the *British Medical Journal*, written by Dr. J. N. Morris and Dr. Margaret D. Crawford, demonstrated that "physical activity of work is a protection against coronary (ischemic) heart disease. Men in physically active jobs have less coronary heart disease during middle-age, what disease they have is less severe, and they develop it later than men in physically inactive jobs."

Also, since the heart is basically a large muscle, exercise will affect the heart and a skeletal muscle in similar ways. That is, training or continued exercise of an endurance nature will increase the number of functioning

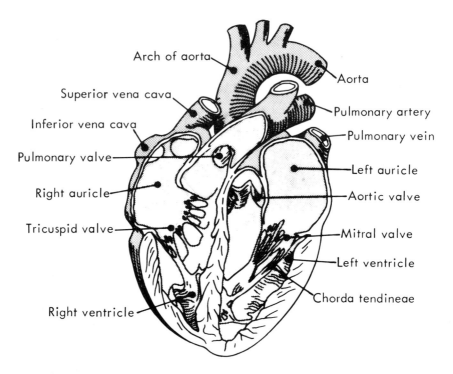

This cross-section drawing of the heart shows the longitudinal front view.

capillaries in the heart as well as in a skeletal muscle. The increased capillarization brings more oxygen to the heart and helps remove the waste products more efficiently. If the work is of a short, explosive nature, the heart will hypertrophy (enlarge the fibers). The ventricles, therefore, will also increase in size and result in more powerful expulsion of blood from the ventricle, thereby increasing the stroke volume. Such activity accounts for the greater stroke volume and lower pulse rate of the trained individual. See ATHLETE'S HEART. In endurance work, the heart is hypertrophied somewhat as a result of increased capillarization.

For more specific information about the circulatory system, its various parts, and ailments, see ANGINA, ARTERIOSCLEROSIS, ATHLETE'S HEART, BLOOD, BLOOD PRESSURE, CHOLESTEROL, CIRCULO-RESPIRATORY ENDURANCE, CIRCULO-RESPIRATORY SYSTEM, DEGENERATIVE CARDIOVASCULAR DISEASE, DIET, EFFECTS OF EXERCISE, HEART DISEASE and ISCHEMIC HEART DISEASE.

CIRCULO-RESPIRATORY ENDURANCE

Circulo-respiratory endurance is the capacity of the entire body to continue muscular exertions for prolonged periods. Those exertions require major adjustments of the circulatory and respiratory systems. Activities such as running, jogging, swimming, cycling, walking and climbing are examples. Quick recovery upon cessation of the activity is an indication of circulo-respiratory endurance. Another sign is an adjustment to the increased activity without undue breathlessness or feelings of distress, fatigue and pain.

Value

Circulo-respiratory endurance is invaluable in many activities, for without a satisfactory level, performance drops off very rapidly, and the ability to continue ceases. The person who has a high degree of endurance can persist in strenuous tasks for a long time. Circulo-respiratory endurance, however, should not be confused with *muscular endurance*. The latter is the capacity of muscles to persist in an activity over a period of time (as in push-ups, pull-ups, and sit-ups). See MUSCLE ENDURANCE.

Circulo-respiratory endurance, moreover, is also an indication of the health status of the circulo-respiratory system. Circulo-respiratory endurance means improved work capacity, increased productivity in daily living and a prevention in the onset of many chronic degenerative cardiovascular diseases.

See ANGINA, BLOOD PRESSURE, DEGENERATIVE CARDIOVASCULAR DISEASE and HEART DISEASE for a more complete discussion.

Exercise and Endurance

Attaining circulo-respiratory endurance is a matter of adjusting to hard work over an extended period of time. Generally, the exercise of workouts must get progressively harder and longer if improvements in the system are expected. After training at a certain level, you will find that your body *adapts* to that level of work. For example, if you are running two miles every day in 18 minutes, in a matter of time, you will find that your body no longer experiences the feeling of fatigue, pain and breathlessness. When that occurs, the run is no longer stressful; for the body has *adapted*. Therefore, you must *progressively* run the two miles in a shorter period of time, say 17 minutes, or increase the distance in 18 minutes. By increasing, you are *overloading* the body again with a new stress. For a more detailed discussion on the principles of training, see TRAINING.

The general procedure for placing stress on the circulo-respiratory system in order to develop circulo-respiratory endurance is to select an activity that will increase the heart rate to at least

140 beats per minute, approximately double the resting rate. See PULSE RATE. The exercise selected should use up 300 to 500 calories in a half hour. Generally, if the activity causes an increase in pulse to around 140 beats per minute, the calories burned up in the body will be in that 300 to 500 range.

It is important, moreover, that the activity be continuous. Activities of short irregular bouts are not effective in the development of circulo-respiratory endurance. Note the stress on irregular session, in effect suggesting the opposite of interval training, an effective technique in developing circulo-respiratory endurance. In interval training, the basic idea is to exercise at a maximum level for a specific time, then to rest for a period, usually until the pulse rate drops to 120, and finally to exercise again for the allotted time. The work and rest bouts are repeated in that manner several times. See INTERVAL TRAINING.

Here's what you can expect from developing satisfactory circulo-respiratory endurance:

Lower resting heart rate.

Lower heart rate during work or exercise.

Higher heart stroke volume during work or exercise.

A faster return to normal pulse after a period of exercise.

Lower blood pressure during work.

Lower oxygen consumption during exercise.

Greater maximum oxygen consumption.

The ability to persist longer in exercise.

See BLOOD, CIRCULATORY SYSTEM and RESPIRATION.

Endurance training will not harm the human organism if the training is progressive and is adapted to the individual. A misconception is that children should not engage in circulo-respiratory endurance training.

Research indicates that provided the child gets adequate sleep and relaxation, has a proper and adequate diet, and restricts sedentary habits, endurance training is not harmful to children over 7 years of age. A normal, healthy heart will not be harmed by exercise.

The best guide to follow in determining the severity of the program is to check to see if the child demonstrates a sudden breathlessness and/or severe fatigue, nausea, palpitation of the heart, sleeplessness, loss of appetite, or unusually high pulse rate. If those occur, the child should terminate the activity for a few days.

The best activities for endurance training for children are obstacle races, circuit training, interval training and continuous rhythmical activities. They are superior to mild games which have only recreational value.

The typical techniques of testing or measuring circulo-respiratory endurance are running and bench stepping. In the laboratory, oxygen intake during exercise is the most valid measure. For a more detailed discussion see TESTS.

CIRCULO-RESPIRATORY SYSTEM

The circulo-respiratory system includes the organs of both the circulatory and the respiratory system. Those systems play a vital role in the transport and exchange of gases within the body and between the body and its environment. A healthy circulo-respiratory system is an indication of good general health, because it means a good work capacity, an efficiency in daily living and a prevention or delay in the onset of several chronic degenerative diseases.

Work Capacity

Work capacity (either exercise or work) is determined by oxygen requirements, oxygen debt tolerance and maximal oxygen intake.

The oxygen requirement is the amount of energy required to perform a specific activity. The more intense the exercise, the more oxygen is required. The tissues demand oxygen for continued action which must be accomplished by the circulo-respiratory system.

See CIRCULO-RESPIRATORY ENDURANCE, ENERGY COST OF ACTIVITIES, METABOLISM and RESPIRATION.

Oxygen debt tolerance comes into play when the circulo-respiratory system can no longer supply the tissues with the necessary oxygen. The tissues may continue to function without oxygen for a while before losing their ability to perform. During that period, the body is functioning with an oxygen deficit. The period of time that a person can continue to work without sufficient oxygen is called oxygen debt tolerance.

After cessation of the activity, oxygen continues to be pumped to the oxygen-starved tissues to replace used oxygen. That is why you breathe heavily after exercise for a period of time. You are repaying your tissues with the necessary oxygen. A person with a greater oxygen debt tolerance is better able to persist at an activity for a longer period of time because he has a greater work capacity. See OXYGEN DEBT, RESPIRATION and OXYGEN INTAKE.

Maximum oxygen intake is the amount of oxygen taken during a specific task. The higher the oxygen intake a person has for a specific task, the slower the accumulation of oxygen debt. A person with a good degree of fitness will have a higher maximal oxygen intake, whereas the reverse is true for a person with low fitness. See OXYGEN INTAKE.

Training improves the work capacity of a person by causing beneficial changes in the three areas of oxygen requirements, oxygen debt tolerance and maximal oxygen intake.

Efficiency in Daily Living

A person's efficiency in daily living is closely related to his work capacity. For if his work capacity is improved, fewer calories will be expended to perform a specific task, thereby making his daily living more efficient.

CLAUDICATION

Intermittent claudication is a leg disorder caused by an arteriosclerotic condition. Usually the iliac or femoral arteries of the legs are affected and result in severe pain on walking. Drugs, operations and cessation of smoking have been the standard treatment.

Recently, exercise has been used effectively in treating intermittent claudication. Two Danish doctors, Andre Larsen and N. A. Lassen of Copenhagen, tested a theory that people with claudication can greatly increase their ability to walk. Their subjects were patients with chronic arteriosclerotic occlusion of the main leg arteries. Each patient walked as energetically as possible for about an hour each day. After 6 months, most patients tripled their walking limit.

CLIMATE

See ENVIRONMENT.

COLLATERAL CIRCULATION

Collateral circulation is the addition or substituting of blood vessels that increase circulation in a tissue area. For example, some of the coronary arteries may become narrowed by the gradual development of atherosclerosis. The narrowing restricts the flow of blood to the heart muscle. To compensate, nearby arteries get wider and open up new branches to the area of the heart that needs it. That collateral circulation often develops at the same time coronary arteries are being narrowed. If collateral circulation is sufficient, the person will not suffer from angina or heart disease because the heart muscle is getting sufficient blood. If the collateral circulation does not develop fast enough, then heart disease or a coronary thrombosis may result.

Collateral circulation is one of the ways the body mends itself after a heart attack.

Effect of Exercise

Regular exercise causes an increase in collateral circulation, for exercise produces the formation of new capillaries within the muscle fibers. Those capillaries increase the supply of blood to the muscle—up to 50% in skeletal muscle. Furthermore, latent capillaries open up as a result of training, thereby increasing blood flow. That effect has an important implication in reducing the possibility of angina and heart attacks, for when an occlusion blocks one coronary artery, cutting off the blood supply to a part of the heart, it may be possible for blood to reach the damaged area through other vessels that have been developed by exercise.

Collateral circulation plays a more important role in rehabilitation. Research has shown that progressive exercise aids in the development of collateral circulation after heart attacks, one of the prime objectives in rehabilitation of cardiac patients.

COMMUNITY FITNESS

The mere mention of physical fitness alone usually calls to mind difficult exercises. But hard exercise and muscular body build, contrary to common opinion, are not necessarily criteria upon which physical fitness is based. To be physically fit is to be in a state of good health, physically and emotionally, to be able to perform daily tasks, and to meet emergencies calling for unexpected expenditures of energy.

The physically fit person is able to think more intelligently in his work,

exhibit greater creativity, demonstrate greater confidence in his abilities, and enjoy life more fully than is the person who gives little attention to total fitness. Some functions of exercise in the fitness program are to help the heart in its work, to strengthen the muscles, to assist in weight control, and to keep the muscles in tone with the bodily processes.

Not everyone needs a hard and long exercise program. The age of the persons involved will determine the type of activity that is proper. Neither expensive equipment nor expansive space is needed. Ten minutes of walking, running and jogging, swimming, or bicycling daily can provide for people of all ages a valuable part of their total fitness program. In addition, bowling, golf, tennis, folk and square dancing, or other organized activities are available in most communities.

Any community can have a high level of physical fitness among its citizens if the proper leadership is available and if the community is willing to work regularly and consistently. The local school or college is staffed with people who have the professional background to work with parents and children.

Summertime Fitness

For year-round fitness, the summer vacation period offers many desirable features. During the summer days, there are excellent opportunities for working with the Red Cross in swimming and water safety programs. Lessons cost nothing, and the school and college pools are often not being used during a greater part of the day. With proper planning, all students can have the privilege of learning correct swimming and water safety skills. As more and more people turn to the great outdoors, that program should receive greater emphasis.

On most college campuses during the summer, there are numerous faculty children eager to take part in whatever fitness programs are available. The children provide good teaching projects for students majoring in physical education. At the same time, as active participants in the fitness program, the children learn many skills that will last a lifetime. Four years old seems to be the proper starting age for both boys and girls. While working with the smaller participants, older children can learn much about safety and accident prevention.

The Vacation Bible school provides another opportunity to work with young people. Often the groups are small, and the group leaders need help during activity hours and play periods. In those situations, boys and girls of a very young age are easily controlled and led in desirable activities. High school students and college students who are prospective teachers of physical education can use leisure hours to help others gain considerable skill and enjoyment.

During the last days of summer, many opportunities are present through newspapers, radio, and other news media for articles and sports announcements of coming fitness activities of the community. It is during that period that many families are taking one last outing or vacation. Because sports are at a virtual standstill, many people if given proper encouragement are anxious to stay active. People in charge of news media need and want interesting projects and activities that concern their public. Pictures and stories of public figures at work in exercise and fitness programs make excellent material. Frequently unusual activities arouse enthusiasm. Fitness and exercise programs on early morning radio and television programs, employing exercise records or instructions, have been enthusiastically received.

School-year Fitness

The first days of the school year are often hectic and demand the best efforts of those whose responsibility it is to establish proper units of intramural competition. Although some work is being done in the public schools, the greatest effort seems to come from the college and university programs. Here trained personnel are in a favorable situation with adequate facilities and possibly hundreds of young men and women anxious to join in group and team activities. While the varsity sports program is meeting the needs of the skilled, hundreds of eager learners need encouragement to enter the wide world of intramural competition, which is bounded only by the imagination of those in charge.

Sports-officiating clinics not only add strength to the intramural and varsity programs but also provide an avenue of activity involving those people who are willing to help others through the application of their own knowledge of the techniques and regulations of the game. At the same time, the neophyte officials are entering into the fitness programs themselves. They learn to enjoy the activities while helping many others to do the same. In most communities, there are qualified officials who are willing to help sponsor clinics and demonstrations. State and local organized officials' groups are looking for techniques and means of adding to their programs by enlisting the aid of new prospects. There never seem to be too many football, basketball, baseball, wrestling, track, swimming and volleyball officials. Many college men and high school boys are earning spending money in that manner while rendering a genuine service to the citizens of the community.

College classes in the theories of play and activities are looking for subjects with whom to work. Many elementary schools need the effort to strengthen their existing fitness programs. Prospective teachers learn much, and at the same time, they are a great aid to the elementary teacher as he attempts to broaden and strengthen the activity program. Effective utilization of the laboratory experience can do much to recruit and maintain physical education teachers. Here in a live situation, future teachers can visualize a rewarding vocation.

Professional physical educators are available to serve as consultants in existing programs at the elementary, secondary and college levels. Those people bring a fresh insight to existing programs and, through consultation and advice, are better able to plan new programs while strengthening existing ones.

The local YMCA, Boys' Club, and Community Center are looking for more participants and more leaders as they seek to upgrade their work. While the professional staff is the guiding force behind the program, there is often room for volunteer and lay personnel to contribute much know-how and effort to making the community more fitness minded. High school and college students make excellent leaders in these community organizations.

The Scout movement always needs qualified leadership to carry out a wide range of fitness projects, including camping, hiking, swimming and sports competition. Young adults as well as older people need to become involved with that recognized agency as it attempts to promote worthwhile living.

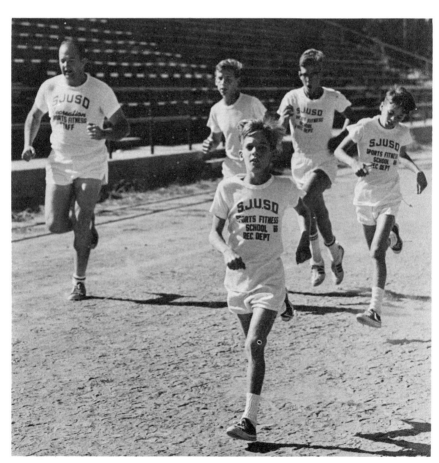

Students and instructor participate in a 600-yard run during a school fitness program.

An outstanding proponent of fitness for living is the Marine Corps and its youth fitness projects. Entranced with all the prestige and glamour of this defense organization, boys are anxious to endure the rigors of exhaustive training periods to win the acclaim of a group they proudly look up to. With the many awards and rewards that the Marine Corps bestows, numerous opportunities for becoming men are made available.

Possible Activities

Many areas are introducing to their citizens new activities in the form of one of the world's most popular competitive sports. Soccer, a game demanding tremendous physical exertion, is being introduced to many elementary and secondary school groups. There is hardly a community without some resourceful person who is willing to serve the community through clinics and demonstrations in soccer and/or other new sports. Angleball may be a partial answer for mass game participation by large groups of young people.

Running is one of mankind's oldest recreative and fitness activities. With just a small amount of leadership, your community can start a cross-country program. Turkey and cake races offer incentive to many young people to want to pay the price for endurance running. Hundreds of boys are being added to cross-country rolls each season, and many continue to run regularly throughout the year. Here is an example of young manpower at its best in an event that requires very little coaching and practically no equipment. Given an opportunity to run, youth may exhibit considerable improvement in stamina and endurance. Running begun early in the school year can lead to a series of spectator events as half-time entertainment at soccer or football games initially and, later, as an event based on its own merits.

For the individual or for the group, volleyball can be the source of relaxation or a strenuous exercise program. Youngsters at the age of 12-14 can begin the sport as an activity that will continue for years. Business men, college students, and high school boys and girls are likely participants. As a part of their fitness drive, military units have for years used volleyball as an indoor or outdoor activity with inexpensive equipment and with limited leadership.

Both boys and girls should be involved in track and field events. Because children love to jump and run, with just a little organization, competition can be developed into an annual event, enhancing greatly community year-round fitness programs. Though ribbons and prizes may be offered, they are not necessary for a solid track and field operation. Many adult women point with pride to their earlier achievements in the sport.

With its continued widespread popularity, softball should be considered an effective agency in community fitness. Girls, particularly, can achieve much enjoyment from that team sport. They are willing to pay the price in order to play on a team that proudly spreads a name across the shirt of the players. Many local businesses support teams in summer recreation programs.

One other area of fitness deserving consideration is work with the mentally retarded. A whole new horizon is opening up in providing fitness for that group. While the work does require a specialized instructor, most communities will provide personnel to do the job if the citizens show concern. Research is available to show that the mentally retarded learn better through physical activity. They can participate in much the same activities as other boys and girls, but they do require some specialized instruction. Volunteers from high schools and colleges are eager to help. Parents and other citizens are also willing to help if given the opportunity.

Local recreational functions such as softball, basketball, volleyball, tennis, bowling, golf, and folk and square dancing can be encouraged by proper leadership of qualified physical educators.

Significant results may be obtained with proper leadership and very little financial outlay. Ample play areas are usually available or can be acquired for most of the suggested games and activities. Scheduling is not an insurmountable problem. The suggested programs and activities make it possible for any community to have year-round fitness for all of its citizens if someone in authority is willing to involve the community resources. Available leadership only need be drawn into play and focused on the citizens. Fitness can be fun. "Fitness for Living" could well be the slogan of every community.—*Garland M. Dickey, Joanne Rowe*

Community Responsibility

Germans in the little town of Münster in Westphalia have a community-sponsored physical fitness park. Basketball baskets and horizontal bars are the only traditional playground equipment found in that park. Instead, the community leaders with the active support of the Federal Republic Sports League have installed special exercise devices such as a "soft" running track, a conveyor-belt ergometer or treadmill, weightlifting equipment supported by strong springs to prevent injuries, and five tree trunks set vertically in a row which participants use to play leap frog. With each piece of equipment comes a point system with scores of between zero and 20 which townspeople can use to measure their level of physical fitness.

The purpose of the fitness park is to get all of the people in the community —especially sedentary adults—involved in an exercise program. According to

the German newspaper *Frankfurter Allgemeine Zeitung,* "The initial response in Münster shows that the general public has accepted the challenge and are cheerfully making use of the facilities." And why not? The park is convenient, free, and open at any time of the day and has a built-in testing element—everyone scores a certain number of points and can see how his performance improves from week to week. For example, in the test of flexibility, the participants jump from a standing start to try to touch a wooden plank with their fingertips. Their height is subtracted from the point they reach on the curved wooden target, and points are awarded on the basis of the height they have managed to jump.

In addition, the park was so designed to enable even the novice exerciser to train without supervision and without fear of injury. To cut down on running discomforts and injuries, the planners devised a soft-springy track made from a mixture of sawdust, peat, and sand over a layer of gravel and loose stones. "It responds so flexibly to the foot that the runner gains all the advantages of running in a forest on a springy bed of pine-needles." The same concept of ease in exercising and protection against injuries has gone into the design of the other exercise devices which measure strength, stamina and agility. For example, the weightlifting equipment which must be hoisted from a shoulder height in one test is firmly lodged in vertical supports and strong springs at shoulder height.

What would it take to get communities throughout the United States to provide similar facilities for their residents? No one would dispute their value, especially since they do provide a community playground that adults can use. Community-sponsored fitness facilities for adults are lacking in most cities and towns. Although many give their residents a choice of municipal tennis courts, golf courses, pools, and the like, few provide anything similar to the Münster park for the average citizen interested in maintaining personal fitness.

There are probably thousands who would jump at the chance to see just how physically fit they are by getting involved in some simple, nonathletic activity. Testing and scoring your agility by climbing up a 13-foot pole is certainly good exercise and good fun. But finding such facilities in the community is another problem. Parks similar to the one in Münster could be one answer. They are relatively inexpensive to construct—Münster's park cost less than $2,000—and can be set up in any park, meadow, forest or vacant lot.

Of course, the problem of potential injuries could be one hurdle which could scare away local communities. However, any person over the age of · 30 just starting a physical fitness program, whether it be in a physical fitness park or in his own home, should have a complete medical checkup before starting that program. The Federal Republic Sports League reports no medical problems among people using the Münster park. The same is true for similar facilities sponsored by local communities throughout Scandinavia.

It will probably be a long, hard struggle before any community will take to the idea of a municipal physical fitness park. Individuals bent on improving their fitness now have a hard time getting school systems to open their gyms, pools, and playgrounds for evening and weekend work outs.

But there are encouraging signs that government is willing to do more in the way of providing fitness facilities. The Secretary of the Interior during the Johnson administration, Stewart Udall, opened four special jogging trails in federal parks in the Washington, D. C., area. It is a pilot program for the nation and shows how every town could stake out markers every 110 yards and every quarter mile, along a park trail. A recent study, *Trails for America*, reports on the *Nationwide Trail Study*, by the Bureau of Outdoor Recreation recommended that communities establish trails close to centers of population. Called a neglected recreational element in America, such trails could provide further notes that the reservoir of potential demand that exists for outdoor recreation in most metropolitan areas is so large that as soon as a trail facility is provided it is overused. Obviously, Americans want readily accessible fitness facilities.—*John Haberern*

CONDITIONING

In most instances, conditioning is used synonymously with training. Some say that training is the technique of progressively exercising the body, whereas conditioning refers to the type of exercise or therapy used. In this book, conditioning and training are synonyms. See TRAINING.

CONNECTIVE TISSUE

Connective tissue is the most abundant type in the body. Some of the connective tissues most affected by exercise include fascia, adipose tissue, tendons, ligaments, aponeuroses, deep fascia, bone, cartilage and hemopoietic tissue.

Fascia is dense fibrous tissue arranged in a sheet and associated with muscle. *Adipose tissue* (fat) affords protection and insulation. *Tendons, ligaments, aponeuroses* and *deep fascia* provide strong, flexible connections between different body parts. *Bone* gives the body rigid support. *Cartilage* acts as a shock absorber between bony parts and makes up the fibrous portions of the nose, ears and trachea (windpipe). *Hemopoietic tissue* is located in the marrow spaces of bone and functions in the formation of red blood cells and other blood constituents. See EFFECTS OF EXERCISE.

The condition of connective tissue depends on factors like nutrition, health habits and exercise. Without the essential nutrients, the formation of connective tissue as well as other body tissues will be adversely affected. See NUTRITION. Postural habits are also important, for poor habits put a strain on the connective tissues that can lead to chronic problems.

The human body functions as an integrated whole. The many organs, tissues and systems are interdependent on each other, and what tends to benefit one part of the organism will also benefit the other parts. Exercise benefits the entire organism.

The effects of exercise upon the circulatory, respiratory and muscular systems are well known. The single most important benefit of regular, intense physical exercise is that it conditions the circulatory and respiratory system to efficiently supply oxygen and nutrients to the cells of the body via the blood. Through exercise the capacity of the blood to carry oxygen is increased. During exercise, the temperature of the blood rises and viscosity (resistance to flow) decreases, making it easier for the heart to move the blood through the vessels. With an adequate supply of blood, the many billions of specialized cells of the body can more effectively perform their specific functions whether they be contraction, protection, secretion, support, connection, or any of the numerous cellular activities.

Muscles are attached to bones by tendons. Pulling of the muscles on the bones causes movement. Ligaments differ in that they connect bone to bone and are important components of all joints. Muscle strength is closely related to the strength of certain connective tissues. As muscles increase in strength so also must the tendons. Muscular strength contributes to joint stability and strength. Exercise helps develop and maintain "muscle tone" (the constant partial contraction evident in healthy resting muscles).

Weak or lazy muscles (those with poor tone) allow the skeletal framework to sag, leading to fatigue of certain connective tissues, particularly the ligaments. Over a prolonged period, muscle weakness or laziness can lead to postural problems. In addition, weak muscles cannot keep joints in alignment during intense activity. When a joint is not in proper alignment, joint injuries most often occur. The majority of injuries that occur in bruises, sprains or strains, damage some form of connective tissue. Strong muscles not only keep joints in alignment but also aid the joints in resisting outside forces that may cause misalignment.

A primary benefit of exercise is that it helps to keep body fat from becoming excessive. A combination of poor eating habits (usually overindulgence and poor selection) and a lack of exercise results in the storage of unused calories as fat. Not only does fat present an unattractive health hazard, but it affects efficient movement.

Cartilage is a unique tissue that provides protection for the articulating surfaces of bones. Under pressure or shock, cartilage compresses slightly and absorbs some of the force. Pieces of cartilage are present between each of the vertebrae and in each of the knee joints. Injuries involving cartilage consist of bruises, displacements, or tears which affect joint motion and stability. Displacements and tears often need surgical repair. The most common cartilage injury occurs in the knee joint. Many experts feel that the incidence of knee cartilage and ligament injuries could be reduced if proper conditioning exercises were employed to strengthen the knee muscles.

Muscles and connective tissues tend to shorten if not regularly stretched. Therefore, stretching exercises should be included in every exercise program. The shortening leads to a loss of range of motion and, if not acted against, can lead to postural or mechanical problems. Muscle weakness coupled with a lack of flexibility is probably the major cause of chronic back problems, particularly in the low back. The usual prescription is light resistive exercises and gradual stretching exercises. See FLEXIBILITY.

CONTINUOUS RHYTHMICAL EXERCISE

Continuous rhythmical exercise is an extensive exercise program developed by Dr. Thomas K. Cureton of the University of Illinois. Perfected over a period of years at the University Physical Fitness Laboratory, the program develops physical fitness for both men and women. Its effectiveness has been demonstrated by experimental and clinical studies.

The basic concept is that since "the law of life is movement, rhythmical continuous movement, the law of exercise should be rhythmical continuous movement." The program has been used by many Y's and physical education instructors throughout the world with great success. In all the programs, there has been modification to meet particular needs and situations, but the basic concept has remained the same —continuous and rhythmical exercise.

The Program

A program is divided into a series of 20 lessons or more, to be completed in 6 to 9 months, depending upon the age and physical condition of the people involved. The program is not binding since each person may progress at his own rate, according to his abilities, from low gear, to middle gear, to high gear. Every lesson regardless of the gear level, begins with (1) an introduction, if taught by a teacher; (2) a period of warm-up; (3) the main body of exercises; and (4) a

tapering-off period involving deep breathing, stretching, massage and rest. During each lesson, it is important to keep work continuous, with a progressive buildup of speed and exertion.

In low gear, which lasts 8 lessons, the primary emphasis is placed on flexibility. The exercises are rhythmical endurance exercises done at a slow pace. Attention is focused on deep breathing. Thirty minutes of the exercises are done at least 3 times a week.

The middle-gear program consists of harder exercises, done faster and for longer periods. Flexibility, muscle strength, muscle endurance, and moderate circulo-respiratory endurance are

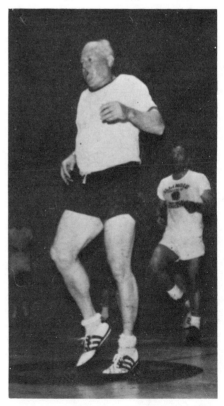

Dr. Thomas Cureton leads a class in a program of continuous exercise.

the objectives. One hour of 4 times a week is the minimum for middle-gear workouts. One day's workout should last beyond 60 minutes.

In the high-gear program, high-speed exercises that place a great demand on the body, are chosen. Those hard exercises are done 5 days a week for one hour, with two days lasting longer than one hour.

Exercises

Every exercise included in the EXERCISE section may be used in Dr. Cureton's program. Below are representative examples of each of the three gear programs. Remember that each gear level demands a different exertion. At low gear, exercises are done slowly, moderately, then fast for a few seconds and finally slower again. At high gear most of the exercises are performed at top speed. A warm-up and tapering-off period must be included in every level.

Representative Workouts for the Three Gear Levels

30 Minute Low-Gear Workout:

Introduction. Do the exercises slowly and deliberately, without interruption. Emphasize deep breathing. Take several deep breaths after each exercise.

Warm-up. Walk and/or jog slowly around the workout area. Walk a lap and jog a lap. When walking or jogging, swing the arms in full circles. Occasionally hold a deep breath.

General Body Exercises
Neck, Arm, Shoulder and Chest Exercises (5 to 10 minutes):
 Neck circles (1 minute)
 Arm circles (1 minute)
 Arm flexors (1 minute)
 Arms back (1 minute)
 Jumping Jacks (1 minute)
Take 10 deep breaths.
Trunk Exercises (10 minutes):
 Thigh flexion (1 minute)

Alternate leg raise (1 minute)
Mountain climber stretch (1 minute)
Leg raiser (1 minute)
Forward bend (1 minute)
Double knees up (1 minute)
Back arch (1 minute)
Stretch (1 minute)
Take 10 deep breaths.
Abdominal exercises (5 minutes):
 Flutter kick (1 minute)
 Chest lifts (1 minute)
 Abdominal curl (1 minute)
 Alternate knee kicks (1 minute)
 Trunk rotations (1 minute)
Take 10 deep breaths.
Legs (5 minutes):
 Toe raisers (1 minute)
 Skip kicks (1 minute)
 Side skip kicks (1 minute)
 Hop on one foot for 30 seconds, then 30 seconds on the other.
Take 10 deep breaths. Then walk a few minutes shaking legs and arms, and gradually massaging the muscles.

That workout may be engaged in by almost anyone without fear of injury. If you feel that your physical condition warrants a more demanding workout, follow the exercises with some continuous activity, like bicycling, walking, or swimming. If your existence has been sedentary, stay with the simple workout. When the lesson is no longer difficult, the exercises should become gradually harder. As you progress, include a rhythmic activity lasting about 10 to 30 minutes after the general part of the exercise.

At about the eighth lesson (not session), the middle-gear workout begins. (To get to the eighth lesson may require several weeks or even months.)

60 Minute Middle-Gear Workout:

Introduction. Prior to middle gear, the emphasis is on slow exercises and proper breathing. In middle gear, the speed is doubled. Begin in the same slow manner as in low gear, but gradually increase the speed. As daily workouts progress, increase the length of time the speed is maintained. Tapering-off is important at middle-gear level.

Warm-up Exercises. Walk one lap around the exercise area. Then run/jog two.

Walk one lap around the exercise area. Then run/jog four.

Walk one lap around the exercise area. Then run/jog six.

Walk one lap around the exercise area. Then run/jog eight.

Walk three laps around the exercise area. Breathe forcibly during the walk/jog laps, which serve as middle-gear warm-ups.

General Exercises. The exercises are the same as those presented under low gear, except that the exercise is started slowly and then accelerated for longer periods. Throughout the workouts more difficult exercises may be chosen, such as push-ups, sit-ups, knee bends, inverted bicycle, etc.

As progress is made through middle gear, endurance activities are included, like walking, jogging, swimming, cycling, running place, skipping rope, or anything of a vigorous rhythmical nature. The activity should take 20 to 30 minutes.

Tapering Off. The tapering off period must last 5 minutes. Walk at will, then slower, and rest.

60 Minute High-Gear Workout:

At lesson 18, high gear is begun. Here, the limits of strength and endurance are tested and pushed.

Warm-up Exercises

Run two laps around the exercise area and walk one.

Run four laps around the exercise area and walk one.

Run six laps around the exercise area and walk one.

Run eight laps around the exercise area and walk one.

Run ten laps around the exercise area.

Walk for 3 minutes.

That warms you up for the following:

General Exercises. Arm and Shoulder:

Push-ups. Perform as many push-ups as possible. Then walk slowly around the exercise area, breathing deeply, stretching and shaking arms and legs. (The walking, breathing, stretching and shaking is to be performed after the end of each exercise below.)

Pull-ups.

Abdomen. Sit-ups (as many as possible in 2 minutes). V-seat for one minute.

Back. Upper body arch for one to two minutes. Flutter kick for one to two minutes.

Legs. Half squat for one minute. Squat thrusts, as many as possible in 20 seconds.

Relaxation. Jog around the exercise area two times and walk once shaking arms and legs.

THEN REPEAT GENERAL EXERCISES AGAIN.

Tapering Off. Jog five times around the exercise area. Walk five times around the exercise area. Walk, breathe deeply and stretch until recovered. Massage muscles, then take a hot and cold shower.

Those are only three of the 20-odd exercise lessons outlined by Dr. Cureton.

Once a person has attained high gear, the program can be modified. The workout need last only 30 minutes, after which a continuous rhythmical activity is selected.

The basis of Dr. Cureton's program is to develop many of the components of physical fitness—organic health, motor fitness and physique.

Numerous studies have been conducted that demonstrate that this program is superior to other forms of exercise as far as achieving optimal fitness levels. It has been shown to be more effective than jogging, 5BX, weight training, golf, tennis, isometrics, lawnmowing, volleyball and calisthenics as a means of conditioning.

COOLING DOWN

See TAPERING OFF

COORDINATION

Coordination is the common denominator of all motor ability components, yet it is the one we know least about. Coordination involves the nervous, skeletal and muscle systems, and the senses of sight, feeling and hearing. Also involved is kinesthetic sense—your awareness of the position and the balance of the body at a given moment.

Dr. Edwin Fleishman has noted that although it is difficult to determine what coordination really is, there are two definite types—multi-limb and gross body. Multi-limb coordination is the ability of a person to coordinate simultaneous movements of two hands, two feet, or a combination thereof, while operating a certain device. Gross motor coordination is a rather nebulous area that is difficult to define or measure. See AGILITY.

Some claim that there are other phases of coordination such as hand-eye coordination used in trying to hit a pitched baseball with a bat or eye-foot coordination used in punting a football.

Precise measurement of gross motor coordination is impossible with present tests, but it is possible to measure and define specific tasks, e. g., hand-eye coordination in hitting a baseball with a bat. Coordination is really the ability to get all the motor abilities (balance, muscle strength, muscle endurance, agility, etc.) working together to make movement efficient, whether it is typing, running, playing sports, writing, driving a car, walking, or whatever. It is a component of motor ability that

is largely inherited, yet it may be inhibited or developed by the environment. The improvement of gross, motor coordination is difficult if not impossible. Through practice, the specific parts of coordination, such as walking, shooting a pistol, hitting a nail on the head, or typing, can be improved.

CORONARY HEART DISEASE

See DEGENERATIVE CARDIOVASCULAR DISEASE, HEART DISEASE and ISCHEMIC HEART DISEASE.

DAILY ACTIVITIES

Whether you know it or not, you perform many different exercises during the day which can assist you in maintaining a minimum degree of fitness. When you push yourself from a chair you do a modified bar push-up. When you bend your knees to pick up something from the floor you are doing a knee-bend.

There are literally thousands of ways in which you can supplement your daily habits simply by being aware of activities to improve fitness. Dr. Arthur Steinhaus has called this technique "Living With Fitness Built In." Here are some of his tips for incorporating exercise into everyday activities:

1. Always stand when dressing and undressing.

2. Park your car or get off the bus or train a few blocks from your destination, and walk at a brisk rate.

3. Avoid using the elevator or escalator to go up or down two or three flights of stairs. If you must take the elevator get off on the wrong floor and walk two or three flights. You may find it invigorating to take two steps at a time.

4. Take a walk around the block in the morning and/or in the evening after work.

5. After coming home from work do

not drop into a chair for the rest of the evening, but become involved in a hobby or do some chores.

6. On your day off wash the car yourself, get out and garden, rake leaves or mow the lawn (walk behind the power mower—don't ride)!

7. If you are a housewife, sweep and dust with brisk, vigorous movements. Reach whenever possible in your housework, whether scrubbing, getting linens or making the beds.

It is important to sit, lift, walk, climb, run and stand properly. See BODY MECHANICS for the proper techniques.

Office Exercises

Here are some exercises that you may perform in the office without drawing attention to what you are doing:

1. Pull in your abdomen when the telephone rings, when you are brushing your teeth, or shaving. Do not hold your breath. That is excellent for firming up abdominal muscles.

2. While sitting, raise your legs. Hold them a few seconds, then lower. This exercise is good for the thigh muscles and abdomen. To place further stress on those muscles, sit on the edge of the chair, being certain the chair does not tip.

3. While filing, bend your knees to file in the lower drawer instead of bending the back.

4. Whenever possible, stretch to get something from a top shelf, a practice that is good for the entire body.

5. When looking up a phone number twist your body to the side. The movement is good for the lateral abdominal muscles and muscles of the lower back.

6. When sitting in your chair, grasp the arms of the chair and push yourself upward then lower yourself back to the chair. Repeat several times. This exercise is good for arm and shoulder muscles.

7. When you answer the phone, grip it tightly as though you were trying to crush the phone. This is good for the muscles of the forearm and hand.

8. Push outward on either side of your desk well with your legs, or place a sturdy waste can between your legs and push inward. Those exercises affect the thighs.

9. When standing, rise up on your toes and drop down on your heels. Repeat several times to benefit the calf muscles.

10. Place your hands on top of your desk and push down with all your might, or place your hands underneath your desk and attempt to lift upward. Those two exercises are good for the arm and shoulder muscles.

11. Put your feet on the desk, and cross one leg over the other. Raise both legs into the air for a count of

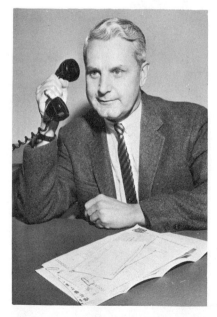

Often you can exercise without anyone knowing. This executive does a grip strengthener after answering a phone call.

five. Then switch legs. This affects the thigh and lower abdominal muscles.

12. Lean against the wall and slide your body down, by bending at the knees, to a sitting position. Hold as long as possible.

13. Stand with your hands behind your back, left fist in your right palm. Press downward with your left arm and upward with your right. Then change hands. This is good for your arm muscles. See BUSINESS and FAMILY FITNESS.

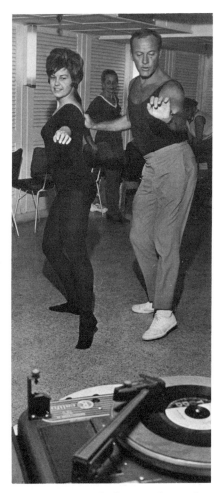

Because it is rhythmic and creative, dancing ranks as an enjoyable activity.

Tension-reducing Techniques

There are several techniques that may be used to aid relaxation, and reduce tension:

1. Wear well-fitting, comfortable clothing.

2. Check yourself frequently for signs of tension, e.g., clenched fists, scowling, strained shoulders.

3. Avoid excessive noise.

4. Stretch whenever you can; then relax completely.

5. Grip you chair or desk tightly and then relax completely.

6. Yawn whenever possible.

7. Roll your head in a large circle.

8. Tense your face muscles, and then allow them to relax.

Specific tensing of various parts of the body and then the sudden "letting go" promotes relaxation. For example, sharply clench your hands and then let them relax. Perform this several times. Then try it with your feet, leg muscles, etc.

In short, as soon as you feel tension building up, relieve it. Just getting up and walking around the desk can be extremely beneficial. See RELAXATION.

The above exercises and techniques must be habitual if you expect them to improve your physical condition. Remind yourself to incorporate them into your daily routine until they become second nature.

DANCE

Dance is a universal expression. It is infinitely varied and without regimentation. There are no known people who do not dance. We are born already attuned to rhythm—it is only some form of inhibition, restraint, or frustration that seems to make a person unrhythmic. It is natural to dance.

But dance, as an art form, uses all lesser forms of dance as its "raw material," includes every way man has ever moved rhythmically to express himself, and trains man to be articulate through patterned, purposeful and rhythmic movement. And a physically literate man should be able to converse through gesture as easily and as naturally as through words, spoken or written. Violent, jerky movements go against nature, and are dull, boring and disliked by the majority. Rudolf Bode, a great German pioneer in physical education, created and used what he called "Rhythmic Gymnastics." Those were always accompanied by music. Thus dance took a step forward for we know that rhythmic movement is easier, more pleasurable, more efficient and more beneficial.

Rhythm

Rhythm (spelled with a capital letter) is one of those big words like Life, Truth, Love, Justice and Art that are almost impossible to define. But Life itself is rhythmic—our breathing is rhythmic, our heart beat is rhythmic, even the peristaltic action of our intestinal tract is rhythmic. When rhythm is spelled with a small r, then it can be defined—for a rhythm, such as waltz, or polka, is made up of the three elements of duration, stress and speed, and there are almost an infinite number of such rhythms.

My definition of physical fitness deviates somewhat from the traditional concept. When I speak of fitness, I mean someone who has not only a strong and healthy body, but one which is articulate and expressive.

It is universally conceded that mankind reached one of its highest peaks of culture during the 5th century B.C. in Greece. Here dance was given a prominent part in the whole range of man's life: it was the chief means of religious ritual. It was used as the most efficient way of training the soldiers—Pyrrlic dances were used to give the soldier every strength and coordination he would need in actual battle. And for hand-to-hand combat, no army was ever so efficient. Famous men danced solo dances in the stadia

to celebrate a great victory—and the highest tribute possible to give a man was to call him "aristoi orchestas"—a superb dancer. For to be a superb dancer, a man had to have a well-stocked mind to draw upon for his subject matter. He had to have a nobility of soul so that the content of his dancing was life—enhancing to the beholders and left them in some way enobled. And if a man had the body, the technique, and the vocabulary, and danced with such spontaneity, it seemed as if the dance was improvised and did achieve the enoblement of his audience.

Self-discipline of Dancing

The physical education systems of most of our educational institutions lean heavily on competitive sports—violent movement which under the stress of wanting to *win* can, and often does, lead to overstrain and injury. In true physical fitness, there is only one person to "beat"—i.e., one's self—to be better at what you do than you were yesterday. This then is the basic way of health—to grow gradually—to evolve from what you were to something finer, more capable, more efficient. This is what dance training in the area of dance as an art form does for the trainee. No movement is ever done in such a way as to cause injury or to overstrain leading to a heart attack: at all times insist on this.

The disciplines of dance training require a more complete use of every muscle in the body than any other form of sport, and, at the same time, require mental discipline, and by use of good music, the performers are exposed to an emotional enrichment in harmony, rhythm and an experience in beauty. And in group training in dance the student learns to take his part in a community enterprise—someone said "It was dance that first socialized man."

You need not, however, even think of performing for a public—for dance is something you can enjoy anywhere. Social dancing requires a place, an orchestra and partners. But then golf, tennis, swimming, and many other sports require special places, special equipment and other people. With dance, a record player, your favorite record, and your own bedroom are enough—although you can extend your dance activities into communal situations if they are available. But you can get the benefits of dance alone and by yourself. Find your own rhythms by experimentation, choose the music that allows you to express the things you want to express, and by that expression release your inner emotional tensions.

Conditioning Programs

Dancing involves every one of the major forms of movement: walking, developing into running, which in turn develops into leaping; swinging movement both of arms and legs, exercises which concentrate on tensing and relaxing every muscle in the body; falling and rising successions, which are wave-like movements passing through the entire body and through parts of the body; torsions and twistings; exercises that develop balance control; jumping, folding and unfolding, shaking and many others.

The dancer has the problem of having to use his own body as his instrument of expression and as the material of his art form. Therefore, the first essential, before the dance, as such, is approached, is to develop and train the body until it becomes instantly and completely responsive to any order the brain gives it. Muscular strength must be built up through the right kinds of exercise—to enable the dancer to leap into the air, and to land without shock or jar; all stiffness must be eliminated, so that fluid movement may pass through all or part of the body like a wave; the rhythmic and ever-present principle of tension and relaxation must be so much a part of the dancer that he can be relaxed at will (*qualities* of movement) and he must even-

tually be able to improvise in movement that is communicative, as readily as he engages in conversation.

Contributions of Dancing to Fitness

Although social and folk dancing are at least a physical rhythmic activity, and thus to that extent good, they are largely confined to exercise of feet and legs. The larger concept of dance requires a completely coordinated body, expressive freedom and fluidity of every part of the body. Some of these successions of the entire body provide flexibility of the entire spine. The pelvic rocks and hip circles, often used in dance, give a resilience and strength to the hip and low back area that may help reduce the occurrence of backaches and sacroiliac slips that can occur as a result of poor development and improper carriage or posture.

Swinging movements which involve the arms stretched high and then swooping down until the backs of the hands brush the ground and a following movement back to vertical are excellent for added flexibility. These movements as well as head rolling to rhythm help relieve the tension of desk work that may cause various stresses and headaches. These are the pragmatic benefits, and only a few of them mentioned.

Everyone gets some satisfaction out of an enjoyable physical activity—even as simple as a good walk preferably in the clean air of the country. Many get this pleasure out of games; but for me, dance goes beyond these and gives release to emotional and mental tensions as no other physical activity does—because it is rhythmic, expressive and creative.

Dance, furthermore, belongs to the entire human race, both sexes and from childhood through old age. Plato, in the *Laws* which was the culmination of his many years of philosophic writings, described an ideal civilization in which he lists dances suitable for people over 80.

As the great English philosopher Havelock Ellis said: "If we are indifferent to the art of dancing we have failed to understand not merely the supreme manifestations of physical life but also the supreme symbol of spiritual life." There cannot be true physical fitness without the radiant well-being also of mind and soul.—*Ted Shawn*

Dance, Social

Social dance is enjoyed by many people in our western culture, especially teenagers. In some cases, it is the only activity that some people get. Therefore, it is very important that its fitness benefits be considered.

Down through the ages social dance has taken on many different forms. It has been used for both recreational and educational purposes. The Greeks included dance as part of instruction because of its mental and physical benefits in the attainment of good posture, agility, health and *esprit de corps*. The cultural hibernation of the arts during the Dark Ages included dance as well as all other physical activity. The Reformation, however, fostered individual participation in leisure-time pursuits which tended to encourage interest in recreational dance.

During the eighteenth century, ministers and the press appeared to attack dance at every opportunity. Laws were written against it. Nevertheless, people continued to enjoy social dance participation, and the unskilled developed a desire to learn. The nineteenth century fostered, however, an independence in the preference of recreational social dances. The exacting *Quadrilles* and class-conscious *Cotillions* bowed out to the nineteenth century couple dances that suited the mood and thinking of Americans. A new foundation was laid for a new breed of recreational social dance that was truly American.

The United States made its first contribution to the field of recreational dance with the Two-Step in 1890. Americans began to cast aside European social dances in favor of their own and those of Latin neighbors. The Cake Walk (1893) and Ragtime music became a national craze by the turn of the century. Those were the most popular social dances until 1910, together with European imports—the *Waltz*, the *Polka*, the *Galop* and the *Schottische*. The "Castle Era" (1910-20) produced the *Turkey Trot* (1911), the *Bunny Hug* (1911), the *Tango* (1912), the *One-Step* (1912), the *Castle Walk* (1912), the *Brazilian Maxixe* (1913), the *Hesitation Waltz* (1913), the *Fox Trot* (1913), and the *Toddle* (1915).

The "Flapper Era" of the Twenties emphasized a strong negroid influence with the *Shimmy* (1920), the *Charleston* (1923), *Dance Contests* (1923), the *Black Bottom* (1926) and the *Varsity Drag* (1927). The *"Depression"* decade during the Thirties brought forth the *Rumba* (1930), the *Big Apple* (1936), *Truckin'* (1936), the *Suzi-Q* (1937), the *Shag* (1938), the *Lindy Hop* (1938), the *Conga* (1939), and the *Samba* (1939). The *Mambo* (1944) was the only off-spring of World War II years of the Forties. The "Fabulous Fifties" fathered the *Bunny Hop* (1953), the *Merengue* (1954), the *Bop* (1955), the *Cha Cha Cha* (1955), the *Calypso* (1958), and the *Madison* (1959). Other than the *Bossa Nova* (1962), the "Sensual Sixties" centered attention on the Discotheque social dances. Included were the *Twist* (1961), the *Mashed Potato* (1961), *Slauson* (1962), the *Watusi*—also known as the *Frug* (1963), the *Swim* (1964), the *Monkey* (1964), the *Pony* (1964), the *Jerk* (1965), the *Shaggy Dog* (1966), and the *Funkie* (1968).

Through the recorded history of civilized man, society has had its dance. A key to man's mode of living and thinking may be found in the manner in which he dances and his reasons for doing so. Popular social dances have had special status and interpretation in the lives of devotees.

Contribution to Fitness

Social dance provides exercise for the feeling of well-being, minimizes the causes of fatigue by sufficient exercise to stimulate body-organ functions, motivates a healthy appetite and restful sleep, and helps to maintain muscle tone, aiding correct posture, balance and coordination.

If done vigorously, social dance may help to develop circulo-respiratory endurance. Such dances as the Polka, the Watusi, the Jerk and the Mashed Potato will aid greatly to achieve that fitness component.

Psychologically, social dance provides an opportunity for relaxation; a cartharsis for stress, mental strain, and pent-up emotions; peer acceptance; creative experiment; self-confidence development; and experience in democratic principles.—*John Youmans*

Since dancing is a moderate to moderate-high energy-cost activity, it may be used to help improve your fitness level, especially your circulo-respiratory and muscle endurance. Below are two dancing programs which take into account the important principles of fitness training.

* POLKA AND OTHER VIGOROUS DANCE PROGRAMS**

Chart 1	Chart 2
1. 10 minutes	1. 55 minutes
2. 15 minutes	2. 60 minutes
3. 20 minutes	3. 65 minutes
4. 25 minutes	4. 68 minutes
5. 30 minutes	5. 70 minutes
6. 35 minutes	6. 75 minutes
7. 40 minutes	7. 78 minutes
8. 45 minutes	8. 80 minutes
9. 50 minutes	9. 85 minutes

* See ENDURANCE and ENERGY COST OF ACTIVITIES for an explanation of these charts.

** Doesn't include rest periods.

Fitness 1

If you achieved a score of poor or low average on the *Harvard Step Test* or a score of very poor or poor on the *12 Minute Run*, start on Chart 1-Level 1 and spend 1 week at each level until you reach Chart 2-Level 9. Try to participate 4 to 5 days a week. When you reach Chart 2-Level 9, 4 days a week is sufficient.

Fitness 2

If you achieved a score of high average on the *Harvard Step Test* or fair on the *12 Minute Run*, start on Chart 1-Level 1. Spend one week on Chart 1-Levels 1, 2, 4, 6, 8, or 9, and Chart 2-Levels 2, 4, 6, 8, and 9. It is recommended that you participate 4 to 5 days a week. When Chart 2-Level 9 is reached, 4 days a week is sufficient.

Fitness 3

If you achieved a score of good or excellent on either the *Harvard Step Test* or *12 Minute Run*, continue your current program or select Chart 2-Level 9 as your level of participation. Four days a week is sufficient.

* SQUARE DANCING PROGRAM

Chart 1	Chart 2
1. 20 minutes	1. 100 minutes
2. 30 minutes	2. 105 minutes
3. 40 minutes	3. 110 minutes
4. 50 minutes	4. 115 minutes
5. 60 minutes	5. 120 minutes
6. 70 minutes	6. 125 minutes
7. 75 minutes	7. 130 minutes
8. 85 minutes	8. 135 minutes
9. 95 minutes	9. 140 minutes

* See ENDURANCE and ENERGY COST OF ACTIVITIES for an explanation of these charts.

Fitness 1

Same as Vigorous Dance Programs.

Fitness 2

If you achieved a score of high average on the *Harvard Step Test* or fair on the *12 Minute Run,* start on Chart 1-Level 2. Spend one week on Chart 1-Levels 2, 4, 5, 7, and 8, and Chart 2-Levels 1, 3, 5, 7, and 9. It is recommended that you participate 4 to 5 days a week. When Chart 2-Level 9 is reached, 4 days a week is sufficient.

Fitness 3

Same as Vigorous Dance Programs.

DANGEROUS EXERCISES

See EXCESSIVE EXERCISE.

DEGENERATIVE CARDIOVASCULAR DISEASE

Types

Two primary types of circulatory disorders may be crippling or fatal.

1. The most common is a blood clot (thrombosis) forming in a blood vessel and blocking, partially or completely, passage of the blood. Sometimes this clot (an embolus) may break off from the wall and lodge in a vital area of the body. Death or serious impairment can result. If a blood clot blocks an artery in the heart, brain, or kidney, a coronary thrombosis, stroke, or uremia can result. Atherosclerosis is the most common cause of this circulatory disorder and occurs when yellowish and whitish spots accumulate on the walls of the arteries. Those small spots protrude into the inner surfaces of the vessels themselves.

At the outset of this disease, these atheromas are very small and may appear to be little more than marks on the inner lining of the vessels. In a period of years, however, the atheromas enlarge substantially until there is little room for the blood to flow through. These atheromas may occur in the arteries of any part of the body.

When the atherosclerosis occurs in the coronary arteries and develops into later stages, a coronary thrombosis with myocardial infarction (heart attack) occurs.

The heart has an extensive network of arteries that supply it with blood. See CIRCULATORY SYSTEM. The left and right coronary arteries, which arise from the aorta and then develop into an amazing capillary network, literally bathe every fiber of the heart with blood and, therefore, provide oxygen for the chemical process of muscle contraction.

In coronary thrombosis with myocardial infarction, the clot blocks the blood supply to one part of the heart muscle. When the supply is blocked, pain may or may not be present. Sometimes the chest pain is very severe and may extend to the neck, arms, or shoulders. In other individuals, however, the pain is virtually nonexistent. But there may be an unexplained weakness, sweating or breathlessness.

Actual Heart Attack

At the point of blockage the "heart attack" has occurred. A pain or ache may persist sometime after the initial blockage, for the fibers of the heart that are not receiving the oxygenated blood stop contracting; then, the fibers become swollen and die. At this point, the pain subsides. The part of the heart that does not receive oxygen suffers an actual injury, and therefore, requires time to heal. The rest of the heart (unless the attack is so severe that the heart muscle is damaged causing death) continues to struggle along in a limited capacity.

Once the attack occurs, the heart begins to repair itself. First, leukocytes are sent to the damaged area to clear away the muscle fibers that are no longer able to contract. The removal must occur before the tissue can heal and form a scar—the process takes about a week. For the tissue to heal, nearby arteries must open up new branches to deliver blood to the area of the heart that needs it. These new vessels that supply blood to the area around the injury produce what is called *collateral* circulation. See COLLATERAL CIRCULATION. If the healing is normal and continuous, the person who suffered a moderate to fairly severe attack may leave the hospital after four weeks. If complications develop, the healing process usually takes longer.

Angina Pectoris

In some cases there is an incomplete blockage that causes a portion of the heart to suffer from an insufficient blood and oxygen supply. The result is a tightness and feeling of pressure in the chest, usually during exercise or

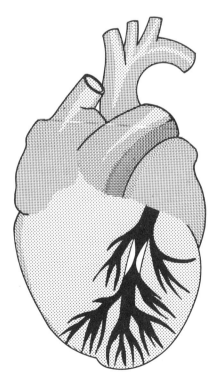

A heart under attack. Because the coronary artery is narrowed, the heart tissue normally nourished by that artery is dying. Regular exercise can offset the effects of many such attacks.

excitement, called *angina pectoris.* Angina is not a disease, but a symptom that a portion of the heart is not receiving an adequate blood supply. There is no damage to the heart when this pain occurs. See ANGINA.

Avoidance of physical activities that cause the pain, more frequent rest periods, loss of extra weight, and reduction in animal and dairy fats in the diet may help to alleviate the occurrence of the pain for some people. Nitroglycerine or some other form of nitrate in pill form may be used to stretch or dilate the coronary arteries whenever the heart muscle is under a stressful situation.

The difference between a coronary thrombosis and angina pectoris is obvious. In the former there is blockage. In the latter there is narrowing of the coronary arteries without a complete blockage. Why some people develop angina, a coronary thrombosis or both is not clear. It appears that in some individuals the atherosclerosis is slow in developing, while in others it is more rapid. Those individuals who have the slower atherosclerosis may realize through attacks of angina that they have a narrowing of the arteries and may make a few modifications in their daily living to arrest the progress of the condition. In the others the disease progresses very rapidly, and the heart attack occurs before they are aware of the disease developing. See ANGINA.

Cause of Strokes

If brain vessels are blocked by a clot, the result is a stroke. When the stroke occurs, a part of the brain is affected, for it is not receiving sufficient blood and oxygen, causing a weakness, numbness or loss of sensation or movement in some part of the body. The extent to which the above occurs depends upon the area and side of the brain and the size of the vessel that is blocked.

Reduction of the blood supply to the kidneys through a narrowing of the vessels that supply these organs will reduce the efficiency of the kidneys as a waste remover. If the damage is severe enough from the blocked arteries, poisons may pile up in the blood stream and produce uremia.

The second general type of degenerative cardiovascular disease is a rupture or lesion of a blood vessel. It results in a loss of blood to a vital area of the cardiovascular system and is caused by a sudden increase in blood pressure often brought about by excitement or unusual exertion.

The brittleness of the vessels is called *arteriosclerosis*, or "hardening of the arteries." The disease is usually associated with old age because the artery walls become too thick and hard and lose their elasticity. The lack of elasticity is a common cause of high blood pressure. Moreover, the diseases mentioned earlier—heart attack, angina, stroke, loss of kidney efficiency—may all be a result of hardening of the arteries. The most common cause of cerebral vascular disease (stroke or apoplexy) is arteriosclerosis.

Prevention

What can be done to prevent and lessen atherosclerosis or arteriosclerosis is the subject of much controversy. Although physicians cannot agree on the best method, several factors appear to be critical in promoting these diseases.

1. *Heredity*

Various studies indicate that heredity is of prime importance in the development and occurrence of cardiovascular disease in certain people. Since heredity has a definite effect on metabolism, nerve function, and general body chemistry, you may be predisposed to coronary heart disease. Although you have no control over your ancestorship, you can do something about the way you live. For if you have or have had a close relative who has suffered from coronary heart disease, you have a clear warning to

watch your diet, fitness and other health habits. Sound health and fitness practices may later contribute toward warding off cardiovascular problems.

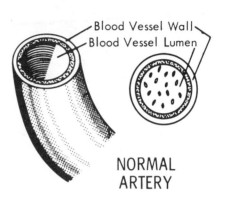

NORMAL ARTERY

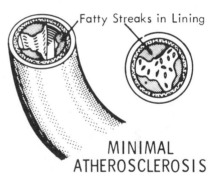

MINIMAL ATHEROSCLEROSIS

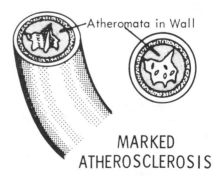

MARKED ATHEROSCLEROSIS

This cross-section of an artery shows progressive stages of atherosclerosis. Properly programmed exercise can prevent and often reverse this condition.

2. Obesity

Obesity is usually the result of too rich a diet and can seriously interfere with circulation, for it places too great a stress on the heart. A person who is more than 20 per cent heavier than his ideal weight is considered obese. Today one-fifth of the population in the United States is in this category.

People who are overweight may have an enlarged heart—an organ that is abnormally large because of excess fat tissue. An athletic heart, on the other hand, is enlarged because of vigorous exercise which makes the heart muscle stronger and more efficient. See ATHLETE'S HEART and LOAFER'S HEART.

Increased fat on the body taxes the heart considerably by making it work harder. The resting pulse rate of an obese person often exceeds a nonobese person's pulse rate by 10 beats per minute or 14,000 beats per day and over 5,000,000 beats per year.

Increased heart and respiratory rates resulting from overweight are undesirable, for the obese person becomes less efficient. During exercise, those rates also increase, but the long-range result is a gradual decrease in both heart and respiratory rates and a general increase in the individual's efficiency. See OBESITY. For more information on the advantages of elevated pulse rates from exercise and the disadvantages of overweight, see HYPOKINETIC DISEASE.

3. Cigarette Smoking.

Excessive cigarette smoking has recently been linked to degenerative cardiovascular disease. Several studies indicate that people who smoke 20 or more cigarettes daily run a greater risk of suffering heart attacks than those who do not smoke. The higher incidence is prevalent regardless of high blood pressure and cholesterol.

When you smoke or inhale, the heart rate and blood pressure rise, the cardiac work increases, and the removal of oxygen from the blood is lowered.

Perhaps the best summary of the value of smoking was presented in an editorial in the 1965 *Medical Tribune* by Dr. Alton Ochsner. He stated:

"In the use of tobacco there is nothing but risk—it is harmful to everyone who uses it—no person has ever benefited by the use of tobacco. It is the only substance for which one pays considerable money to produce disabling illness and premature death without any advantage to be derived from it." See also SMOKING.

4. Stress

Stress has been associated with cardiovascular disease for several years. Dr. Hans Selye has noted that psychological stress of long duration produces a syndrome that can cause excessive hypertension, colitis, gastric ulcers, chronic diarrhea and death if it is not removed or released.

Stress is apparent in many walks of life. It occurs in individuals who put in long hours, are pressured to meet deadlines, are confronted with demanding jobs and domestic obligations, or have a driving type personality. The latter is the individual who is aggressive, conscious of deadlines and never relaxes. He is the person who squeezes twenty-five hours into a twenty-four hour day. He is the person who has intense desire for recognition and a profound sense of obligation. He is unable to relax during his leisure hours because he has a feeling of guilt that he should be doing something.

Stress, whether it is the result of fear, anxiety, frustration, fatigue, or hostility, produces an increase in heart rate, blood pressure and blood cholesterol. Those increases are attributed to the release of adrenalin. Then the central nervous system is affected. If the stress and resulting release of adrenalin continue repeatedly over extended periods, the heart muscle and blood vessels are affected. See STRESS.

5. *Diet*

The relationship between high blood cholesterol and high fat (butter, eggs, meat fats) has finally been established. Yet, the diet of the typical American contains more fat than ever. In fact, it is estimated that the typical American's diet is 40 to 45 per cent animal fat, which means that 40 to 45 per cent of the calories ingested are composed of hard or saturated fats.

The *kind* of fat is as important as *how much* fat is ingested. Many studies have been conducted in recent years which show that individuals who maintain a high fat (saturated) diet have a greater tendency to suffer high cholesterol than those who maintain a low monounsaturated or polyunsaturated fat diet. Researchers have also indicated that ½ to ⅔ of fat diet should be monounsaturated or polyunsaturated.

All medical experts do not agree, however, that saturated fats are the sole culprit in the diet which cause cardiovascular disease. Those who disagree maintain that excessive calorie consumption or sugar intake may also play critical roles in the development of cardiovascular disease. See DIET and NUTRITION.

6. *Age*

An increase in age brings a greater risk of degenerative cardiovascular disease. Statistics reveal that after the age of 45 cardiovascular disease accounts for 45 per cent of all deaths, after the age of 65, 61 per cent. See AGING.

7. *Sex*

The American male is more prone to develop degenerative cardiovascular disease than the American female. First, housewives tend to be more active than their husbands because they must keep a house in order and raise children. Second, women have a tendency to be more weight conscious than men because of their interest in maintaining their figure and wearing the latest fashions. And third, women appear to be protected by the estrogen sex hormones. Those hormones seem to have a regulating effect upon the development of serum cholesterol. Why then don't more women suffer from degenerative cardiovascular disease after menopause? The accumulation of cholesterol in the arteries takes men years. Since women are protected from that build-up during menstruation, they actually reach menopause with an insignificant cholesterol count. Men, on the other hand, get a "head start" on this disease by developing atherosclerosis in their twenties and thirties while most women do not start until their forties or later.

8. *Race*

The white American male has a higher incidence of degenerative cardiovascular disease than the negro American male. Likewise, the negro American female has a lower incidence of this disease than the negro male, but a higher incidence than the white American female. The reasons for the latter occurrence are not clear, although it has been speculated that there is a tendency for the negro female to be a bit heavier than the white female.

9. *Sedentary Life*

Lack of activity appears to be strongly related to degenerative cardiovascular disease. According to recent research, regular participation in suitable exercise and the degree of body fitness appear to have significant importance in preventing and reducing this disease and in aiding recovery. Numerous studies have been conducted to compare sedentary occupations and their relationship to the incidence of heart attack and cardiovascular disease.

A study in England classified 2,500,000 people according to occupations, sedentary or nonsedentary, and compared the percentage of deaths from heart attacks in each. The findings revealed that people engaged in occupations requiring only light physical work had a much higher percentage of deaths from coronary disease than people engaged in heavy physical work.

Another study compared the incidence of that disease among several hundred adult men living in Ireland to its presence among brothers who had migrated to the United States and settled in Boston. The Irish-Americans were less active and heavier than their Irish brothers. It was found that the Irish-Americans had a much higher incidence of coronary disease even though they had the same hereditary background.

Other studies on London employees revealed that (1) Conductors who frequently walk around the double-decker buses and continually climb stairs have a lower mortality rate and higher recovery rate from heart attacks than the bus drivers have. (2) Postmen delivering the mail have a significantly smaller percentage of heart attacks than have postal executives, whose work is very sedentary.

A lack of activity appears to have a decided relationship to degenerative cardiovascular disease, for it contributes to obesity, high blood pressure, and stress. The sensible path to follow is regular participation in vigorous exercise.

Importance of Exercise

Studies have indicated that the collateral circulation of the blood increases with exercise. That is, the number of capillaries and the elasticity of the existing blood vessels increase. If an artery, especially a coronary artery, is blocked by a clot and sufficient blood is not able to get to the rest of the heart via that artery, the other vessels developed by exercise can take over, thereby keeping the damage to a minimum. R. W. Eckstein conducted an experiment on dogs that involved deliberately restricting and narrowing their coronary arteries. The dogs, through surgery, had several of their small arteries supplying the heart tied so that blood flow was re-

stricted, and some tied off completely. The dogs were then split into two groups. One group was exercised 4 times daily while the others were kept inactive for 6 to 8 weeks. At the end of the experiment the exercised dogs had very few scars on their heart muscle. It was concluded from the investigation that physicians should prescribe exercise for both preventative and remedial medicine for poor circulation of the heart muscle See COLLATERAL CIRCULATION.

Experiments have also been conducted that show that the blood of people who perform regular vigorous exercise have a slower blood clotting time than those individuals who are sedentary. The slower clotting time is important in preventing the formation of a thrombosis in critical areas of the body. See BLOOD.

DIET

Cholesterol, Calories and a Prudent Diet

A prudent diet is essential to good health. The development and maintenance of the body depends on the proper chemical constituents which can be used to build tissue and supply energy. Those substances must come from dietary intake that can be used directly or be converted into new substances within the body. Because the body isn't able to chemically prepare all the materials needed, the diet must meet certain requirements.

The indispensable nutrients for body structure are (1) proteins, often combined with other substances, which build tissues; (2) minerals, which build the bony framework and a number of special organs and chemicals in the body, and (3) vitamins, which are essential to the building of catalytic agents called enzymes. Enzymes perform the functions of both construction and energy release.

Fats and carbohydrates serve as fuel and are, therefore, consumed and destroyed in the process of living. They provide the necessary energy for body function. When those substances are not available, the tissue must use its protein to produce energy. That process deteriorates the body structure and weakens its resistance to disease.

Variety Necessary

Your diet should include a variety of foods. Protein can be supplied in quality and quantity by meat, fish, poultry, eggs, soybeans and dairy products. Large amounts of calcium and phosphorus are found in meats, eggs, whole grains and vegetables. Special consideration must be given to iron, which is likely to be lacking in a child's diet. Meat, particularly liver, has considerable iron, with smaller quantities in eggs, leafed vegetables, whole and enriched grains and certain fruits. Most of those foods will furnish one or more vitamins. Since cooking is likely to destroy vitamin C, oranges or tomatoes should be supplied in liberal amounts. Vitamin B is found in whole grains, fruits and vegetables; Vitamin B_2 in meat, eggs and milk; Vitamin A in carrots, some dairy products, sweet potatoes, eggs and green leaves; Vitamin D in fortified milk or a Vitamin D concentrate. Proper elimination is usually assured by a daily diet of two fruits, two vegetables and whole grain products; the liquid requirement for elimination is furnished by milk, water, or fruit juices.

Food requirements change from the growing child, who needs more structural materials, to that of the adult; and the value of large quantities of milk in the diet of the adult is dubious. A great deal of additional work is needed to relate proper diet and good health, particularly in certain diseases. A great deal of individual difference occurs in ability to digest and utilize food, and the time necessary to establish dietary habits makes objective research very difficult.

There is no scientific evidence to support the concept that physical fitness or performance can be improved by modifying a basically sound diet. It is true that a more active individual will have greater dietary demands than a sedentary person. But most of the dietary notions that have been proposed by athletes and trainers are more traditional than factual. It is important to remember that individual differences exist and that what is good for one person may not be good for another. Enzymatic systems vary considerably and affect the digestion and absorption as well as utilization of substances within the total organism.

Basic Diet for the Physically Fit

A physically fit person should follow a few basic guidelines: (1) Use fruit and fruit juices for dessert. They furnish calories while contributing their share of vitamins and minerals. (2) Don't allow coffee, tea and alcohol to take the place of more nutritious foods; they don't add to the diet and may cause undesirable effects such as decreased muscular efficiency. (3) Avoid fatty foods. They slow peristalsis and hinder gastric action and they are not as efficient as carbohydrates in producing energy. (4) Make every effort to eat two servings of fresh fruits and four servings of vegetables daily. The fruit should include citrus or tomato and the vegetables should include leafy greens, roots and tubers. (5) Spread the dietary intake over the entire day. Three meals are recommended, with more if weight gain is desired. (6) Drink at least three glasses of water daily to maintain body function. (7) In case of extreme temperature or heavy work, additional water is needed, along with salts to replace those lost in perspiration.

As a rule, the physically fit individual needs more calories per day than his sedentary counterpart. For that reason, it is necessary to include a higher caloric intake in the diet. If the supply is not adequate, the body will utilize structural tissues and impair the functions of the organs from which the tissues came. Furthermore, physical efficiency is lower when body tissues are used as fuels. The total daily energy requirement for an active man ranges from 3,000 to 8,000 calories depending on his size and physical condition, as well as the severity of the work performed. The sedentary individual uses considerably less, meaning that he must eat less or increase his body weight. Both inactivity and an excess caloric intake tend to produce obesity. A greater caloric expenditure does not necessarily elicit a greater desire for food, and for that reason the active individual generally has less adipose tissue. If you wish to reduce the percentage of body fat, eat less and/or exercise more.

The body can be likened to a balance sheet. If the caloric expenditures are greater than the intake, the body loses weight. If the caloric expenditures are less than the intake, it gains weight. A balanced intake and output is, of course, most desirable. Our current population has had problems obtaining it. That has initiated a greater concern and a greater need for a proper diet and activity. The caloric expenditure at rest is approximately 1.25 calories per minute, 75 calories per hour, or 1,800 calories per day. Comparing this with 10 calories or more per minute during heavy work, or at least 600 calories per hour, you can easily see the effect of exercise on total body weight. The daily output at that level would be staggering, and you would not be able to work at that level for that length of time. Some of our more rigorous workouts while training for athletic competition do put that kind of demand on the caloric expenditure and should be compensated for in the dietary intake.

Cholesterol and Health

Generally, we consider diet as a means of providing the proper materials for optimal physical development and function. The reverse is also true

in some cases. For example, atherosclerosis is accompanied by a rise in blood levels of cholesterol. The actual cause of this abnormal plasma level has been a point of discussion for some time. An evaluation of current research indicates that it is a function of dietary intake. For that reason, cholesterol-free diets have been used to reduce plasma levels and as a precautionary measure for those who have vascular problems.

Cholesterol is a large molecule in the family of lipids or fats. This compound is usually found in the presence of other large molecular substances consisting also of protein material, called lipoproteins. The high levels of cholesterol and lipoproteins may represent altered fat metabolism. They bear a direct relationship to the development of atherosclerosis. The effects of atherosclerosis become apparent in middle age, as evidenced by the number of coronary heart attacks and deaths. Usually men are affected more frequently than women until the latter are past childbearing age. That implies that the female sex hormones are a protective factor. Heredity also seems to play a role, some families having a greater incidence of the disease than others.

Obesity and sedentary living undoubtedly also have a share in the development of atherosclerosis. Life insurance statistics show a far greater incidence of death resulting from that condition. It is possible that the decreased physical activity affects not only the development of overweight but also may directly influence blood flow and the depositing of fatty plaques in the blood vessels. Obesity and sedentary living also have been associated with higher cholesterol and lipoproteins in the plasma. It is rather evident that a combination of those factors has increased the incidence of coronary disease.

Animal fats, such as butter, meat fats, egg fat and some hydrogenated vegetable fats, all of which contain a large proportion of saturated fatty acids, increase the blood levels of cholesterol and lipoproteins. On the other hand, vegetable oils such as corn, cottonseed, sunflower and soybean oils, which contain a higher percentage of polyunsaturated fatty acids, particularly linoleic acid, tend to lower the levels of cholesterol and lipoprotein in the blood when taken in fairly large amounts.

The finding of increased cholesterol levels in the blood of patients with atherosclerosis inaugurated a period of low cholesterol diets, in the hope that such restriction would lower blood cholesterol levels. When researchers realized that cholesterol is synthesized by the liver as needed, that form of dietary control was largely abandoned. However, recent work seems to indicate the dietary intakes of cholesterol may indeed affect blood cholesterol levels and that the cholesterol content of the diet should be kept below 300 to 400 mg. per day. See NUTRITION and WEIGHT CONTROL.—*Wayne H. Osness*

DIGESTIVE SYSTEM

Food in its natural state cannot be used by the body. It must undergo certain physical and chemical changes before it can take part in the metabolic processes of life. It is the function of the digestive system to change food into a usable form, a process referred to as digestion.

Effects of Exercise

A. J. Carlson studied the effects of varying intensities of exercise on hunger contractions of the stomachs of dogs and men. He found that moderate exercise stimulated muscle tone and hunger contractions, or left them unchanged, while exhausting exercise led to inhibition of gastric muscle activity. Many are aware of the discomfort that follows intense physical exertion shortly after a large meal. One

cause suggested for that is a lack of blood in the smooth muscles of the stomach as a result of the blood being detoured away from the stomach muscles to the voluntary skeletal muscles engaged in the activity. Intense exercise closely following a meal results in a delay in gastric emptying time.

The secretory phase of the stomach function includes the secretion of previously mentioned substances (enzymes, hydrochloric acid, mucous). Control of these secretions is via the vagus nerve, which is stimulated by taste, smell and anticipation of eating. An increased amount of digestive juice is present in the stomach just before, during and after a meal.

The results of studies done on the effects of exercise on gastric secretion indicate that moderate exercise before or after a meal either has no effect or causes a slight increase in secretory action. Exhausting work was almost always found to depress secretion. A full stomach seems to crowd the heart and lungs and possibly hampers breathing. The stomach, being just below the diaphragm, resists the diaphragm's downward movement during inspiration. Some individuals experience difficulty when trying to take a deep breath following a large meal.

Other studies involving other organs of the digestive system have proved inconclusive. Attempts have been made to show that exercise increases the propulsion of food through the small intestine.

J. Barcroft and H. Florey studied the effect of exercise on the large intestine of dogs and concluded that running *per se* had no effect on colon function. In another study done on dogs, six minutes of treadmill running caused a temporary increase in muscular activity in the large intestine in most cases. That increase was usually followed by a prolonged period of decreased muscular activity. Those findings, however, are not conclusive.

Strenuous exercise does affect gastric emptying time and, therefore, may temporarily slow the overall digestive process. As far as the other organs of the system are concerned, no definite statement can be made as to the effect of exercise on their function. The idea that daily exercise aids regularity seems to have no scientific basis.

Available evidence indicates that the absorptive phase of digestion, despite a slowing of gastric emptying, goes on at close to a normal rate during exercise.

Why Exercise Affects Digestive Function

Any effect exercise may have on digestive function is the result of a combination of several factors. Some of these include (1) reduced blood flow to digestive organs during exercise, (2) rise in body temperature, (3) changes in the composition of the blood, (4) nervous reflex changes.

The psychological aspect of exercise compounds the problem of studying the physiological effects of exercise on digestive function. Emotions play an important role in triggering digestive activity. Aggressiveness has been found to stimulate the stomach as though it were going to receive food. Digestive juices are secreted, and blood flow to the stomach wall increases. Emotions such as fear and depression have been found to cause the

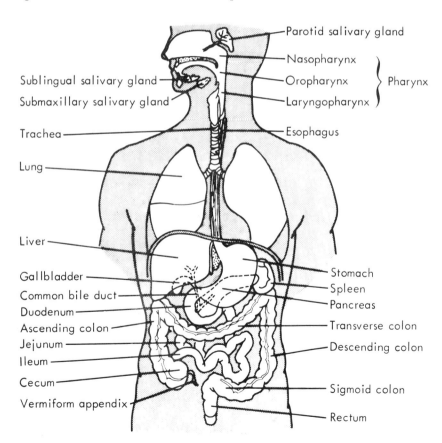

A cross-section of the digestive system.

opposite reaction. Emotions and the physical exertions they lead to are difficult to separate with respect to the digestive changes they may cause. An important consideration is what causes the changes, the emotions or the exertion? Also, the same emotion may not excite the same physical response from two different people. In a natural competitive situation emotions play an important part in preparing the body physically, while the laboratory situation may be almost devoid of emotion. Before a competitive effort the psychological phenomenon known popularly as "butterflies" helps to initiate physiological adjustments (changes in body chemistry) in anticipation of a physically or mentally stressful situation.

A common affliction among middle-aged businessmen is ulcers, a digestive disorder resulting from excess stomach acid which, when no food is present in the stomach, will actually begin to digest the stomach wall. Emotions are a highly suspect cause of this malady. An attempt has been made to show that regular exercise may offset the unfavorable changes that occur as a result of certain emotions. Many persons with ulcers are those who keep their emotions "bottled up" inside. Exercise is a healthy outlet for certain emotions.

The study of the effects of exercise on digestive function is a complex problem since the many variables are difficult to control. Much is known about the effects of exercise on digestive function, and a good deal more is yet to be learned.

DRUGS

Since the 1890's, more than 1,000 studies have been made on how drugs affect performance. Most of them have dealt with clinical populations in the treatment of physical and mental illnesses. Several nonclinical studies, on the other hand, have attempted to determine the actions of the popular drugs—amphetamine, caffeine, lysergic

acid diethylamide (LSD), glutamic acid, benadryl, hyoscine—on both men and lower form animals. Unfortunately, the results have often been inconclusive because of limited numbers of subjects, crude statistical design, single dose levels, failure to establish baseline performance levels, and various other experimental faults.

The effects of these drugs on performance of athletes and the average population have been mainly ignored. Many reports indicate that amphetamines and caffeine can *change* performance. However, there is variation in conclusion about whether they improve or hinder performance or are neutral in their effect. The most heavily documented subjective effect of amphetamine is the relief of the feelings of fatigue developed by prolonged work. Certain types of psychomotor, physical, and mental performance have been improved after or during bouts of activity by the use of that drug. Other studies report no effects on performance, and some report deleterious effects when drugs are used in an effort to restore performance to baseline levels.

The basic question of whether the central nervous system stimulants improve or retard physical or mental performance has not been conclusively answered.—*Bill W. Lovingood*

LSD has been reported to cause some very damaging effects: chromosome changes, elevated blood pressure, bizarre feelings, impulsive behavior, personality changes, suicidal attempts and flight. As a result the drug is usually taken under supervision. However, even that is risky. For accidents have occurred under the restrictive measures, personality change cannot be controlled, and some reactions to the drug are delayed for days, weeks, or months. Hence a person may experience an LSD reaction a considerable time after taking the drug.

Although we do not know whether drugs enhance or inhibit performance, we do know that drugs and physical fitness are not compatible, for fitness requires a constructive effort, and drugs can only destroy.

Types of Drugs

Drugs cover a large spectrum, ranging from simple kitchen spices to highly sophisticated addictive killers. The 5 basic categories of drugs are (1) narcotics, (2) sedatives, (3) tranquilizers, (4) stimulants, (5) hallucinogens.

Narcotics are drugs which produce insensibility because of their depressant effect on the central nervous system. Included are opium, opium derivatives (morphine, codine, and heroin) and synthetic opiates (meperidine and methadone). Sedatives such as barbiturates have a depressant effect on the nervous system, while tranquilizers are used to counteract tension and anxiety without producing sleep or impairing normal physical or mental function. Two such tranquilizers are meprobamate and chlordiazepoxide. Stimulants directly activate the central nervous system, the best known being caffeine. Other popular stimulants include amphetamine and cocaine. Hallucinogens, last of the five big drug categories, cause distortions of perception, dream images and hallucinations. They include mescaline, LSD and chemically distinct marihuana.

Dangers in Drug Abuse

Although many of those drugs have medical application they are currently being used indiscreetly by many people in our society. The result is drug abuse.

Abuse of drugs may lead to serious physiological and psychological consequences. Abuse of morphine (narcotics), for example, can result in physical or psychological dependence. Other highly undesirable effects are elevated blood pressure, increased breathing rate and elevated body temperature.

Overuse of depressants, such as barbiturates, can also result in psychological and physiological dependence, which may lead to death. Withdrawal from the drug is very painful.

Abuse of tranquilizers may or may not result in physiological and/or psychological dependence. If one is addicted, withdrawal is painful. The abuse of tranquilizers is not as prevalent as that of other drugs.

Stimulants, such as amphetamine, do appear to produce physical dependence. When the drug is withdrawn, however, mental depression and fatigue set in. Abuse of the drug can cause a blackout from exhaustion and schizophrenic symptoms. Some users have become highly susceptible to pneumonia and malnutrition as a result of going for long periods without food. Other possible effects are high blood pressure, abnormal heart condition, heart attacks and brain damage.

Hallucinogens, such as marihuana and LSD, are not habit forming. To date, there is little evidence that overuse of marihuana has any physical effect, but its psychological effect cannot be discounted. People on this hallucinogen experience a feeling of euphoria and exhaltation. They experience a free flow of ideas. Senses of time, distance, vision and hearing are distorted. Once a user has established the amount of marihuana he needs to get himself "high," he will notice that he needs more marihuana or something stronger to achieve the desired feeling. As a result, marihuana is considered to be a stepping stone to more powerful and more dangerous drugs.

DUAL-RESISTANCE EXERCISES

Dual-resistance exercises are those in which a person strains against resistance supplied by another. The partner acts as a weight to be lifted, moved, or resisted as the other partner pushes or pulls. If body movement is involved, the exercises are isotonic. If no movement occurs, they are isometric.

There are various advantages of dual-resistance exercises. They require no equipment and little space, develop muscle strength and endurance, improve specific muscle areas of the body, provide interesting competition and encourage many participants.

Conversely, there are some disadvantages in that type of exercising. There is no objective method to determine the amount of resistance experienced in each effort. Therefore, it is difficult to determine progression. Those exercises develop only two of the many components of physical fitness (muscle endurance and strength). They cannot be performed without a partner. Although the following dual-resistance exercises may be performed isometrically, performing them isotonically may be more beneficial since there is no possibility of losing flexibility because of restricted movement. The ready position for each isotonic and isometric exercise is the same. The only difference is in the action. Unless you want to develop some specific area, select exercises that involve all parts of the body. Keep in mind that your partner should have about the same amount of strength. Take turns doing the exercise.

Difference between Isotonic and Isometric Exercise

In the isotonic action of the exercise the resister should resist for 8 to 10 seconds (8 to 10 counts) before the performer completes the required movement. Perform 3 to 4 repetitions.

In the isometric action of the exercise the resister should push against the performer's hand, arm, leg, etc., so that the performer cannot move. Hold for 6 seconds, relax for 1 to 2 seconds, and hold for the final 6 seconds.

A possible variation in the isometric exercise is to place the part of the performer's body in the various positions it would have been in if actual movement occurred. Then you are able to exercise the muscle groups in various positions, thereby reducing the likelihood of flexibility loss.

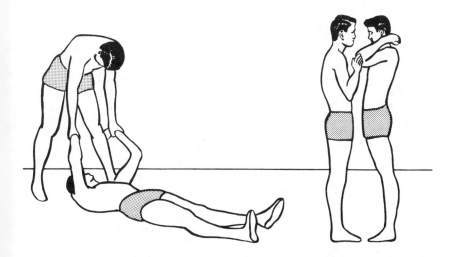

Two dual resistance exercises. The supine press (left) and the elbow push down.

Shoulder Exercises

The muscles affected are the deltoids, pectoralis majors, latissimus dorsi, teres majors, rhomboids.

1. *Elbow Push-Down*—Ready position: Face your partner. Bend your elbows, and place your hands on his shoulders with your elbows pointing toward him. Your partner places the palms of his hands under your elbows.

Isotonic Action: Force your elbows downward toward the sides of your body. When the elbows are next to the body, your partner should force your elbows back to the original position.

Isometric Action: Attempt to force your elbows downward toward the sides of your body, while your partner resists and does not permit movement.

2. *Supine Press*—Ready Position: Assume a reclining position on the floor or mat with your arms flexed and elbows against your sides. Hold your hands, palms up, near your shoulders. Your partner should stand behind you and lean forward, grasping your hands.

Isotonic Action: Slowly force your hands upward until your arms are completely extended. Be sure to keep your hands directly above your shoulders. Once arms are completely extended, your partner should force your hands back to the starting position.

Isometric Action: Attempt to force your hands upward, while your partner actively resists so that no movement takes place.

3. *Supine Pull Over*—Assume a reclining position with your arms extended over your head. Your partner assumes a kneeling position behind your head and then grasps your hands.

Isotonic Action: Move your arms upward to a vertical position. Keep the elbows locked throughout the movement.

Isometric Action: Attempt to move your arms upward to a vertical position, while your partner prohibits any movement. This exercise is a perfect example of how you can place the arms in various positions so that the muscle groups are exercised in their full range of motion.

4. *Arms Across Chest*—Assume a supine position with your arms at right angles to your body, and your palms facing upward. Your partner kneels with his legs straddling your head and places his hands (palms downward) on your wrists.

Isotonic Action: Raise your arms to a vertical position over your chest as your partner resists. Then your partner forces your arms back down to the original position.

Isometric Action: Attempt to force your arms upward, while your partner restricts movement.

5. *Reclining Backward Push*—Lie on the floor face down, legs extended, with your arms extended along side your body (palms up). Your partner should straddle your legs and place his hands on your wrist.

Isotonic Action: Squeeze your shoulder blades together and push your arms upward as far as possible. Keep the elbows locked throughout the movement.

Isometric Action: Attempt to push your arms upward, while your partner prohibits movement. Keep your chin on the floor and the shoulders pinched together.

Arm Exercises

The exercises involve muscles of the upper arm (flexors of the forearm): biceps brachii, brachialis, brachioradialis, and pronator teres.

6. *Front Curl*—Face your partner. Stand with your arms against your sides with the palms facing forward and upward. Your partner places his fist in your open palms or against your wrists.

Isotonic Action: Forcibly raise your forearm to your shoulders, being certain that your upper arms are against the sides of your body as the movement is made. As soon as your partner's hands touch your shoulders, he should force your hands back down to the starting position.

Isometric Action: Place your forearm at waist height—upper arm and lower arm form right angle. Attempt to raise your forearms while your partner actively resists and permits no movement.

7. *Reverse Curl*—In this variation of the front curl, take the same position as for the front curl except face your palms toward the floor as your partner grasps the backs of your hands or wrists.

Isotonic Action: Same as for the front curl.

Isometric Action: Same as for the front curl.

8. *Rowing*—Face your partner. Bend at the waist so that your upper body is parallel to the floor and your arms hang down in front of your body. Your partner grasps each of your wrists.

Isotonic Action: Slowly pull your hands toward your chest against sufficient resistance. When your hands touch your chest, your partner should slowly pull them back to the original position.

Isometric Action: Attempt to pull your arms upward, while your partner does not permit movement.

Muscles of the Upper Arm

9. *Resistance Push-up*—Assume a push-up position with elbows bent at a 90-degree angle. Your partner straddles your hips and places his hands on your shoulder blades.

Isotonic Action: Execute a push-up until your arms are extended while your partner slows your movement. When your arms are extended, your partner pushes you back to the starting position.

Isometric Action: Attempt to straighten your arms as you would in a push-up while your partner resists.

10. *Elbow Extension*—Stand in front of your partner facing the same direction. Raise your arms directly over your head with the elbows bent slightly behind the head. Bend the knees for balance. Your partner grasps your wrists.

Isotonic Action: Extend your arms upward over your head, while your partner slows the movement. Once your arms are completely extended, your partner pulls them back down again.

Isometric Action: Attempt to raise your hands above your head, while your partner actively restricts movement.

Back Exercises

These muscles of the upper back are developed: trapezius, latissimus dorsi, rhomboids, and teres major.

11. *Prone Back Lift*—Assume a prone position on the floor with your arms extended at your sides at a 90-degree angle, thumb pointed toward the ceiling. Your partner should straddle your lower back or hips and place his hands on your wrists.

Isotonic Action: Raise your arms as high as possible, as your partner resists and slows the movement. When your arms reach the maximum height, your partner pushes the arms back down.

Isometric Action: Raise the arms as high as possible. Your partner attempts to push your arms down, allowing no movement.

12. *Shoulder Flexion*—Assume a prone position on the floor, with your arms overhead to an angle of 45 degrees. Keep your elbows straight and place the back of your partner's hands towards the ceiling. He kneels in front of you and places his hands on your wrists.

Isotonic Action: Push your arms upward as far as possible keeping your forehead on the ground. Your partner slows the movement. When your arms reach their maximum height, he gradually pushes the hands back down again.

Isometric Action: Raise your arms as high as possible. Your partner should attempt to push them down.

13. *Lateral Arm Depressor*—Sit on the floor with your arms extended above your head and your palms touching. Your partner stands or kneels behind you and grasps your wrists.

Isotonic Action: Keep your arms straight and slowly force downward, laterally. When your arms touch your sides, your partner slowly forces them back to the starting position.

Isometric Action: Keep your arms straight and attempt to force them downward, while your partner does not permit any movement. The arms may then be placed at shoulder level.

Muscles of the Lower Back

14. *Prone Arch*—Assume a prone position, with your fingers interlocked behind your head. Your partner straddles your calves and places one hand between your shoulder blades. He may aid the exercise by holding down the lower part of your legs.

Isotonic Action: Slowly raise your chest off the floor as far as possible as your partner resists. When you get as high as possible, your partner should push you slowly back down to the floor.

Isometric Action: At the beginning of the exercise lift your chest off the floor, while you maintain that position.

15. *Straight Leg Raise*—Assume a prone position with your arms at the side of your body, palms up. Your partner kneels beside your heels.

Isotonic Action: Keeping your entire leg straight, slowly raise your *entire* leg upward. When you reach maximum height, your partner pushes the leg down to the ground.

Isometric Action: In the ready position, lift your leg off the ground as high as possible, keeping the knee straight and both hips on the ground. Your partner attempts to push your straight leg to the ground, while you

resist. A variation of this exercise is to have the knee cap barely off the ground.

16. *Body Arch*—Assume a prone position, arms next to your body. Your partner kneels beside you and places his one hand slightly below your shoulder blades and the other hand on the calf muscles of the legs.

Isotonic Action: Slowly raise your chest and legs off the floor (simultaneously). When you achieve maximum height, your partner slowly pushes you to the original prone position.

Isometric Action: Assume an arch position (chest and thighs off the floor). Your partner attempts to push you back to the floor, while you resist.

Abdominal Muscles

The muscles affected are the iliopsoas, rectus abdominus, internal and external obliques, and transversus abdominus.

17. *Bent Leg Sit-Up*—In a supine position bend the knees so that your heels are drawn up near your buttocks. Lock your fingers behind your head. Your partner kneels next to you with one hand on your chest and the other hand on your knees.

Isotonic Action: Slowly curl your upper body until the trunk comes to an erect position. Then your partner slowly forces you into the starting position.

Isometric Action: Assume an upright position. Resist as your partner attempts to push you down to a supine position. A variation is to attempt a sit-up as your partner resists. Or you can assume a 45-degree angle as your partner attempts to push you down.

18. *V-Sit-Up*—Ready Position: Raise both legs and upper body simultaneously, keeping the legs straight and arms out straight for balance. Your partner kneels beside you and places his one hand on your chest and his other hand on your shin or calf.

Isotonic Action: Your partner slowly pushes your back and legs to the floor.

Then you slowly raise both legs and back off the floor to the starting position.

Isometric Action: Your partner attempts to push your back and legs to the floor while you resist.

19. *Lateral Sit-Up*—Assume a right-side lying position, with right arm across the chest. The left arm is raised to the side for balance. The resister sits straddling your thighs. His left hand is placed on your right hand, and he grasps the extended left hand with his right.

Isotonic Action: Raise your upper body off the floor laterally as high as possible. When this point is reached, the resister slowly pushes you down to the ground, after which you return to the side upright position. After the three or four sets are completed, you should be on the left side.

Isometric Action: Raise your upper body off the floor laterally or as high as possible. The resister attempts to push you down. The exercise must be performed on both sides.

20. *Straight Leg Sit-Up*—Assume a supine position with legs straight, fingers behind your head and elbows pointed forward. The resister straddles your knees and places his hands on your elbows.

Isotonic Action: Perform a sit-up as your partner offers slight resistance. When you reach an upright position, he pushes you back to a supine position.

Isometric Action: Assume a half sit-up position. The resister attempts to push you to a supine position.

Hip and Leg Exercises

The muscles of hips and thighs, abductors and adductors (Adductors longus, brevis, magnus, gluteus medius, and minimus) are affected.

21. *Side Leg Raising*—Assume a right-side lying position, and bend the right leg slightly for stability. Place the left hand across the chest. Your partner kneels behind you and places his one hand on your shoulder and the other on your ankle.

Isotonic Action: Raise your top leg as high as possible, without bending the knee. Your partner slows the movement. When your leg is raised as high as possible, he pushes the leg back to the starting position. Perform the exercise on both sides.

Isometric Action: Raise your leg to little less than a 45-degree angle, and rotate it inward slightly. Your partner attempts to push the leg downward while you resist.

22. *Legs Apart*—Assume a supine position on the floor with your legs extended and apart 12 inches at the knees. Your partner kneels between your legs and places his hands *inside of the knees.*

Isometric Action: Attempt to bring your legs together as he resists this movement.

23. *Hip Adduction* (Hips and Knees Bent)—Assume a supine position with your knees bent and feet flat on the floor. Put your arms beside your body. Your partner kneels next to your hips and places one hand on one of your knees.

Isotonic Action: Slowly pull the two knees apart while he resists. Once the knees are pulled apart, slowly close them as he resists.

Isometric Action: Open your knees slightly in the ready position. Your partner attempts to push open the legs while you resist.

Muscles of the Hips and Thighs
(Flexors of the thigh)

These muscles are the iliopsoas and rectus femoris: (extensors of the lower leg and quadriceps).

24. *One-half Squat*—Stand with your partner mounted on your back. He wraps his legs around your waist and drapes his arms over your shoulders, clasping his hands.

Isotonic Action: Slowly execute a knee bend to a ½ squat position. Then return to an erect position.

Isometric Action: Hold a ½ squat position for six counts with your partner on your back.

25. *Hip Flexion* (Straight Leg Raising)—Assume a supine position with your knees straight and your arms at your side. Your partner kneels beside your hip and places his one hand on your ankle.

Isotonic Action: Slowly raise your leg until it is perpendicular to the floor, as your partner slows that movement. When the leg is perpendicular to the floor, he pushes the leg back down to the floor as you resist.

Isometric Action: Place your leg at a 45-degree angle. At that point your partner attempts to push the leg down, as you resist.

26. *Knee Bent Flexion*—Sit on a table with a towel rolled under your knees for comfort. Place your hands on the outside of the knees for stability. Your partner stands in front of your legs and clasps his hands on top of one of your knees.

Isotonic Action: Slowly raise the resisted knee toward the ceiling, being certain that the knee is kept bent. Once the knee reaches its maximum height, your partner slowly pushes the leg back to the table. Exercise both legs.

Isometric Action: Attempt to raise the knee while your partner resists that movement. A variation is to start the knee at the point of maximum height.

Muscles of the Hips and Thighs
(Extensors of the thigh)

The gluteus maximus and biceps femoris, hamstring muscles are developed.

27. *Thigh Extension*—Assume a prone position with your arms at your sides, palms up. Your partner kneels beside you and places one hand on your heel.

Isotonic Action: Slowly raise the resisted leg as high as possible. At that point your partner slowly pushes the leg back to the ground.

Isometric Action: Place your leg at maximum height at the beginning of the exercise. Your partner attempts to push the leg to the ground.

28. *Leg Curl*—Lie in a prone position with your legs together. Your partner kneels beside your thighs, placing his one hand on your ankle and the other on your back thigh.

Isotonic Action: Slowly curl your lower leg upward while your thigh is held down. When the lower leg is curled as far as possible, your partner slowly pushes your leg back to the starting position. Exercise both legs.

Isometric Action: Partially curl your leg. First your partner attempts to push the leg to the upper thigh as you resist. Then, with your leg at a half-curl position, he attempts to push the leg back to the prone position.

Muscles of the Lower Leg
(Extensors of the foot)

These muscles are the gastrocnemius and soleus.

29. *Heel Raise*—Assume a standing position with your partner mounted on your back. Then stand on one foot (the toe of the other foot may be slightly touching the floor for stability).

Isotonic Action: Slowly raise your heel from the floor by standing on your toes. Then stand on the other foot.

Isometric Action: Start out by standing on the toes of one foot, while your partner is mounted on your back. Repeat the process for the other leg.

30. *Wrist Flexion*—The two partners sit on chairs facing each other. Drape your hands over your knees, palms facing upward. Your partner places his palms in yours.

Isotonic Action: Your partner slowly pushes your hands as far down as possible. Then you slowly raise your hands upward as far as possible, and repeat.

Isometric Action: Your partner attempts to push your hands downward while you resist.

31. *Wrist Extension*—The two partners sit on chairs facing each other.

Drape your hands over your knees with the back of your hands facing upward. Your partner places his palms on the back of your hands.

Isotonic Action: Your partner slowly pushes your hands as far down as possible. At that point, slowly raise your hands upward as far as possible, and repeat.

Isometric Action: Your partner attempts to push your hands downward.

32. *Neck Exercises*—If you want to develop the neck flexors, your partner places his hand on your forehead. If you want to develop the neck extensor muscles, he places his hand on the back of your head. For lateral muscle development he places his hand on the side of the head.

Isotonic Action: Slowly press your head toward the resistance.

Isometric Action: Press your head into your partner's while he resists, allowing no movement.

EFFECTS OF EXERCISE

What usually happens when you exercise vigorously? Some of the more noticeable changes are deep breathing, profuse sweating, a throbbing sensation in your head and, of course, a heavy pounding in your chest. Other changes such as increased rate of metabolism and increased size of the capillaries are not so obvious. All these adjustments are called *immediate* or *acute effects* of exercise. These temporary changes occur whether you have been continually exercising for a period of weeks or months, or have just undertaken an exercise program. After the exercise ceases, those immediate changes reverse and in a period of minutes or hours, return to their normal resting state.

If you continue to exercise vigorously day by day and week by week, other changes take place very gradually. Those changes occur as a result of the body adapting to the exercise. They are called the *chronic effects of exercise* and occur when you engage

in regular vigorous exercise over a period of approximately 6 weeks or more. The long-term exercise is called training.

Although exercise affects almost the entire body, some areas benefit more than others. Below is a summary of the immediate and chronic effects of exercise on the major systems of the body.

The Cardiovascular System

The cardiovascular system consists of the heart, arteries, veins, arterioles, and capillaries. It is the function of the system to supply circulating blood to the various systems of the body. The blood in turn furnishes the tissues with oxygen and food materials necessary for energy and removes the waste products that have accumulated. The heart is the pump that provides the force to circulate the blood.

When you exercise vigorously, your heart rate increases. The increase begins immediately after the start of exercise or even before the beginning of exercise in anticipation. Along with that increase there is an increased contracting force of the heart which results in a greater amount of blood being expelled from the heart with each contraction (stroke volume). The increased stroke volume and heart rate result in an increase of blood flow to the muscles, and consequently more blood is pumped by the heart per minute.

The capillaries in the muscles increase in size (dilate) during exercise, which allows an increased amount of blood to flow through them. Because of the dilation, the muscles are supplied with the necessary oxygen and food for increased energy requirements. The waste products are also removed more efficiently because of the dilation, thereby allowing the muscles to work relatively long periods of time without becoming fatigued. There is also an increase in the number of circulating red blood cells.

Vigorous exercise also increases the peripheral heart action causing the muscle cells that surround the capillaries to contract and force the blood out of those capillaries and into the veins. When those cells relax, the fresh blood is then pushed into the cells as a result of the vacuum created by the blood pushed into the veins. The action, therefore, increases the flow of the blood back to the heart, thereby sending more blood to the muscles.

Blood pressure is also affected during vigorous exercise. The systolic pressure is increased so that more blood may be forced into the capillary beds (a maze of capillaries). The diastolic blood pressure is affected in one of two ways. If you have a poor level of fitness, your diastolic blood pressure will be increased—there will be an increase in the resistance to the blood flow. If you have a good or high fitness level, your diastolic blood pressure will drop—there is a decrease in the resistance of blood flow.

Vigorous exercise also increases the flow of blood to the circulatory system of the heart. The heart, since it is a muscle, must also have arteries, capillaries and veins. Vigorous activity, naturally, increases the rate of circulation for this muscle as it would for any other muscle.

During training or long-term exercising, there is a slow but consistent reduction in the resting heart rate but an increase in its stroke volume. Since more blood is pumped during each stroke, the heart does not have to beat as rapidly as before to supply the body with blood. The lowered heart rate and the increased stroke volume allow a greater rest for the heart between beats.

When a trained person exercises, it appears as though the pulse rate increases almost the same number of beats, perhaps slightly less, than for the untrained person. The former, however, has a lower pulse rate during exercise because of a lower resting rate. As a result of the lower resting and exercise rate, the trained individual's heart has a greater opportunity to

rest. Training also reduces the length of time required to return the heart rate and blood pressure to resting level, thus enabling a quicker recovery from physical stress.

Vigorous, regular exercise will increase the number of functioning capillaries of the heart. They will provide the heart with a more nourishing supply of blood, thereby making it a more efficient organ.

There will also be an increase in the number of functioning capillaries in the muscles. The result in the skeletal muscles is similar to what occurs in the heart muscle. Blood, rich in oxygen and food materials, will reach more parts of the muscles, thus increasing muscle endurance and efficiency.

Long-range exercise will produce four other important changes. (1) The elasticity of the artery wall will be increased, enabling a person to recover more quickly from sudden stress. (2) The red cell count will rise, increasing the internal supply of oxygen. (3) The clotting time of the blood will be increased, therefore decreasing the formation of blood clots. (4) There will be a decrease in fatty lipids in the blood. The decrease will lower the possibility of fat deposits accumulating on the walls of the blood vessels (atherosclerosis). See CIRCULATORY SYSTEM.

The Digestive System

The digestive system consists of the mouth (mastication and salivary glands), esophagus, stomach, and small and large intestines. Directly related to the system are the liver, gall bladder, pancreas and spleen. Those organs and tissues work together to mechanically and chemically break down food so that it may be absorbed by the blood.

Exercise can affect the digestive system. For example, the blood that should be supplying the digestive tract with the necessary nutrients is being diverted from that area to the muscles being exercised.

The intensity of the exercise, however, determines to what extent the digestive system is affected. In light exercise, such as leisurely walking, there are practically no effects. In moderate exercise, such as fast walking or jogging, digestion may be retarded, and the stomach may not be emptied as quickly as it normally would. Vigorous exercise such as endurance running or sprinting, may stop digestion altogether until the exercise is completed.

After mild, moderate, or vigorous exercise there may be an increase in appetite. But after exhausting exercise there may be a decrease in the appetite. Scientists are still searching for an answer to that phenomenon. See APPETITE.

The effect of training on the digestive system has not been scientifically established. It can safely be stated, however, that a higher level of physical fitness, with good muscle tone and better circulation, will result in a more active digestive system. See DIGESTIVE SYSTEM.

The Endocrine System

The endocrine system is one of the major regulatory systems of the body, accomplishing its regulation through the secretion of hormones. A hormone is a chemical substance that has been formed in one part of the body and is carried in the blood stream to another organ or tissue and excites it to activity, thereby affecting the metabolic processes of the tissue.

Generally speaking, the endocrine system has a role in the maintenance of physical activity, for an increase in exercise results in an increase in the secretion of adrenalin. That secretion enables functioning at a higher metabolic rate.

Exercise conducted over a long period, 6 weeks or more, helps to normalize the basal metabolic rate. Basal metabolic rate refers to the minimum energy needed to maintain the normal processes of the body at rest. Training, therefore, may reduce ten-sion in people who have a high basal metabolic rate and also reduce the lethargy in people who have a low basal metabolic rate. See ENDOCRINE SYSTEM.

The Excretory System

Technically, the excretory system is composed of the kidneys, skin, respiratory system, and digestive tract and is concerned with the removal of waste products. The kidneys filter the blood and excrete water, excess materials, and waste products (urea and uric acid). The skin eliminates water and, to a small degree, carbon dioxide. Most of the carbon dioxide, however, is removed by means of the lungs. The digestive tract removes the waste products of digestion (feces).

During exercise, blood flow to the kidney is reduced, allowing less blood to be filtered. Therefore, less urine is produced, and the reduced excretion aids in the prevention of dehydration.

Vigorous exercise also produces profuse sweating through the skin, which may be misinterpreted to mean that the skin is removing much of the waste material. Although some waste may be removed, the main reason for the increased sweating is that it cools the body surface and keeps the body temperature down.

Although vigorous exercise may slow down the digestive process, the increased activity may necessitate a bowel movement, especially if the intestines have not been voided for some time. The activity of the abdominal muscles may aid in pushing the waste material along the intestines.

Training appears to have little effect on the excretory system, except that finely conditioned, strong abdominal muscles may aid in evacuation. See EXCRETORY SYSTEM.

Muscular System

The muscular system has several responsibilities: (1) The muscles produce movement of the body or any of its parts. (2) The muscles are responsible for producing a great deal of the body heat. (3) The muscles hold the body in the upright position. (4) The muscles give contour and shape to the body.

During vigorous physical exertion or exercise there is a temporary increase in the muscle size. The increase in size is a result of the energy materials being sent to the muscles and the removal of waste products. The muscle has, in effect, become a dynamic factory.

Exercise will increase the amount of heat produced. As a result the temperature of the muscles is raised as high as 8 to 10 degrees Fahrenheit. The increase in temperature causes a decrease in the viscosity of the muscle —the resistance of the molecules of the muscle to internal movement. The viscosity phenomenon can be likened to a cold jar of molasses—it hardly pours —but warming the jar allows the molasses to pour more readily.

A vigorous amount of exercise will increase the utilization of energy. If a muscle is to function, energy is required, and the more activity, the greater the need for energy. For that reason, exercise will create a demand for more energy for utilization.

Exercise will increase the peripheral heart action of the muscle. As a person exercises, the muscles contract and relax. The contraction of the muscle presses down on the capillaries that lie within it, pushing the blood out of the capillaries and into the veins. The relaxation of the muscle opens the capillaries and allows the fresh blood to rush into the empty capillaries. The major veins of the body lie between the various muscles so that the alternating contractions and relaxations of the various muscles milk the veins (milking action) and aid in returning the blood to the heart from the veins.

Long-range Exercise

Regular, vigorous exercise has a profound effect on the muscular system.

There will be an increase in the size of the muscle fibers (the connective tissues that bind the muscle fibers together thicken and strengthen) called hypertrophy resulting in increased muscular strength. Muscle tone will also improve, producing an improved appearance. Muscles used in respiration will increase in size, for a more efficient functioning of the respiratory system.

Training will also produce an increased blood supply to the muscles. More capillaries are utilized, and more capillary beds are created. The increased blood supply permits a greater amount of nutrients to get to more parts of the muscle. Because of the increase, the muscle is more efficient, and the muscular endurance is increased. See MUSCULAR SYSTEM.

The Nervous System

The nervous system includes the brain, the spinal cord, and a network of nerves that spread from these two structures to every part of the body. The *central nervous system* is the brain and spinal column. Both of these structures are encased in a bony protection. The *peripheral nervous system* is comprised of all the nerves outside of these structures. These are not two separate systems, but rather two parts of the same system. Certain functions of the body, such as running, speaking, or writing are under the conscious control of the body. There are, however, certain functions over which we have no control, such as digestion, blood pressure, or heart rate. The part of the nervous system that is responsible for conscious control is called the somatic system, whereas the autonomic nervous system controls those parts of the body over which we do not have any conscious control.

The autonomic nervous system is broken down further into two separate portions, the sympathetic and the parasympathetic. These two portions generally either slow down or speed up the various organs. The sympathetic opposes the activity of the parasympathetic system, for the sympathetic nervous system acts to prepare the body for responding to an emergency situation. All of the functions mentioned depend upon the ability of the nerve cells to transmit impulses from one part of the body to the other.

The nervous system is the basis of all exercise, in fact, all body movement. It initiates, coordinates and directs exercise. Furthermore, the sympathetic and parasympathetic autonomic nervous systems have a profound effect on the regulation of the body for exercise. Both of these systems affect adjustments to the various body functions to make exercise possible.

Training has two critical effects on the nervous system: improvement in specific neuromuscular coordination and reduction of tension. If you practice a particular skill repeatedly, you will undoubtedly improve because you will establish the correct pattern for performing the skill via better neural control and will become more efficient by eliminating unnecessary muscle contractions. Moreover, enjoyable exercise can divert the mind and direct it toward new horizons. This diversion helps to eliminate emotional stress that may develop from daily activities. See NEURO-MUSCULAR SYSTEM.

Respiratory System

The respiratory system contributes to the exchange of gases between the individual and his environment and involves the exchange of oxygen and carbon dioxide between the body cells. The former function is called *external respiration* and involves the process of bringing air into the lungs, where oxygen is absorbed by the blood and carbon dioxide is released from the blood. The latter function is called *internal respiration* where energy is released for work and production of heat.

With the onset of vigorous exercise there is an increased rate and depth of breathing. The increase makes more oxygen available for production of fuel and helps to remove carbon dioxide.

Training or regular, vigorous exercise improves the efficiency of the respiratory system by affecting several important changes.

1. There is an enlargement of the muscles used in respiration, providing more efficient breathing.

2. An increase in the size and number of the capillaries in the lungs occurs, enabling more oxygen to be absorbed.

3. There is an increase in lung capacity, thereby permitting more oxygen to be inhaled.

4. The air sacs or alveoli become more functional, permitting greater transfer of oxygen and carbon dioxide.

5. There is a deeper respiration movement providing greater availability of oxygen.

6. The breathing rate returns to normal more quickly after exercise, allowing a quicker recovery from physical stress. See RESPIRATION.

The Skeletal System

The skeletal system consists of approximately 200 bones of various shapes and sizes that give support and protection to the body. The bones also serve as a storehouse of essential materials. Those bones are bound together by strong fibrous tissues, but the junctions (joints) between many of the bones allow limited movements.

Many people consider the bones of the body to be composed of a dead, lifeless substance. Such is not the case. The bone is a dynamic factory that has its materials constantly being dissolved and passed into the blood and replenished by the blood stream with food. Vigorous exercise has an immediate effect on the skeletal system—an increased blood supply to the bones for better nutrition of the skeletal system.

Over a period of weeks, vigorous exercise increases the size and thickness of the bones, thereby giving greater strength to the skeleton. That increase in size may be lost if the exercise is discontinued. See BONES.

Summary

As a result of regular exercise, the body is able to recover more quickly from a physical strain. Since the systems of the body are operating more efficiently, the body is able to do more work with less effort and quicker recovery. The trained person will feel better during and after exercise as a result of his better physiological condition.

The chronic effects of exercise related to all areas of the body will continue to occur only if you continue to exercise in a regular vigorous manner. If you do not progressively add to your present exercise level, a decrease in the chronic effects may occur—some more rapidly than others. Continued, progressive, vigorous exercise is necessary for maintaining and improving physical fitness.—*Clint E. Bruess*

EMPHYSEMA

Next to heart disease, emphysema disables more working men than any other disease. More men die of emphysema than from tuberculosis, and current evidence reveals that the incidence of emphysema is increasing rapidly.

Smoking, polluted air, infection, and unknown factors are all causes of this disease. Chronic bronchitis, with a chronic cough lasting 3 months or more, often precedes emphysema. Wheezing and shortness of breath, especially after exertion, are the next steps. During that exertion your skin may turn bluish. Another sign is that you cannot blow out the flame on a match from 4 inches away with the mouth wide open.

Emphysema causes an increase in the size of the alveoli of the lungs and a destruction of capillaries. Because of the size of the alveoli, the total lung capacity volume is increased. However, the effective lung volume and vital capacity are reduced because of the loss of pulmonary capillaries (less aeration of the blood) and restricted exhalation.

Anatomy of the Lungs

The lungs are composed of many small clusters of air sacs that hang from bronchial tubes, similar to grapes on a vine. Those clusters are very small—so small, in fact, that dozens can be placed on the head of a pin. The sacs, only one cell thick, have their own capillaries with walls so thin that carbon dioxide passes from the blood right through them.

Impurities brought in from the air are filtered and strained by the tiny hairs pointing upward in the bronchial tubes. The impurities are gradually expelled after being trapped. However, some impurities like tobacco tars and chemical fumes are too fine to be expelled. They cling to the walls of the tubes and irritate the tissues. That irritation may cause the bronchial tubes to tighten and interfere with exhalation. As the chest expands, the internal air will enter the lungs, through the tubes. The chest expansion causes a partial vacuum. Once the air is inside, however, the passages close, trapping the air inside making it difficult to release the air.

The irritation invites infection by bacteria from the air or blood and damages many of the tiny glands in the bronchial tubes which keep them moist and lubricated, thereby drying up the affected area and blocking the passage. As one section of the lung is shut off, another area expands to fill the area. Fortunately the body has plenty of lung tissue, but there is a limit.

The onset of emphysema is insidious. The cause is progressive and often deceptive, particularly if therapy is absent. As mentioned previously, emphysema is diagnosed by shortness of breath, coughing (without phlegm), wheezing, tiredness, feeling of tightness in the chest and dizziness. But special tests are required to make a definite diagnosis—for other ailments have similar symptoms.

Treatment and Therapy

Several techniques can be used to alleviate emphysema. Naturally, some are more successful than others, depending upon the person and ailment.

1. Reduce the possibility of infection, particularly in cold weather. If you do have a flare-up, your *doctor* may recommend an antibiotic.

2. Special medications may be used. A bronchodilator (drug) helps to open up the bronchial airways. A chemical is administered to break up the accumulation of phlegm that may have thickened and obstructed the bronchi. Intermittent Positive Pressure Breathing is also used. That oxygen therapy is used to enrich the oxygen supply and to improve ventilation.

3. Many times bronchodilators and detergents do not release obstruction so that postural drainage is necessary. Here the physician teaches you to allow gravity to aid in draining bronchial secretions through the windpipe and the mouth. Since the affected bronchi twist in many directions, one position is not sufficient. Many postures must be assumed, such as sitting and leaning forward, backward, and to the side, lying in various positions, including on an incline, on the side, or over the edge of the bed. These exercises are done at least twice a day.

4. Breathing exercises are also helpful, especially to reduce the stresses and strains of physical exertion. These exercises help you to breathe properly and efficiently, and the basic principle is to learn to breathe by moving the abdominal muscles and not the chest muscles.

With the onset of emphysema the diaphragm and the abdominal muscles do progressively less and less in respiration, while the chest muscles become more active. The breathing exercises are merely an attempt to reverse that action and get the abdominal muscle back into action.

To accomplish that breathing technique, use a progressive program involving learning to relax. Force the abdomen out as you breath in (through the nose) and draw the abdomen in and up as you breath out through the mouth with only a small opening in your lips. To feel the action, place the hands on the chest and abdomen. Another technique is to place a weight, such as a sandbag or book, on the abdomen while doing the exercises. Wrapping a towel around the waist is also used to learn the breathing action while sitting, standing, or walking.

Another recommended exercise is to blow at the flame of a candle with pursed lips using the abdomen muscles. At first, place the candle 5 to 8 inches away. The distance is gradually increased until after a certain number of sessions the flame can be blown from 3 feet away.

5. Another point to be considered in the treatment of emphysema is proper living habits. Temperature plays an important role—avoid dry or humid environments and excessively cold or hot temperatures. Smoking, fumes and similar irritants must also be avoided. Diet is important, primarily to keep the weight down. Frequent coughing helps remove foreign objects from the bronchial tubes. It is only when the coughing is violently exhausting that medication is prescribed to suppress that reflex.

6. It is very important to visit and consult with your doctor. His examination will determine the extent of the condition and the methods to alleviate or retard it.

Role of Training

Both abstinence of activity and overexertion are dangerous. Abstinence will make you greatly dependent upon others, while overexertion will make breathing excessively difficult and frightening. A happy medium must be achieved.

Regardless of the activity selected, it is important to master breathing techniques and to establish a reliable pace. Although still somewhat controversial, exercises have been used successfully in the treatment of chronic obstructive, pulmonary emphysema patients.

For example, Dr. Lazlo Ambrus and his co-workers at the Veterans Administration Hospital in California have experimented with a combined exercise program involving breathing, relaxation, postural and general conditioning exercises. The breathing and postural exercises were similar to those described previously. For relaxation, the patients contract and relax their muscles while sitting or lying down. These first three phases are the traditional approaches that have been followed in emphysema therapy. Dr. Ambrus added the new element of exercise training.

His program involved special trunk exercises and progressive resistive exercises for the upper and lower extremities done twice daily in the gymnasium. Wall pulleys, a treadmill, a rowing device, N/K Table, a shoulder wheel, and weights were used intermittently for a change of pace. Progressive walking and stair climbing were done daily.

At the beginning of the program, the 43 male subjects were tested for grade of dyspnea (labored breathing), breathing function, and various activities, i.e., walking, stair walking, treadmill walking, etc. They were then placed on a 6-week training program as described above. At the conclusion of that period the men were retested. The findings revealed:

1. Less reliance upon the intermittent positive breathing aid.

2. A more efficient respiratory pattern, which may indicate a reduction of the energy cost of breathing.

3. Changes in the weight of patients. The underweight and normal weight patients gained, while the overweight lost.

4. Thirty of the patients showed positive changes in dyspnea while 20 showed improvement in ventilatory (breathing) function.

5. Endurance increased as measured by the ability to walk for longer periods of time, from 3½ minutes to over 7 minutes. The ability to climb stairs, exercise on the Exer-Rower, and walk on the treadmill all improved significantly.

6. Strength, as measured by grip strength, improved.

7. Eighty percent of the patients maintained or even improved their functional level at 3-6-9 and 12 months after discharge.

8. The patients subjectively stated they felt better, enjoyed the exercise program and increased activity, breathed easier, and worried less about their condition. They even claimed that their food tasted better, and their outlook on life improved. The improved natural state may be the most important result of the study.

The authors concluded that a combined and supervised exercise program is an important supplement to the medical treatment of the chronic obstructive pulmonary emphysema patient. See ASTHMA.

ENDOCRINE SYSTEM

Connected with intense exercise are certain neural (nervous) and hormonal responses that occur in the body. These changes represent the body's adjustment to stress, a condition caused by physical and/or emotional strain. Stress tends to upset the body's homeostatic balance while the neural and hormonal adjustments strive to maintain that balance.

A stress reaction is initiated by receptor nerves which stimulate secretion of certain hormones. Among these hormones are ACTH (adenocorticotrophic hormone), STH (somatotrophic hormone) and TSH (thyroid stimulating hormone). These secretions as well as other mechanisms affect the following physiological changes: increased heart rate and stroke volume (the amount of blood pumped per stroke), increased rate and depth of breathing, increased body temperature, changes in the composition of the blood and other changes.

Changes in heart function during exercise are controlled by a combination of complex nervous and chemical mechanisms. Accelerated heart rate is caused in part by an increased amount of adrenalin which has been secreted into the blood. Upon reaching the heart, it causes a response from the heart muscle. Quite often, particularly in competitive situations an increase in heart activity occurs before the actual physical exertion begins. Emotions have been cited as a cause of this. Although emotions do elevate the production of adrenalin, several other factors are likely involved in emotional response to competitive situations.

Aside from an increased need for oxygen, the cells involved in prolonged or intense activity demand more glu-

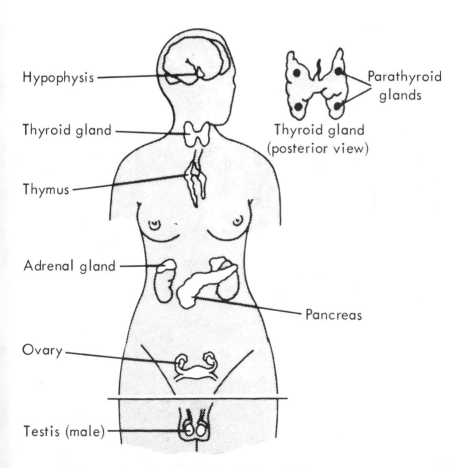

Location of the endocrine glands.

cose, the fuel that provides the energy for the cells to carry out their specific functions. When needed additional glucose is secreted by the liver. Physical stress acting via the pituitary gland results in increased secretion of *ACTH* (*adenocorticotrophic hormone*) which stimulates the adrenal cortex to produce glucocorticoids. Glucocorticoids are responsible for stimulating the process of gluconeogenesis, which causes an increase in the blood sugar level (amount of glucose in the blood).

Changes occur in the amount of urine produced, and, correspondingly, the amount of water retained by the body during varying intensities of exercise. Whether or not water is removed or retained by the filtering action of the kidneys is essential in the maintenance of the constancy of the body's internal environment (homeostasis) during times of physical stress. The amount of water reabsorbed is controlled by secretion of the anti-diuretic hormone. During exercise more blood is shunted to the active muscles leaving less blood for the kidneys to filter. In this situation the kidneys produce less liquid waste. This in part makes up for the increased fluids lost through the skin via the sweat glands. See EXCRETORY SYSTEM.

These are a few of the adjustments to physical stress affected by certain hormones of the endocrine system. There are also numerous other internal changes that occur in response to stress. Understanding of endocrine mechanisms connected with exercise is by no means complete. Much research is presently in progress to expand man's understanding of endocrine function.

ENDURANCE

Endurance is the ability to persist in submaximal physical activity and the ability to resist physiological fatigue. It is one of the most important components of physical fitness, for it helps to indicate the state of health of the circulatory, respiratory, nervous and muscular systems of the body. Endurance is a term that is often misinterpreted, possibly because there are two types of endurance, i.e., muscular (local) and circulatory (circulorespiratory, cardiovascular, or general). Muscular endurance refers to the involvement of one or several localized muscle groups in exercise, and the fatigue or resistance to fatigue of these muscles. The second type, circulorespiratory, involves the whole body and its ability to continue in physical activity. They are closely interrelated and at times difficult to differentiate.

Two extremely important psychological elements play a critical role in endurance: the one is motivation, and the other is willingness to endure pain. See CIRCULO-RESPIRATORY ENDURANCE; MOTIVATION, MUSCLE ENDURANCE; and TRAINING.

A Word About the Exercise Programs

Many of the activities classified as moderate high, high, and very high energy cost have been placed into exercise programs that permit a training effect on the body, especially the circulo-respiratory systems.

Each program is progressive and allows adequate time for the body to adapt, taking into account the important principle of training. See TRAINING. The programs are designed for the average citizen, not for the athlete and are based on the energy cost of each activity (calories burned per minute).

At the outset the program is very easy but as you progress, your activity level increases appreciably so that a training effect occurs on the body.

Before you embark on a program, check with your doctor. Then proceed with either the *Harvard Step Test* or *12 Minute Run* as described under TESTS. Your achievement on the test(s) determines your starting level. A score

RUNNING PROGRAM

Chart 1	Chart 2
1. Walk-Run ¾ mile in 10 minutes	1. Run 2 miles in 22 minutes
2. Walk-Run ¾ mile in 9 minutes	2. Run 2 miles in 21 minutes
3. Walk-Run 1 mile in 12 minutes	3. Run 2¼ miles in 24 minutes
4. Run 1 mile in 11 minutes	4. Run 2¼ miles in 23 minutes
5. Run 1¼ miles in 14 minutes	5. Run 2½ miles in 26 minutes
6. Run 1¼ miles in 13 minutes	6. Run 2½ miles in 25 minutes
7. Run 1½ miles in 16 minutes	7. Run 2¾ miles in 28 minutes
8. Run 1½ miles in 15 minutes	8. Run 2¾ miles in 27 minutes
9. Run 1¾ miles in 18 minutes	9. Run 3 miles in 30 minutes

Fitness 1

If you achieve a score of poor or low average on the *Harvard Step Test* or a score of very poor or poor on the *12 Minute Run*, start on Chart 1-Level 1 and spend 1 week at each level until Chart 2-Level 9 is reached. It is recommended that you participate 4 to 5 days a week. When Chart 2-Level 9 is reached, 4 days a week is sufficient.

Fitness 2

If you achieve a score of high average on the *Harvard Step Test* or fair on the *12 Minute Run*, start on Chart 1-Level 2. Spend one week on Chart 1-Level 2, 4, 6, 7, 8, and 9, and Chart 2-Levels 1, 3, 5, 7, 8, and 9. It is recommended that you participate 4 to 5 days a week. When Chart 2-Level 9 is reached, 4 days a week is sufficient.

Fitness 3

If you achieve a score of good or excellent on either the *Harvard Step Test* or *12 Minute Run*, continue your current program or select Chart 2-Level 9 as your level of participation. Four days a week is sufficient.

---

of poor or low average on the *Harvard Step Test* or a score of very poor or poor on the *12 Minute Run* will place you in category "Fitness 1." A score of high average on the *Harvard Step Test* or fair on the *12 Minute Run* will place you in category "Fitness 2." A score of good or excellent on either

the *Harvard Step Test* or *12 Minute Run* will place you in category "Fitness 3."

Once you achieve Level 9 on Chart 2 you will be able to jump from one activity to another, provided you select Level 9 of Chart 2. But because of the training principle of specificity (see SPECIFICITY), and other factors you may experience some difficulty. For example, other muscles may be used, and more flexibility may be required. As a result you must allow almost one week for adjustment to take place. Otherwise, muscle soreness and/or labored breathing may occur.

Below is the running program as a sample.

ENERGY COST OF ACTIVITIES

Many people lead a life that requires little physical activity. This sedentary existence has been blamed for various degenerative ailments that plague modern man. As a result, physical activities of all types have been recommended as a means of reversing the trend so as to prevent those degenerative disorders. But most of our activities today do not place a sufficient stress on the human body. The normal circulo-respiratory systems, in particular, need considerable external physical stress, for those systems play a critical role in preventing many degenerative diseases, especially coronary heart disease.

Research has demonstrated that in order to improve the circulatory and respiratory systems, exercise needs to raise the pulse rate to 140 beats per minute for a period of time and to burn at least 300 calories in one-half hour, or about 11 calories per minute. Generally, an exercise that burns more than 300 calories in one-half hour will result in a pulse rate of about 140 beats per minute. If the activity is of longer duration, the intensity of exercise decreases so that approximately 600 calories should be burned up in one hour—10 calories per minute for an hour, or approximately 1,000 calories in two hours—8.3 calories per minute in a two-hour period.

Of course, many activities make a significant contribution to actual fitness but may not develop optimum levels of circulo-respiratory endurance. Weight training, for example, is an excellent means of developing muscle strength and muscle endurance but does little to improve circulo-respiratory endurance.

Furthermore, all activities regardless of their low level of intensity can be helpful in weight control. If you are currently balancing your caloric intake (food) with calorie outgo (activity), you are not gaining or losing weight. But if you are 20 pounds overweight, selecting almost any additional activity will help you lose weight. If you select gardening as your daily activity (220 calories per hour) and garden 4 days a week, in one week's time the total is 880 calories; in a year that would be 45,760 calories. *To burn one pound of fat requires using 3,500 calories.* Therefore, in one year's time 13+ pounds would be lost merely by gardening. See APPETITE, CALORIES and WEIGHT CONTROL.

The following chart includes a series of activities ranging from low to very high energy cost activities. They are presented in average calories burned per minute for the typical person. Also included are the calories consumed in

one-half hour and one hour if the activity is continued for that period of time.

Traditionally, activities have been classified by calories consumed per hour. The problem with that classification is that some activities can be done for only a short period of time, such as sprinting, while others, such as mountaineering, are done at a steady rate for a long period of time. It is ridiculous to compare sprinting and mountaineering in terms of calories burned per hour. People do not sprint for an hour, and certainly mountaineers would not get anywhere unless they climbed for hours. Therefore, the activities are more efficiently compared in terms of calories burned per minute, which gives you a more realistic appraisal of the intensity of exercise. You may ski two hours, but you may be actively skiing downhill only 20 minutes. The remainder is spent on the lifts or in resting. Using calories burned per minute in the chart gives a better evaluation of exercise intensity.

The calculations are approximations based on numerous studies, and there is considerable variation from one person to another depending upon size, body type, age, fitness level, skill level, nutrition and environmental conditions. The chart is quite important as a general exercise classification indicating the intensity of exercise and as a guide for establishing an exercise program.

Recently, exercise physiologists have been comparing physical activity in terms of liters of oxygen used per minute because it is more accurate. We've used calories burned per minute here because this measure is more popular with the public. Energy expenditure in calories per minute is calculated from the oxygen intake per minute. See METABOLISM for a closely allied discussion.

If you are not in good physical condition, you can't undertake an activity that has a very high energy cost rating. Select one that is not nearly so de-

ENERGY COST OF ACTIVITY (In Calories)

Intensity of Exercise	Hour	½ Hour	Per Minute
Low	70-150	35-74	1.17-2.49
Mild	150-299	75-149½	2.5-4.99
Moderate	300-449	50-224½	5.0-7.49
Moderate High	450-599	225-299½	7.5-9.99
High	600-749	300-374½	10.0-12.49
Very High	750+	375+	12.5+

	Hour	½ Hour	Minutes
LOW	70-150	35-75	1.17-2.15
Sleeping	70	35	1.17
Lying Quietly	80	40	1.33
Sitting	100	50	1.67
Mental Work—Seated	105	52½	1.75
Standing	110	55	1.83
Sitting (Handwork)	120	60	2.00
Driving a Car (Pleasure)	140	70	2.33
Sailing (Calm Water)	141	70½	2.35

	Hour	½ Hour	Minutes
MILD	150-300	75-150	2.5-5.0
Pool	162	81	2.7
Horseback Riding (walk)	170	85	2.83
Airplane Flying	175	87½	2.91
Walking 2 mph	192	96	3.2
Motorcycling	204	102	3.4
Bricklaying	205	102½	3.41
Hiking—40 lb. Pack 1 mph	210	105	3.5
House Painting	210	105	3.5
Gardening	220	110	3.67
Carpentry	230	115	3.83
Canoeing	230	115	3.83
Horseshoes	230	115	3.83
Bicycling 5½ mph	240	120	4.0
Dancing (mod.)	250	125	4.1
Golf	250	125	4.1
Lawn Mowing (Power)	250	125	4.1
Domestic Work	250	125	4.1
Walking 2½ mph	256	128	4.27
Bowling (Continuous)	270	135	4.5
Hiking—40 lb. Pack—2 mph	270	135	4.5
Mowing (Hand)	270	135	4.5
Softball-Baseball (Not Pitcher)	280	140	4.67

	Hour	½ Hour	Minutes
MODERATE	300-449	150-224½	5.0-7.49
Rowing 2½ mph—Pleasure	300	150	5.0
Fencing	300	150	5.0
Hiking 2½ mph (20 lbs.)	300	150	5.0
Walking 3 mph	300	150	5.0
Swimming Crawl 20 yd./min.	300	150	5.0
Breast 20/yd min.	300	150	5.0
Back 25 yd/min.	300	150	5.0
Archery	312	156	5.2

ENERGY COST OF ACTIVITY (In Calories)—*Continued*

Intensity of Exercise	Hour	½ Hour	Per Minute
Hiking 3 mph—20 lbs.	312	150	5.2
Walking 3½ mph	315	157½	5.25
Weeding	336	168	5.6
Hiking 3 mph—40 lbs.	348	174	5.8
Walking 4 mph	348	174	5.8
Badminton (Recreational)	350	175	5.83
Volleyball (Recreational)	350	175	5.83
Skating (Leisure) Ice & Roller	350	175	5.83
Table Tennis	360	180	6.0
Hiking 3½ mph—20 lbs.	380	190	6.33
Baseball Pitcher	390	195	6.5
Pick and Shovel	400	200	6.67
Horseback Riding (Trot)	415	207½	6.93
Canoeing 4 mph	420	210	7.0
Square Dancing	420	210	7.0
Swim Crawl 30 yd/min.	420	210	7.0
Tennis (Recreational)	426	213	7.1

	Hour	½ Hour	Minutes
MODERATE HIGH	450-599	225-299½	7.5-9.99
Chopping Wood	450	225	7.5
Swimming Breast 30/min.	450	225	7.5
Back 30/min.	450	225	7.5
Hiking 40 mph (20 lbs.)	450	225	7.5
Walking 4½ mph	480	240	8.0
Sawing	480	240	8.0
Farming, Planting, Hoeing, Raking	480	240	8.0
Water Skiing	480	240	8.0
Digging & Shoveling	500	250	8.33
5 BX—Chart 1A	510	255	8.5
Hiking 40 lb. 4 mph	540	270	9.0
Polka Dancing	540	270	9.0
Swimming Back 35/yd	540	270	9.0
Side 30/yd	550	275	9.17
Boxing (Sparring)	550	275	9.17
Skiing (Downhill)	594	297	9.9

	Hour	½ Hour	Minutes
HIGH	600-749	300-374½	10.00-12.49
Badminton (Competitive)	600	300	10.00
Hill Climbing	600	300	10.00
Handball	600	300	10.00
Swimming Breast 40/min.	600	300	10.00
Mountain Climbing	600	300	10.00
Orienteering	600	300	10.00
Soccer	600	300	10.00
Tennis (Competitive)	600	300	10.00
Volleyball (Competitive)	600	300	10.00
Basketball	608	304	10.13
Football (Playground)	611	305½	10.18
Squash	612	306	10.2
Fencing	630	315	10.5

ENERGY COST OF ACTIVITY (In Calories)—*Continued*

Intensity of Exercise	Hour	½ Hour	Per Minute
5BX–Chart 2A	640	320	10.67
Skating (Vigorously)	640	320	10.67
Walking 5 mph	660	330	11.0
Bicycling 13 mph	660	330	11.0
Running 5.5 mph	660	330	11.0
Swimming Side 40/yd	660	330	11.0
Back 40/yd	660	330	11.0
Rowboating 3.5 mph	660	330	11.0
Jogging	660	330	11.0
Swimming Crawl 45/yd	690	345	11.5
Parallel Bars	710	355	11.83
Running 7.2 mph	720	360	12.0
Skiing on Level 5 mph	720	360	12.0
Swimming Butterfly Stroke	720	360	12.0

	Hour	½ Hour	Minutes
VERY HIGH	750+	375+	12.5+
Wrestling & Combatives	790	395	13.17
Swimming Back	800	400	13.33
Running 8 mph	825	412½	13.75
Swimming Crawl 55/min.	840	420	14.0
Sculling Racing	840	420	14.0
Running 8.7 mph	900	450	15.0
5BX–Chart 3A and 4A	960	480	16.00
Rowboating (Racing)	970	485	16.17
Rowing Machine Very Vig.	972	486	16.2
5BX–Chart 5A and 6A	1080	540	18.00
Cross Country Skiing	1200	600	20.0
Running in Place 140 counts per min.	1500	750	25.00
Swimming Crawl 65 yd/min.	1600	800	26.67
Running in Place 160 counts per min.	1800	900	30.0

manding, i.e., a low or moderate activity. You could also engage in a high-intensity activity but only for a few minutes rather than the stipulated half hour.

As your condition improves, you can move up the scale selecting more demanding activities. Most of the high, moderately high, and very high energy cost activities have a graduated exercise program to help improve physiological functions. Several of the activities have methods for progressing from one level to another. See individual entries for the chart demonstrating a progressive training program.

ENVIRONMENT

Introduction

Until recently there was little attention directed toward the effect environment has upon exercise, performance and fitness. But certain events —the 1968 Olympic games in Mexico City (el. 7,347 feet), the 1967 NFL Championship in −13° F. temperature, the increased interest in winter sports, and the transporting of athletic teams throughout the country—have triggered concern about the effect of climate and altitude on human performance and the attainment of physical fitness.

Climate

Heat loss and gain are important factors in climate's effect on physical fitness, for they both regulate and prohibit the amount of exercise that can be done in a particular geographical area.

How Heat is Lost

Conduction: Heat loss by conduction occurs when the body comes in direct contact with something colder than the skin. The rate of exchange, naturally, is determined by the temperature difference between the body and other substances. An example of conduction is immersing the body in a pool of cold water—the body loses heat.

Convection: Heat loss by convection is the process by which heat is transferred from the body by a moving liquid (usually water) or gas (usually air). An example of convection is the movement of air by a hand fan to cool off a person when he feels warm or hot.

Radiation: Radiation transfers heat by way of electromagnetic waves. All warm bodies emit these waves, and the human body is constantly gaining and losing more heat by radiation. In normal environments (temperate climate) the loss of heat exceeds the gain and constitutes the most important method of heat loss. In a hot desert environment, however, where a person is exposed to the sun, there may be an increase in heat due to radiation. Radiation also explains why people may be comfortable skiing in high mountains with a minimum of clothing.

Evaporation: Heat loss by evaporation or vaporation refers to the process of converting liquid to a gas state. For example, the evaporation of sweat on the skin cools the skin by taking from it the necessary heat to vaporize the water of the sweat. Sweating cools the skin, but *only* when the water is evaporated.

How Heat is Gained

Heat can be gained from one of two sources, environment and metabolism. In a comfortable environment temperature heat gain is due entirely to metabolism. Metabolic heat production increases in exercise; likewise, metabolic heat production increases during exposure to cold by shivering—a type of muscle contraction.

If the body is exposed to intense sunlight or some type of artificial heating device, such as a stove or heat lamp, it may gain heat by radiation. Or if the body is exposed to a substance of a high temperature, such as hot water, it may gain heat by conduction.

Exercise in Cold Environments

A number of sports events are carried on in cold environments. Skiing, skating, tobogganing and curling are activities that depend upon snow and ice. Likewise, many activities such as football, soccer, and even track and field meets are occasionally performed in very cold weather.

Generally, a cold environment poses no real problem because of increased metabolic heat from the activity or the clothing that may be worn to help retain the body heat.

One problem that seems to plague many people is preventing a sudden change in temperature of the body (chilling) which usually occurs during periods of rest. Many times a person will be running for quite a distance in cold weather and will experience no chilling while running. But when he stops, there is a sudden change in temperature (decreased metabolic heat), and a chill sets in. That chilling may be prevented by putting on a warm garment immediately or by tapering off the activity gradually so that the decrease in temperature is not so rapid. If you have participated in some physical activity during cold weather you will undoubtedly remember that you didn't feel cold during the exercise. That is because metabolic rates may increase up to 25 to 30 times the resting metabolic rate. In fact, during intense exercise in very cold weather you will sweat profusely.

Natural Body Protectors

The body is protected from exposure to the cold by a phenomenon called *peripheral vasoconstriction.* That phenomenon is a reduction of blood circulation in the cool areas of the body and an increase in the metabolic heat production through increased muscle contraction (shivering). Humidity and air movement, called convection, increase the rate of loss of body heat in a cold environment. When fatigue from the exercise occurs, the heat production of the body will fall, and the heat loss of the body will occur rapidly—resulting in a drop in body temperature.

Body build and fat tissue play an important role in the ability of a person to withstand cold. Generally, the person with a greater proportion of fat is better able to withstand the cold than the thin person, for the fat acts as an insulation against heat loss. The reverse is true in hot weather; the thin person is better able to get rid of heat and remain cooler than is the heavy-set person.

Your ability to adapt to cold weather may be partly mental. Studies show that ability to acclimate to cold may be a combination of the physiological and psychological. That undoubtedly accounts for the wide variation of cold tolerance from one individual to another.

Efficiency in Work and Cold

Unless you have adequately adapted to the cold environment or made the necessary adjustments (extra clothing, etc.), you will find that your efficiency is reduced. When you work in a cold environment, your hands will become cold and will have difficulty in performing tasks that require finger dexterity. If you catch a football or baseball with cold hands, they will "smart" from the impact. Cold feet retard efficiency and may prevent you from moving quickly.

A person who is inadequately clothed will start to shiver. The purpose of shivering is to raise body metabolism. That increase in body metabolism will bring about an increase in calorie consumption. When you shiver most, your basal metabolism rate may be increased about seven times. P. F. Iampietro and others mention one other aspect of loss of efficiency because of cold. They discuss the possibility of your being unable to concentrate on the task at hand. When chilled you become more concerned with keeping the body warm than with performing the necessary task.

How to Improve Efficiency in Cold Weather

Clothing: For you to exercise well in cold environments, wear several layers of light clothing that are easily removable. Then you can adjust the amount of clothing according to the rate of work. Those layers will enable the moisture-laden air that is accumulating because of sweat to be dissipated away from the body and keep the clothing dry. Keep your hands and feet warm—they are first to get cool when the entire body is being exposed to the cold.

Diet: If you will repeatedly be exposed to extremely cold temperatures, you will find it advantageous to see that the proportion of fat in your diet is high. Keep the amount of protein rather low. Eat several small meals rather than just a few large ones. Below are some further guidelines.

1. Concentrate on the thickness of insulation. Thickness is equal to warmth. The type of material you use to clothe yourself is insignificant. Don't be swayed by manufacturers who suggest that one style of material will protect you better than another. Even

newspaper of the sufficient thickness will keep you warm, although you wouldn't want to hike in a coat made of paper.

2. Keep the torso warm. Then your body will send the excess heat to the less well insulated parts of the body. But if your torso is poorly insulated, the extremities of your body will be even colder.

3. Avoid sweating. That can best be done by ventilating to bypass your insulation before you even start to sweat. The sweating will lower your body temperature.

4. Be certain that your insulation is sufficiently protected from wind or rain by an outside covering. Many products for warm weather include an outer covering of weather proofing adhering to the insulation.

5. Keep your head covered to heat your hands and, especially, your feet. Although it may sound facetious, wearing a hat will keep your feet warmer. The head is a primary radiator of excess body heat because of the rich blood supply and the fact that it has muscular surfaces next to the veins and arteries.

6. If you are buttoned up and still cold, increase your metabolism. That can be done by exercising or rapid movement. If that is not possible, employ isometrics to speed up metabolism.

The following table taken from the U. S. Army Quartermaster data shows the amount of insulation needed to stay warm at different temperatures. If it is windy, it may be necessary to add additional insulation.

Exercise in Hot Climate

Exercise in a hot climate is a much more difficult problem than exercising in the cold. In a cold environment man can aid himself by putting on more clothing. In a hot environment, however, adjustment is difficult. In a cold climate the increased metabolic heat production, as a result of exercise, helps to keep the body warm. In a hot environment, however, the environment and the increased metabolic heat production combine to increase the body temperature. The problem is compounded when environmental temperatures approach the skin temperature; then heat loss through convection and radiation slowly ends. The only means of heat loss then is through evaporation of sweat.

Sweating is extremely important in keeping the body cool, but *only if the sweat evaporates*. Sweat that simply rolls off the body is rather ineffective since no cooling occurs. In a dry environment (low humidity) the sweat evaporates very quickly and helps to cool the body. However, in a wet environment (high humidity), the reverse is true. The sweat does not evaporate, and very little cooling takes place.

Hot and Dry Environment

When you work or exercise in a hot and dry environment, the skin is cooled by the evaporation of the sweat. The rate of evaporation is high because the air can absorb the moisture.

When cooling the outer body, it is important to cool the internal portions

INSULATION REQUIREMENTS

Temperature	Sleeping	Light Work	Heavy Work
40°F	1.5″	.8″	.20″
20°F	2.0″	1.0″	.27″
0°F	2.5″	1.3″	.35″
−20°F	3.0″	1.6″	.40″
−40°F	3.5″	1.9″	.48″
−60°F	4.0″	2.1″	.52″

as well. That is done when exercise increases the flow of blood through the skin and subcutaneous tissues. The increased flow results in a greater volume of blood moving at a slower rate near the skin, thereby allowing a better transfer of heat.

The cooling-off process places an extra load on the circulatory system. Since a considerable amount of blood is needed in the exercising muscles and near the skin, the heart rate must increase. Therefore, exercise in hot and dry environments can place a very severe load on the cardiovascular system. Exercise in that type of environment can also cause dehydration, since the process of cooling depends upon elimination of water through perspiration. For that reason, water intake during exercise is imperative. See WATER CONSUMPTION DURING EXERCISE.

When a person exercises or works in a hot, humid environment, the perspiration is not evaporated because the moisture-laden air cannot absorb the additional water. Since heat dissipation cannot occur, the body temperature rises. If the temperature continues to rise, death will occur (106-108°F.).

When you exercise in a hot and humid environment, you will encounter the same problems as you will experience in a hot and dry environment—increased cardiovascular load, and dehydration—except that the situation is more serious because of the inability to cool the body.

Effects of Heat During Exercise

Body Temperature: Research has demonstrated that when you exercise or work, your body temperature starts rising. If the work load is not too severe (within the capacity to adjust) and the temperature is not too high, your rising body temperature will level off after about 30 minutes or so. The new temperature will range from 1 to 4°F. higher than resting temperature. However, when the work load is too

severe, and/or the temperature and humidity are too high, the body temperature will not level off but will continue to rise until exhaustion occurs.

Dehydration: Although there is considerable variation among individuals on their rate of water loss, a person may lose several pounds of water during exercise. Dr. P. V. Karpovich has reported that 6 to 13 pounds of water may be lost from the body in a day.

It is not uncommon to observe athletes who have lost 8 to 15 pounds in a strenuous two-hour workout.

Salt Loss: Along with that water loss a good deal of salt is also lost. The amount of salt (sodium chloride) in sweat ranges between .2 to .5 per cent. Theoretically that means up to 35 grams of salt a day could be lost through sweating. Actually that is not the case, for in profuse sweating, even under the most severe conditions only about 16-17 grams of salt are needed. Since the normal daily intake is about 10 to 12 grams, the exerciser should be more cautious about his intake of salt, both naturally and as a supplement.

A deficiency in salt, according to Drs. L. E. Morehouse and A. T. Miller may cause a person exercising to lose more weight (water), drink more water, and sweat less. Pulse rates and body temperature will be higher. Poorer cardiovascular adjustments will be evident. Other problems may be dehydration, nausea, vomiting, tachycardia (rapid heart action), hypotension, vertigo, cramps and collapse.

Several techniques may be used to supplement the salt intake. One, salt tablets may be taken. A considerable amount of water should be taken with these tablets to avoid nausea. Second, add ½ teaspoon of salt to each four glasses of drinking water every day, provided the amount is not disagreeable. Third, liberally sprinkle food with salt at mealtime. Fourth, maintain an adequate diet. See SALT TABLETS.

Pulse Rate: For the same amount of work, the pulse rate is higher with an increase in environmental temperature. The heart needs to do more work because the amount of blood circulating through the skin increases greatly. Research studies have also shown that exercise in a hot room, as compared to the same exertion in a cold room, will result in a heart output increase per minute of 1 to 4 quarts.

Efficiency and Fatigue: If you exercise in a hot environment, you will discover a drastic effect on your efficiency and fatigue level. H. M. Vernon, reporting in *Physiological Reviews,* made observations on over 100 miners. Under the most desirable conditions of temperature and humidity the miners rested only 7.3 minutes per hour. But when the temperature and humidity rose to an uncomfortable degree, they rested 22 minutes per hour.

Generally it is considered that the most efficient work occurs in temperatures between 40°-75°F. Above 75°F. man's efficiency drops off gradually. The most favorable conditions for work are 68°F. and 50 per cent humidity.

Other Considerations

At times you may have to exercise under conditions that are undesirable. Below are a few techniques that may be employed to help you.

Acclimatization: When you are first exposed to a hot environment you will experience a sharp decrement in performance in work or exercise if the activity places a heavy demand on your cardiovascular system. However, you will start to be acclimated on the first day of exposure to the heat and continue to develop to the fourth and fifth day and into two weeks or more. The acclimatization progresses rapidly. Several noticeable changes occur when you become acclimated to the heat. The flushing of the face and head will start to disappear or modify during exercise, the body temperature and heart rate are lower, and blood pressure is more stable.

Partial acclimatization will occur if you just rest in the heat. If you do some exercises in the heat and progressively add to the exercise, the acclimatization will occur more rapidly and efficiently. You should not expect to reach full acclimatization within a day or two. Several days, even weeks, are required. In fact, if you overwork on the first day you may find that it will take several days to recover, thereby slowing down the acclimatization. The acclimatization is retained for about two weeks.

A man in good physical condition will suffer less than those in poor condition when first exposed to heat and will retain his acclimatization longer. A significant amount of acclimatization can be brought about artificially by workout sessions in hot rooms.

Diet: A decrease of protein in the diet may be helpful, because protein digestion causes more heat formation than other foodstuffs. Include foods with high water content, i.e., fruits and salads. Since a great deal of vitamin C is lost through sweat, be sure to provide for it in your diet.

Clothing: Clothing, no matter how light in weight, will hinder the regulation of temperature in a hot and humid environment. It is best that the clothing be loose and lightweight in a hot environment to allow for evaporation, yet to protect the body from heat absorption by radiation.

Altitude

Although over one-half billion people in the world live at an altitude of over 6,500 feet, the effects of altitude on physical performance have recently become a topic of international interest. That concern—and in some cases—alarm—was sparked by the decision to hold the 1968 Olympic Games in Mexico City, at an altitude of 7,347 feet. Man has frequently experienced ill-effects, usually transitory, during the first few days at a moderately high altitude. The terms "altitude sickness" and "mountain sickness" are commonly used to describe the condition which is characterized by weakness, headache, vertigo, nausea and mental confusion. Although there is a great deal of variability among individuals as to altitude tolerance, some people suffer from mountain sickness at an altitude of 7,000 feet or less.

A more serious condition is high-altitude pulmonary edema. It typically occurs in cases where persons travel rather rapidly (within a day or two) to altitudes of over 9,000 feet. A dry cough, dyspnea (labored breathing), pain in the chest, and sometimes nausea and vomiting are the usual initial symptoms. Later wheezing and rattling sounds are heard in the respirations, and frequently there is coughing and spitting of blood mucous. Collapse, coma, and amnesia are among the symptoms in the more severe cases; and of course at very high altitudes, such as in mountain climbing, acute pulmonary edema is sometimes fatal.

In any case, the ill-effects of altitude are brought about much more rapidly when the person is exercising vigorously than when he is sedentary. It is this fact that induced the widespread concern regarding the well-being of the Olympic contestants in Mexico City. Consequently, many studies have been conducted recently pertaining to the performance of athletes at varying altitudes and the medical aspects of such performance. An International Symposium on the Effects of Altitude on Physical Performance was held at Albuquerque, New Mexico, in March, 1966. The event was co-sponsored by the United States Olympic Committee, the Lovelace Foundation for Medical Education and Research, and the University of New Mexico. The collection of papers presented at the symposium was published in 1967.

Effect on Physical Performance

Physical performance is directly related to the ability of the body to supply a sufficient amount of oxygen to the working muscle tissues. That, of course, is the reason why performances requiring endurance are impaired much more than are short performances. In the altitude studies involving track and field, swimming, and various laboratory performance activities, strength, reaction time, sprints, and other efforts of short duration have not been adversely affected. In other words, the reduced percentage of oxygen in the air at moderately high altitudes (for example, seven to eight thousand feet) is not detrimental to performance which is accomplished to a large extent anaerobically. As a matter of fact, theoretically the reduced atmospheric density should be a slight advantage in certain events.

There can be no doubt, however, that activity that involves sustained effort of over two minutes duration is definitely impaired at altitude. Not only is there a decrease in work efficiency, but longer periods of recovery are needed following exercise. The consensus is that persons who are physically fit are able to function more effectively and to tolerate the effects of altitude better than individuals who are in a poor state of fitness. The person in the fit state is better able to resist the deleterious effects of lactic acid build-up and hypoxia deficiency of oxygen reaching the body tissues) during work because of better peripheral oxygen distribution. Although the physically fit person can do more work at altitude than the unfit person, he is by no means immune. The percentage of performance decrement in the well-conditioned individual is about the same as for the unfit individual. Nevertheless, physical conditioning, especially endurance training, does improve work efficiency at altitude and assists in altitude acclimatization.

Adjustment Efforts of the Body

The debilitating effects of decreased oxygen intake are the most acute on the second and third day at altitude. There are several physiological processes through which the body attempts to become acclimatized to the reduced oxygen intake at altitude. Some of those adjustments are (1) an increase in the number of red blood cells and the hemoglobin content in the blood; (2) an increase in myoglobin, which is the oxygen carrying pigment in the muscle; (3) increased lung ventilation resulting from the need to breathe more air to get the same amount of oxygen; (4) decreased cardiac output and increased heart rate for submaximal work loads; and (5) probably improved vascularization in the lungs and muscle tissue.

The acclimatization process takes time. Of course, it will vary in accordance with the type of work to be performed, individual differences in altitude tolerance, and the state of physical fitness. In addition, one should not overlook the psychological factors. If an individual is fearful that he will be adversely affected at altitude, his performance will undoubtedly suffer. Attempts to objectively analyze physiological manifestations are frequently complicated by the possible effects of suggestion.

Regardless of the time spent for the purpose of acclimatization, whether it be three or four weeks that have been recommended as a minimum for strenuous athletic competition, or whether it be months or even years, an individual's performance at altitude in an event requiring endurance will be inferior to his performance in that event at sea level. The unacclimated person must learn to pace himself more and allow for much longer periods of recovery.

So much for moderate altitudes, ranging from approximately 6,000 to 9,000 feet. Obviously, the higher one ascends, the more serious the problem of decreased maximum oxygen consumption becomes. In aviation, unless the aircraft's cabin is pressurized, personnel are required (or advised) to breathe supplementary oxygen when flying at altitudes above 10,000 feet. At extreme altitudes, such as 30,000 feet and above, the average unacclimatized individual even at rest will become unconscious in a matter of seconds.

Although certain physical performances are hampered by decreased maximum oxygen consumption at high altitudes, man is truly remarkable in his ability to adjust. There are large differences among individuals in that adjustment. Generally speaking, persons can function safely at altitudes up to 10,000 feet. Everyone requires a period of time for the acclimatization process. The length of time is largely dependent upon the individual and upon the type of work the person is going to perform. Individuals have to learn to pace themselves more at altitude than at sea level in physical performances of long duration. Also more time must be allotted for recovery after hard work. Finally, persons who are in good physical condition have an advantage over those less fit at altitude just as in any environment and in almost any situation.—*Jack K. Nelson*

Altitude and Fitness Buffs

What about us ordinary Joes who jog wherever we are, who golf in the Alps and ski in the Andes and hike in the Himalayas? Experts say we should watch our rest, our food, and our activity, as follows:

1. When visiting a high-level city such as Denver or Mexico City, get at least 10 hours sleep at night.

2. Avoid gas-producing foods, such as cabbage, okra, asparagus and cauli-

flower. Lessened air pressure outside the body sometimes allows internal organs to swell to painful proportions.

3. Before going on a high-level business trip or vacation, get in shape. Tests show that a fit man adjusts more quickly and almost never suffers from mountain sickness.

4. After arrival, give yourself two or three days before undertaking golf, jogging, or tennis.

5. When you begin active exercise, hold your speed down by about ten per cent.

6. Don't go for a long swim alone. If exhaustion hits you, as it probably will, you might be in serious trouble.

7. Don't walk or jog on the roads after dark. Don't try to drive, either. Thin air cuts your night vision by about 50 per cent.

8. When you get back home, tackle your favorite sport with renewed vigor. If you're a jogger, slip into your shoes and run your favorite mile route against time. Remember, you are a better man, according to science. Your blood is redder and richer, your nerves are steadier, your endurance is increased. Who knows, maybe you will join the legion of those who have come down the mountain to find wings on their heels.

Such achievements may look like small dividends but consider the ultimate. What is important is that so much Olympic research which involves physicians marks a turn. Traditionally, medical men have been healers, germ-fighters and bone-setters. Suddenly the job has become too big for them. Many of them are realizing that they must deal first with the human body, not with disease, and that they must teach mankind how to grow in health and hardiness.

The body's use of oxygen is fundamental to the life process. To improve that is to improve health. Physicians who work with athletic teams are learning such things. That field is sometimes called sports medicine. But it looks toward a greater goal than winning games.

To send a victorious team to the Olympics is a worthy objective, no doubt, but to create a generation of truly fit men and women, that would be a stroke of genius.—*Curtis Mitchell*

EQUIPMENT

Family fitness trips to the local gymnasium can be lengthy and frustrating. The preparation that is involved in rounding up the family and getting them ready can puncture your good intentions. An ideal solution is to set up a room at home for your personal workout or to utilize the backyard. See BACKYARD FITNESS.

The development of a home fitness room with equipment can be quite expensive if little planning is done, or if equipment is bought without first attempting to see what you really want and need, what should be purchased or made from another piece of equipment.

Finding a Room

Size up your home to find an available area that you can reclaim for your workouts. Maybe you can rearrange the furniture to make available an unused portion of the basement or family room. A vacant bedroom upstairs is ideal. The most important thing is not being held back by lack of space. A patio or breezeway is fine during the summer months. But if your scheme of family fitness is going to take root, you'll have to make provisions for exercise bouts on rainy days or during the winter. That means an indoor workout room.

A room 20 × 15 feet is excellent, but you'll probably have to content yourself with a smaller area, at least in the beginning. You may be lucky enough to have a portion of the house that can use a little "redesigning." If you have a hankering to install permanent pieces of exercise equipment, a section of the house that has old walls or ceiling—like the basement— should rank near the top of your selection list. A key point to keep in mind is that the room environment is only secondary. The finest-looking and most elaborate exercise area is no good if it gets only sporadic use. It is better to have a less elaborate corner of the house that can provide full-time service.

Try to select a place that has adequate ventilation with a sink or washtub nearby for easy cleanup. Be sure the room is accessible to all members of the family.

How to Start

At the beginning it's best to concentrate on simple, strength-building activities. Although strength is not the only by-product you should expect, strength activities are the easiest to set up and get started. A chinning bar may make a simple enough beginning. Commercial *chinning bars* fit neatly

into a handy doorway or between exposed studs. Costing around $8.00, they are really a good investment. If you don't want to invest until you see whether your family will use it, why not take an old piece of pipe (about 1 and ¾ inches in diameter) and nail it securely to the cellar joists. Be certain that it's firm and can support more than it has to. Nail it above a much-traveled line of traffic and you'll find that everyone will want to grab it and swing as they pass. It's just an easy step from there to chin-ups and some degree of upper torso strength and muscle endurance. And don't neglect the more elaborate built-in chinning bars that can be bolted to your walls. Some have adjustable heights so that all ages can benefit.

A natural offshoot of the overhead chinning bar is the *overhead ladder.* It's possible to nail up several chinning bars spaced about two feet apart to form a walkway on the ceiling. Of course, it would be easier to simply

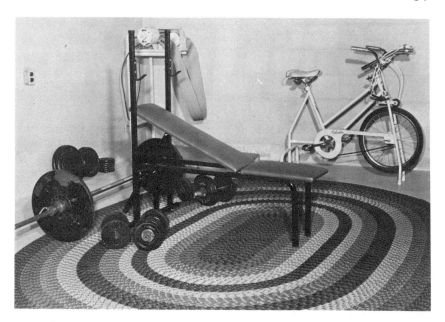

Developing your own home fitness room could be the first step toward a sensible, regular program of family exercise.

take an old, unused, but still reliable wooden ladder with circular rungs and secure a portion of it to the basement ceiling—if possible. Walking with your hands by swinging from rung to rung will speed up muscle strength fast.

If that bit of basement reconstruction gets past the "family censors," you should have no trouble fastening strands of rope to the ceiling for rope-climbing workouts. The rope should be heavy duty and wear resistant and be at least an inch in diameter. And you don't have to have a high ceiling. Even a stairwell makes a neat place for rope activities.

What if a child should fall climbing rope? Put a thick, folded blanket underneath the rope or invest in a home-type gym mat. But don't try to prevent climbing. It's as natural as any other act for growing children. Try to make the fall as painless as possible.

Advanced activities include a spread rope climb, which is done by keeping the legs at a 90-degree angle during the climb, or a double rope climb—two ropes side by side, ascending with one hand on each rope.

Another strength builder to add to your fitness room is the *peg climber,* or peg board. That is a vertically mounted board containing rows of holes spaced about a foot apart. In those holes fit pegs which you use to pull yourself up the board. Place a peg in the hole and then lift yourself up to a position where you can pull the peg out and insert it in the next higher hole. The device is great for the arms, shoulders and upper torso. Although it's possible to build your own out of heavy-duty wood, there are many kinds available commercially.

There are other items you'll want to include in the strength-building section of your exercise room. For example, a *weight training* routine is ideal for building strength. You should have at least 50 pounds of weights to start. A *bench* or *weight rack* makes a handy asset. The racks make a convenient

storage area, and the bench can be used in many lifts—like the bench press.

Circulo-Respiratory Fitness

Incorporating into your exercise room routines or devices which condition the heart and lungs may be a bigger task than providing for strength-building activities. The maneuvers which provide for cardiovascular fitness usually require a larger area. Fast walking, jogging, bicycling, stair climbing, and swimming are many of the sports that keep the heart, lungs, and respiratory systems in good shape. Trying to provide room for activities that will improve your wind might seem an impossible task. But it isn't.

A great gimmick for your exercise room and one that doesn't need the space of a quarter-mile track is *rope skipping.* A level floor and about a 6-foot area for swinging the rope are all that's needed. The family might take to a rope skipping contest. Keep a chart and record of the number of consecutive steps you can make successfully. Dr. Carl K. Ware Rodhl says that most people under 50 years should be able to skip at least 25 consecutive times without missing. But don't stop at 25.

Then, too, if there's room to stand, there's room to run in place. Skipping and running in place are excellent for fitness of the circulatory and respiratory systems. Of course those exercises can be done almost anywhere. Having a room for your exercise, however, provides an added incentive to do them.

Walking is healthy and convenient, but the weather may often force you indoors. When lack of space is a problem, you might consider any one of the several commercial *walking machines* that are available. Consisting of a treadmill-like incline, the walking machines can increase the normal benefits that outdoor walking always provides. Because of the slight incline, walking is slightly more difficult and, therefore, more beneficial.

As the use of your exercise room becomes more frequent, you'll want to add other standard pieces of equipment. Those include *electric cycling-type devices, stationary bicycles, spring tension pulls, Indian clubs, rowing machines, sweat suits* (rubber and cotton), *isometric devices and ropes, hand or grip exercisers,* and other items that fit your interest and needs. Having a specific room is basic to using these products and getting your money out of them.—*Glenn F. Johns*

For more specific details on equipment see BACKYARD FITNESS.

ERGOGENIC AIDS

The recent realization of the importance of physical fitness for a functional and efficient life has resulted in a parallel emphasis of many "ergogenic aids" by people legitimately and illegitimately connected to the health and physical education profession. These aids supposedly assist in the improvement of muscular strength and endurance, and likewise increase the amount of stress that an individual is capable of overcoming. By definition, ergogenic aids simply refer to those foodstuffs, materials, or methods of approach which are capable of improving physical work performance. It is obvious that an ergogenic aid could consist of substances which directly affect the physical body, or it could be some method or technique of mental stimulation which could ultimately improve physical performance.

Perhaps you would immediately classify ergogenic aids in the area of drugs, such as can be used in "doping" a race horse or a track runner. Most certainly, epinephrine and cocaine may have some ergogenic effect; but, the inclusion of such materials is hardly practical and often illegal in your attempt to improve the physical fitness level. The following substances mentioned are more practical and can possibly be included in your daily regimen. The validity of some of these aids is sometimes questioned in recognition of the lack of research evidence in controlled experimental situations.

Diet Control

Much has been written about what an athlete should eat and why he should eat such food. It is most important that you have an adequate diet for growth requirements and for the added expenditure of energy demanded by a physical activity schedule. Dr. T. B. Van Itallie and his associates summarized the diet research quite appropriately when they stated that "the performance of an athlete can be impaired significantly by a faulty or inadequate diet. But, the manipulation of an already adequate diet does not enhance performance."

Wheat Germ

Experimentation with wheat germ, soybean oil, and corn oil has been conducted in the past. It has been claimed that with the extended use of wheat germ, the body builds up a glycogen reserve. Most certainly, if deficiencies are present, wheat germ can assist in partial correction. D. O. Nelson has stated that there is little evidence to support food supplements. Also, even if the diet is inadequate, the money would be more profitably spent on proper food rather than "shot-gunning" vitamins and minerals with the hope of fulfilling some unknown inadequacy.

Vitamins

It would seem logical that a vitamin deficiency can impair physical fitness and performance. That deficiency can be overcome by an adequate diet which provides not only the vitamin needs but other physiological necessities which seem to correspond with vitamin deficiency. The value of an extra supply of vitamins for increased fitness has been experimentally shown to be insignificant in most instances.

Sugar Foods

Since simple sugar furnishes the fuel needed by muscles for their work, it has been assumed that extra amounts of sugar will result in better perform- ance. Various experiments show that in endurance activities sugar does add to performance. It is doubtful if it affects short-duration performance. You should get enough carbohydrates in your regular diet to provide the reserve needed to persist through regular physical activity. Of course, if you do not have the reserve supply readily available, added quantities of sugar foods may help. Dr. J. Mayer and Bullen state that sugar feeding during a long exhausting contest does improve performance. They further state that glucose pills, pieces of sugar or honey, tend to dehydrate the organism. Mayer and Bullen thus recommend the ingestion of strongly sweetened tea with lemon to overcome the difficulty. Athletic coaches frequently recommend candy, soft drinks, and other sugar foods at the half-time break of athletic contests. The psychological effect and improved performance justify their use even if little physiological adjustment actually occurs.

Liquid Nutriments

Liquid diets are used mainly as a means of supplementing regular diets and as a pre-game meal for athletes who experience nausea caused by precontest emotional stress. The value of liquid nutriments is similar to that of other food supplements in that their effectiveness is related to the adequacy of the existing diet and nutrition.

Salt and Water

Physical fitness requires some exercise, which probably results in profuse perspiration. Excessive water loss reduces the water and salt level to the point where exhaustion occurs quite rapidly. Some athletic coaches have expressed their opinion that salt tablets can improve performance. Dr. P. V. Karpovich has stated that the addition of salt to the diet is only a precautionary measure to maintain the normal amount of energy output, which may be lowered if an excessive loss of salt occurs. Obviously, it may be a wise practice to drink water during exercise.

Coffee and Tea

Initially, small amounts of caffeine, as found in coffee and tea, tend to stimulate the central nervous system and the contractile power of the heart. During this initial stimulation, muscular performance may possibly increase. Three to four hours following ingestion, coffee and tea may have a depressing effect and thus could somewhat reduce efficient physical performance levels.

Milk

Athletic coaches often suggest that their players carefully control the intake of milk during days of competition. They state that milk causes difficulty in breathing, produces gas in the stomach, and is high in fat content. Research evidence tends to discount the theory since controlled studies of physical performance one hour following milk consumption showed no significant difference in performance.

Other Erogenic Aids

There are many other physiological aids that may have a "work-producing effect." Most of them are not practical, and some are considered dangerous. You can find experimental evidence related to work output on substances or methods such as hypnosis, oxygen, alcohol, benzedrine, hormones and numerous others.

Psychological Aids to Physical Performance

The majority of the work-producing substances and materials mentioned previously are questionable when you wish to explicitly explain the actual effects on the body organs. However, it would be foolish to completely disregard these aids to performance. Many athletic coaches justifiably use many of these gimmicks because young athletes in the past have obviously responded to them and improved their level of performance. A psychological effect occurs in many people when they eat a dextrose tablet or drink a soft drink before a contest. Mental preparedness for physical activity can offset some strength and endurance limitations, thus producing an effective performance in a game. The use of placebos (an inactive substance) in experimental research often results in a competitor improving his physical performance when he unknowingly believes that he has taken some powerful strength-producing substance. Thus, the psychological advantage of substances which supposedly improve performance are often of great importance.

Other psychological aids which have proved to be valuable are pep talks, cheering, music, signs, slogans, trophies and rewards, and other outside stimulation.

Summary

The previously mentioned ergogenic aids to improve physical fitness are quite illogical when separated from a daily program of physical activity. The search for the easy way to physical fitness must be expected in this sedentary world. Unfortunately, if you are looking for the short-cuts, only one remedy exists; a regular physical exercise program and dietary control. A more meaningful and qualitative life of optimum mental and physical vigor requires a daily regimen of intelligent body discipline.—*Murray Vincent* See ALCOHOL, DIET, DRUGS, NUTRITION and OXYGEN SUPPLEMENT.

EXCESSIVE EXERCISE

"Too much exercise is a bad thing; it wears you out, puts a dangerous strain on your heart and lungs, overdevelops your muscles, leads to heart attacks, causes athletes to die younger and burns up extra energy." Even though these comments are quite familiar, today's trend is away from condemning exercise. Vigorous, progressive exercise is good for the human body. But what about excessive exercise? Is too much exercise dangerous to the body? How much in exercise is considered excessive?

Excesses Can Be Fatal

Pushbuttons, elevators, automobiles, power mowers, power tools, golf carts, all combine to rob the typical American male of the exercise he needs. The pace of life in our time seems to demand that he play hard when he has the time. Heart specialists, however, warn of strain put on the entire body, particularly on the arteries and heart, by men *who seldom exercise* and then violently. It can be fatal.

Theodore Irwin canvassed a representative group of medical men on the effects of overstrain, and the verdict is unanimous. For the rare person who is in perfect physical condition, for the professional boxer, the distance runner, the gymnast, overstrain is not harmful. He can push strength and endurance a notch higher. But for the typical citizen the occasional overstrain can be very dangerous. Irwin's consultants report that most of 5,000 fatal cardiac cases investigated occurred at the beginning of the week, immediately after a period of likely overstrain. The circulatory system needs to be conditioned, worked gradually to the point where it can cope with a 100-yard plus sprint around the bases, a run of three miles, or an hour or two of tennis. Massive loads put on hearts, unconditioned to such effort, are foolhardy.

Doctors agree also that women are less prone to heart disease than men, possibly because of exercise. Despite the rash of labor-saving devices introduced into the home, the average housewife and mother still is on the move all day long. In reality the ladies' children and household chores keep them from degenerative ailments. Also, few women feel compelled to be a weekend athlete.

Exercise Sensibly

The answer, doctors suggest, is not "don't exercise," but "exercise sensibly." A little exercise every day is good; a lot once a week is very bad. Likewise, once the decision is made to exercise regularly, a moderate and gradual approach is best, for years of sedentary living may have softened you more than you realize. The next morning you may find it virtually impossible to get out of bed because of the aches and pains. Go slow at first. You can't rebuild in a day or two what you have allowed to deteriorate over a period of years.

The best way to get started is by walking. Many heart specialists recommend that technique. It's single, safe and enjoyable. Dr. Herman K. Hellerstein of the University Hospital of Cleveland walks six miles every day. Dr. Theodore G. Klumpp, president of Winthrop Laboratories, advises, "One, walk three times as much as you're walking now. Two, walk three times that much, three times as fast." Dr. Paul D. White, heart surgeon for the late President Eisenhower, recommends walking but prefers bicycling for himself. All three stress that the walk should be brisk but that the beginner should build up to his own proper rate of walking.

Success is not achieved overnight; it will take the average person 6 to 8 weeks to demonstrate a significant improvement in fitness and 6 months to achieve a high level of strength and endurance. Following the principles

set forth under CONTINUOUS RHYTHMICAL EXERCISE and TRAINING will help you greatly in establishing your exercise program. When high levels of fitness are achieved, the dangers of overexertion are not so great.

Detrimental Exercises

There are several types of popular exercises that are to be avoided because of the possibility of their doing more harm than good. There is a great deal of controversy over the use of the following exercises; but we feel that, on the basis of the current research and reasoning, they should be avoided. There are other exercises that can be used just as effectively to accomplish the same results without causing damage to the body.

1. *Toe Touches*—Any exercise that involves a trunk bend with the legs straight either standing or sitting can be detrimental. The traditional exercises are standing toe touches and sitting and bending from the waist with the legs straight, such as trying to lower the forehead to the knees.

These exercises place undue force and strain on the discs of the spine in the small of the back, causing disc rupture and tissue damage. Many times these exercises are done to improve the muscle tone of the abdomen. In reality, however, they do not. Their prime function is to stretch the hamstrings of the leg (back leg muscles) and the muscles of the low back. Other exercises just as effective and yet not so dangerous are high kicks for hamstrings and sit-ups with the knees bent for the abdominal muscles.

2. *Deep Knee Bends*—Any exercise that makes a person assume a forced squat position is dangerous, especially with weights or with one leg.

Although these exercises are great for building strength of the leg, they cause a stretching of the medial and lateral collateral ligaments and anterior cruciate ligaments of the knees. Abnormal pressure is placed on cartilages.

Since the ligaments are the first line of defense in knee stability and function, the above exercises are considered dangerous and should be modified.

Half squat or one-leg squats should be used. Several isometric and weight training exercises can also be used effectively. See KNEE.

3. *Leg Lifts*—Avoid exercises involving leg lifts in a reclining position, especially those elevated 6 to 24 inches and held. Until recently leg lifts were recommended for abdominal strengthening. But careful analysis of the anatomy of the trunk muscles reveals that the muscles from the pelvis to the thighs (internal muscles) do the most work. These hip flexors, as they are called, pull the front of the pelvis down and the back up. In effect, the pelvis has rotated. This rotation can place pressure on the lower back, thereby aggravating the low back area. Leg lifts can be beneficial for the highly trained person because he is able to stabilize the pelvis.

4. *Straight Leg Sit-ups*—These exercises have also been used to strengthen the abdominal muscles. But like the leg lifts they too cause a rotation of the pelvis, aggravating the lower back and causing low back pain. Again, the finely conditioned person may be able to perform the exercise without injury.

In the place of the leg lifts and straight leg sit-ups do the abdominal contraction, the curl-up and the V-seat. All three of these exercises may be done without danger of injuring the lower back, yet they contribute greatly to the abdominal strength.

5. *Prone Arch*—The prone arch has been used to strengthen the muscles of the lower back. But a sedentary person performing this exercise may develop a lower back injury rather than the desired back musculature. The prone arch can be performed, but it should be done gradually. Instead of raising your chest and legs such a distance from the floor, start out by raising the chest only a few inches and gradually progress from that point.

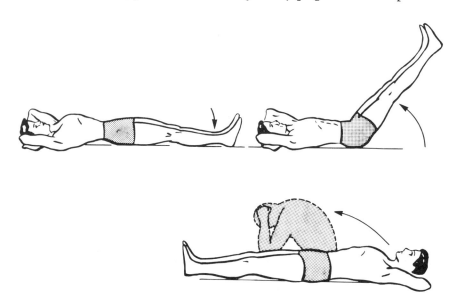

These exercises *will* hurt you. Both the reclining leg lift (above) and the straight leg sit-up (below) rotate the pelvis and place pressure on the low back area.

Signs of Excessive Exercise

The overall axiom is that if you feel other than pleasantly tired following exercise and are fatigued the rest of the day, ease up. There are certain definite signs indicating that your exercise level is execessive for your current physical condition.

1. Marked fatigue following exercise, rather than a relaxed feeling.

2. Insomnia as a direct result of the exercise.

3. Hang-over fatigue the next day and the inability to get going.

4. Higher resting pulse rate.

5. Very sore muscles. There will be some degree of soreness; but when the pain is great and restricts proper movement, then the exercise is excessive.

Summary

It has often been stated that exercise can not harm the healthy heart. However, today many hearts are not healthy because of sedentary living and rich diets. It is necessary to consult your family physician before engaging in an exercise program to determine your current health status. It is also a good idea to discuss your intended exercise program with him.

Once your exercises or activities are selected, try to engage in them at least 4 times a week. Avoid exercising only on weekends. Take some time off during the week, or set some time aside for regular, vigorous exercise, thereby avoiding excessive weekend exercise. Remember that common sense is your best guide in exercising. Use your own judgment to slow up or even stop when you show signs of excessive fatigue or physical distress.

Exercise is an excellent preventative measure against cardiovascular disease, but be certain that your program does not defeat its purpose. Keep your program moderate, progressive and enjoyable. See INTENSITY OF EXERCISE, PRETRAINING, PULSE RATE and ENERGY COST OF ACTIVITIES.

EXCRETORY SYSTEM

The major organ in the excretory system is the kidney. The kidneys filter the blood (about one fourth of the blood is filtered per minute) and excrete water, excess materials, and waste products, such as urea, uric acid and creatinine.

Dr. Laurence G. Wesson, Jr., noted that during exercise blood flow to the kidneys is reduced, therefore filtering less blood. The reason for the reduced blood flow is that the body adjusts to the exercise by taking blood away from the organs that can spare it, in order to give exercising muscles extra blood for more efficient movement. The blood flow to the kidneys is reduced in proportion to the severity of the exercise; sometimes more than one-half. Since less blood is sent to the kidneys, less urine is formed. Urea, creatinine, and phosphate excretion are decreased moderately because of decreased glomerular filtration. Sodium chloride decrease is more marked as a result of the filtration.

After cessation of exercise, blood flow and glomerular filtration return to the level prior to exercise. In moderately severe exercise the process may take an hour. Urea, creatinine, and sodium chloride excretion also return close to the normal level in the same period of time. The phosphate excretion, however, rises markedly immediately after exercise but returns to normal after an hour or so.

The rate of urine flow after exercise increases measurably, especially if the person has taken on water. Protein substances may also be present in the urine but the condition is not permanent. See ALBUMINURIA.

EXERCISE

THE PHYSICAL FITNESS ENCYCLOPEDIA might appropriately have been called the ENCYCLOPEDIA OF EXERCISE because of the main interest in exercise and its contribution to the attainment of physical fitness. But exercise, no matter how important, is not the panacea for all your ills. You need a happy balance between rest, relaxation, work and exercise. You need to know, understand and apply diet and nutrition to daily living. You must learn that you cannot divorce one part of the body from the other. Your mental, social, moral and physical being is wrapped up into one big package. Each is just as important as the other, each affecting and directing the other. You are a total being, not a series of compartments that can be nicely separated for microscopic examination.

Exercise plays a major role in the attainment of physical fitness, for through the complex mechanisms of the body, it affects all the body systems. In our mechanized society, however, man has exercised less and less through the ages. Today he is no longer the vigorous being he was created to be.

As a result, many new ailments arc plaguing man that at one time were of trivial importance. Tremendous strides in science have been made to help man live better, but he is still surrounded by diseases that cut his life short and rob him of his vigor.

We can draw an analogy from the wild animal that is captured and placed in a zoo. When it arrives, it is a vigorous, muscular animal. When it dies, it is sluggish and fat. Man, too, is like that caged animal. At one time he had to fight for his existence physically —for protection and for food. Today our mechanized society has robbed him of any physical challenge. The tragedy is that man's body has not changed. It is still the same basic organism it was 4,000 or more years ago when man walked to work or toiled in the fields; yet his activity level, in Western society, at least, has dropped to almost zero.

Man has not yet devised a solution or an artificial substitute for the many benefits of regular exercise. The body is geared for vigorous action; and use, not disuse, is of paramount importance. Without it the organism will decay.

See BENEFITS OF EXERCISE, EFFECTS OF EXERCISE, HYPOKINETIC DISEASE and PHYSICAL FITNESS.

EXERCISES

Introduction

Whether you realize it or not, you exercise in some way every day. You do knee bends or toe touches to pick something off the floor, perform stretching exercises to reach the top shelf, do a modified form of bar dips to get up from the desk, execute a form of bench stepping when climbing stairs, and perform many other exercises too numerous to mention.

The fact is, however, that because of a sedentary, automated way of life you do not do enough of the stooping, bending and stretching to fulfill certain physiological functions. Specific exercises, on the other hand, can provide you with an opportunity for active movement so necessary to help maintain good physiological performance.

Types of Exercises

There are two types of general exercises that may be performed by an individual. The first type is *free exercises* or *calisthenics*. These are the exercises that are associated with one's "daily dozen" or warm-up. The second type is performed with apparatus and often associated with gymnastic stunts, such as pull-ups. See also WEIGHT TRAINING and ISOMETRICS.

Calisthenics or Free Exercises

Free exercises have been performed for many centuries dating back to early Egypt and China. Perhaps the only development of those exercises through the years has been the knowledge of man to classify certain exercises with areas or muscles of the body and to determine that some exercises are not as beneficial as others or that some may be harmful.

Calisthenics or free exercises have different meanings to various people. To some they are a drudgery or a waste of valuable energy, to others a tension release and/or an exhilarating experience, and to still others something to be endured for getting into and remaining in good physical condition.

Advantages and Drawbacks of Calisthenics

We should recognize, however, that calisthenics are a convenient and economical means of establishing an exercise program, since no equipment is necessary, and the space required is at a minimum.

As with any exercise program, the reasons why people select free exercises as a means of developing physical fitness vary considerably. Some of the reasons are (1) calisthenics are relatively easy to learn and to perform; (2) very little equipment and a minimum of space are required; (3) vigorous workouts can be established in a short period of time; (4) almost all muscles or muscle groups can be developed; (5) free exercises can be performed alone or with a group.

The major drawback of calisthenics is that if they are used for a long period of time, the performer may become bored and find them monotonous. Furthermore, he may find it difficult to overload a muscle group for development of muscle strength with some of the exercises.

Variance of Skill and Muscle Endurance

Dr. Donald F. Mapes at Western Illinois University has devised a simple technique for helping a person utilize the overload principle with calisthenic exercises. The major problem with calisthenics is that we all have varying

degrees of strength and muscle endurance. As a result, when we are told to do 10 push-ups we all have a different response to the exercise. For some, it is too easy, and the gain is little; for others it is just right, or for still others it is too difficult, even impossible. To help combat this inequality Dr. Mapes has used a rather simple technique for overloading the muscles with calisthenics.

The illustration that we are using here is the push-up, but any exercise might serve when using calisthenics to develop muscle strength. See MUSCLE ENDURANCE and STRENGTH.

To execute the traditional push-up, lie prone on the floor with your feet together and your hands underneath your shoulders. Keeping the body straight, extend the arms until you are supporting your body with only your hands and your toes. Then return to the starting position. Your chest is to touch the floor. Most of you know about this push-up, but there are many more, all of which can be placed in a logical progression to allow development of strength.

The secret is using your body weight and using it correctly. The basic idea is that if you are unable to do a regular push-up, you are to support more of your body weight with your legs than with your arms and shoulders. Conversely, if you find the traditional push-up easy, you are to support more of your weight with your arms and shoulders than with your feet.

The simplest push-up is the *wall push-up*. Stand facing a wall and lean against it with both hands. Push yourself away until your hands leave the wall, then fall back toward the wall until your face is about an inch away. Your feet are to be 24 inches away from the wall. If you can't do 10 push-ups at this level, do not do any other type of push-ups until you can. Remember if you can do more than 10 you are then starting to build muscle endurance rather than muscle strength.

To help assist you in your strength development it is a good idea to do the exercises in sets. In this instance 10 repetitions represent one set. You should be able to do 3 sets of 10 repetitions before progressing to the next push-up.

The next exercise is also a wall push-up, only a little more stress is placed on the arms and shoulders than was placed on these muscles for the first push-up. Stand about 30 to 36 inches away from the wall. The same procedure as before is followed—3 sets of 10 repetitions must be performed before you are allowed to progress to the next level. Some people will find that it will take them several weeks to progress from one level to the next. Gradually you lower the body until you are in the traditional push-up position. Once you are there and are able

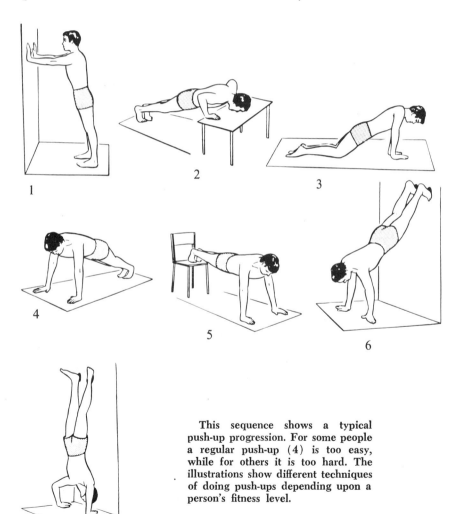

This sequence shows a typical push-up progression. For some people a regular push-up (4) is too easy, while for others it is too hard. The illustrations show different techniques of doing push-ups depending upon a person's fitness level.

to do 3 sets of 10 push-ups, then it is time to place greater emphasis on the arms and shoulders. With each step less weight is placed on the legs and more is placed on the arm and shoulder musculature. The hardest push-up of all is the hand-stand push-up. The figures below show a logical progression of push-up for strength development. Note that at the outset almost all the weight is on the feet. Gradually, the weight shifts until all the weight is on the arms and shoulders. The figures are only a few of the many push-ups. Dr. Mapes has reported that one of his students devised 100+ types of push-ups.

The above procedure can also be applied for muscle endurance. But instead of doing 3 sets of 10, do 3 sets of 30.

All the exercises listed in the following calisthenics section may be modified for both strength and muscle-endurance performance. Some are more readily adapted than others, but adjustments can be made. Do not think that since only 46 calisthenic-type exercises are presented, these are the only ones to be performed. We are all individuals with different abilities. Adapt the exercise to your needs.

There are literally hundreds of free exercises that you can choose from to establish your exercise program. Although many of these exercises are excellent, some leave something to be desired. Furthermore, exercises that may be beneficial for one person may be harmful to another. Care is important in the selection of exercises. The description of the exercises presented at the end of this section are some of the better free exercises. The criteria used to select these exercises were popularity, simplicity, usefulness and convenience in classification. An individual appraisal is necessary, however, before you select any of these exercises.

Free exercises are classified according to purpose, i.e., flexibility, muscle endurance and strength, and circulo-respiratory endurance; and to body areas, i.e., neck and shoulder. Flexibility exercises are those that involve bending and stretching to increase the range of motion of various joints. Strength exercises involve repetitive movements of the various muscle groups. The circulo-respiratory exercises feature rapid movements of the limbs over an extended period of time.

Guidelines to Follow

When performing calisthenics, follow several guidelines to achieve the optimal benefit from the exercises.

1. Always follow correct form.
2. Perform a variety of exercises (at least 10 to 15).
3. Follow a definite rhythm or cadence.
4. Increase systematically to ultilize the overload principle.
5. Initially, exercise the various parts of the body in turn, i.e., one set of exercises for the neck, the shoulders, etc. Later on, when a higher level of fitness is achieved, exercise specific areas extensively with a series of exercises.
6. Evaluate yourself to determine if you have any physical handicaps that may limit the performing of some exercises.
7. Increase the intensity of the free exercises. Merely doing more exercises or a greater number of repetitions of a certain exercise is not the only means of increasing the intensity of the exercise. For example, you may try to do a limited number of exercises in a certain amount of time, and literally race against the clock as a runner would in attempting to lower his time; or modify the exercise so that it is more difficult. See CIRCUIT TRAINING, INTERVAL TRAINING and PROGRAMS.

Calisthenics—Flexibility

Neck:
1. Head Flexor—Assume a standing position with your arms at your sides.

Flex the head forward by dropping the chin to your chest. Then extend the head backward as far as possible.

2. Head Circles—In a standing position tilt the head backward and then turn it to the left side, front, right side, and back again. Attempt to turn the head as far as possible. Be careful to avoid injury. Do the exercise gradually.

Shoulder and Upper Back:

3. Arm Circles—Standing with your feet slightly apart, rotate your arms backward in full circles, first with your right arm, then your left. For variation rotate the arms forward or perform the circle while bending from the waist. Start either exercise with small circles and gradually increase.

4. Arm Flexors—Stand with your feet almost a foot apart and arms flexed at the elbows and shoulder height. Force the elbows backwards for three counts; on the fourth count, extend the arms as they are thrown backwards. Then start the count over again.

5. Arms Over—Assume a standing position with the arms at the sides of the body. Gradually raise the arms at right angles to the body and move them above the head until the hands meet. Arms are to be kept straight throughout the entire movement. Palms may be turned either in or out.

6. Arms Back (1)—Assume a standing or reclining (face down) position on the floor. Extend the arms above the head so that the arms are straight. Push the arms backwards as far as possible.

7. Arms Back (2)—Assume a standing position, arms at the sides of the body. Push the arms backward and upward, keeping them straight. A variation is to bend at the waist while performing the exercise.

Wrist:

8. Wrist Flexion-Extension—Assume a standing position with the arms extended to the sides and the palms facing forward. Extend the wrist as far as possible and then flex the wrists. Although the wrist flexion-extension exercise is a relatively easy one, don't neglect it.

Trunk: (hip area)

9. Thigh Flexion—Lying flat on the floor, bend the left knee toward the chest and wrap the arms around the flexed knee, pulling it to the chest. Keep the right leg flat on the floor and then change legs. You can also stand to do this exercise, but be certain to keep the back straight. Thigh flexion also aids leg flexibility.

10. Alternate Leg Raise—Lie face down on the floor, with the arms on the outside of the thighs, palms up. Raise the right leg as high as possible. Return, then raise the left; continue alternating. During the exercise keep the chest and hips on the floor.

11. Bouncer—Assume a push-up position. Arch the back by pressing the hips toward the floor. *People with low back trouble must not perform this exercise.*

12. Sprinter's Stretch—Assume a sitting position with the right leg extended in front of the body and the left leg bent at the knee. The lower left leg should be extended backwards. Bend forward from the waist and try to come forward as far as possible. Repeat with the left leg stretched out in front and the right leg in back. This exercise also contributes to low back flexibility.

13. Mountain Climber Stretch—From a squat position place both hands on the floor, arms outside the knees. Extend the left leg backwards keeping the knee and back straight. The right knee remains bent. Push the left knee toward the floor so that a pull is felt in the groin area. Repeat several times then change legs.

14. Leg Raiser—Assume a left-side lying position, the left arm extended above the head with the head resting on that arm. Place the right arm in

front of the waist for stability. Raise the top leg (right) upwards as high as possible. Return. Repeat on the other side.

Low Back:

15. Forward Bend—Sit on the floor with the legs stretched out in front. Keeping the legs straight and flat on the floor, bend forward as far as possible. Arms may be locked behind the head, but that's optional. The forward bend also aids leg flexibility. People with low back pain should perform this exercise with caution or avoid it entirely.

16. Double Knees-Up—Lie flat on the floor, face up. Keeping the small of the back on the floor, curl the knees up to the chest. Lock the arms around the shins and try to draw the knees up to the chin. *Keep the small of the back on the floor.*

17. Back Arch—Assume a kneeling position with the hands on the floor. Arch the back toward the floor, then hump the back as an angry cat would do. Return to the original position.

Legs:

18. Stretch—Standing straight, fold both arms across the chest. Cross the right leg over in front of the left. Bend over as far as possible. Repeat with the other leg. People with low back pain should not perform the exercise unless checked by a physician.

19. Toe Raise—Assume a standing position with the left leg in contact with the floor and the right leg bent at the knee. Raise up on the toes as high as possible and return. On the way down bend forward slightly. Repeat and change legs.

20. Ankle Stretch—Assume a standing stride position with the left foot about two feet in front of the right foot. Bend the left knee and lean the body forward. Keep the right leg straight with the heel on the floor. You should feel tension on the calf muscle. Reverse the position and repeat.

Muscle Strength and Endurance

Shoulders, Chest, and Arms:

21. Push-up—Assume a prone position on the floor with the feet together and the hands underneath the shoulders. Keeping the body straight, extend the arms and return to the starting position.

22. Side Leaning Leg Raiser—Assume a position in which the left foot and the left hand support the body in a side position. Then raise the right or top leg upward as high as possible. Return. Perform on the other side.

23. Forearm Press-ups—Lie face down, arms fully extended with the forearms on the floor. Keeping the body straight, press upward until only the toes and the forearms touch the floor.

Back:

24. Upper Body Arch—Lie flat on the floor, chest down with the hands beside the body. Lift the upper body from the floor so that the rib cage is completely off the floor. Return.

25. Body Arch—Assume the same position in Exercise 24. Then raise the chest and legs off the floor so that only the pelvic area touches. Return.

26. Flutter Kicks—Assume the same position in Exercises 24 and 25. Kick the legs straight and the upper body on the floor. Vary the speed of the exercise.

27. Heel Slide—Lie flat on the back with the fingers interlocked behind the head. Pull both knees to the chest. After the legs are drawn up, gradually lower the legs and straighten them at the same time.

28. Chest Lifts—Assume a position in which the heels and the hands support the body. The back faces the floor and the body is kept straight. Bounce the midsection up and down vigorously.

Abdomen and Hip Flexors:

29. Abdominal Compression—Stand

or lie on the floor with the arms at the sides of the body. Contract the stomach muscles as much as possible, so that you feel as though the stomach is going all the way to the backbone. To make the exercise more difficult, exhale as you draw the stomach in and inhale as you release.

30. Abdominal Curl—Lie flat on the back with the lower back touching the floor. Curl the head and upper part of the body upward and forward to about 45° angle. At the same time, contract your abdominal muscles. Return slowly to the starting position. For extra benefit on the abdomen, bend your knees.

31. Curl Down—Start from a sitting position with the knees bent and the hands placed behind the head. Slowly lower the upper body to a 45° angle. Hold that position and return.

32. V-Seat—Sit on the floor with the hands interlocked behind the head, the legs off the floor and the body resting on the buttocks. Hold a V-position and return.

33. Sit-up—Interlace the fingers behind the head while lying on the back. Put the heels close to the buttocks with the knees together. You may need assistance to hold the feet down. Attempt to sit up and touch the right elbow to the left knee and return. Repeat with the left elbow to the right knee. If the exercise is too difficult, do not bend the knees as much. Another technique is to do the sit-ups with the legs straight.

34. Rowing Curl—Lie flat on the back with the arms extended overhead. Curl the head and upper body forward. At the same time bring the arms forward and bend the knees.

Note: In Exercises 30, 33 and 34 be certain that the back is curled up, so that the lower back is not aggravated.

Sit-ups are done many times on an incline board. The board positions the body so that additional stress is placed on the abdominal muscles during exercise.

35. Alternate Knee Kicks—Sit with the legs extended and the hands resting on the floor next to the hips or on the hips. Lift the right leg slightly off the floor and bend the leg so that it almost touches the buttocks; return. As you return the right leg, start to bring the left leg toward the buttocks.

36. Trunk Rotations—Either sitting or standing place the hands behind the head. Twist the upper part of the body to the left as far as it can go; then rotate to the right.

Legs:

37. Half Squat—Assume a standing position with both hands on the hips or locked behind the head. Bend the knees and drop to a half-bent knee position; return. To make the exercise more demanding, stand on the left leg and extend the right. Then do a ½ knee bend with the left leg. Return. Repeat with the other leg.

38. Scissors—Lie flat on the back with the arms perpendicular to the body. Keeping the legs straight throughout, touch the right foot to the left hand; return, and then touch the left foot to the right hand.

39. Toe Curls—Stand with the hands on the hips and feet about one to two feet apart. Pretend that you are attempting to crumble a newspaper with your toes.

40. Inverted Bicycle—Lie flat on the back and raise both legs up into the air. Place the hands at the small of the back to give support. The entire body weight is supported by the head, the shoulders, and the back of upper arms. In that position, vigorously pedal your legs as you would a bicycle.

For other leg exercises see the circulo-respiratory exercises below.

Circulo-Respiratory

The circulo-respiratory exercises, in general, involve the entire human organism. Some may be more vigorous than others; but they all involve gross body movements that dramatically increase pulse and breathing rates.

41. Running-in-Place—Run in place lifting the feet at least 4 inches off the floor. For greater stress lift the knees higher to waist height.

42. Jumping Jacks (Side-Straddle Hops)—Start by standing erect, feet together, arms at the sides. In a single motion jump off the ground spreading the feet and raising the arms. Land with the feet about 3 feet apart and the hands above the head. Return by reversing action.

43. Mountain Climbers—Assume a push-up position. Bring the right leg up underneath the chest with the knee bent. Extend the left leg backwards. Then switch legs and continue alternating.

44. Squat Thrust (Burpee)—Assume a standing position. Then squat down with both knees, placing the hands between the knees. On the next count extend the legs backwards, so a push-up position is assumed. On the third count bring the legs back up to the squat position. Then stand. If you have knee difficulty, avoid the exercise.

45. Squat Jumps—Stand with one foot forward and one foot back and hands resting on top of the head. Lower to a full squat, keeping the back straight. From that position jump upward by straightening the legs. Switch the legs in the air. Come to a standing position. Then repeat. If you have knee difficulty, avoid the exercise.

46. Bear Hugs—Stand erect with the feet comfortably apart, hands on the legs. Step diagonally with the right foot, taking a long step. Bend the trunk toward the right knee and wrap both arms around the right thigh. Keep the left leg on the floor. Return to the standing position. Repeat to the other side. See CALISTHENICS.

Exercises With Apparatus

Exercises with apparatus involve such equipment as ropes, rings, side horse, horizontal bars, parallel bars, horizontal ladders, peg boards and climbing poles. For the most part these exercises are concerned with developing the musculature of the arms and shoulder girdle, an area of the body that is often poorly developed in modern man.

These exercises are often more difficult than the free exercises and may require more time to learn. Take care to learn elementary stunts before the more difficult. Spotting and assistance is necessary, especially in the early stages.

Hanging Exercises

The hanging-type exercises develop the musculature of the upper arms, shoulders and upper back.

You may feel that you do not have sufficient equipment to perform all these exercises. A little ingenuity, however, can help overcome that obstacle. See BACKYARD FITNESS EQUIPMENT and FAMILY FITNESS for some ideas of what may be done with odds and ends around the house.

Note: In all of these exercises place a mat or some other soft substance on the ground to prevent injury in case of a fall.

Ropes:

47. Climbing Ropes—Climbing rope develops a strong grip together with musculature of the upper arms, shoulders and upper back.

There is a logical progression to follow in climbing a rope. Begin by using a *leg lock*. Start out by grasping the rope with both hands in an overhead position; stand with the rope between the leg. Wrap the rope around the right leg and cross it over the instep of the same foot. Then flex the hips and draw the legs upward, allowing the rope to glide around the right leg and foot. Step with the left foot on the right instep. Straighten the body and flex the arms. At the same time, cross the hands over one another. Repeat until the desired height is reached. Reverse the procedure for coming down. The next step is to use the *foot lock*. Here assume the same stance as before but place the rope on the outside of the right leg. Put the rope under the right foot and over the instep of the left. The movements are the same as in the leg lock except that the knees are held out in front of the body when they are flexed. Also squeeze the sole of the right foot against the rope and the instep of the left foot.

The third step in the progression is the *scissors*. Here the rope is trapped between the thighs, calves, or feet. The other movements are similar to those of the leg lock but they require more strength of the arms and shoulders.

Finally, attempt the *hands only* climb. Grasp the hands in an overhead position and jump upward, pulling with both hands and flexing the arms as much as possible. Then release the bottom hand and grasp the rope above the top hand. Repeat in that fashion.

Rings:

Exercises on the rings may be of a hang or support-type nature. Generally, the hanging activities are easier and should be attempted first.

Hang-Type Exercises:

48. Hang and Swing—Jump up and grasp the rings; hang in an extended position. Now, by flexing and extending the leg, swing back and forth, keeping the arms straight.

49. Inverted Hang—From a hanging position swing the legs upward so that the legs are above the head between the rings and rope.

50. Chin-up—From a hanging position, flex the arms and pull yourself up so that the chin is above the bottom of the rings.

51. Skin the Cat—Grasp the rings and swing the legs up. Rotate your legs between your arms and into an extended position behind you, until your toes are pointing down. Then reverse the steps.

These are but a few of the hang-type ring exercises that may be attempted.

Support-Type Exercises:

These exercises develop the triceps muscles and the muscles of the shoulders, chest, upper back and abdomen. They are usually extremely difficult.

52. Support—Jump up until you are supporting all your weight with your straight arms, which are near the sides of your body.

Side Horse:

The side horse is a difficult piece of apparatus. Remember that while performing the arms should be extended and the shoulders should remain over the hands of support.

53. Front-Support Position—Place the hands on the pommels of the horse, jump up to a support position.

54. Single-Leg-Half-Circle—From a front-support position, with the thighs resting against the horse, swing both legs to the left. On the return swing, swing the extended right leg to the right, raise it, and bring it forward over the end of the horse. Release the right hand, bring the right leg in front of the center of the horse, and regrasp with the right hand. Then reverse the action to get back.

55. Double-Leg-Half-Circle—From a front-support position swing both legs to the right. On the return swing keep the legs together and pass them over the side of the horse as was done in the Single Leg, except that both legs move around. Once the legs are over the horse, regrasp and hold in a rear-support position. Reverse to get back.

Parallel Bars:

Parallel bars utilize either support or hang-type activities.

56. Support—Stand at the end of the parallel bars and place both hands on the bars. Then jump to a support position. Your body should be perpendicular to the bars.

57. Forward-Backward Hand Walk —Assume a support position (straight-arm cross-support) as described above. Then keeping the body straight, alternately move the hands down the bars. When you are at the end, return by coming backward.

58. Dips—Assume a support position. Flex the arms, lower the body as low as possible, and then raise until the arms are extended. Repeat as often as possible.

59. Half-Lever—Assume a support position. Keeping the arms straight, raise the legs to a right-angle position. Hold for several seconds and return.

Horizontal Bar:

The horizontal bar is placed parallel to the floor, one to two feet above your reach. For the more advanced stunts, start out with the bar at chest height.

60. Flexed Arm-Hang—Place both hands, palms away, on the bar and pull yourself to eye-level, arms shoulder-width apart. If you cannot pull yourself up, have someone put you there. Hold that position as long as possible.

61. Pull-up—Place both hands on the bar, palms away. By flexing your arms pull yourself upward until your chin is above the bar; lower yourself till your arms are fully extended.

A variation, called a chin-up, has the palms facing you when you execute the action. Here the grip must be wider, and as you come up thrust your head forward so that the back of your neck touches.

62. Belly Grinder—Grasp the bar, palms away, and hang beneath the bar. Pull yourself upward by flexing the arms. At the same time, raise the extended legs to the bar, flexing the hips. Extend the head backward, continue to pull upward, and slide the legs up and over the bar until a front-support position is reached.

Exercises done on the rings such as skin-the-cat may also be attempted.

Horizontal Ladder:

Like the horizontal bar, most of the horizontal ladder activities are of the hanging type. The ladder is mounted parallel to the floor, one to two feet above your grasp.

63. Ladder Walk—Jump to a hanging position. Then move hand-over-hand from one rung to another.

64. Half-lever—Jump to a hanging position. Then raise the legs to an L position. Hold for several seconds and return.

Peg Boards:

A peg board is a vertically mounted board that contains two or more rows of holes which are spaced from 6 to 18 inches apart. The holes are about one to one-and-a-half inches in diameter. Two removable wooden pegs are placed in these holes.

65. Peg Climb—With arms and legs straight, grasp a peg in each hand. Then pull yourself upward and attempt to hold yourself in that position with the right hand as you pull the other peg out of its hole and into one above the right peg. Then pull up with the left hand, take the right peg out, and place that in the hole above the left peg. Continue upward in that manner to the desired height. Then return by reversing the pattern.

In all of these exercises it is advisable to work in pairs, one person performing and the other spotting and assisting.

Summary

Free exercises have no particular superiority over exercises on apparatus. You may select either method or a combination of the two depending upon your needs, interests, abilities, and/or facilities. The exercises presented here should serve as a guide for you to select exercises for the development of certain areas of the body, and should provide you with a reference point for the performance and evaluation of other exercises.

EXTENSION

The body's 600+ muscles are really cables which pull on the bones to move the body. For movement to occur, the muscles must contract; and to make motion efficient and smooth, the muscles work in pairs. For example, one muscle may contract to pull a bone forward, while the opposite muscle will contract to pull the bones backward.

Extensor muscles are those muscles that cause extension at any joint when any body segment is moved in a front to back plane. Extensors increase the angle of a joint between the front surfaces of the bones. For example, if you are standing in what is called an anatomical position (the position of the body hanging from a hook, with the arms and legs dangling freely and the palms of the hands facing forward), the body limbs would be in extension. Assuming that the knees had been brought to the chest, the movement of straightening the legs would be called extension. Some of the more well-known extensors of the body are the trapezium and the latissimus dorsi, which extend the upper arm; the triceps brachii which extend the lower arm; the gluteus maximus which extends the thigh; the quadriceps femoris group which extends the lower leg; the gastrocnemius and soleus which extend the foot; and the sacrospinalis which extends the back. The opposite of extension is flexion. The muscles that reverse the movement of the extensors are called *flexors*. See FLEXION. For a related discussion see ABDUCTION and MUSCLES, SKELETAL and ADDUCTION. The total movement of muscles is controlled by the brain and spinal cord. See NEUROMUSCULAR SYSTEM.

FACE AND HEAD

Women are very much concerned about their facial appearance. They apply all types of creams, lotions, and make-up to help make their face more beautiful. They use all kinds of straps and aids to help remove or prevent wrinkles. Every year billions of dollars are spent on facial cosmetics and similar aids.

The same women, however, fail to realize that facial exercises can aid them greatly in improving their facial appearance.

Exercise and Facial Appearance

The appearance of your face is highly dependent upon the muscles of the face. If your facial muscles are unused, they become loose and sag. The exercises that follow will aid in firming those muscles and help make lines and wrinkles disappear. But for these exercises to be effective they must be

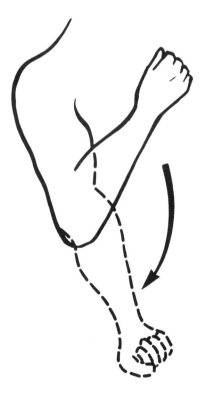

Extension is the straightening of a joint in a back to front vertical plane.

done every day. Try to get into the habit of doing them several times a day, and soon they will become part of your daily routine.

The principal muscle of the scalp is the occipitofrontalis. It is a broad sheet that covers the upper part of the head from the eyebrows to the back of the head. The muscle is considered to have two functions: (1) the occipitalis tends to fix or tighten the sheet covering the head, (2) the *frontalis* wrinkles the forehead.

Here is the exercise that helps to smooth out wrinkles of the forehead and to stimulate the scalp muscles. Raise the eyebrows and forehead as high as you can, so that you feel the movement of the scalp. Then frown by bringing your eyebrows down as

far as you can. Repeat vigorously 15 to 25 times.

The orbicularis oculi is composed of muscle fibers that circle the opening of the eyelid. That muscle is located in the upper and lower eyelids, and its function is to close the eye. The *levator palpebrae superioris* opens the eye by pulling the eyelid up. There are also several internal muscles of the eye.

If you want to smooth the wrinkles or lines around the eyes, or to strengthen the internal muscles of the eyes, look straight up, then down without moving your head. Then look left and right as far as you can without moving your head.

Closely allied is a second exercise that entails making slow circles with your eyes, first to the left and then to

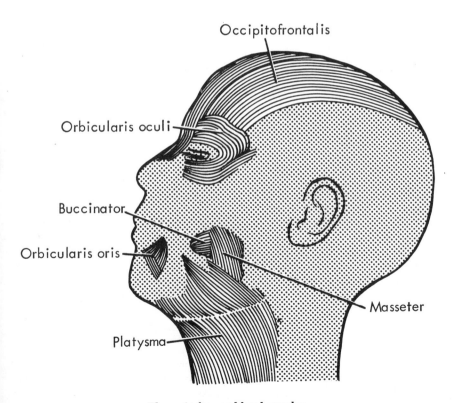

The main face and head muscles.

the right. At first do these exercises only a few times. Then gradually increase to 10 or 15 times.

The *orbicularis oris* is a circular muscle that closes the mouth opening. It acts with other muscles and enables you to whistle or to draw your lower lip upward to pout. There are several muscles attached to the outer fibers of the oris muscle which allow you to open your lips.

The *buccinator*, or trumpeter's muscle, is the principal muscle of the cheek, that pulls the lip and cheek against the teeth.

The *masseter* raises the lower jaw, and therefore, cooperates with other muscles in chewing.

There are several exercises that can be used to tighten the muscles of the mouth, cheeks and nose. One that will strengthen and firm the cheek muscle as well as stimulate the circulation of the face is to lift the right side of the mouth and cheek so that the right eye is closed. Then repeat on the left side. Each movement should be done 10 times.

To develop more attractive lips, suck against the heel of the hand with the lips slightly parted.

Are your cheeks too full? Perform this exercise with the mouth closed or the teeth slightly apart: Suck the cheeks between the teeth. Relax and repeat. Ten to 15 times is sufficient.

To strengthen and firm the muscles around the nose, cheeks, mouth and chin, keep the mouth closed and draw it upward by wrinkling the nose. Then, since the mouth is puckered, draw the mouth downward as far as you can. Repeat 10 times.

Another good exercise for your facial muscles is to try a soundless scream. Open your mouth and eyes as wide as you can. Attempt to stretch every muscle in your face. Then try to squeeze your face together by closing your eyes and mouth tightly.

FADS AND FITNESS

Many sportsmen, games players, and coaches are gullible people because they are so easily swayed by fitness fads. Some fads are psychological crutches. Others are downright dangerous. Often they take the form of a ritual which must be followed to win. They may have the backing of a grain of truth, or they may have no supporting evidence whatsoever.

In essence many fads are intended short cuts to fitness. There is, in fact, no substitute for hard work if you aim to be fit.

Water Fads

There are a number of fads associated with water. It is considered almost a crime for a boxer to do more than gargle the water that is forced past his lips between rounds. It is also a fetish with the boxing fraternity that during the period between rounds—supposed to be a time for recuperation—the boxer must try to acquire the skill of drinking from a bottle with a narrow neck. This is not an easy one at any time, and becomes a painful, hazardous operation during a boxing match. And having managed to force some water into the boxer's eager mouth, the trainer immediately urges his charge not to swallow it. The film of the World Bantamweight Championship fight, February, 1968, shows fighting Harada, defending World Champion, tackling this problem, while Rose, the challenger, and the eventual winner, is given a normal drinking vessel. Even though it is unwise to take part in vigorous physical activity with a full bladder, there is no evidence to indicate that drinking water (except in huge quantities) during training or during intervals in competition adversely affects performance. On the contrary it has been established that dehydration leads to decreasing efficiency and ultimate collapse under certain conditions. See WATER CON-SUMPTION DURING EXERCISE.

Water is often considered as something to be avoided during training and prior to competition if it is heated and run into a bath. Likewise for some obscure reason many boxers, track and field men, and games players imagine that swimming somehow interferes with the performance of their major sport. A long hot bath just prior to a contest obviously would not be stimulating, and a long hard swim just prior to a 440-yard track race would expend energy that could not be afforded; but cleanliness and recreational swimming are both recommended.

Dietary Fads

The athlete's daily intake of food is beset with fads and fancies. Different types of foodstuff enjoy popularity for varying periods—blood to make one ferocious, crushed lion's teeth for vigor, steak for strength, glucose for speed, vitamins for endurance, alkalis to offset fatigue. None of these things are likely to do a great deal of harm except where the athlete learns to rely on one or the other and is then forced for some reason to do without. His "let down" may be catastrophic. In reality the athlete's diet—in balanced content and energy value—is no different from that of a man doing heavy physical labor, such as men used to do on farms, in industry and at roadwork. If through training and competition energy expenditure is increased, then energy input in the form of food and drink must be augmented. If the diet is well balanced then the intake of all types of nourishment will be increased automatically, and there should be no need to take in additional quantities of vitamins and minerals. See ERGO-GENIC AIDS and NUTRITION.

Many athletes indulge whims immediately prior to competition. A glucose tablet or glucose drink just before a one-hundred-yard sprint is a particularly useless practice, especially if the reserves of sugar in muscles and liver are adequate, as they undoubtedly should be. Insistence upon a thick juicy steak as the pre-competition meal has no particular value, although steak is a good source of protein and, for some, the basis of a pleasant dish. The growing boy or girl needs relatively more protein than the fully grown man or woman. However, protein in any form which is eaten in excess of the organism's requirements will be excreted and will throw unnecessary strain on the normally hard-working kidneys.

Other athletes favor beer, bread and cheese, while still others prefer a sip of wine. The truth is that there are no magic foods or drinks—one man's meat is another's poison. The important thing is to eat what you enjoy, preferably something which will be far along the digestive system before competition is joined.

Massage, Bandages and Oxygen

Associated also with pre-competition dietary fads are the fads of massage and bandages. Pregame massage —often performed by an unqualified, untrained person, usually against the flow of blood—is a pleasant enough pastime for the competitor but has little value. The stimulation to blood and lymph circulation and the heat generated are as nothing compared with internally generated heat through muscular activity and the concomitant stimulation of heart, lungs and blood vessels. And the many bandages and strips of strapping placed around players' ankles are useless for support but may give a feeling of comfort and false security!

From time to time there is an upsurge of interest in oxygen, which develops into a fad for swimmers, games players, and sportsmen who suck away at an oxygen mask. *Oxygen cannot be stored in the human organism!* Certainly if equipment is developed which enables endurance athletes to take in oxygen *continuously during* competition, then improved performance is assured. At present the trappings of transportation—harness, heavy cylinder, mask—make taking oxygen during a contest an unprofitable exercise. The fad of the prerace, pregame or half-time whiff of oxygen, is, however, a very fine way of spreading any respiratory infection that *one* of the competitors may have. The one advantage oxygen has to offer is quicker recovery after exertion. There are no competitive events, however, whose nature and organization make provision for oxygen between bouts of activity a worthwhile procedure. Indeed, a competitor who was in such condition that he needed oxygen for recovery between sessions ought, in fact, to be in the hospital. See OXYGEN SUPPLEMENT.

Commercial Exploit

Commercial exploiters of exercise and diet are prone to create fads. "With my course (or my special equipment, or my special dietary supplement) you too can have a body like mine—and yet live." Such claims ignore the fact that no two people react identically to the same type of exercise (the current world-wide fad is for "isometrics" and therefore for special isometric apparatus), certain exercises, a certain magical number of repetitions, and consumption of certain wonderful foodstuffs at certain times. There are no magical foods, exercises, or numbers of repetitions. Certainly there is no one type of exercise—least of all isometric muscle training—which can lead to the development of all the components of fitness. Those who subscribe to the isometric fad may, in fact, find that the results lead to worsened, not improved performance. See MECHANICAL DEVICES.

Weight control is an area which appears to lend itself to the development of fads, special exercise regimens which build up or slim off, and special foods which build bulk or shed fat. Weight control is, in fact, largely a matter of balance between input and output, a judicious adjustment of both diet and exercise.

Drugs

The most dangerous, most recent, and most undesirable fad of all is undoubtedly "doping." It is all the more deplorable in that not only do highly trained, superbly fit, dedicated, young athletes suddenly die as a result of drug taking, or degenerate speedily into human flotsam, but many competitors and officials fail to or refuse to differentiate between "doping" for the sole purpose of giving a boost to the organism—nervous and/or circulatory systems especially—in order to win an event, and taking medicine or a dietary supplement to restore health or make good a dietary deficiency.

On the opening day of the Olympic Games in Rome, 1960, a 23-year-old Danish cyclist, Knud Jensen, collapsed during a road race and died within a few hours. On July 13, 1967, Tom Simpson, a world champion road cyclist, collapsed as he negotiated a bend approaching the summit of Mont Ventoux in Provence, during the Tour de France. He also died shortly afterwards. Post-mortem examinations showed that each of these young men had taken drugs. At least one physician was appointed in 1964 to ensure that all girl swimmers in an Olympic team should compete unhindered by menstruation. Hormones are available to delay the onset of menstruation. However, some hormones of male origin that interfere effectively with the menstrual cycle will equally and effectively produce personality changes and the development of male sex characteristics. That fad must be eliminated if honesty and morality are to be restored to games and athletic competition. Neither fitness nor happiness can be achieved in that way. See DRUGS.

Personal Idiosyncrasies

Most high-performance athletes have personal fads—idiosyncrasies—too often of superstitious origin. These, of course, usually harm no one. However, they may well be a potential hazard to the individual athlete. If, for example, he is distracted during his prerace preparation and later recalls that he violated his routine—perhaps put his left sock on before his right—and there is no time to repeat his actions in correct sequence, he may be adversely affected. Other seemingly childish fads may develop into gamesmanship and may well annoy officials, spectators, and those competitors who do not subscribe. "Being last to strip" is a typical example of this type of fad, and some swimmers and track and field competitors are prone to play this ad nauseum.

This book, in its entirety, establishes many things in relation to fitness; the most important is undoubtedly the fact that there is no substitute for hard work when fitness training is considered. Thus the individual who aims at fitness would be well advised to adopt only those procedures which can be justified by science or common sense.—*Albert W. Willee*

FAMILY PHYSICAL FITNESS

Exercising in a group is the best way to stay on an exercise program, and exercising as a family is the best form of group exercise.

Research indicates the necessity of the family unit doing things together, including mom and dad. Too often, however, dad runs off to play golf while mother goes to the health club to "shimmy and shake" her excess pounds away. That system has its drawbacks—golf and mechanical vibrations are not efficient ways of getting into shape. Both are expensive, and the family suffers.

A child's attitudes toward exercise and activity are established by the parents' attitude towards exercise and activity patterns. Parents must also be aware that the more active child learns more because he experiences more objects, body positions and movements. His brain and nervous system are stimulated, thereby enhancing his learning experiences. A parent does a grave injustice to his child if he keeps him in a crib or play pen all day long. That child needs activity and explorative movement— NOT restraint!

Gimmicks and Techniques

The list of gimmicks and techniques to enhance family-oriented physical fitness is virtually unlimited. A family physical fitness room can be built. See EQUIPMENT. The backyard can be playscaped for activity. See BACKYARD FITNESS. Walks, hikes, backpacking and camping may be enjoyed by all members of the family. Specific exercise programs such as isometrics, weight training, calisthenics, and dual-resistance exercises may also be a great asset for family activity. Learning a new sport together is a thrilling, enjoyable experience. Take along children who are too small to engage in a sport activity. Put kiddie seats on the back of bicycles, or invent piggyback child carriers for hikes and walks. If you play tennis, for example, put the children in walkers on the tennis courts. They love to scoot around on the smooth surface. How about using the older preschoolers as ball boys? The opportunities are unlimited.

Some families have developed other techniques for family fitness. For example, one family jogs together three times a week, early in the morning before the children go to school and dad goes to work. Another family has a "No Car Day." On that day the car is locked in the garage, and the children walk or ride a bicycle to school. Dad does the same for work. Even mom uses her legs to go shopping. The hardest part is fending off remarks by friends and passersby. A similar idea is a "Y" Day. On that day the entire family goes to the local Y or club for two hours or more of activity. They make it a ritual and fight any encroachment on their time. Still another approach is to build fitness

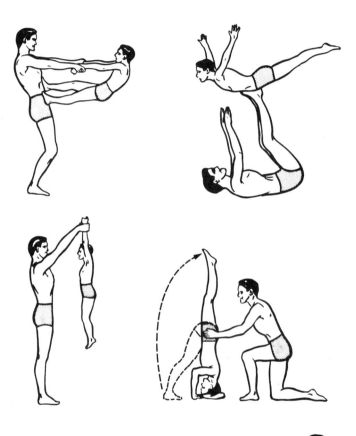

Some exercise routines can benefit both child and adult.

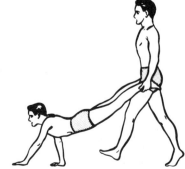

through daily activities. See DAILY ACTIVITIES.

Everyday Exercises

Set a time aside in the evening for free play. Turn off the television to allow for thirty minutes of gymnastic, tumbling-type activities or family wrestling. The elementary school children will probably take over with ideas they learned in their physical education classes. Although they are designed for children, mom and dad and even big brother and sister will find them great fun. Below are a few ideas:

1. Mountain Climbers—Stand and face your child. Clasp his wrists. Tell him to put one foot on each of your knees. Then have him walk up your body as far as possible. To assist him you must lean backward to balance his weight. Then let him walk down.

2. Swan—Remove your shoes and lie on your back. Bend your knees and draw them to your chest. Have your child place his abdomen on the bottom of your feet. Grasp hold of his wrists. Slowly straighten your legs and release the hands. Continue until the legs are practically straight. Your child should then extend his arms as he would in a swan dive. Keep your hands up for protection. A more advanced skill is to do the exercise with one leg.

3. Arm Lift—Stand and face the child. Have him stiffen his arms so that there is no bending at the elbows. Grasp his wrists firmly and raise him off the floor. Keep your arms rigid. Perform this exercise carefully and gradually. As a variation have your child grasp your thumbs. Then pull him up to shoulder level.

4. Head Stand—Have your child place his head on a pillow on the floor, with the rest of the body in a crouching position. Assume a kneeling position in front of him and have him place his hands slightly in front of his face with his head and two hands forming a triangle. Then tell him to kick his legs toward the ceiling for a head and hand stand. Assist his movement upward. Hold him in the position for several seconds. After a series of practices, slowly attempt to remove your hands so that he maintains balance by himself.

5. Wheelbarrow—Have your child lie face down on the floor. Stand behind him and ask him to raise his body until his arms are straight. Bend down and grasp his ankles. Straighten your body until you are erect. Have him walk forward with his hands, while you walk along with him.

Other activities include having your child imitate animals. For example, ask him to jump like a kangaroo, scurry like a crab, slither like a snake, move like an inchworm, or act like a lame dog. When your family gets the idea they may make up animal walks, animal ailments, or even animals. The children will amaze you. Don't be bashful. Try some of them yourself—they'll love you for it. Don't be afraid to have them jump off the bed or chair and don't pamper their activity. Give them a real opportunity to grow physically.

Family physical fitness is the epitome of fitness, for it develops the person not only physically, but also emotionally and socially. The family activity gets the family back together, something that has been lacking in our mechanized, specialized society. The opportunities and benefits of family exercise are limited only by your lack of interest and imagination.

For years psychologists and sociologists have been urging us to recognize the necessity of the family as a unit in both work and play. Don't refuse your children's companionship. They will be more than willing to join in any activity with you.

FARTLEK

Fartlek originated in Sweden, and its best known teacher was the great Swedish coach, Gosta Holmer. As

National Coach, he was the main power behind the development of the Swedish athletes Gundar Hagg, Arne Andersen, Lennart Strand, all of whom ran world records, and Ericson and others who won Olympic medals.

Fartlek, liberally translated, means speed-play. The idea is to get away from the regimentation of the running track to the enjoyment of the woods, the lakeside and the mountains.

However, as the English interpretation suggests, fartlek is no easy jogging through the forests or over the grassy plains. It implies speed; high-speed runs whenever possible. Easing up occurs only to recover on those sections of the paths where it is impossible to run fast.

So, in the extensive woods of Sweden, beside the many lakes and up on the flatter lands of the mountains where grassy undulating plains extend for miles, the Swedish athletes had their huts and camps. From these places they would run for many miles, for as long and as fast as the terrain permitted.

How does fartlek differ from cross-country running? The paths and running terrain in England vary considerably from the paths and terrain in Sweden. For that reason, the English missed the vital principle of fartlek. In fartlek there are no fixed distances as in cross-country training. Fartlek also calls for greatly varied speed efforts joined by easy efforts to recover. Cross-country training requires continuous running at a fixed pace.

Whatever the training and the conditioning may be, whether through the woods and forests, over the plains and on the mountains, the primary consideration is attention to considerable variation in pace and the avoidance of the customary steady plodding effort. The human organism must be intermittently subjected to exhaustive efforts followed by recovery periods if the highest expression of human endeavor is to be demonstrated. Fartlek introduced to the world the importance of intermittent efforts under a condition of motion, as opposed to the stereotyped program or schedule associated with training only upon the running track.

Contribution to Fitness

Fartlek makes for variety, for spontaneity, for variation, for expression. In the conditioning and formative period of any athlete, it must be considered a basic and essential part of his development. Fartlek can be considered the foundation upon which future world records, like most of the past records, will be built. It must be considered an integral part of the science of athletics.

You can use fartlek in your fitness program. Some joggers after they have achieved reasonable levels of fitness incorporate speed play or fartlek into their routine. It is a great technique for fighting boredom. Some joggers will start out with an easy pace to gradually warm up their bodies. Then, they will break into a fast sprint for a considerable distance or until fatigue will not let them continue. After that they again fall back into a slow jog to recover. For the most part fartlek is most effective through woods, along streams, up hills and the like.—*Percy Wells Cerutty*

FATIGUE

Although fatigue implies tiredness and the inability to continue, it is a difficult term to define. The most common definition given is that fatigue is the decrease in work capacity as a result of work itself. Fatigue, then, is the result of work, and not drugs, illness, or lack of incentive. Those factors may also reduce work capacity, even though no work is accomplished.

Different types of exercise produce different types of fatigue, i.e., after a 50-yard dash or during 18 holes of golf. The level of training also influences the level and onset of fatigue.

Types of Fatigue

Basically, there are two types of fatigue—mental and physical. Mental fatigue is the result of mental work and is often due to boredom or lack of interest. Physical fatigue, on the other hand, is caused by physical or muscular work. It is very difficult to separate mental and physical fatigue, since mental activity is often associated with physical activity, especially in the form of concentration of performance and emotional conditions. Furthermore, muscular work may cause mental weariness.

Levels of Work and Fatigue

D. B. Dill notes that there is a distinction between the fatigue of moderate, hard and maximal work, based upon metabolism (the individual's capacity for supplying oxygen to his tissues).

Moderate work requires an energy expenditure of about three times the resting metabolism (basal) rate. That energy expenditure is equivalent to most eight-hour work days involving white collar and some blue collar work. The expenditure of energy is so small that after a day's work the worker usually can enjoy such hobbies and activities as golf, gardening and dancing. Many times, however, uninteresting moderate work may lead to boredom, and therefore, mental fatigue. Care should be taken by the employer and employee to balance working and social conditions to avoid the occurrence of fatigue and boredom.

In hard work, the use of energy ranges somewhere between three and eight times the basal metabolism rate. An average of eight times the basal metabolism rate is the maximum rate that can be maintained for an eight-hour day, meaning up to that level the circulatory and respiratory systems

of the body can successfully provide the body with the necessary oxygen. In both moderate and hard work, only minor blood changes occur; lactic acid concentrations and alkaline reserves are apparently unchanged, and the heart rate, respiratory volume, and circulatory rate remain in direct relationship with the metabolic rate.

In maximal work the energy expenditure exceeds eight times the basal metabolism rate, which means that a person enters the "overload" zone and that a steady state can no longer be maintained. Hence, there is a breakdown, and the individual is no longer able to continue. What has happened is that the circulo-respiratory system is not able to meet the oxygen requirements of the tissues.

The breakdown is not immediate, however. Since oxygen is not actually required for muscle contraction but is involved only in the removal and conversion of waste products resulting from contraction, a considerable amount of work can be accomplished in spite of the lack of oxygen. Obviously, you cannot continue to exercise endlessly with a lack of sufficient oxygen. The level which the deficit can reach before you can no longer continue working, however, depends upon the *oxygen debt tolerance*. Debt refers to the fact that following the completion of a task, oxygen continues to be delivered to the tissues in amounts above resting levels until the deficit is eliminated.

The deficit is usually eliminated by resting or slowing down the work load to less than eight times the basal rate. The rest or slowing down is called the recovery period in which the oxygen debt is being repaid. Heavy breathing occurs at that time. See OXYGEN DEBT and ENERGY COST OF ACTIVITIES.

Other terms have been used to define or clarify terms of moderate, hard and maximal work; these are aerobic (with oxygen), partially anaerobic, and anaerobic (without oxygen) respectively. See AEROBIC EXERCISE and ANAEROBIC EXERCISE.

Symptoms of Fatigue

There are many signs of fatigue, some subjective and others objective. Some of the most common indicators of fatigue are tired feeling in the head, feeling of sleepiness, pain in the upper or lower back and soreness of muscles. The standards of performance falter, the sense of timing fails, and errors and accidents begin to occur. In the more advanced stages of fatigue the more refined skills are lost, and only the most prominent gross skills are retained. Generally, fatigue is relieved when sleep, rest and relaxation are adequate. When those factors do not relieve fatigue, the person is experiencing chronic fatigue or staleness. The most prominent symptoms of staleness are a feeling of tiredness, loss of interest in work, a loss of weight, poor appetite, increase in resting pulse rate, lowered blood pressure, tremor of the hands and poor color. See STALENESS.

Sites of Muscular Fatigue

The term muscular fatigue refers to the muscles' inability to respond to a stimulus. It is possible that the fatigue is centered in one of three places: (1) the muscle itself; (2) the nerve; or (3) the muscle-nerve junction. There is conflicting evidence as to where the true site of fatigue is, although it is generally accepted that the location of fatigue is not in the muscle tissue itself. When a muscle is repeatedly stimulated through its motor nerve, it will eventually stop contracting (fatigue). But when an electrical stimulus is applied to the supposedly fatigued muscle, it will contract.

Since the muscle tissue is not the site of fatigue, then either the nerve fiber or muscle-nerve junction must be. Dr. Peter V. Karpovich rules out the possibility of the nerve fiber being the site of fatigue with the following experiment and comment: "This fiber is relatively indefatigable. That may be demonstrated by an old laboratory experiment which consists of blocking the transmission of nerve impulses to a muscle either by passing a galvanic current through a small segment of the nerve or by placing a piece of ice on the nerve near the muscle. The nerve is then stimulated continuously for hours at some point on the side beyond the muscle and the block. If, now, while the nerve is still being stimulated, the block is lifted, the muscle is found at once to be responsive to the nerve, and immediately proceeds to produce a typical performance curve. Thus, the seat of fatigue in our nerve-muscle preparation was neither in the muscle tissue itself *nor in the motor* nerve. It must, therefore, be in the motor end plate."

Physical Fitness and Fatigue

In vigorous exercise, the degree and rate of fatigue depends upon your state of physical fitness. Research has demonstrated that during exercise the heart rate, respiratory rate, and blood lactate levels are not as high in men in good physical condition as compared with those in poor physical condition.

Furthermore, those with a high physical fitness level have a higher maximal oxygen intake, thereby slowing down the accumulation of an oxygen debt and increasing the oxygen debt tolerance. Therefore, the work capacity of the person will be increased.

An unfit person has a higher energy cost for the same task performed in the late afternoon as compared with the early morning. The fit person, however, seems to maintain his efficiency throughout the day.

Fatigue Prevention

The National Safety Council has prepared a list of techniques for reducing fatigue. The principles can be applied to many situations for planning programs of work and sport so that many of the effects of fatigue can be reduced or eliminated:

1. Job selection should include considerations of the applicant's physical and mental competence and his interest in the work.

2. Heavy muscular work tires the nervous system more quickly than the muscles; therefore, don't require a combination of heavy muscular work and mental work performed simultaneously.

3. Arrange for work of great intensity to be of short duration.

4. Arrange for work which must be carried on for long periods to be of low intensity.

5. Use hoists and conveyors where the weight of the material is a factor. A workman who must move a heavy weight every ten minutes will be tired at the end of the day.

6. Arrange loads to be lifted from the floor in a compact form. Plan the job so that the lifter will not have to twist. Provide ample room for good footing, and a clear path for the carry.

7. Carry loads as close to the center of gravity as possible.

8. Lower loads as close to the center of gravity as possible. See BODY MECHANICS for discussion of proper techniques.

9. Precede work of great intensity either by a warming-up period of work progressive in intensity from low to great, or begin at a reduced rate, load or range of movement, and then gradually increase.

10. Simplify work to adapt to the structure (physical dimensions and space requirements) and functions (strength, speed and accuracy) of the human body.

11. Employ principles of motion economy, utilizing momentum—easy and natural rhythm; arrangement of work, place, chair, materials and controls; and positioning of levers to achieve greatest mechanical advantage.

12. Avoid muscular and ligamentous stresses and strains in positions at work and movements, such as carrying, pulling, pushing and lifting. Perform those movements with the glottis open to avoid sudden alterations in blood circulation. See VALSALVA PHENOMENON.

13. Rhythm (the regular repetition of a group of motions) regularizes work labor, makes it easier, lightens it and enlivens it.

14. When a worker can set his own rhythm, there is less fluctuation in his rate of work; there is a greater interest and satisfaction in the work; and he feels less tired than when working with an imposed rhythm.

15. Synchronize the speed of the worker's machine with the worker's customary rhythm.

16. Where a group of machines is operated by a single prime mover, adjust the speed of the machines to the ability of the workers to keep pace with it.

17. Transfer workers who are not adept at high speed or cannot keep up with the average pace to jobs requiring a slower pace.

18. In non-machine operations, don't place a worker among others who have superior strength, skill and speed. It may encourage him to attempt to keep up with the swift pace and may lead to injury. He should work alongside those with a similar or only slightly faster pace.

19. In a job assignment consider advantages and limitations resulting from different structures and functions in different ages, sexes, races and body builds.

20. Arrange for frequent and regular exercise to relieve fatigue from office work requiring close concentration.

21. Conduct periodic physical examinations to aid in the early detection of diseases such as tuberculosis,

diabetes and cardiovasculo-renal conditions.

22. Correct weaknesses in vision and hearing, poor posture habits, foot trouble, and chronic infection such as tonsillitis and tooth infections.

23. Achieve and maintain physical fitness in terms of the muscular strength, cardio-respiratory endurance, and joint flexibility required for easy performance of the task.

24. Provide for comfortable and clean housing so workers have pleasant surroundings and facilities for relaxation and entertainment.

25. Relieve sources of worry arising from fears of loss of employment or reduction in wages and, in hazardous occupations, death or serious injury through the publicizing of personnel policies and through improved protection against accidents.

26. Be concerned about social and economic conditions at work and at home and see that they provide incentive and security.

27. Plan and promote recreational activities which provide for the active participation of everyone through an employees' association, supervised and coordinated by a trained recreation director to obtain their maximum values.

28. Offer frequent attention, encouragement, and expression of appreciation to the worker to keep him highly motivated.

29. Provide a change of activity, especially during periods when work output falls off.

30. Provide for a midafternoon snack when work has been continuous throughout the day.

31. Provide rest periods from 5 minutes' duration at hourly intervals in moderate work to 45 minutes in strenuous work, such as between running races in track.

32. Realize that a greater work output can be achieved by working steadily for short periods, and then resting, than by working steadily without rest periods.

33. Workers voluntarily take rest periods ranging from 3 minutes an hour in light work to 12 minutes an hour in heavier work. When such rest periods are authorized, the worker is able to relax without tension.

34. Improve accuracy of mental work requiring close concentration by providing a rest period of 5 minutes at the beginning of each hour.

35. Allow rest in a horizontal position, preferably with the legs elevated, between bouts of strenuous work. Teach relaxation techniques if the worker is incapable of voluntary, complete relaxation.

36. Provide broadcasts of music and entertainment through a public address system during periods when work output ordinarily falls off, except in work requiring intense concentration in which the broadcasts would be distracting.

37. Rest is generally much more effective if taken in a quiet rest room instead of in the workshop, because noise is inseparable from most industrial work.

38. Inform workers that they should get 8 hours of sleep nightly, preferably in a comfortable bed in a dark, quiet, cool room.

39. Provide a work area with ample space for free movement and vision, air-conditioned if necessary to achieve comfort in temperature, humidity, ventilation, and clean air free from dust, fumes and undesirable odors. The light source should illuminate the work surface providing about 100 foot-candles of illumination without glare, and noise and vibration should be reduced.

40. See that machine design provides for normal postures and positions.

41. Determine the height of the work bench and chair by the kind of work to be performed.

42. Diet should provide essential

elements of nutrition and should be in sufficient quantity to maintain normal body weight.

43. Food intake at mealtimes, especially at breakfast, should be adequate to support subsequent activity.

44. Midmorning and midafternoon snacks increase work output.

45. Separate lunchrooms from the workrooms where hot nourishing food can be eaten in an inviting and cheerful atmosphere.

46. Avoid overindulgence in alcohol and tobacco.

47. Be sure work at high altitudes is progressive in intensity to allow for acclimatization. Supplementary oxygen during work is useful at altitudes above 8,000 feet.

48. Restrict the use of drugs to allay sensations of fatigue to very severe emergency situations.

49. Follow exposure to extreme fatigue, to very high altitudes, to great depths by ample periods of rest to promote full recovery and prevent progressive deterioration resulting in excessive aging.

FEATS OF FITNESS

To reach the unreachable height, to beat the unbeatable foe have always been man's historical goals. He has always strived to excel beyond anyone else, to have a lasting monument to his existence. Those efforts have in turn become goals for other people to achieve. That continual striving toward excellence is reflected in our abundance of good literature, the advances made by the sciences, and our increasingly high standards of living. It is especially evident, however, in the athletic world. Great team efforts have enabled underdogs to upset champions. Even greater, however, are individual feats of fitness, which often pass unnoticed or fade quickly from the glare of the publicity which temporarily surrounds them.

Fasting, Hiking and Body Efficiency

One of the most unusual feats of fitness was combined with complete fasting. On June 1, 1926, George Hasler Johnson set out to walk from Chicago to New York without eating along the way. Hardly a big man, Johnson was 5 feet, 6 inches tall and weighed 157 pounds. He undertook the hike to prove that the body can operate efficiently for long periods of time while subjected to complete fasting.

In his account of the trip, Johnson said that he traveled all sorts of roads in all kinds of weather. He was followed by his personal physician, who checked his condition daily. He also said that he was never alone because he was constantly observed to make sure that he did not hide any food on his person and that he was not given any food while he was on the hike.

Johnson walked 500 miles, still going strong as he passed Pittsburgh. Approaching the mountains past Greensburg, however, he began to experience difficulty. His feet were sore because most of the fat had been used to keep his body going and the bones of the metatarsal arch no longer had the pads of fat which usually cushion them. Nevertheless, he pressed on through the Pennsylvania mountains. He climbed the long 4½-mile hill to the top of the Tuscarora summit. But by the time he arrived in Chambersburg, he had to quit. According to his physician, he was in fine health and good spirits, but his feet were too sore.

What Johnson accomplished on his 20-day walk is a feat that still stands. He had covered a total of 577.88 miles—almost 30 miles a day over the rough terrain and primitive highways of the day. After his walking with fasting, Johnson regained his weight rapidly, putting on 23 pounds in the first week.

There are many other walking and running records in the annals of sport. Some of the more interesting ones are 50 miles in 6 hours, 13 minutes, and 58 seconds by E. W. Lloyd in 1913; 100 miles in 13 hours, 26 minutes by Charles Rowell in 1882; 200 miles in 35 hours, 9 minutes, and 28 seconds by Charles Rowell in 1882; 300 miles in 58 hours, 17 minutes by Charles Rowell in 1882; 400 miles in 84 hours, 31 minutes by James Albert in 1888. Even longer distances have been recorded. Edward Weston, at the age of 70, walked from New York to San Francisco in 105 days. An even greater feat of fitness was performed by John Ennis, who walked from the surf at Coney Island to the surf in San Francisco, about 4,000 miles, in 80 days and 5 hours, a distance of about 50 miles a day!

Swimming and Rowing

Swimming and rowing records offer equal testimony to the stamina of physically fit individuals. Aside from the people who swim the English channel, there are other little known endurance records. In 1914, Henry Elionsky started a swim at 189th Street and the Hudson River. He swam to Winburne Island in the lower bay, then to Ft. Lee in New Jersey, and ended his swim at the Woolworth building. The officials who judged the swim estimated the distance to be over 60 miles! An interesting sidelight of the swim that has nothing to do with endurance is that, although this swim was made in 1914, Elionsky said he swam most of the way through debris and oil, still a problem in the Hudson River.

Today, most boating enthusiasts who feel that they are physically fit and have a seaworthy craft take to the raging Colorado River and "shoot the rapids." With the introduction of powerboats, which some people now use in favor of rafts and canoes, that activity has lost some measure of the adventure once associated with it. At one time, however, rowing records were popular, although little is heard of them currently. C. A. Barnard rowed 50 miles in 8 hours and 55 minutes in 1877. Bob Hoffman, the publisher of well-known fitness magazines, rowed from Conneaut Lake, not far from Lake Erie, nonstop to the Pittsburgh Aquatic Club in Pittsburgh. He covered the distance of 150 miles in 26 hours and 32 minutes, shattering the two-man record for that distance in the process.

Although most feats of fitness are aimed at shattering records which have already been established, some are done just for the fun of it. One such feat is the marathon water-skiing trip during which a group of girls ranging in age from 12 to 25 skied from Florida to Expo '67 in Canada. In another feat six British youngsters, whose average age was 13, swam the English Channel. Those tests of endurance and physical stamina were not aimed at establishing any records. They were done because the participants reveled in the joy of being physically fit.

Not all feats of fitness, however, are surrounded by such casual circumstances. Many require strenuous training and preparation. In training for the first four-minute mile, Roger Bannister had to cope with criticism of his training program by his fellow countrymen because of his performance in the 1952 Olympics. Bannister remained unimpressed by the insults leveled against him and continued training. Then, on May 6, 1954, the long months of training paid off. Crossing the finish line, Bannister was clocked at 3 minutes, 59.4 seconds, a seemingly impossible time. Others have done better since, and the current record is held by James Ryan of the United States, who ran the distance in 3 minutes, 51.3 seconds.

Unusual Endurance Feats

The fun of doing, the hope of breaking a record, or the sheer exhilaration of participating in athletics do not surround all feats of fitness. Some have been done in fear. Such is the case of the Russian athlete who ran and walked across the Asian continent in a successful attempt to escape the iron curtain. This performance was greeted by skepticism until investigation revealed that he had, indeed, escaped by crossing the entire continent on foot!

Although usually not considered feats of fitness by sports-minded individuals, some unusual records of endurance have been set in such things as dance marathons and equally unusual events. Perhaps one of the most unusual is that of Charles M. "Mile-A-Minute" Murphy, who kept up with a Long Island Railroad car pulled along at 60 miles per hour. His time for the mile was 57.8 seconds. He ran on a board surface between the rails. Years later, in 1941, Alfred Letourner set a record of 33.05 seconds for the mile, racing in the wake of a midget racing auto at the rate of 108.92 miles per hour.—*Thomas Puschock*

FEET

Although the musculature of the foot, in general, resembles that of the hand, the foot does not have as much flexibility and is specialized to support the body.

At the bottom of the foot is the plantar surface, which is a heavy sheath of connective tissue that lies underneath the skin in the sole of the foot. Above the tissue lies the *flexor digitorum brevis*, whose function is to act as a flexor of the toes and to help support the arch of the foot.

There are also four layers of plantar muscles. These muscles from the most superficial to the deepest are (a) *abductor hallucis, flexor digitorum brevis,* and *abductor digiti minimi;* (b) *flexor digitorum accessorius lumbricales; (c) flexor hallucis brevis, adductor hallucis, flexor digiti minimi brevis,* and

(d) *interossei.* In most instances, the action of the muscles of the feet are described by their name. For example, the abductor hallucis abducts the big toe, and the adductor hallucis adducts it. The most important functions of the foot muscles are to support the arches and to steady the toes for firm support.

An exercise that may be used to strengthen the foot muscles is to stand erect and attempt to curl your toes underneath your foot. Then relax. Repeat several times, making sure you accentuate a high arch.

A second exercise is to walk on your toes. Make sure that you take short steps. Take about ten steps and return. Then walk on your heels, take ten short steps and return.

For an exercise that you will find relaxing, remove your shoes as often as possible, stretch out your toes, flex your arches, and rotate your ankles.

FEMININITY

Although women are experimenting with exercise and finding that it is compatible with femininity, there are those who avoid physical activity by using the excuse that exercise gives a woman big muscles and a masculine manner. That's nonsense! There are as many masculine looking women in art and music classes, in orchestras and other cultural endeavors as there are in physical education classes or on the athletic field. Feminine masculinity is a matter of genetics and attitude much more than the result of stimulating or sustained physical activity. Linda Lee Mead, Miss America of 1960, says exercise and sports helped her become Miss America. For several years prior to her becoming beauty queen of Mississippi and the nation, she had been very active in sports. Later as a professional model she continued to enjoy water skiing, bowling, horseback riding, fencing and calisthenics.

Another widely held misconception is that women should exercise only in their youth. The physically active life should be a stage from which a girl passes into a cultural stage and leaves the physical behind like the disposable section of a space vehicle. Nine years ago I interviewed a young woman who in high school had been a basketball player and loved sports. At the time I saw her, she had been out of school and sports for several years and was working as an assistant in a doctor's office. She also complained of severe back pains. Last fall I interviewed her again and learned that her back pain had become so severe that major surgery was necessary. She offered this explanation: "At that time of my life (9 years ago), I was convinced that sports were of no importance whatever. All I was interested in was music and culture." However, her life and outlook changed. She told how her surgeon insisted she take up sustained exercise programs for rehabilitation of her back following surgery. Even after she had totally recovered, she stuck to the exercise program, changing it from time to time as a particular program became monotonous for her. "Now," she said in a jubilant voice, "even though my life is more demanding than it has ever been and I have gone through a series of severe difficulties, I feel 200 per cent better than I ever have in my life!"

Your Normal Work Is Not Enough

One of the most subtle deterrents to a woman's physical development is the assumption that if you are physically active in your work, there is no need for a physically recreative outlet. Nurses, for example, walk miles of halls, pull, push and lift patients, and use their hands, feet and back in ways which demand dexterity and energy. It is easy for them to claim that their work provides all the exercise they need. A physical therapist at a large state medical center once told me that her co-workers were constantly amazed by the amount of work she could turn out. "I could do more work every day

in less time than any of the other therapists who usually were dragging by the middle of the afternoon. Yet they criticized me for playing tennis during many of my lunch hours," she explained. "They can't get through their heads that it isn't a question of working so hard that I'm too tired to play, but a question of playing so as to build up the energy I need for my work."

Whether a woman is a nurse, a dancer, a farmer's wife, or a typical urban housewife and mother, she needs physical activity that is not associated with work to recreate her vital energies and sustain both her physical and emotional health. A ballet dancer in New York City told me that in spite of the wonderful physical workout ballet gives a woman, most of the dancers in her corps complained of various ailments and illnesses. She herself, however, had no such complaints and believed that it was due to the fact that she was the only one who supplemented her dancing with extra exercise. "I spend my vacations skiing in the Alps and the Adirondacks."

One of the hardest working farmer's wives in the West told me that she still does thirty minutes of calisthenics every day of her life. She started 20 years ago. A hard working mother of 4 children in Michigan spoke of her weekly volleyball workout as "my mental salvation." A former college campus beauty queen in Ohio maintained her vitality and spirit by "30 minutes of calisthenics and 40 minutes of dancing every day and wrestling with my husband once a week."

Regular vigorous and interesting physical activity throughout your life is an indispensable asset in providing a foundation for intellectual, artistic, cultural and social activity. It will help to prevent physical and emotional ills and breakdowns and serve to sustain you in your efforts to be an effective wife, mother and citizen.—*Thomas Boslooper*

FENCING

Why not consider fencing as one of your routes to fitness? You'll develop a new skill with only a minimum investment in equipment and time. Forget about serious competitive events in the beginning. Those bouts demand years of learning and experience, coupled with the guidance of a good instructor.

Equipment Needed

Getting started takes little equipment. A foil (around $6-$10), a mask ($5-$8), a fencing glove ($3) and sneakers or other rubber-soled shoes. As you progress and find someone with whom to practice, you will add a fencing jacket ($10) and pants ($8). The pants and jacket are made of firm white canvas. With a sweatshirt under the jacket they provide more than enough protection. But until you develop your skill and interest to a point where you round up a fencing partner, you can practice quite well with a full-length mirror.

In competition the field of action is limited to a rubber strip 40 feet long, and 6 feet wide. That accounts for the grace and control you see in a match. (No throwing chairs or swinging from chandeliers permitted.) So you may be wise in marking off a limited area even when practicing by yourself.

There are three basic fencing weapons. The foil can be used by men and women and is by far the most popular weapon. The épée is a heavier weapon and requires electrical equipment used in scoring. The third is the sabre, perhaps the most dramatic and exciting of the three. It requires the greatest strength and speed and is not usually thought of as a beginner's choice.

While different in appearance and execution, all three weapons require the same basic training and conditioning. All begin from similar "on-guard" positions. The lunge that carries the attack is the common denominator for all three weapons.

The Basic Position

Actions begin from the on-guard position. That will be your basic position. From it you will either advance, retreat, or launch your attack. So be sure you feel comfortable and balanced in it. To take the on-guard position, first place your feet at right angles,

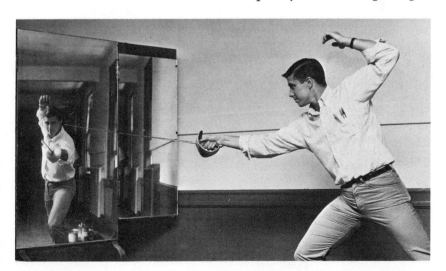

In a solo workout, a large mirror offers a chance to practice the basics of fencing.

then step forward with your right foot around 18 inches in the direction of your opponent (or the mirror). Bend both knees so that the left knee is above the left toe and the right knee over the right heel. The left arm is bent over the left shoulder with your hand a little higher than your head. Your right arm is relaxed with your blade lined with your forearm. Your body should lean slightly forward from the hips with your weight equally distributed.

At first you may feel a little stiff in that position, but as you practice, the on-guard stance becomes as second nature as sitting down. From there you move forward by stepping out with the right foot then bringing up the left to the on-guard position. Be sure to lift, not slide your feet. When perfected that advance is like one fluid motion. You step back by reversing the procedure. But again, remember to lift your feet.

From your on-guard position you move to your basic attack, the lunge. When seen in a match, the lunge appears as one graceful motion, but it is actually two parts. First extend your arm swiftly from your shoulder to the target. Then launch your body forward by extending your left leg. Your right foot lifts forward until the left leg is extended. Your left arm is straightened and brought down above the extended left leg.

You recover from a lunge by bending the left knee while pushing off from the front foot. Remember to skim your right foot just above the floor as an awkward recovery opens you to your opponent's attack.

Having mastered the basics of the on-guard and lunging positions you are ready to go into the various attacks and defenses necessary for competitive fencing. For that it is almost necessary to find a local YMCA or club offering fencing lessons. There are several good books, especially *Sports Illustrated's* "Fencing" (J. B. Lippincott, Phila.

and N.Y. 1962) and "Sword and Masque," (F. A. Davis, Phila., 1967) that have easy-to-follow drawings and illustrations that can be a big help to the beginner.

Fitness Benefits

But even if your early fencing activities are confined to the basics of lunging, advancing, and recovery you get several fitness plusses. The bending and movement is a great conditioner for the legs. The short, quick strides so essential to proper fencing technique build up leg strength quickly. You also build stamina, coordination and wrist strength and flexibility. But the big benefactor in a fencing routine is the heart-lungs complex. The thrusting and driving, the attack and withdrawal are only effective when done quickly. Consequently, you'll become somewhat winded in fencing, and you'll be getting the benefit of aerobic exercise that has lately become much publicized. In fact, even the warm-up prior to a fencing workout is a good conditioner in itself.

In his book "Sword and Masque," fencing master Julius Palffy-Alpar suggests the following workout to prepare and warm up the muscles for fencing. Any calisthenics are useful, but be sure to choose exercises that strengthen and loosen up the muscles of the arms and legs, and avoid those which tend to stiffen your muscles. Some exercises are essential before every lesson, practice session, or competition. These are:

For the legs

(a) Half knee bends
(b) Hopping in half knee bends
(c) Stretching the legs in half knee bends (Russian dance)
(d) Skipping and bouncing on toes
(e) Lunging from half knee bend and returning to half knee bend
(f) In lunging, the stretching and bending of the right knee
(g) Knee bends in "on-guard" position

For the arms

(a) Swinging the arms around the shoulders

(b) Bringing the fists close to the shoulders and describing circles with the elbows

(c) Swinging the arms from front, sidewards and upwards, and back

(d) Bending the arms in front of the chest with tearing-like movements

(e) Stretching the arms in front and grasping the fingers

Once you have mastered the art of fencing it will continue to pay dividends long after more demanding sports would have put you on the sidelines. Danish fencer Ivan Ossier competed in the Olympics in London in 1908 and was back in London when the games were held there again after World War II. Along the way he gained a silver medal at Stockholm in 1912. No Olympic competitive span can compare to this fencer's remarkable 40 years.—*Robert Teufel*

Associations

Amateur Athletic Union (AAU). See ORGANIZATIONS.

Division of Girls' and Women's Sports (DGWS).

National Collegiate Athletic Association (NCAA). See ORGANIZATIONS.

Amateur Fencers League of America (AFLA), 33 62nd Street, West New York, New Jersey 07093.

Intercollegiate Fencing Association (IFA), Hotel Manhattan, New York, New York 10036.

Since fencing is a high-energy-cost activity it may be used to help improve your fitness level, especially your circulo-respiratory and muscle endurance. Below is a fencing program that takes into account the important principles of training.

If you desire to improve your strength and power for this activity see WEIGHT TRAINING and ISOMETRICS. The weight training and isometrics exercises may also be used to prepare your body for athletic competition.

° **FENCING PROGRAM**
(Competitive) ° °

Chart 1	Chart 2
1. 5 minutes	1. 28 minutes
2. 10 minutes	2. 29 minutes
3. 13 minutes	3. 30 minutes
4. 15 minutes	4. 32 minutes
5. 17 minutes	5. 35 minutes
6. 20 minutes	6. 36 minutes
7. 23 minutes	7. 37 minutes
8. 25 minutes	8. 39 minutes
9. 25 minutes	9. 40 minutes

° See ENDURANCE and ENERGY COST OF ACTIVITIES for an explanation of these charts.

° ° Doesn't include rest periods, time outs, etc.

Fitness 1

If you achieved a score of poor or low average on the *Harvard Step Test* or a score of very poor or poor on the *12 Minute Run*, start on Chart 1-Level 1 and spend 1 week at each level until Chart 2-Level 9 is reached. It is recommended you participate 4 to 5 days a week. When Chart 2-Level 9 is reached, 4 days a week is sufficient.

Fitness 2

If you achieved a score of high average on the *Harvard Step Test* or fair on the *12 Minute Run*, start on Chart 1-Level 1. Spend one week on Chart 1-Levels 1, 2, 4, 5, 6, 9, and Chart 2-Levels 1, 3, 5, 7, 9. It is recommended that you participate 4 to 5 days a week. When Chart 2-Level 9 is reached, 4 days a week is sufficient.

Fitness 3

If you achieved a score of good or excellent on either the *Harvard Step Test* or *12 Minute Run*, continue your current program or select Chart 2-Level 9 as your level of participation. Four days a week is sufficient.

FISHING (Angling)

Fishing is an ancient sport that still generates a great deal of enthusiasm.

Over 30 million people, men, women and children, in the United States participate every year.

You may fish for sport, food, or business. The sport fisherman is called an angler, for he fishes for the sport rather than food, despite the fact that he usually eats what he catches. His prime concern is the catching of fish.

Sport fishing is normally done from the stream bank, lake shore, dock, or anchored boat. Unless the angler decides to stalk after his fish, his fitness program doesn't benefit. Occasionally, the fisherman may be required to go to a rural area and then walk several miles to the best fishing area. Once he has found the desired location, he may have to walk up and down the stream, river, or lake shore for quite a distance. Fishing in that way offers fitness benefits similar to hiking. See HIKING.

Casting requires a special kind of rod and reel to throw an artificial lure or natural bait into the water. It is retrieved by cranking the reel and pulling the line back to the fisherman. The lure simulates live action, because it moves as a result of the various maneuvers on the pole made by the angler. That movement causes the fish to strike. The most common types of casting are fly, bait, spinning and spin casting. If the fisherman remains in one spot, he places little physiological stress on his body. If, however, he walks considerably from one spot to another, the fitness benefits will increase in proportion to the amount of walking.

Surf casting or *surf fishing* is a variation of casting. Here the fisherman stands along the ocean shoreline (generally in the water) and casts into the surf. Since many game fish feed close to the shore, surf casting is a rather productive means of fishing. In surf fishing there is less walking than may be found in the other forms of casting, but the fitness benefits achieved are great because of the weight of the pole used, the fish caught, and the long period of standing in the generally rough surf. The muscles most affected are the anti-gravity muscles from the prolonged standing and the muscles of the arm (flexors) from the repeated pulling in of the bait.

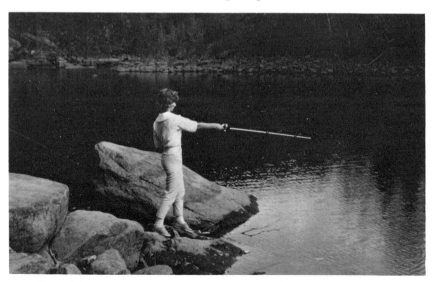

It often takes a brisk hike to reach the better fishing spots. Once there, casting and working mountain streams mixes healthy exercise with great fishing.

To learn accurate casting requires a great deal of practice, for a good fisherman will want to place the lure or bait at an exact spot. Sidearm casting is easier for a beginner, but the overhead cast is considered to be more accurate and is used by most experts.

Trolling is fishing from a moving boat by dragging the bait or lure behind the craft. Trolling may be done at a fast or slow speed depending upon the type of fish being sought. When the fish is hooked, the boat is stopped until the fish is brought into the boat or lost. Fitness benefits achieved from this type of fishing are very low. Trolling in the deep ocean waters requires heavy rods and reels. That type of fishing is called *deep-sea fishing*. Little fitness benefits are achieved from this type of angling. However, a moderate to high degree of arm and shoulder strength and circulo-respiratory endurance are needed to pull in a big fish. A bout with a fish may last for an hour or more. When the fish being caught puts up that much of a fight, a very high degree of arm and shoulder strength and endurance is mandatory.

There are other kinds of sport fishing: *ice fishing*, *spear fishing*, *tickling* and *snagging* with nets or loops of wire.

Few fishermen engage in any type of conditioning program for their sport, other than practicing the cast. The angler wants to perfect each cast so that he can control the placement of his bait. In the "off season" anglers often duplicate their sport with a game called *skish*, formally called *fish-o*. In skish, targets about 30 inches in diameter are placed at random distances from the caster, who attempts to cast his lure into the target. Many times the caster can set up his own targets at home with old tires.

Conditioning Programs

Although few fishermen engage in any type of training program other than accuracy casting, it would be advisable if the angler would spend as much time with his body as he does with his equipment. The fisherman merely sits on the bank and lets the fish come to him, and has little need to exercise. But the angler who stalks his quarry and walks several miles, will find it to his advantage to start walking 6 to 8 weeks prior to the opening of the fishing season. Occasional jogging may be interspersed with the training. The additional training will allow the fisherman to get to that extra spot, not to fear overexertion, and to enjoy the fishing expedition. The surf fisherman should perform some weight training exercises such as barbell curls, reverse curls, shoulder shrugs and forward raises with the weights. Push-ups, upper back arches, and half squats with regular exercises will be very helpful.

The deep-sea fisherman who expects to put up a long battle with a fish needs a special program. Because the battle with the fish may last for some time, he should condition the circulo-respiratory system with walking, jogging and cycling. He should undertake the exercise program 6 to 8 weeks prior to fishing. Some deep-sea fishermen may not see the value in engaging in the circulo-respiratory endurance training because of long sitting. The important thing to remember is that when a big, fighting fish strikes, the entire upper body is put into vigorous action. As a result the heart beats faster to pump more blood to the exercising muscles. The bout may last for a long time, placing a great deal of stress on these systems. It is imperative, therefore, that the body be trained for such action.

Injuries

The injuries most common to fishing are:

1. Pricking or puncturing the skin with the fish hook.

2. Burns from the line rubbing

against the skin. That injury is particularly prevalent in deep-sea fishing where the line may be pulled out very quickly by the fish.

3. Sunburn, especially in surf and deep-sea fishing.

4. Sunstroke, especially in deep-sea fishing.

Associations:

American Casting Association (ACA), P. O. Box 51, Nashville, Tennessee 37202.

International Game Fish Association, A. I. duPont Building, Miami, Florida 33132.

FLEXIBILITY

Flexibility is the ability to move the body parts through their full range of motion at their joints. Your muscle system, including ligaments, the bones, and the joints, is critical to the degree of flexibility you possess.

Dr. Edwin Fleishman recognizes two areas of flexibility—extent (static) and dynamic. Extent flexibility is the ability to move or stretch the body, or some part of it, freely in various directions. The person who is often mistakenly called "double jointed" would score well in extent flexibility tests.

Dynamic flexibility, on the other hand, involves the ability to perform repeated flexing or stretching exercises. In short, it is the ability to move a

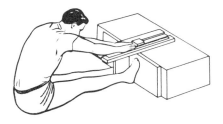

The Wells Sit and Reach test measures back and leg flexibility.

joint through various ranges of motion at varying speeds.

Flexibility is specific to a joint or a combination of joints. For that reason you may have adequate ankle joint flexibility but not arm and shoulder joint flexibility. According to F. L. Hupperich and P. O. Sigerseth it would be incorrect to call you a "flexible" individual.

Tests for Flexibility

Extent

There are two basic methods that may be used to measure extent flexibility—direct and indirect. The direct measurement, used primarily in the laboratory situation, involves measuring the angle of the joint at both ends of its movement range (goniometry) and determining the range of movement.

The indirect method, on the other hand, refers to the measurement of the joint angles, by determining how closely a body part can be brought into opposition with another body part. There are several tests that are commonly used to measure "flexibility." One of the most popular is the "Sit and Reach Test" that was designed by K. F. Wells and E. K. Dillon to test back and leg flexibility. In that test you assume a long sitting position and then slide your hands forward on a table (shoulder height) to the limit of your reach. The distance reached by the fingertips is the score on the test.

Another test included is Cureton's "Trunk Flexion Forward." Assume a long sitting position, with the hands behind your neck. The feet are 18 inches apart. Then bend downward and forward, attempting to get your forehead as close as possible to the floor. The distance of the forehead from the floor is the score on the test.

Fleishman believes that one of the best measures of extent flexibility is the "Twist and Touch," a test which evaluates how far you can rotate your spine.

Assume a standing position with the nonpreferred side toward the wall on a line drawn perpendicular to the wall. A horizontal scale is extended on either side of a line on the wall perpendicular to the line drawn on the floor. The horizontal scale is marked off from 0 to 30 inches, with the 12-inch mark being bisected by the perpendicular line. The action of the test is as follows: keeping the feet in place, twist your back around as far as possible, and touch the wall with the preferred hand, keeping your hand at shoulder height with the palm facing the floor. An assistant can aid in this test by placing his own foot against your foot. The score is recorded as the farthest point on the scale reached and held for at least two seconds.

Dynamic

In describing dynamic flexibility, Herbert de Vries says, "This method, developed by Wright and Johns, (Physical Factors Conceived with the Stiffness of Normal and Diseased Joints, *Johns Hopkins Hospital Bulletin,* 106:315-31, 1960), to measure the 'stiffness' of normal and diseased joints, uses laboratory devices to measure the forces (torque) needed to move a joint through various ranges of motion at varying speeds. Although this method has not yet been applied to research in physical performance, it seems to have distinct possibilities for such use. It seems highly probable that this measurement can tell us more about potential performance in speed events than can static flexibility."

Degree of Flexibility

The degree of flexibility is quite important. A lack of adequate flexibility is often associated with low back pain and muscle and joint injuries, regardless of the degree of physical activity in which you engage. A lack of flexibility also restricts graceful movement.

If you participate vigorously in sports, your degree of flexibility plays a critical role in performance level. Good flexibility increases the ability to avoid injuries. Since there is greater range of motion of the joint, the possibility of ligaments and muscle fibers being torn is reduced. Possession of a good degree of flexibility enables you to change direction more easily and fall properly, with less likelihood of injury. In short, a good degree of joint flexibility means better adaptation to the many physical stressful situations that occur in sports.

Controversy over Flexibility

There is a great deal of controversy concerning flexibility exercises and tests. Many people feel that they are harmful to the spinal column. (See EXCESSIVE EXERCISE.) The current thinking is that flexibility exercises are to be gradual, rather than a forceful, ballistic movement. Nevertheless, if you experience pain, stop.

Some people discount flexibility as an important aspect of fitness. But since adequate flexibility is necessary for the prevention of injury, it is a fitness component that should not be neglected. See TESTS and TRAINING.

It is a matter of common observation that there is a great variation in the flexibility of different people and of the same people at different ages and in different parts of the body. The term "flexibility" conjures up the

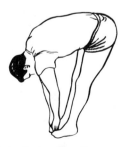

It's not short arms that prevent you from touching your toes, but a lack of flexibility in the back of the legs.

idea of folding-up or bending but a more meaningful term would be mobility, which would imply movement in all directions, bearing in mind the anatomical limitations of various parts of the body. The concepts of mobility can be satisfactorily defined as range of movement in joints.

Factors Limiting Mobility

A number of factors are believed to be responsible for determining the mobility of joints; skeletal structure, muscles, ligaments, soft tissues, temperature and post-injury adhesions. Although opinion appears to differ concerning what factors actually limit the range of movement in joints, it is obvious that each is involved to a greater or lesser extent, depending upon which joint is studied. The movement possibilities of a joint are determined by the shape of the bones, the disposition of muscles, ligaments, and other soft tissues, such as joint capsule and cartilage, and the way in which they fit together. The type, direction, and extent of movement are uniquely determined for each joint by a complex interweaving of the above factors. See TESTS.

The lack of precise knowledge in this area has led Munrow to select the term "joint-complex" to refer to "the anatomical joint or joints involved in a movement, together with the overlying soft tissues involved."

Movement in the human body can be produced by externally applied forces, including gravity, and by internally applied forces of the muscles. However, muscles not only cause motion; they also limit movement. If you raise the lower limb with a bent knee, the range of movement is considerably greater than when you raise the limb with a straight knee. In order to increase the range of motion with a straight knee, you must stretch the hamstrings group of muscles (*biceps femoris, semitendinosus, semimembranosus*). It is, however, extremely unlikely that muscle fibers can be stretched. They have to be made to relax more fully in order to increase the range of movement.

The size of the muscles or the presence of fat may also affect the range of movement in some joints. For example, the amount of flexion in the knee joint may be limited in some well-muscled or fat individuals as the surfaces of the calf and thigh come together. The effect of an increase in muscle bulk, associated with weight lifting, has led to the allegation that weight lifters are muscle-bound and consequently restricted in their range of movement. That limitation might occur in both elbow and knee joints, but such a reduction would not affect the functional performance of the individual.

The stability and security of many joints in the human body depend to a large extent upon the ligaments, as well as the muscles. The collateral and cruciate ligaments of the knee joint play an important role in checking the extent of, or completely preventing, motion in some directions.

Ligaments can become relaxed and lose their elasticity if exposed to excessive or continuous stress. Joint stability can be adversely affected in such circumstances. For example, the collateral ligaments of the knee joint serve to check excessive sideway movement (abduction and adduction) but persistent or excessive stress, or even prolonged immobilization, can result in an unstable or "wobbly" knee.

Colson has indicated that an uninjured joint immobilized because of a nearby injury stiffens "slowly and progressively from the time of immobilization by shortening of its capsule, ligaments and contracting muscles, and by the formation of adhesions."

Maintaining and Improving Mobility

Exercise can increase the range of movement of joints, but it appears that the type of exercise is of crucial importance and that lack of exercise (or movement) results in a reduction in the range of motion.

Extreme ranges of motion are achieved by hurdlers, high jumpers, gymnasts and ballet dancers who perform highly specific exercises. However, when these exercises are no longer practiced, the gains are lost and the range of movement becomes restricted.

In considering the problems of maintaining and of increasing the range of movement in joint-complexes, Munrow discussed:

Movements in which the limbs or other moving parts go to the extreme end of the range of movement. Such a limb in movement may be moving actively or passively. Active movements are those achieved by active contraction of the protagonists throughout the range. Passive movements are defined as those in which the limb or section of the body, in the final range of travel, is not being moved by active contraction of protagonistic muscle.

Munrow recommends moderate-speed movements in which conscious effort is made to reach the end of the range of movement and short movements or presses in the end position. He points out the possibility of injury occurring with passive exercises in which the movements are not under the control of active muscle contraction, particularly "fast swinging movements in which the momentum achieved towards the end of the movement is considerable." The value of passive exercises in the end position, where the amount of external force is carefully controlled, is recognized especially for remedial work.

Steinhaus reports in an article entitled "A New Way to Increase Range of Movement and the Problem of Muscle Boundness," how Dr. Schmitt, a Chicago physician who specializes in physical medicine, tackled one of the most common ailments of older people—limitation of the range of movement in joints. Schmitt assumed that in the absence of any bone defor-

mation, loss of motion can be caused by changes in the connective tissue of the joint capsule, of the muscle itself, and of the superficial fascia. He found that those changes could be reversed by physical and mechanical means. Consequently, he devised a machine, known as a motorvator, which "imparts 1,140 sine-wave strokes per minute through a rubber applicator to the tissue over which it is held." That machine performed the same function as manual procedures but without the demanding physical exertion on the part of the manipulator. Steinhaus reports that increases in the range of movement in the joints of the right upper extremity occurred after 6, one-half hour periods of motorvation (two per week).

Normal Range of Motion

Without doubt, the normal range of motion is extremely wide, varying from subject to subject and from joint to joint. Dr. Wells reports the range of motion in selected joint movements, using twenty-four young women as subjects:

(a) *Flexion at the shoulder joint.* The subject sat on a bench with the head and back braced against the edge of an open door and raised both arms forward-upward as far as possible, keeping them shoulder distance apart, with the palms facing each other and the elbows fully extended. The angle between the upper arm and the vertical was measured with a plumb line protractor.

    Range = 161° to 186°
    Median = 172.5°

(b) *Horizontal extension at the shoulder joint.* The subject lay on her back on a narrow bench with her knees drawn up and feet resting on the bench. The arms were extended sideward at shoulder level, then lowered toward the floor as far as possible. Care was taken to see that the bench was narrow enough so as not to interfere with free movement of the shoulder joints. The angle between the upper arm and the horizontal was measured with a plumb line protractor.

    Range = 20° to 57°
    Median = 44°

(c) *Hip flexion with straight knee.* As a measure of hip and ham-string flexibility, hip flexion was measured with the knee kept in complete extension. The subject lay on a narrow bench and raised the right leg from the hip as far as possible, keeping the knee and the ankle fully extended. The angle between the midline of the lateral aspect of the thigh and the horizontal was measured with a plumb line protractor.

Range　$= 53°$ to $114°$
Median $= 92°$

Relationship of Mobility and Athletic Performance

No one has determined what constitutes a satisfactory range of joint movement for normal living or athletic performance. Although evidence is available to show that some athletes

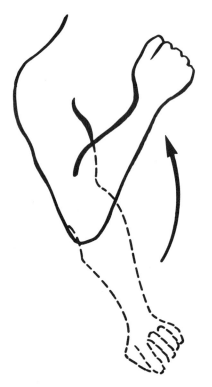

Flexion is the bending of a body segment at a joint in a front-to-back plane.

have greater range of motion in some joints than normal individuals, there is no evidence to show the effects of changes in the range of joint motion upon athletic performance. Leighton, however, has compared the flexibility characteristics of specialized skill groups of athletes (baseball players, basketball players, swimmers, shot putters, discus throwers, weight lifters, gymnasts and wrestlers). His findings indicate that different specialized skills require extreme range of motion in different parts of the body. His final comment is particularly apt and valid today: "Apparently the field of bodily flexibility has hardly been scratched. An extensive research program is needed."—*E. R. Sandstrom*

FLEXION

When the body's 600+ muscles move the bones of the body, the movement is smooth and efficient because the muscles work in pairs. For example, one muscle may contract to pull a bone forward while the opposite muscle will contract to pull the bone backward.

Flexor muscles cause flexion or bending at a joint when a body segment is moved in a front-to-back plane. A few examples of flexion are: bringing the calf of the leg toward the abdomen (hip flexion); bringing the forearm up toward the upper arm (forearm flexion). Some of the more well-known flexor muscles are the pectoralis major, which flexes the upper arm; the biceps brachii and the brachialis, which are flexors of the forearm; the iliopsoas and the femoris rectus, which are the flexors of the thigh; the hamstrings, which are flexors of the leg; and the rectus abdominis and iliopsoas, which are flexors of the trunk.

The opposite of flexion is extension. The extensor muscles reverse the movement of the flexors and work in close harmony with them. See EXTEN-

SION. For a related discussion, see ABDUCTION, ADDUCTION and MUSCLES, SKELETAL.

The movement of the muscles is controlled by the brain and spinal cord. See NEUROMUSCULAR SYSTEM.

FUTURE OF ATHLETIC RECORDS

The rash of new records in sports during the past decade has caused people to wonder where all the record breaking will end. How far can man go? Does he actually have a psychological or physiological limit?

In 1952 Parry O'Brien put the shot over 60 feet, a feat once considered impossible. Today the record stands at over 70 feet. Roger Bannister first cracked the four-minute mile in 1954 with a time of 3:59.6. In the past 15 years his time has been consistently lowered, until in 1968 the record reached 3:51.3. Progress in the pole vault is another phenomenon. For years Cornelius Waterdam's record of 15 feet, 7¾ inches was tops. Now the record is well over 17 feet, and vaulters are setting their sights on 18-foot heights.

Similar achievements are being made in swimming, where records fall every time a major swimming meet is held. The record performances are not limited to these sports, however. You have only to look at the morning sports page to realize that records are tumbling in every sport.

A second outstanding aspect of the onslaught on records is the many athletes involved in record-breaking performances. After breaking the four-minute mile in 1954, Roger Bannister predicted that there would be a rash of sub-4-minute miles. His words were prophetic. Today, few important outdoor miles are won at Roger Bannister's time. In fact, in one meet eight runners bettered four minutes in a single race! The same has been true in the pole vault. After Waterdam broke the 15-foot barrier there were only a handful of participants during the 1950's who reached the 15-foot vault—such as Richards, Bragg and Gutoski. Now, if a vaulter does not reach 16 feet in a major meet he has little chance of winning or even placing.

Johnny Weissmuller set a 100-yard free-style swimming record of 52 seconds in 1927. Today over 100 college swimmers in the U. S. alone can match or better that time; and several women are challenging that one-time magical figure.

A third startling aspect of the phenomenon of record breaking is the age of the record setters. At one time the world record holder for the mile was in his twenties, and it was recognized that he would not reach his prime until his late twenties. When Jim Ryan set the mile record (1966), he was only 19 years of age. Even more outstanding are the performances of young swimmers. For more information on age see AGE AND ATHLETIC PERFORMANCE, AGING.

The breaking of records is not new, for records have been broken ever since the first measurements of athletic performance were recorded in the 1860's. What is new, however, is the rate at which the records are broken and the increase or decrease in the record. For example, 19 years elapsed before Bob Gutoski eclipsed Cornelius Waterdam's record by a little more than one inch. Today, however, pole-vault records are being set every year, and sometimes every week. The increases are often more than an inch, sometimes 6 inches or more. Likewise, before Roger Bannister broke the 4-minute barrier athletes crept closer and closer to that obstacle by tenths of a second. In 1966, however, Jim Ryan smashed the existing world record by almost two seconds! In fact, the past 12 years' record for the mile has dropped 8.1 seconds. But in the 17 years before Bannister's breakthrough the record dropped only 5 seconds. Why are there such phenomenal improvements? Here are several reasons: better general health, newer training techniques, improved equipment, more participants and psychological attitude.

Better General Health

Despite hunger in some parts of the world and failure to obtain an optimal diet by many people in the most affluent societies, man is bigger, stronger, and healthier on the whole than he was 50 or 100 years ago and because of his increased strength and size, is better equipped for record-shattering performances. Improvements in medicine also contribute greatly to a healthier human organism. Well-balanced diets (including ample calories) are necessary to achieve peak performance and more athletes are maintaining the optimum diet throughout life in order to reap maximum benefits.

Newer Training Techniques

In times past an athlete would get out on the track and doggedly run numerous laps around the track to get "into shape." Swimmers, likewise, would methodically swim many laps through the water. Weight training was taboo, for it made the athlete muscle-bound. Furthermore, there was a great fear that the athlete would go "stale" if he trained too hard. A great deal of the training was based upon traditional rather than scientific principles.

Today all those concepts have changed. Intensive training is now the word. One of the first to practice this technique was Emil Zatopek, the great Czechoslovakian distance runner of mid-century. Despite the weather, Zatopek rigidly stuck to running mile after mile with weighted boots. Prior to Zatopek few athletes would adhere to such a schedule. Vladimir Kutz and Herb Elliott were also proponents of exhausting workouts. Both Kutz and Elliot would run until they dropped from exhaustion. Elliot also trained with weights, a practice virtually unheard of for milers.

Specific training techniques such as Fartlek, Interval Training, Repetition Training, and Over and Under Training have been used with great success. Interval training, for example, consists of swimming or running a series of repeat efforts at a given distance with a controlled amount of rest and effort. The rest interval allows partial but not complete recovery of the heart rate to normal. For a more specific discussion of Interval Training and the various other techniques, see the respective entries. See also TRAINING.

Weight training and Isometrics are two other training techniques that have been used effectively by athletes in all sports, because they allow controlled building of muscle strength.

Improved diet and a higher standard of living have made man better developed and more powerful and better able to endure those grueling methods. Today, he knows more about his body and its limitations, how it can be trained, and how it can be refreshed through food, rest and care.

Improved Equipment

Equipment over the years has improved greatly. The use of starting blocks in track has improved performance. Prior to those aids, athletes dug shallow holes in the dirt tracks. Jesse Owens, a prestarting-blocks Olympian, has remarked that these blocks were worth "a tenth of a second or two" in the hundred. Track surfaces have changed. No longer are they made of dirt and cinders, but of synthetic surfaces that permit more efficient movement and faster times.

The most publicized track and field innovation was the fiber glass pole. For years 16 feet was an insurmountable barrier. Then with the advent of this special pole 16 feet was no longer the barrier, but 18 feet. If timed properly with the force of the vaulter, the pole actually helps whip the athletes over the bar, giving them extra lift and height.

In swimming, backwash gutters and heavy lane markers help keep the water smooth despite 8 swimmers racing through the water.

And the improvements are not confined to track and swimming. A livelier baseball and bat have been credited with aiding Roger Maris in hitting 61 home runs. Livelier golf balls and improved golf clubs enable pro golfers to drive 275-300 yards, a distance at one time reserved to just one or two. Improved kicking shoes have improved greatly the accuracy of the kicking specialist in football.

Another equipment technique, and one not often heard about, is cinematography (photography). Through the use of films, the athlete and coach are able to analyze movement very carefully. They can study form and movement, timing, coordination and critical errors.

Electromyography, the study of muscle actions by electronic recordings, is another aid to the scientific study of sports.

More Participants

At one time sport was the privilege of a few wealthy people. Today sport is for the masses. Until very recently sport was primarily the prerogative of Western man. Slowly, the people of the African and Asian countries (especially the Red Chinese and their 800 million inhabitants) are getting involved in the more popular sports. With those additional people the trend toward record breaking will be even greater.

Psychological Aspects

The psychological aspects of effort have been one of the major forces behind the world record-breaking phenomenon. At one time, athletes felt

there were barriers. Today they do not. It took years for man to break the 4-minute mile, the 60-foot shotput, and the 16-foot pole vault. Yet today athletes do with amazing regularity!

Athletes and coaches used to overemphasize that prolonged effort would cause staleness. Today staleness is not a great problem, for it can be recognized and eliminated. See STALENESS.

Many sports enthusiasts feel that mental barriers are the only barriers to hamper performance. Once those mental blocks are overcome, the records will be changed even more. Some people feel that tolerance of pain and the ability to suppress or endure it is the most important aspect both for training and performance. When that hurdle is vaulted the performance usually rises considerably.

Other Factors

Other factors such as drugs have been used to improve performance. A great deal of controversy has arisen over their value. The important thing to remember, regardless of whether performance improves or not, is that drugging an athlete is a highly unethical practice. It endangers the health of the performer and promotes competition on an uneven basis.

How far and how high will man go? Millions ask that question. Will man continue to improve at his current rate indefinitely as he has for the past 100 years? Will he continue to improve but slow down as he approaches his psychological and physiological limits, never quite reaching his potential but advancing by tenths and hundredths of seconds? Or will he improve until he reaches his potential and remain at his level, only to improve as new equipment is devised?

Most researchers agree that man will continually approach his psychological and physiological potential but never quite reach his maximum performance. Improvements will come based on better training techniques, new equipment, new diet aids, and a better understanding of man and his body. Eventually the progress may be measured only in tenths, hundredths and even thousandths of a unit. But it will undoubtedly continue at a much faster pace for some time.

GARDENING

I know I must exercise but I like to be able to breathe easy while I'm doing it. Give me a garden to take care of while I'm keeping this 60-year-old chassis functional and in shape. You can keep that smog-bound, over-crowded city gym. I'll take the digging, hand cultivating and the pushing of the lawn mower. And I'll walk my way to health behind the tractor and the tiller. Here's one of my typical weekends.

**A Four-Mile Workout
with Tiller and Mower**

Last Saturday and Sunday I walked 3½ miles behind the mower, and did another half-mile behind the new rotary tiller after I uncrated it fresh from the factory and assembled it. As usual, I found wrestling with the tiller quite strenuous. But again as usual, I found myself thriving on both chores, and really felt keen and alive working up a sweat and then leaning into the freshly fragrant country breeze while I caught my breath.

I'm not at all sure that a workout in a city gym could give me the all-around physical workover imposed by my garden chores. In addition to running the tiller, I used the two-handed axe, the small hatchet and pruning shears, the hoe, rake and wheelbarrow, and finally the "pump-action" hand grass shears which really call for a lot of hand "pumping."

Besides getting the new tiller ready and giving it a thorough test, I scheduled two big spring jobs—planting the potatoes in hay, and hauling in a new supply of firewood after clearing up the yard to make room for it.

Ever plant potatoes in hay?—you need plenty of bales for it. I belly-bucked fifteen 40-pound bales about 40 feet to the potato patch, broke them open, and then spread them around in a fluffy planting layer 6 inches deep. After carefully setting the seed spuds in place—lots of bending there!—I took more hay and this time spread a fluffy layer 18 inches deep over them to keep the sunlight off the tender plants. That's how you plant potatoes in hay—less scab and disease when they're not in the soil—and it calls for plenty of arm, back and stomach work, lots of limbering, shaking and bending—much more fun than simply working with the weights and barbells.

Sunday morning I was over at my friend's place, busy loading sawed-off chunks of two-foot-thick apple and willow. When I got back home I took one look at the 3 piles of late winter sapling cuttings and just knew I'd have to make room for the bigger stuff. So, out came the axe, the hatchet and the pruning shears, and I went to work swinging, hacking and shearing the inch-thick middlings into neatly uniform and easily stacked lengths. By the time I got through hauling, pulling, dragging, cutting and piling, my hands were rough and tingling, and the sweat was running easily and pleasantly down my face and back. You can't ask for a better workout. You're building personal health while fixing up the homegrounds!

**Walking and Mowing
Your Way to Health**

Although I never seem to get through cutting the grass on my place, mowing the lawn does have its own set of rewards and virtues. It keeps me walking for 90 minutes at a time, stretching the legs and breathing deeply. It not only seems to open up the lungs, but it also gives the chest, shoulders and upper back muscles something to do when I swing around a close turn.

Walking an Acre Into
3½ Miles Is Easy

If you're conscientious, you can stretch an acre of mowing into 3½ walking miles. Here's how I figure it. An acre is a plot of land 200 feet long by 200 wide. What with overlapping and misses, my mower cuts a two-foot swath—that's 100 trips back and forth along the 200-foot length. Multiply 100 × 200 and you come up with 20,000 feet, which divided by 5,280 feet (that's a mile) gives you a walking tour of 3.78 miles!

Yes, you can get a great workout cutting the lawn, exercising the arms and shoulders as well as the legs. Don't talk to me at age 60 about riding mowers—I'm keeping myself alive by stimulating my circulation and digestion with clean outdoor work, and I think that walking while mowing is about the cheapest and easiest way to achieve that goal.

The Sweet Science of
Rotary Tilling

Everything I've said about mowing goes double for rotary tilling. I can't think of any piece of apparatus, any vibrator or massaging machine that will take you apart and then put you back together again better than a vigorously pulsating rotary tiller.

It's a bucking bronco and sparring partner combined. I like to work mine on an uphill grade, giving the tiller its head until I get used to its pace and tendency to lurch and leap. Going downhill I try to throttle back and throw in the reverse on turns. I watch my footing carefully at all times—this means stepping nimbly. This, I submit, is a workout for a man who wants to shake all the twists and bends out of his carcass down from the neckbone clear to the anklebone!

Another Good Workout—
Shredding In The Row

Shredding is an organic gardening operation which does exactly what it says—it literally shreds vegetable tissues and fibers into small bits so they are more easily handled as mulch or reduced to compost or humus. Although generally the shredder stays in one place, and you bring the material to it, sometimes we wheel the machine —it weighs a good 250 pounds—out into the garden where the work is and trundle it along the planting rows.

It's hard to beat that kind of exercise which makes demands on the entire body—arms, legs, trunk, hands, feet. By the time you've shredded two or three 30-foot rows—hauling the shredder uphill and down, and then stooping, bending, lifting and raking— there's nothing in the gym that can take the place of the shredder, which, again, gets something done while it gives you a workout!

Exercising by gardening is not a private matter but a universal custom that has been going on for a long time —ever since men stopped living in caves and trees. What has been reported here is neither new nor particularly original, but it is something which should be reported and stressed because we all-too-frequently take good things for granted and overlook them.

Nothing really unusual or special took place over my gardening weekend. I did two things—built fertility in the soil and improved my health by doing so. It's hard to get a better bargain today at the existing rates of exchange.—*Maurice Franz*

Contributions to Physical Fitness

Since gardening is a moderate-high-energy-cost activity it may be used to help improve your fitness level, especially circulo-respiratory and muscle endurance. Below is a gardening training program that takes into account the important principles of fitness. See WORK for a closely allied discussion.

Fitness 1

If you achieved a score of poor or low average on the *Harvard Step Test* or a score of very poor or poor on the

* FARMING, PLANTING, HOEING PROGRAM

Chart 1	Chart 2
1. 30 minutes	1. 90 minutes
2. 40 minutes	2. 95 minutes
3. 50 minutes	3. 100 minutes
4. 60 minutes	4. 105 minutes
5. 70 minutes	5. 110 minutes
6. 75 minutes	6. 110 minutes
7. 80 minutes	7. 115 minutes
8. 85 minutes	8. 120 minutes
9. 90 minutes	9. 120 minutes

* See ENDURANCE and ENERGY COST OF ACTIVITIES for an explanation of these charts.

12 Minute Run, start on Chart 1-Level 1 and spend 1 week at each level until Chart 2-Level 9 is reached. It is recommended that you participate 4 to 5 days a week. When Chart 2-Level 9 is reached, 4 days a week is sufficient.

Fitness 2

If you achieved a score of high average on the *Harvard Step Test* or fair on the *12 Minute Run,* start on Chart 1-Level 1. Spend one week on Chart 1-Levels 1, 3, 4, 6, 7 and 9, and Chart 2-Levels 2, 4, 6, 7 and 9. It is recommended that you participate 4 to 5 days a week. When Chart 2-Level 9 is reached 4 days a week is sufficient.

Fitness 3

If you achieved a score of good or excellent on either the *Harvard Step Test* or *12 Minute Run,* continue your current program or select Chart 2-Level 9 as your level of participation. Four days a week is sufficient.

GOLF

From early spring to late autumn and even early winter golfing buffs dot the nation's fairways and greens chasing that ever-elusive "par." Probably no other sport has such devoted participants as golf. And for good reason. Golf is a stimulating, relaxing recreational activity enjoyable at all age levels. It provides a degree of physical activity commensurate with the needs of the individual involved, AND may be played singly or with a group. A handicap system allows people of varying ability to compete on an equal basis; golf makes an absorbing demand on the player involving mental self-discipline, complete analysis of each situation, and skill. It is a game that rewards sound strategy and accurate shots.

Contribution to Physical Fitness

You do not have to attain a high level of physical fitness merely to enjoy a round of golf. You can ride a golf car from hole to hole, walk the same distance leisurely, walk briskly, or actually run the course. Thus, the effect golf has on circulo-respiratory endurance depends on how the sport is played and, more important, on how you set the pace.

Don't expect to significantly increase muscular strength, power, or endurance through golf play. Those components of fitness are essential for long, powerful drives, a fluid performance and stamina; but you will have to supplement the actual golf play with practice and an exercise program to improve them. Such an approach will help alleviate unnecessary fatigue and muscle soreness and stiffness brought on by inadequate physical preparation.

To make golf a "fitness" activity you must play in pairs or singly and carry your own clubs. Your walk from the tee to the hole must be brisk—at least 4 miles per hour.

Conditioning Exercises

1. General Exercises
   a. Jogging. See JOGGING
   b. Walking
   c. Wrist Flexion—Extension
   d. Squeezing rubber ball in both hands
   e. Trunk Bends
   f. Upper Body Arch
   g. Body Arch

h. Flutter Kicks
i. Chest Lifts
j. Push-ups, Chin-ups, and/or Shoulder dips
k. Club swinging with weighted head covers.

2. See WEIGHT TRAINING for exercises with weights.

3. Isometric Exercises

Several isometric exercises are valuable, particularly those that involve the back, the arms, and the trunk. Do not neglect leg exercises.

The single best isometric exercise is to place the club head against a door jamb. Exert a maximum force as though you were trying to hit a golf ball. Hold for three seconds and release. Repeat three times and gradually increase to 6 seconds. Don't exert a maximum effort until after the first week or two to avoid unnecessary muscle soreness.

Physical Qualities Needed

A sufficient degree of hand-eye coordination is an important attribute in golf. Also, you will need to possess certain minimal levels of muscular strength and endurance and circulorespiratory endurance before you will be able to concentrate on the more intricate aspects of the game.

Associations:

National Collegiate Athletic Association (NCAA) Suite 206, Fairfax Building, 11th and Baltimore, Kansas City, Missouri 64155.

Professional Golfers Association (PGA) Box 12458, Palm Beach Gardens, Lake Park, Florida 33403.

United States Golf Association (USGA) 40 East 38th Street, New York, New York 10016.

Ladies Professional Golf Association (LPGA) Public Relations Office, 220 South Fifth Street, Box 80, Quincy, Illinois 62303.

National Federation of State High School Athletic Associations (NFSH-

SAA).—William H. Zimmerli. See ORGANIZATIONS.

GOVERNMENT

Until recently, governments were not greatly concerned with the physical fitness of youth or adults. During past wars the interest often increased as a result of the number of rejects for military service. But with the end of the war the interest soon diminished, only to be rekindled with the advent of another military conflict.

Increased Concern for Physical Fitness

Today, governments throughout the world have become more concerned about the fitness status of their entire population, particularly in those countries where a great proportion of the population is sedentary. The concern is most evident in Western countries, where the societies are so highly mechanized. Research has demonstrated that exercise is vital to delay or reduce the onset of many degenerative dis-

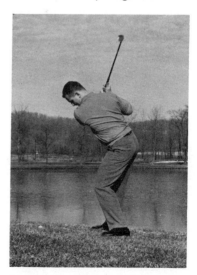

To get the most from golf go alone or with only a few partners. That will allow you to spend your time walking and swinging rather than standing and waiting.

eases, and that it adds to the emotional well-being of the population. Gradually, governments have come to recognize that the vitality of their country is directly dependent upon the vitality of its people—a vitality that cannot be maintained or developed without physical, mental, or moral fitness.

Programs in Other Countries

The steps the various governments have taken are many. Russia uses exercise breaks, instead of coffee breaks. Periodic health check-ups at clinics often diagnose possible hidden ailments; the Russian government also sponsors recreational facilities for the worker and his family in the evening. Several communist and non-communist European countries have developed reconditioning centers. Those centers, run by governments, businesses and other interested organizations, provide periodic "rests." Here the patients spend several weeks in pleasant surroundings going through emotional and physical retraining. The program consists of relaxation, vigorous outdoor exercise, hobbies and proper diet. At those centers particular attention is directed toward a lifetime fitness program.

For 40 years, Sweden has offered official awards to citizens who are able to meet certain physical standards. One million Swedes now wear the coveted national sports badge. Germany has had a similar awards program for 30 years and now gives out almost one million such awards each year.

U. S. Programs

The United States government entered the area of physical fitness during the 1950's. A series of tests (Kraus-Weber) administered to the youth of America demonstrated the poor physical condition of our children. In 1956 the President's Council on Youth Fitness was established to help combat

that low level of fitness in our youth. But progress was slow. The real impetus did not come about until the administration of President Kennedy. Then the Council's title was changed to the President's Council on Physical Fitness, so as to include the entire population. More recently, the title has been changed to the President's Council on Physical Fitness and Sports, a change that has been met with mixed emotions. There is some fear that the council may overemphasize the sports aspect, thereby adding to the tragic situation in many schools where prime emphasis is placed on the 10 per cent of the children who participate in inter-school sports, rather than on the entire school population. The trend that the government takes, however, will depend upon the general population.

The Council was not intended to be another vast Washington agency. The original idea was that the prestige of the Presidency could be used to clarify to citizens the desirability of fitness as a personal goal. That method continues to be the technique used by the Council. Using persuasion and counsel instead of muscle and money to convince a variety of organizations—including other government bodies—its executive staff of five people acts as a public relations arm of the Executive Department, for the purpose of motivating the American people toward better fitness.

Results of Programs

Since the President's Council was formed, there have been improvements in youth fitness. Many schools have intensified their physical education programs, and average scores on fitness tests given to children have markedly improved. The President's Council points with pride to the 50,000 American children who have qualified for its fitness awards. It also has set up special programs in selected elementary schools, which serve as models for other schools. Its goal is to have one such demonstration center school in each state, but at present there are only 25. The old public relations program of the Council encouraged school boards to open their athletic and playground facilities for more hours each day, primarily for community recreation. Its slogan was "Don't fence me out!"

The primary efforts of the Council have been in the schools, because of the easy way to contact and work with people. V. L. Nicholson, ex-Director of Information for the President's Council, has said that the council's assignment is vague and general and that its resources are limited. Plans are being made to extend the Presidential Physical Fitness Awards to boys and girls in the 10 to 17 age group. If the program works here, it will extend to college and universities and perhaps eventually include adult award programs. Mr. Nicholson made it clear, however, that fitness awards for adults would depend on success in creating or finding ways to do the necessary testing. They may never materialize.

Adult Fitness

Physicians seem to agree that adult fitness is now a more critical problem than youth fitness, particularly because of the rising rate of coronary heart disease. The coronary disease process begins in youth and probably can be stemmed by physical conditioning of young people. But the biggest saving of lives today would come from cardiovascular training of adults, through such activities as brisk walking, jogging, cycling, swimming and vigorous sports. However, the amount of such conditioning that is being done is pitifully small and is largely being spurred by individual enthusiasts and private organizations like the YMCA.

What Should Government Do?

The regimentation of children is an accepted fact of life in almost all so-cieties and civilizations, and it is through regimentation that children now receive their physical education. Children are instructed to do exercises and learn physical skills; adults, however, can't be forced into fitness. Even the most totalitarian governments would have difficulty requiring each of their citizens to go through a prescribed routine of exercises each day. In America, it would be unthinkable. Fitness is rightly considered a private matter, even though it has many public implications.

What does that leave for the government to do? Although the actual enforcement of fitness standards is obviously beyond the authority of government, there remain many avenues for federal, state and local action. The example set by leaders is all-important. Many of today's programs and activities owe their birth and even their continuation to John F. Kennedy and his legend. Obviously, present leaders at all levels of government have similar opportunities to stimulate their interest in personal fitness.

Facilities and Research

Creating facilities for fitness activities is also an important function of government. Parks, trails, sidewalks, wilderness areas and sport installations are a public need, and are rightly made available by way of government. So is education, but so far little has been done by government to provide physical education for adults. Research is another great need, now largely unfulfilled. The President's Council has no money available for grants. Although fitness is a less complicated subject than many health and disease problems, scientists still lack even a universally accepted definition of it. More research could help lay a foundation for adult fitness programs that would have stronger scientific backing.

Motivation—by way of official awards—is the simplest and most obvious route for government to enter the fitness picture, as has been done with successful adult programs in other countries. Perhaps some day there will be such adult awards in America.

Structure of the Council

The members of the President's Council on Physical Fitness and Sports are the secretaries of each of the departments in the President's cabinet. Apparently, however, the cabinet-level secretaries never meet to discuss fitness. They delegate representatives to an interagency advisory group, which holds only occasional meetings. Offices of the President's Council are in the Department of Health, Education and Welfare; and its budget is channeled through that department.

A significant part of the Council's work is the distribution of copy for public service advertisements, which are run free by many publications and TV stations. Those ads and commercials are prepared on a volunteer basis by an advertising firm.

There seems to be little question that the nation is getting good value for its $315,000 annual investment in the President's Council on Physical Fitness and Sports. But the fact remains that the great majority of American adults are physically unfit. And those who seek to attain fitness do so largely through their own efforts, providing their own facilities, and bucking the prevailing public attitude that adult fitness is something a person achieves only if he takes time from more important pursuits.

If Americans are ever going to become fit in significant numbers, there will have to be a tremendous increase in fitness facilities and a big change in the general attitude. A force larger than the President's Council on Physical Fitness and Sports, as presently constituted, is necessary to create an achievement of that magnitude.—*Robert Rodale*

GRASS DRILLS

Introduction

Grass drills condition you for the knocks and bumps you may receive when participating in an athletic event. A secondary objective is to develop certain components of physical fitness: agility, speed of movement, certain neuro-muscular skills, and to a certain degree, balance, flexibility and circulo-respiratory endurance.

Grass drills are generally performed on a soft grass area and include agility activities, calisthenics and various types of running. Isometric exercises and tumbling may also be included.

Using Grass Drills

1. Prior to engaging in grass drills, warm up sufficiently with stretching exercise, running, and/or light calisthenics.

2. There should be little or no pause between the various activities in the drill.

3. The minimum length of time is about one minute, the maximum about five minutes. When you engage in a grass drill continuously, the first day drill should last about one minute and the drills increase about 30 seconds daily, until the five-minute maximum is reached.

4. The grass drill may be performed individually or as a group.

5. If you have a chronic joint injury, be cautious and avoid activities that place undue strain on that joint.

6. The techniques for overloading in grass drills are

    a. Increase the speed of movements

    b. Increase the number of activities

    c. Increase the number of repetitions

    d. Decrease rest time between activities

    e. Increase the number of more difficult activities

See OVERLOAD PRINCIPLE for a discussion on how to make activities more stressful

7. Grass drills are usually more effective when a leader gives the necessary commands, so that you may move smoothly from one activity to the next.

Basic Positions

1. UP—This is the most basic position. Assume a standing position in which your legs are slightly flexed and shoulder-width apart. The trunk is flexed slightly forward with your arms flexed beside your body.

2. BACK—Assume a supine position on the ground. Your legs are straight, and your arms are beside your body.

3. FRONT—Assume a prone position on the ground. The entire front of the body is on the ground. The arms may be next to your body or tucked under your chest.

4. SIDE (left or right)—Lie on your side with your underarm either next to your body or stretched out above your head.

Note: To get into the back, front, and side positions from the up position, squat first and then assume the desired position.

5. RUN—In the up position run in place lifting your knees to waist height and pumping your arms vigorously.

6. RUN AND GO—In the run position sprint forward as fast as possible.

7. RUN AND BACK—Merely run backwards.

8. SHUTTLE (left and right)—From the up position run first to your left and then to your right, changing direction frequently. You may include the run and go, the run and back, and the shuttle.

9. STOP—Regardless of the position or activity, stop on command and do not move until the next signal is given.

Grass Drill Exercises

Many of the activities suggested in the calisthenics, guerrilla drills, and isometric sections may be used in the grass drill routine.

1. BICYCLING—Assume a supine position on the ground. Raise your legs in the air, so that only your shoulders, upper back, neck, head and upper arms touch the ground. Place your hands on your hips, with the elbows resting on the floor for support. With feet in the overhead position, move your legs as if pedaling a bicycle.

2. ROLLS—A forward or backward roll from squat position.

3. ROLL RIGHT or LEFT—On the proper command roll left or right.

4. RUSSIAN KICKS—Assume a full squat position with feet about 6 inches apart, weight on the balls of the feet, and hands on the hips. Kick the left leg out to full extension, just touching the heel to the ground. Then return the leg to the starting position and alternate. If you have a history of a knee injury, do not perform this exercise.

5. SCISSORS JUMPS—Stand with your hands on hips. Then leap into the air, moving your legs in a scissors movement.

6. SQUAT JUMPS—Assume a squat position. Separate the legs and place your hands on the ground between legs. From that position leap up reaching upward with your hands. On the way down assume the squat position.

CAUTION—A forceful squat may cause a knee injury. Therefore, use caution when performing the exercise. If you have a history of a knee injury, avoid it.

Many other activities may be substituted or added to the lists above.

Grass Drill Example

The following is a typical grass drill program:

1. Up (Basic starting position)
2. Front
3. Back
4. Side
5. Up
6. Run (5 seconds)

7. Run and Go (3 seconds)
8. Front
9. Back
10. Run (5 seconds)
11. Run-Back (3 seconds)
12. Stop (1 second)
13. Shuttle Run (10 seconds)
14. Front
15. Back
16. Sit-ups (15 seconds) (Calisthenics)
17. Bicycling (10 seconds)
18. Forward Rolls (3 times)
19. Backward Rolls (3 times)
20. Russian Kicks (10 seconds)
21. Scissors Jumps (10 seconds)
22. Squat Jumps (10 seconds)
23. Push-ups (10 seconds) (Calisthenics)
24. Mountain Climbers (15 seconds) (Guerrilla Drill)
25. Roll Right or Left (10 seconds)
26. Front
27. Front Rolls (10 seconds)
28. Up
29. Run and Go (5 seconds)
30. Stop (1 second)
31. Shuttle (10 seconds)
32. Stop

The object is to move rapidly from one activity to another. Be certain that the exercises are performed correctly. In fact, it is better if you perform the exercise carefully in the beginning until you have mastered the correct techniques and the required movements.

GROWTH

Human growth is a complex but orderly process involving the interaction of heredity and environment. Heredity, or the genetic endowment of the individual, determines the potential for growth. It is frequently viewed in terms of a number of interrelated and interacting factors including the constitutional type of the individual, his ultimate size, the rate at which that size will be attained, and the timing of the growth processes. Environment, on the other hand, determines to a large extent the degree to which the genetic potential is achieved. A wide variety of environmental forces can affect the growth of any individual. One well-known factor is nutrition, for the growth processes require essential building components—the proteins, carbohydrates, fats, minerals and vitamins.

Homeostasis and Growth Balance

Optimal growth presupposes some sort of balance between the genetic and environmental components. This balance resides in what W. B. Cannon called the "wisdom of the body," homeostasis, the maintenance of the internal environment of the body. That balance, however, is not completely fixed or stable. Rather, it is a condition which fluctuates within narrow limits.

It is within that delicate internal balance that the processes of normal growth operate and manifest themselves. Any force which disturbs that balance will cause adaptive physiological responses in the body until the homeostatic balance is restored. Those adaptive responses, in turn, may favorably stimulate or retard the growth processes.

Disruptions of Homeostatic Balance

Intensive physical activity, exercise, or sport is an agent which temporarily disturbs the homeostatic balance, producing a variety of physiological adjustments in the body. The rigors of vigorous physical exercise subject the bones, muscles, and connective tissues to tensile or compressive forces. Circulatory, respiratory, metabolic and chemical responses are also produced. Physical educators believe that the above adaptive responses generated by vigorous physical activity will induce chronic changes and thus favorably influence the growth of the individual. They contend that a consistent and well-balanced program of physical activity will enhance growth during the growing years and will develop the functional powers of a person during the adult years.

Much of the research dealing with the exercise effects on growth in general and on growth of specific bodily tissues has been concerned with the influence of relatively brief exercise and inactivity periods. The results of those studies indicate a favorable role for physical activity in bone and muscle development. There are, however, only a few studies in which exercise has been applied over a sufficiently long time during the growing years.

Influence of Extended Exercise on Growth

One such study, conducted in 1932 by Dr. H. H. Donaldson and Dr. R. E. Messer, investigated the influence of extended exercise on the growth of albino rats followed through seven generations. The animals began the exercise program on the 56th day of life and continued it for 170 days, thus exercising regularly over a period equivalent to the span of 4.5 years to 19 years in man. The findings showed no overall increase in length resulting from exercise; that is exercise did not stimulate linear growth. The exercised animals, on the other hand, showed an increase in muscle tissue, a decrease in fat, an increase in the weights of the heart, kidneys, superadrenals, and gonads, and a decrease in the weights of the thyroid and liver. None of the exercise-induced changes were inheritable through the seven successive generations. An earlier study conducted by S. Hatai in 1915 that also involved albino rats revealed that participation in a strenuous physical activity regime from the third to the sixth month of life (7 to 14 years in man) increase most of the vital organs from 20 to 30 per cent in weight relative to body weight but produced no increase in body length. The body weight of the animals was also increased because of the hypertrophy of muscle tissue. The greatest gains were shown in the weight of the heart and kidneys. In addition, several animals, exercised for only a one month period, showed proportionately smaller increments.

Exercise in Different Stages of Growth

In an attempt to investigate the effects upon growth of exercises beginning at different points in the growth cycle, Dr. Donaldson subjected one group of albino rats to a 31-day exercise program at an age of 25 days (corresponding to 2.1 years in man) and a second group to a 90-day program at an age of 200 days (16.6 years in man). From his results, Donaldson concluded that the response to exercise was the same regardless of the age of its initiation.

Dr. Henry J. Montoye and his coworkers used a different approach. Albino rats were restricted in their physical activity during the growth period and then subjected to a three-month exercise program. Beginning the exercise program when the animals were fully grown, influenced body and organ weights very little. These results would seem to suggest the importance of initiating an exercise program earlier in life, perhaps when the growth impulse is the strongest. However, just when the impulse to optimal growth is the strongest has not yet been determined with any certainty.

Influence of Induced Activity

Donaldson and Messer also investigated the influence of induced inactivity on a small group of growing rats previously exposed to a strenuous exercise program. In general, the findings showed an acceleration of organ and tissue growth during the exercise regime and a regression of organ weights with inactivity. After the inactivity period, however, the organs of the exercised animals were slightly heavier, thus suggesting a somewhat chronic effect of exercise on the growth of rats. The evidence presented clearly indicates a favorable influence of a protracted exercise program on the growth of rats. But the effects of such programs on human growth, is still somewhat uncertain because of the inability to carry on controlled studies

More recently, Dr. E. Simon investigated the influence of physical training on the morphological and functional development of two groups of 14 to 15 year-old children. One group received daily physical training while the other received training twice a week over a 6-month period. The following figures summarize Simon's results:

GAINS AT THE CONCLUSION OF THE EXPERIMENT

	Daily Group	Twice Wk. Group
Body length	.43 in.	.47 in.
Chest circumference	1.92 in.	.39 in.
Respiratory amplitude	2.17 in.	1.36 in.
Difference in upper arm circumference with elbows flexed and extended	.59 in.	.31 in.
Thigh circumference	.91 in.	.59 in.
Shoulder width	.95 in.	.55 in.
Body weight	12.76 lbs.	17.16 lbs.

over the course of the growing years. Nevertheless, there is, some fragmentary evidence which suggests a beneficial influence of exercise on growth. Dr. E. H. Adams, for example, compared the anthropometric measurements of 100 Negro women, 17 to 21 years of age, who had experienced a childhood of strenuous physical labor with the measurements of 100 women of the same age who had experienced no such labor during the growing years. Without exception, the women who did manual labor during the growing years were taller, heavier, and larger in muscle girths, chest breadth and depth, hip width and knee width. Adams attributed the size advantage of the working women over the nonworkers to the program of heavy physical work. P. Godin reported the results of his observations on the growth of gymnasts and nongymnasts from 14½ to 18 years of age. The gymnasts were slightly taller, heavier and larger in thoracic and forearm measurements. Godin attributed those observations to the gymnastic exercises ("exercises with the fixed bar").

It is apparent from these figures that physical training stimulates growth in body bulk but does not lead to an acceleration of growth in body length. The results also illustrate an advantage in favor of the more intensively trained children. Similar changes were also noted in functional measures of running, jumping and throwing performance. In a similar study, Dr. J. B. Wells, Dr. J. Parizkova and Dr. E. Jokl examined the effects of five months of daily physical training on 34 adolescent girls as compared to an equal number of control subjects. The findings showed a definite change in body composition; that is, a significant increase in active tissue (lean tissue) and a corresponding reduction in fatty tissue in the exercise group. No such changes were observed in the control subjects. An improvement in physical efficiency was also noted with training. According to the authors, this improvement ". . . is to be considered a functional equivalent of the tissue changes under reference."

Studies of specialized use of one portion of the body also provide a means of examining some of the chronic effects of exercise. Dr. E. R. Buskirk, Dr. K. L. Anderson, and Dr. J. Brozek, for example, made a comparison of the dominant and non-dominant forearms of seven nationally ranked tennis players and eleven non-tennis playing soldiers. The dominant forearm of the tennis players showed significantly greater muscular development than the non-dominant member. Similar but non-significant muscular differences were observed in the preferred hand and arms of the non-tennis players. Since the tennis players used in that investigation had played extensively during their teen years, the authors attributed the differences to the effects of exercise on the bone "growth apparatus" during the adolescent years. The above findings as well as those of Godin rather definitely suggest that an extended exercise program does stimulate growth in the body regions specifically exercised.

Permanence of Exercise-Induced Growth

In a study of weight training and physique, Dr. J. M. Tanner found increases in anthropometric measures after four months of training. The greatest increment was in upper arm and forearm, which increased significantly in almost all subjects (average increment in the upper arm was 2cm). However, measurements taken four months after the training program ended showed that almost all measures had reverted to the pre-training values. Those results clearly indicate the favorable influence of exercise on muscle growth, but more importantly indicate the need for continued exercise to maintain the exercise-induced changes.

The available information, therefore, indicates a growth-stimulating effect of muscular exercise on bone tissue, skeletal muscle, linear growth of the upper extremity, and changes in breadth and girth. Exercise regimes have little if any influence on total growth in body length or height. Some evidence, rather, suggests that excessive pressures from activity may even retard long bone growth.

Changes produced as a result of short-term physical exercise programs are not permanent but are dependent upon continued activity for their maintenance. In contrast, long continued specializations and training result in the more chronic changes.

Care must be used in drawing conclusions relative to the effects of exercise on growth, for the available evidence is far from conclusive. *It appears that a certain minimum of physical exercise is necessary to support normal growth and to maintain the integrity of bone and muscular tissues.* Just what this minimum is or should be, and just what effects more extended exercise programs have on human growth, remain to be completely answered.—*Robert M. Malina*

GUERRILLA EXERCISES

Introduction

Guerrilla exercises and drills were developed during World War I to condition soldiers for combat. The exercises enable a group to work out in a short period of time, without using any special equipment. When properly conducted, the exercises make a contribution to the development and/or maintenance of agility, balance, flexibility, neuromuscular skill, muscle endurance, muscle strength and cardio-respiratory endurance. In a guerrilla drill almost the entire body is involved.

Guideline for Guerrilla Exercise

Dr. Donald R. Casady, Dr. Donald F. Mapes, and Dr. Louis E. Alley have presented several excellent guidelines for people who participate in guerrilla drills, whether alone or with a group. Below is a resumé of their suggestions:

1. When a group is performing a guerrilla drill, the leader should dem-

onstrate the next activity while the rest of the group runs in place. After the demonstration, the group starts the next exercise and continues until the leader tells them to stop, at which point they run in place while the leader demonstrates the next activity.

2. If at all possible, intersperse individual exercises with dual exercise.

3. Progressively increase the intensity of the guerrilla drills. Here's a typical program

First Day—Three individual exercises and one dual exercise.

Second Day—Five individual exercises and one dual exercise.

Third Day—Six individual exercises and one dual exercise.

Fourth Day—Six individual exercises and two dual exercises.

4. Besides progressively increasing the number of exercises performed, you can overload or progressively add to the guerrilla drill by:

(a) increasing the speed of movements, and

(b) performing the dual exercises with heavier partners. A third possibility is to combine steps A, B, and step 3.

If you have a weak joint or are prone to injury, avoid those exercises that will put a particular strain on that joint.

Exercises—Individual

1. *All-Fours Run*—Assume an all-fours position with hands and feet touching the ground. Flex the legs slightly. Maintain that position while running forward, backward, or sideward, depending upon the instructions of leader.

2. *Broad Jump*—Perform successive standing broad jumps. The action of the broad jump is to have the arms extended and pointing downward and backward; the body is in a crouched position. Leaning forward, swing both arms forward in a rapid, vigorous movement. Extend the legs forcefully.

3. *Cart Wheels*—Advance your left foot and raise the arms above your head; then flex your hip and place your hands (fingers to the left) on a line directly from your left toe, which is pointing straight forward. At that point, swing up your extended right leg and follow it with your left. As the weight travels from the left to the right, the right foot comes down near the hands.

4. *Crab Walk*—Assume a sitting position with legs extended. Place your hands, fingers pointing towards the feet, behind you on the floor. Raise the buttocks from the floor, and flex your knees slightly. Then move forward, backward, or sideward depending upon the instructions received.

5. *Crouch Run*—Flex your legs and hips and then bend forward until your chest is parallel to the ground, holding at that position, run forward, backward, or sideward.

6. *Fast Walk*—Assuming an upright position, walk forward as fast as you can—always keeping one foot in contact with the ground. This is a walk, not a jog.

7. *Giant Step Walk*—In an erect position take elongated steps forward or backward.

8. *Gorilla Walk*—Flex your knees and bend at the waist so that your upper body is at least parallel to the floor. Hang the arms downward so that the fingertips touch the floor. Then walk or run forward.

9. *Hand-Kick Walk*—Assume an upright position and walk forward. With each step kick an outstretched hand, first with the left leg, then the right.

10. *Inch-Worm Walk*—Assume an all-fours position with the legs extended and the arms outstretched and directly under the shoulders. First walk your feet up to your hands, which remain stationary. Then walk forward with your hands while the feet remain stationary. When your arms are directly under your shoulders, start the entire process again.

11. *Hop on One Foot*—Hop on one

foot with your hands on your hips, then on your head, and finally outstretched.

12. *Hop on Two Feet*—Same as above except use both feet.

13. *Jumping, Forward Hand Kick*—Crouch and then jump off the floor, attempting to touch your toes with your fingertips. To do that you must flex your legs at the hips. Land in a semi-crouched position, and immediately jump off the floor again.

14. *Knee-Raise Run*—Run in place or forward. With each running step raise the thighs so that your knees are waist high.

15. *Lame-Dog Run*—Assume an all-fours position and raise your left leg behind you. Then run on the three supporting limbs with your head facing in the direction of movement. The "lame" leg does not touch the ground. A variation of this drill is to use the other leg or one of the arms.

16. *Mountain Climbing*—Assume a push-up position. Then bring one leg to your chest—a position somewhat similar to that of a sprinter; and alternate legs.

17. *Shadow Boxing*—Assume a boxer's stance, left foot forward, elbows bent, and arms in front of the body with the fists clenched. Alternate punches aimed at an imaginary opponent. Include a dancing motion in the shadow boxing routine.

Dual Exercises

Use a partner of similar size and weight.

1. *Arm Carry*—Facing your partner's side, bend forward and place one arm around your partner's back and the other arm under his thigh. The partner clasps his hands together around your neck. Straighten up, support your partner's weight and walk forward or backward depending upon the instructions issued.

2. *Back to Back Run*—Both partners act as performers. Stand back to back, lean against one another, and bend the knees. On the command, your partner walks forward, while you walk backward. For a variation try a sideward movement.

3. *Fireman's Carry*—Face your partner's right side. Bend forward and place your right shoulder against his chest or stomach. Place your right hand underneath your partner's crotch and grasp his right arm with your right hand. Straighten up with your partner resting on your right shoulder. Then grasp the left wrist of your partner with your left hand.

4. *Leapfrog*—Both partners are performers in this drill. Assume a semi-crouched position with your head flexed forward and your hands on the ground. Your partner takes his position directly behind you. He places his hands on your upper back and vaults over you, pushing with his hands and straddling with his legs. He immediately assumes the semi-crouched position, and you repeat the vault that he just performed. Continue to leap frog over each other as you move forward.

5. *Piggy Back*—Crouch slightly and stand with your back to your partner. Your partner mounts you, dropping his arms over you and squeezing his thighs against you. He places his arms around your thighs. For more security the partner may wrap his arms around your chest. Run or walk forward or backward depending upon the instructions.

6. *Two-Man Forward Rolls*—Both partners are performers in this drill. Have your partner lie on his back with his head toward you. His knees should be bent, with his feet near his buttocks. Stand with your feet against his shoulders. He then grasps your ankles while you lean forward and grasp his. Make certain that your partner's feet are firmly planted on the floor, then tuck your head and execute a forward roll. Your partner starts to sit up as you roll. The action is continuous. Hint: both partners must keep their heads tucked at all times.

Sample Guerrilla Program

1.	All-Fours Run	15 seconds
2.	Broad Jump	10 successive jumps
3.	Hand-Kick Walk	15 seconds
4.	Hop on One Foot	30 seconds (15 on each foot)
5.	Knee-Raise Run	30 seconds
6.	Mountain Climbing	15 seconds
7.	Shadow Boxing	15 or 30 seconds
8.	Giant Step Walk	15 seconds
9.	Arm Carry	15 seconds (each partner)
10.	Piggy Back	30 seconds (each partner)
11.	Wheelbarrow Run	15 seconds (each partner)

7. *Wheelbarrow Run* (Front and Back)—Both partners are performers in this action. Your partner assumes a standing position. He then grasps your ankles when you are in a push-up position and raises legs to waist height. On the command start to walk forward. As a variation the performer in the push-up position may assume a face-up position.

HANDBALL

You can learn skills necessary to enjoy participation in handball in a short time. That doesn't mean that the game is so simple there is no challenge. The advanced skills and strategy required for top competition demands a great deal of practice.

There are three types of games in handball: four wall, three wall and one wall. Rules are basically the same for all three games. The major difference is in the one-wall game where a screened shot is considered good strategy. In the four-wall game it is a foul and must be played over. Although the serve is important in all three games, it is considered to be a most important part of the one-wall game. Volleys will be much shorter in one- and three-wall games because of a greater number of passing shots.

Handball may be played by two persons (singles), three persons (cutthroat), and four persons (doubles). Cutthroat is played with the two defensive players working as a team against the one offensive player. Play-

ers rotate each time the offensive player fails to return the ball legally. Singles is more demanding physically, and doubles requires teamwork.

The game is started by the server standing between the short line and service line. The ball is bounced on the floor. On the rebound, the ball is hit with the hand to the front wall so that it hits the floor behind the short line on the rebound. The opponent must return the ball so that it hits the front wall before hitting the floor. Only the server can score, and he continues to serve as long as he returns the ball legally. When the server fails to return the ball, his opponent serves. The first player or team to reach 21 points wins the game. It's legal to hit the ball with either hand, but only with the hand, and only with one hand at a time.

Very little equipment is needed for handball: a pair of gloves, a regulation ball, regular gymnasium clothing including shorts and T-shirt, and a pair of tennis shoes. You may want to wear a sweat suit to aid in warming up.

Contribution to Physical Fitness

Handball ranks high in developing circulo-respiratory endurance. Because of the nature of the game, the entire body is involved—the arms deliver force to the ball, the legs move you rapidly across the court, and the back and abdomen muscles bend and stretch in retrieving balls. Excessive strength is not essential, although the strong muscles of the arms and shoulders do receive benefit from playing.

Conditioning Programs

Since handball involves the use of the total body, develop a conditioning program that will aid and involve each portion. Give special attention to developing the weak or non-dominant side of the body.

General exercise should include running in place, body bends and turns which involve the abdomen, leg stretching to develop flexibility, knee bends, practicing sudden starting and stopping as well as rapidly changing direction from side to side and forward and backward. Weight training will assist in developing strength. Push-ups and pull-ups will develop the muscles of the chest, arms and shoulders used in hitting the ball. A series of full arm swings followed by throwing the ball to the front wall using an underhand, sidearm and overhand motion is beneficial. Start the warm-up early, play slow and easy, increasing the power and length of play as conditioning develops.

A common problem is the tendency

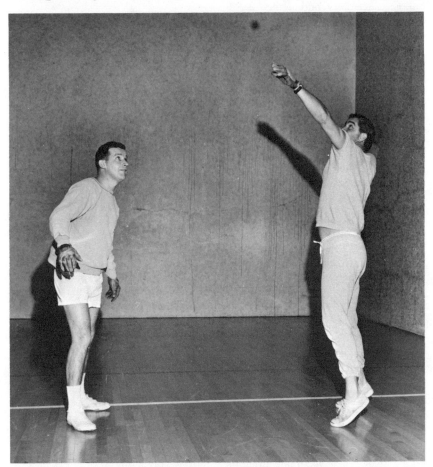

When played strenuously and vigorously, handball can make an important contribution to cardiovascular fitness. Most people supplement it with other activities.

for the hands to become bruised from striking the ball. Soaking the hands in hot water prior to play and using padded gloves may aid in alleviating that problem.

Physical Qualities Needed

Physical size has little if any bearing on success in handball. It can be played by persons of all ages since the pace is determined by the participants. The game involves both sides of the body, the arms, the shoulders, the legs, the feet and the waist. A better than average level of circulo-respiratory endurance, flexibility and agility is required. Eye-hand coordination with the ability to use either hand is essential.

A handball palm is a contusion of the palm that frequently occurs. The palm is painful to touch. The pain is a result of a contusion of the soft tissues of the hand. Soaking the hand in cold water may provide some relief during the initial stages of the injury. Complete rest is best and will speed recovery. Apply heat during the later stages of recovery. Massage, however, should not be attempted.

To protect or at least reduce the possibility of developing a handball palm, you should toughen your hands gradually before engaging in prolonged bouts of handball, or wear gloves. Once the injury has occurred, you may find that it is necessary to pad the palm prior to play.

Associations:

U. S. Handball Association, 4101 Dempster, Skokie, Illinois 60076.

Amateur Athletic Union (AAU). See ORGANIZATIONS.—*Norman L. Sheets*

Since handball is a high-energy-cost activity it may be used to help improve your fitness level, especially your circulo-respiratory and muscle endurance. Below is a handball program that takes into account the important principles of training.

If you desire to improve your strength and power for handball, see WEIGHT TRAINING and ISOMETRICS.

*HANDBALL PROGRAM

Chart 1	Chart 2
1. 10 minutes	1. 38 minutes
2. 15 minutes	2. 40 minutes
3. 18 minutes	3. 43 minutes
4. 20 minutes	4. 45 minutes
5. 23 minutes	5. 50 minutes
6. 25 minutes	6. 53 minutes
7. 30 minutes	7. 55 minutes
8. 33 minutes	8. 58 minutes
9. 35 minutes	9. 60 minutes

* See ENDURANCE and ENERGY COST OF ACTIVITIES for an explanation of these charts.

Fitness 1

If you achieved a score of poor or low average on the *Harvard Step Test* or a score of very poor or poor on the *12 Minute Run*, start on Chart 1-Level 1 and spend 1 week at each level until Chart 2-Level 9 is reached. It is recommended that you participate 4 to 5 days a week. When Chart 2-Level 9 is reached, 4 days a week is sufficient.

Fitness 2

If you achieved a score of high average on the *Harvard Step Test* or fair on the *12 Minute Run*, start on Chart 1-Level 2. Spend one week on Chart 1-Levels 2, 4, 6, 7, and 9, and Chart 2-Levels 2, 4, 5, 6, 7, and 9. It is recommended that you participate 4 to 5 days a week. When Chart 2-Level 9 is reached 4 days a week is sufficient.

Fitness 3

If you achieved a score of good or excellent on either the *Harvard Step Test* or *12 Minute Run,* continue your current program or select Chart 2-Level 9 as your level of participation. Four days a week is sufficient.

THE HANDICAPPED

The handicapped person is one who, because of a physical, mental or emotional complication, cannot engage fully in a standard educational or physical fitness program.

Types of Programs

A number of names have been used to identify programs for the handicapped: corrective, remedial, rehabilitative, modified and adapted. The latter two are most popular because they suggest more closely what is being done in special programs to help the handicapped—the modification and adaption of regular programs to meet the needs and abilities of the handicapped.

Adapted physical education as defined by the AAHPER is "a diversified program of developmental activities, games, sports and rhythms suited to the interests, capacities, and limitations of students with disabilities who may not safely or successfully engage in unrestricted activities of the general physical education program."

Interest in helping the handicapped arose early in this century as a result of an infantile paralysis epidemic in 1916 and World War I. A desire to help the disabled victims of these two tragedies created a new attitude toward the handicapped. Traditionally, in many societies the handicapped were believed to be best treated with suspicion and fear. The handicaps were considered to be created by Satan, and those afflicted were regarded as evil. Since the early days of concern for the handicapped, programs for them have evolved from the baby-sitting type of service to well-planned programs designed to better the lot of the handicapped person in society.

The mentally handicapped, or retarded, have been described by the President's Panel on Mental Retardation: "The mentally retarded are children and adults who, as a result of inadequately developed intelligence, are significantly impaired in their ability to learn and to adapt to the demands of society." One important characteristic of the handicapped is that they do not display behavior patterns which are considered normal— that is, behavior patterns exhibited by the majority of society and which are most widely accepted.

Causes of Handicaps

Most handicap afflictions are a result of accidents and illnesses. Diseases that frequently result in a physical handicap include poliomyelitis, cerebral palsy, nutritional or metabolic disorders, cardiac conditions and others. Serious accidents can leave one with paralysis of, or loss of, one or more limbs. Mental handicaps can arise from complications before or during birth, as well as from post-birth accidents and illnesses. Complications which bring on retardation affect perception, association, abstraction judgement and other mental functions. Deficiencies in any of those areas affect one's ability to learn and retain what he experiences.

The most obvious shortcoming in the handicapped child or adult is his inability to achieve what are considered normal standards for physical and mental tasks. One of the biggest obstacles for the handicapped person to overcome is the psychological feeling of inadequacy that develops when he becomes aware that he cannot perform on a level with the so-called normal person. A basic human need is to achieve and the handicapped person is frustrated by his inability to achieve. That conflict poses an adjustment problem. Frequently, symptoms such as withdrawal and disruptive behavior make up part of the handicapped person's adjustment behavior patterns. Those reactions are particularly true among many of the mentally retarded. A person working with the

HANDICAPS OF SCHOOL CHILDREN

Handicap	Per Cent of School Population Involved
Low Physical Fitness	4-5%
Poor Body Mechanics	4-5%
Nutritional Disturbances	1-2%
Visual Handicaps	3-5%
Auditory Handicaps	1-2%
Cerebral Palsy	Less than 1%
Cardiopathic Conditions	1%
Arrested Tuberculosis	Less than 1%
Diabetes	Less than 1%
Anemia	Less than 1%
Asthma and Hay Fever	4-5%
Hernia	Less than 1%
Dysmenorrhea	25-30% of females

handicapped must be aware of the psychological implications of each individual's incapability.

Establishing Physical Education Programs

In establishing a program for the handicapped, one of the first considerations must be each individual's needs, interests, abilities and limitations. The program must be geared so that they may achieve objectives and gain self-confidence. An important part of the program is the establishment of goals for each individual that are within his reach but that, at the same time, are challenging and provide for the needed improvements. Indications are that between five and ten per cent of the school-age population suffer

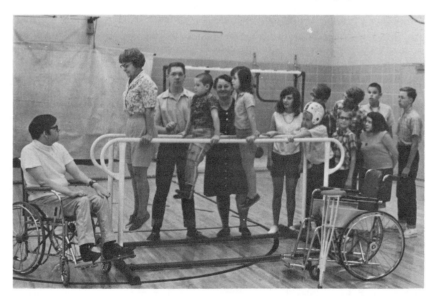

Like more fortunate people the handicapped find appropriate physical activity to be a mental and therapeutic aid. Here handicapped youngsters imitate their instructor.

from some type of physical or mental deficiency which may benefit from an adapted program.

Hollis F. Fait has estimated the percentage of handicapped students in need of adapted physical education.

Problems confronting the establishment of an adapted physical education program include scheduling, securing skilled teachers, acquiring enough space, planning program content, making health reports, keeping records, obtaining the special equipment, grading and providing satisfactory evaluation.

Dr. Fait has listed the following objectives of an adapted physical education program.

(1) develop optimum physical fitness
(2) develop skills in the basic motor movements
(3) develop a variety of sports skills for participation in sports as a worthy leisure-time activity
(4) develop a desire for continuous physical improvement
(5) promote an understanding in the student of the nature of his handicap and its limitations, while emphasizing the potentialities which may be developed
(6) give the student a feeling of value and worth as an individual, regardless of his handicap

Benefits of Exercise

Exercise will afford the handicapped the same benefits it does the normal person. Therefore, physical fitness for the handicapped cannot be overlooked. *Everyone needs exercise.* Obviously many handicapped persons cannot be expected to make achievements that parallel those of normal people but items such as improved body mechanics and efficiency, increased strength and endurance are all important phases of fitness which can become available to them. The handicapped are aware of their disadvantage but in struggling to overcome it, they can develop new levels of physical skill and endurance. That attainment is a pleasurable experience whether one is handicapped or not. According to the American Association of Health, Physical Education and Recreation, the mission of those who work with the handicapped "is not to make champions or even talented athletes and performers, but to use the full impact of physical education and recreation to enable each individual to become better prepared physically, mentally, emotionally, and socially to make his place in society as a self-sustaining adult who is capable of living the fullest, most satisfying and worthwhile life possible within the limitations of his impairment." Although that objective is proposed for teachers of mentally handicapped, it also serves as an objective for those dealing with individuals with any kind of handicap.

HARVARD STEP TEST

See TESTS.

HEALTH

As a practicing physician interested also in the history of man in education and in scientific research, I have observed very intimately the reaction of man to all the remarkable advances that have so altered our lives. While applauding and congratulating the ingenious and brilliant minds of our inventors, engineers, and research scientists, I deplore the fact that we have been unable to avoid, or correct, the difficult health situation in which we find ourselves today.

The Body

The most important change in a period of 75 years was in our diet. Small numbers of almost every country's population have for hundreds or thousands of years been prosperous enough to overeat, a natural temptation of the great majority of the members of the human race. But in the case of primitive countries, very few people are able to gorge themselves with food more than once over a long period of time. Today, in many countries, we all, with rare exceptions, have gotten into the natural but bad habit of eating too much food all the time, and much of this food has been too rich. *Calories do count,* and especially the animal fat calories, despite occasional remarks to the contrary.

Our family in my boyhood was not prosperous enough to eat rich food, although we ate enough to grow up and to carry on a lively program. We did have butter, but we used much less of it. Ice cream we made ourselves in our interesting old freezer about 3 or 4 times a year, especially on holidays, and although we had plenty of milk to drink to help, along with cod liver oil, to protect ourselves from tuberculosis, we did not in our teenage drink the enormous quantities of milk which the teen-agers and even the 20-year-olders of yesterday and today drink simply because they like it. That, along with other overeating and often with underexercising, may very likely be at least partly responsible for the high degree of atherosclerosis (rusting of the intima or inner lining of their important arteries, especially their coronaries) at an early age. In the last few decades I have myself examined hundreds and hundreds of young and middle-aged men sick with coronary heart disease long before their time, following and quite likely resulting from their gain of 30 or 40 pounds of adipose tissue in 20 or 30 years after they had reached their fighting weight.

But perhaps the greatest difference of all in our way of life in my boyhood from that of today was in our transportation. Healthwise we were very lucky indeed without realizing it. We quite naturally walked much of the time to get from one place to the next, even miles away. In the city there were, of course, horse cars. Electric cars were beginning to appear, but these were usually overcrowded and often inconvenient. As for automobiles, we saw and sampled the very first primitive ones. But we gave them up early because of their unreliability and expense, and returned to shanks' mare and our bicycles. Father tested a few, but returned to his horse and buggy. I did finally get a model T Ford when I was 28, but I learned to walk early in life and I still do.

It is not only the automobile, however, that has deprived us of the use of the large muscles of our body which we were born to utilize infinitely more than we do today. Life is often just too easy and soft for our proper health. We should walk upstairs more and use elevators less. We should, except as professionals, use our saws and lawn mowers and shovels with our own muscles much, or at least some of the time. We shouldn't sit to watch television more than one hour at a time. Get up and walk or run a bit. Or use a standing bicycle for at least two minutes once every hour when you are sitting or standing still. That will help to avoid stasis of blood in your legs from gravity, and the danger of clots in the leg veins. Those clots could be pumped as emboli to the lungs, often with serious consequences.

There are three additional reasons why the vigorous use of the leg muscles, which are the largest in the body, is so important for health. The first is physiological. Their contraction squeezes the leg veins which are supplied by nature with valves so that the blood when compressed by the muscular contraction will be pumped up against gravity to the heart and thence to the brain. Our brains are our most important organ and may be poorly supplied with blood if we just sit all day. The second reason is psychological—vigorous leg exercise is the best antidote for nervous or emotional stress that we possess, far better than tranquilizers or sedatives to which, unhappily, so many are addicted to-day. And the third is that in some way, not yet determined, vigorous muscular metabolism helps to prevent or to retard the atherosclerosis or rusting process in our important arteries, especially the coronaries.

Although it matters little, or not at all, how the leg muscles are exercised—by walking, or running, or bicycling, or swimming, or golf without a cart, or tennis, or skiing, or hill-climbing—it should amount to more than a mile walk daily. I have suggested that a minimum of an hour a day of fast walking or comparable exercise is absolutely necessary for one's optimal health, including that of the brain. More would be better.

The Mind

I remember the mental hardships of my youth, or, if one prefers, blessings, depending upon the point of view. I was so fortunate as to be accepted at the Roxbury Latin School, which required intensive study both at school and at home, undistracted by radio or television, which didn't exist then. Although I am one of the first to congratulate those who have organized various educational programs of the highest order, the radio and television should be kept in proper relationship to required reading, group discussions and teaching sessions. At the Roxbury Latin School we studied in the same year English, French, German, Latin and Greek, along with history, mathematics and the sciences. It was a stiff curriculum but it didn't hurt us. And although this eased up a bit in college, it was good preparation for the medical school and for a medical career which has been very demanding of time and energy.

The brain, our most important organ, is kept supplied with the freshest blood by the beating of our heart, which we should regard not as the center of all our life but as the handmaid to all other parts of our body.

The brain is, of course, the site of our mind, which physically is a remarkable computer full of hundreds of thousands of tapes of memorized recordings to be called upon as needed. If the arteries feeding our brain become rusty, our mental processes (our thoughts, which are secretions of our brain), become slowed and defective, as they do when we take too much alcohol or hallucinatory drugs. Many little strokes are fundamentally due to unhealthy habits of health.

The Spirit or the Soul

Much has been written and said about psychosomatic physiology and psychosomatic diseases. Take peptic ulcer, for example. Ulceration of the duodenum, that is, of the first part of the small intestine, may be initiated or even repeatedly precipitated by emotional stresses of one kind or another in a susceptible individual. It is not, however, adequately appreciated that the somatopsychic relationship is equally potent. We are still animals with the physiology of animals and not simply brains with minds and souls. The brain, in which are located both mind and soul, and they can't be anywhere else, needs to be well-fed with oxygen and other chemicals, and its waste products removed. Only the blood can do that. For its optimal function, therefore, the brain must have a good fresh blood supply which is delivered by a good heart and good blood vessels, which should be kept in the best of condition. It is of course, possible for individuals with crippled brains, for example, to have remarkable minds and souls, but that is true despite the disease, very very rarely because of it.

It is not necessary or wise to espouse or endure either extreme of silks and satins or the hair shirt, cakes and ale or a crust and water, the soft life or the hard one. There is to be found and practiced a middle of the road. But a return to at least some of the rugged life and virtues of our ancestors—physical, mental and spiritual—is long overdue.

For physical fitness, I recommend a minimum of a 4-mile walk each day, which should take you about an hour, or 7 hours a week. If on some occasions you can't work in an hour, on certain days a good substitution is 12 miles on a bicycle, whether indoors or out, or the equivalent of swimming, or tennis, or golf, or working in the garden, on a farm or on trees.—*Paul Dudley White*

Exercise and the Skin

There is some evidence that exercise is beneficial to the skin. Dr. Fred E. Abbo in January, 1966, reported an experiment conducted at the Veterans Administration Hospital at Iowa City, Iowa. Men who exercised three times a week with weights produced more of the male hormones known as 17-ketosteroids than did the men who exercised by running, swimming, playing handball, or doing calisthenics. Dr. Abbo stated that "preliminary results suggest that there may be a connection between weight lifting and the ability of the body to continue to produce certain hormones which decline as age increases." The 17-ketosteriods help to regulate skin growth, keeping it tight and smooth, and also help control muscle and bone structure.

Dr. Louis Wexler, chief of Dermatology at Beekman-Downtown Hospital in New York City, at a press seminar sponsored by Winthrop Laboratories and under the approval of the New York City Board of Education, reported that exercise and sports are good for the skin and for skin conditions, such as acne. He said that profuse perspiration loosens sebaceous plugs (black-heads) and encourages a freer flow of sebum. He warned, however, that the beneficial effects of perspiration are counteracted if, after working up a sweat, the individual doesn't wash properly to remove dried

perspiration and superficial bacteria which have accumulated on the skin. He advised bathing or showering after engaging in athletics, preferably with an antibacterial soap or cleanser containing hexachlorophene.

He noted, moreover, that thorough washing and drying of the skin, followed by an absorptive powder, are important in preventing and treating other common conditions affecting people engaged in exercise and athletics. This method reduces such conditions as chafing, skin rashes, athlete's foot and related infections.

HEART

See CIRCULATORY SYSTEM, DEGENERATIVE CARDIOVASCULAR DISEASE, HEART DISEASE and ISCHEMIC HEART DISEASE.

HEART DISEASE

Today when you hear someone speak about "heart trouble," he is probably referring to coronary heart disease. That form of heart disease is one of the most common illnesses that plague American society today.

Actually, a heart attack is not primarily a disease of the heart muscle. It is really the result of a condition in the arteries—the coronary arteries—that supply the heart muscle with blood. Some people have the mistaken impression that the heart receives its blood supply from the blood that it pumps constantly. The heart, just like any other muscle, receives its blood supply through arteries and not from the blood that flows through it.

In the anatomy of the human heart, an extensive network of arteries grows out from two main trunks, the right and left coronary arteries. These main coronary arteries branch in much the same way as a tree. Every branch is smaller than the main trunk, and each one soon subdivides into smaller branches. Those in turn divide into still smaller ones, very like tiny twigs on a tree. Every part of the heart, no matter how small, is supplied with blood and oxygen through this system of coronary arteries.

Terminology

In order to understand coronary heart disease, it is important to become familiar with the following terms:

Arteriosclerosis—a general term for various types of arterial illness. The phrase "hardening of the arteries" is often used synonymously with arteriosclerosis. It is associated with a gradually increasing brittleness of arteries.

Atherosclerosis—a slowly developing disease process of the coronary arteries. In atherosclerosis, the passageway through the arteries becomes roughened and narrowed by fatty deposits that harden into patches along the inner lining of the artery. Consequently, the channel is gradually narrowed, and there is less room for blood to flow through.

Coronary occlusion—a severe narrowing of some coronary artery to the point that blood can no longer pass through.

Coronary thrombosis—a coronary occlusion caused by the formation of a blood clot (thrombus) which completely blocks the flow of blood to some part of the heart muscle.

Myocardial infarct—the condition when the blood supply to a portion of the muscle is blocked, causing the muscle directly around the blocked artery to die.

Angina pectoris—commonly called "angina," an uncomfortable sensation of pressure, tightness, or pain in the center of the chest. The discomfort often spreads to the left shoulder, arm, or hand, where it may be felt as a sensation of numbness. This feeling is a sign that the heart is not getting enough oxygen through its blood supply. Angina may occur in people who have recovered from a heart attack, in people who are going to have a

heart attack, and in some people who will never have a heart attack. See ANGINA.

Collateral circulation—the opening of new arteries and the growth of new branches to offset the effects of atherosclerosis. It is fortunate that the coronary system is able to grow and repair itself. When some of the coronary arteries become narrowed by gradual development of atherosclerosis, nearby arteries get wider and even open up tiny new branches to bring blood to the area of the muscle that needs it. Collateral circulation explains why many people who have narrower arteries do not have a heart attack and also accounts for some of the excellent recoveries from heart attacks. See COLLATERAL CIRCULATION.

Loafer's Heart—a term coined by Dr. Wilhelm Raab to describe the weakening of the heart muscle as a result of a lack of exercise. It is not the so-called *athlete's heart,* which should not be considered abnormal, for it is a strong and well-developed heart. It is instead the degenerating, inadequate *loafer's heart* which is a cause for concern. See ATHLETE'S HEART and LOAFER'S HEART.

Factors Causing Heart Disease

There are a number of factors associated with a high incidence of heart disease. Those include overweight, heredity, faulty diet, emotional stress, cigarette smoking and lack of suitable physical exercise. It is not yet possible to say which of these factors are the primary ones, and it is not known to what extent those factors interrelate with each other. Many people seem to possess all of those factors, yet still do not have a heart attack. Other people seem to be living a life devoid of those factors but eventually suffer a heart attack. *There are always exceptions to any situation,* but, in general, the six factors make a person more prone to heart disease. With this knowledge in mind you must govern your life accordingly.

It is, of course, impossible to change your hereditary background. However, that factor is the only one that you cannot influence. Therefore, by controlling your weight, avoiding cigarettes, selecting a good diet, participating in daily exercise, and eliminating tension problems, you may be able to prevent coronary difficulties.

Physical Fitness and Heart Disease

Physical exercise is not a cure-all for heart disease. Neither prevention nor recovery can be guaranteed despite the extent of exercise. But there is a strong relationship between poor physical fitness and the elimination of heart trouble.

Exercise reduces the incidence of heart disease. Population studies have shown that in numerous instances they compared the extent of heart disease in physically active and relatively sedentary people, especially people employed by the same company, but in different types of jobs. For example, mailmen were compared to postal clerks, and streetcar drivers to the conductors. The findings? Those engaged in the more physically active jobs had fewer cases of heart disease, less severe cases, and better recovery from the cases that did occur.

Exercise strengthens the heart muscle. When you exercise muscles of the arms or legs in certain ways, they become stronger. The same thing happens with the heart muscle. In walking, running, swimming, bicycling and many other activities, the heart gets stronger because it is being used. For example, the pulse rate of a person in good physical condition is *lower* than when he is in poor physical condition. Therefore, the heart is doing its job more efficiently. It needs fewer beats per minute to get the same job done. A stronger heart will enable the person to better enjoy physical activities and be more resistant to heart disease should it occur.

Exercise helps prevent narrowing of the coronary arteries. Since coronary heart disease is caused by an occlusion in a coronary artery, it only makes sense that if you prevent the narrowing of the arteries you will greatly reduce this disease. Exercise, in general, tends to help the coronary arteries remain open and retain their elasticity so that they can do their intended job with a minimum amount of interference.

Exercise aids the development of collateral circulation. Collateral circulation is important in the recovery from coronary-artery disease. If one artery is blocked, the blood supply must have new ways of getting to the given area of the heart muscle. Exercise enhances the development of that circulation and, in that way, speeds the recovery from a heart attack. This fact is one of the reasons why today exercise has widespread use as therapy for patients who have suffered from coronary artery disease. It also explains why some active people may have a heart attack and never know it because collateral circulation can sufficiently carry the load.

Exercise accelerates the clearing time of fat. Exercise, in general, causes fatty substances to be cleared from the blood in less time than it would otherwise take. That removal helps prevent the buildup of fatty deposits on the walls of the coronary arteries (atherosclerosis) and results in lower fat levels in the blood. This occurrence will reduce coronary-artery occlusion because there will not be as much fat available to narrow the openings of the arteries.

Exercise helps maintain the proper neuro-hormonal balance. A certain amount of physical activity is needed in order to maintain a balance between the parasympathetic and sympathetic nervous systems. They establish the rate and metabolism of the heart and control it through the release of chemical transmitters. A lack of exercise appears to upset this balance and make one more prone to heart disease. *Exercise aids recovery and helps prevent further coronary-artery disease.* Since exercise strengthens the heart muscle, aids collateral circulation, helps prevent the narrowing of the arteries, accelerates the clearing time of fat, and helps maintain the proper neuro-hormonal balance, it aids recovery from a heart attack in most cases. But it would be sheer folly to begin an unsupervised exercise program after a heart attack. However, under a doctor's supervision, exercise is likely to be one of the necessary methods used during and after the recovery period. See CIRCULATORY SYSTEM and ISCHEMIC HEART DISEASE.—*Clint E. Bruess*

HEART STRAIN

Many people claim that the heart can be strained and permanently damaged by strenuous exercise and cite cases to prove their point. What such claims fail to mention is that the heart of the injured person had been weakened by some previous disease, such as myocarditis or rheumatic fever. The healthy heart of an adult *cannot* be injured by physical training. See ATHLETE'S HEART, CIRCULATORY SYSTEM, HEART and LOAFER'S HEART.

HEREDITY

According to the British biologist P. B. Medawa, there are two types of heredity—*internal heredity* (*endosomatic*), and *external heredity* (*exosomatic*). Internal heredity refers to biological heredity (chromosome make-up), while external heredity refers to that which is handed down from generation to generation by education and training.

In an effort to determine whether internal or external heredity influences athletic participation and performance,

Professor Luggi Gedda of Italy studied 220 Italian national champions who came from families in which two or more members had attained distinction. The genetic influence was more revealing in some sports. Fencing, boxing, and shooting indicated the highest influence, while gymnastics and soccer revealed the lowest. It can be assumed from the study that fencing, boxing, and shooting may be of genetic influence, while the soccer and gymnastics performers may have been influenced more by training.

Gedda ran a comprehensive study on 1,195 twin-pairs at an Institute in Rome. He investigated both identical and non-identical twins. They were assigned to three groups—those in which both twins participated in sport, those in which only one participated, and those in which neither participated. The investigations revealed that there were virtually no differences in sports participation of identical twins. Either they took part in athletics, or they did not. Conversely, the non-identical twins did not show that relationship. In fact in 85 per cent of the non-identical twins there was a discrepancy regarding participation in sports. Further analysis of the twins revealed that there was an exceedingly close relationship between the identical twins and the sports that they selected, a relationship that didn't show up in the non-identical twins. If the non-identical twins were inclined towards sports selection of that sport and their individual abilities varied greatly. Performances of the identical twins were similar, and they played similar positions on team sports.

From those findings by Gedda and other investigators, it is apparent that, despite many differences in genetic endowment, athletic talent and *potential* are inherited.

The secondary factor is external heredity. Here the parents, or some other member of the family, set the attitudes toward participation. But the motivation can "push" the person only as far as his genetic make-up will allow him to go.

Chromosome Combination and Female Athletes

More recently with the emphasis on sex determination in the Olympics, investigations have been made to determine whether an athlete is really a female or a male. Previously, a gross anatomy examination was sufficient. Recently, however, researchers have attempted to evaluate chromosomes. The technique is to scrape a few cells from the inside of a person's cheek for a chromosome count. A normal woman has 22 pairs of non-sex chromosomes plus two X chromosomes to determine femaleness. A normal man has 22 non-sex chromosomes plus one X chromosome and a Y chromosome to establish his maleness.

However, some people have one chromosome too many. In women who have an XXY combination, there are external male genitalia and poor, nonathletic talent. If, on the other hand, a female has some XYY cells and others containing only single X and nothing else, she will be endowed with all female traits plus super athletic potential. An example of this phenomenon has been demonstrated in the recent Sports Medicine evaluation of the female athletes to determine their sex and "fitness" for competition with other women. One such woman is Ewa Klobulowska of Poland. A co-holder of the 100 meters world record for women (11.1), she was declared ineligible for women's competition because she had one chromosome too many.

Although not all women with super powers have a mixed-up genetic endowment, some people may be superior to others because of heredity.

Heredity and Fitness

We can make these observations about heredity and its effects on the fitness seeker.

1. Each person is different and will achieve a different level of fitness depending upon his genetic endowment and motivation, and each will progress at his own rate depending upon his inherited abilities. Thus it is extremely important that you compete against yourself for fitness achievements as you get older. You need not "beat" the man next door in physical activities or even select similar conditioning programs.

2. You must learn to judge yourself to determine what your capabilities are. Genetic endowment may put limits on your physical talents, but you can always try a little harder to achieve.

3. Teachers must be aware of individual differences among children. Some are physically incapable of performing the task, may take more time in finishing, or may be better motivated in one activity than in another.

4. Finally, in the future, science will provide methods of determining our potential for fitness and athletic ability. Some inroads have been made in that direction, but a great deal more must be learned. Hopefully, a simple test will be devised to adequately measure our potential in athletic fitness. For a discussion of some of the current techniques available for measuring present and potential fitness, see BODY TYPE and TESTS.

HIKING AND CAMPING

It is possible to hike without camping or to camp without hiking, but the two are usually closely linked. The resultant activity is often referred to as lightweight mobile camping, or backpacking, because the hiker carries his camping equipment on his back.

Lightweight Camping

Essentially lightweight camping is a recreative activity in which the hiker carries, as does the tortoise, his house on his back. That basic requirement determines many features of the activity and the equipment required for it. Quality and lightness become of paramount importance when selecting equipment. The hiker/camper must be able to eat and sleep and must carry suitable lightweight food and cooking equipment, an adequate tent, groundsheet and sleeping bag. Because he must transport that equipment, he also needs a suitable rucksack.

Loads carried and distances walked vary according to the experience, fitness and age of the participants. Tentative suggestions were put forward in a 1954 issue of *Mobile Camping* which indicated that 13-year-old boys should walk no more than an average of 10 miles per day. That, of course, will vary depending upon the terrain and the climatic conditions. The boys should not carry over 25 lbs. nor the girls over 20 lbs.

The Effects of Walking with a "Load" upon Fitness

H. Harrison Clarke, writing in *Muscular Strength and Endurance in Man*, reported on the changes in muscular strength and physical fitness occurring as a result of walking with loads varying from nothing to 61 lbs. The men took part in seven marches, one per week for seven weeks, and walked at a rate of 80 to 95 yards per minute.

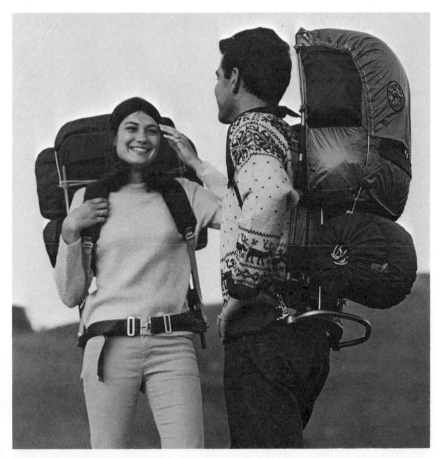

Most modern hiking equipment is constructed so that the load's center of gravity is as high and as close to the body as possible, making for easier carrying.

The length of each was 7.5 miles.

As a result of walking 52.5 miles spread over seven weeks, the men showed significant improvement in a battery of six tests of physical fitness. They also showed significant increases in strength in the following muscle groups: trunk extensors, trunk flexors, shoulder elevators, hip flexors and ankle plantar flexors.

It has been shown that walking with very light loads of 9 lbs. at a speed of 2.5 m.p.h. for durations of approximately 10 minutes has resulted in increases in minute ventilation, pulse rate, and oxygen consumption.

The same workers also showed that the method of carrying the bag with its center of gravity close into the body, and as high as possible, resulted in less energy expenditure. Most rucksacks are constructed with that in mind.

Most Common Injuries

Although there is little risk of injury while hiking and camping, there are a number of common injuries which, of course, vary tremendously depending upon the terrain, the nature of the expedition, etc. John Hunt reported that walking accidents in Britain, during the years 1957 and 1961, amounted to forty per cent of the total accidents as recorded by the British Mountain Rescue Committee.

Apart from minor injuries such as blisters, the most common injuries involve the ankle, the lower leg and the knee joint.—*B. Nettleton*

See CAMPING, MOUNTAINEERING, ORIENTEERING and TRAMPING.

Backpacking

In the United States the combining of hiking and camping is called backpacking. The idea behind backpacking is to carry some or all of life's necessities in your pack on your back. Backpacking is an exciting and pleasurable way for modern man to get his feet back on the ground—to become acquainted with his heritage as a human being.

The most important item needed is a well-chosen pack, which can be of the basket, knapsack, rucksack, or pack-frame style, so long as it distributes the load over the shoulders, back and hips without throwing you off balance.

Contribution to Fitness

Hiking, or backpacking, may range from a mild to high-energy-cost activity depending upon the speed at which you walk or the weight that you carry. The activity becomes more difficult if the pace is stepped up, the weight of the load is increased, and the terrain is more rugged. Most hiking is done on mountain trails that are moderately rugged. Walking on a flat terrain but with different surfaces makes significant differences in the energy cost of walking and, therefore, increases its contribution to fitness. Using a 20 pound pack as a piece of standard equipment while walking on various surfaces will demonstrate the point. Hiking at 3.5 miles per hour on a hard-surfaced road will result in 5.6 calories consumed per minute or 336 calories per hour. Walking on a grass-covered road at the same pace will burn up 6.3 per minute, or 380 calories per hour. Walking on a rougher terrain, such as a plowed field, at approximately the same speed will burn up 7.0 calories per minute or 420 calories per hour. Finally, if you are hiking on a harrowed field at about the same speed or slightly less you will burn up 10.0 calories in a minute or 600 calories in an hour.

See ENERGY COST OF ACTIVITIES for a comparison of the various speeds of walking and hiking. Hiking or walking can be made relatively mild or very demanding. Because of that adaptability, it is one of the best fitness activities, for it allows you to pace yourself according to your own fitness level and to enjoy the great outdoors.

*HIKING PROGRAM
20 lb. pack

Chart 1	Chart 2
1. Up to 1.5 miles in 30 min.	1. 5.4-5.7 miles in 95 min.
2. 1.6-2.0 miles in 40 min.	2. 5.8-5.9 miles in 100 min.
3. 2.1-2.5 miles in 45 min.	3. 6.0-6.2 miles in 100 min.
4. 2.6-3.2 miles in 60 min.	4. 6.3-6.6 miles in 105 min.
5. 3.3-3.7 miles in 70 min.	5. 6.7-7.0 miles in 110 min.
6. 3.8-4.1 miles in 75 min.	6. 7.1-7.3 miles in 110 min.
7. 4.2-4.5 miles in 80 min.	7. 7.4-7.6 miles in 115 min.
8. 4.6-4.9 miles in 85 min.	8. 7.7-7.9 miles in 120 min.
9. 5.0-5.3 miles in 90 min.	9. 8 miles in 120 minutes

See CAMPING, HUNTING, MOUNTAIN CLIMBING, TRAMPING and WALKING.

Association:

National Campers and Hikers Association (NCHA), 7172 Transit Road, Buffalo, New York 14221.

Since hiking can be a moderate-to-high-energy-cost activity it may be used to help improve your fitness level, especially your circulo-respiratory and muscle endurance. Below are hiking programs that take into account the important principles of training. Also included is a hill-climbing program. If no pack is used, the length of time is similar to that of walking. See WALKING.

Fitness 1

If you achieved a score of poor or low average on the *Harvard Step Test* or a score of very poor or poor on the *12 Minute Run*, start on Chart 1-Level 1 and spend one week at each level until Chart 2-Level 9 is reached. It is recommended that you participate 4 to 5 days a week. When Chart 2-Level 9 is reached, 4 days a week is sufficient.

Fitness 2

If you achieved a score of high average on the *Harvard Step Test* or fair on the *12 Minute Run*, start on Chart 1-Level 2. Spend one week on Chart 1-Levels 2, 3, 4, 6, 8, and 9, and Chart 2-Levels 2, 4, 6, 8, and 9. It is recommended that you participate 4 to 5 days a week. When Chart 2-Level 9 is reached, 4 days a week is sufficient.

Fitness 3

If you achieved a score of good or excellent on either the *Harvard Step Test* or *12 Minute Run*, continue your current program or select Chart 2-Level 9 as your level of participation. Four days a week is sufficient.

*HIKING PROGRAM
40 lb. load

Chart 1	Chart 2
1. Up to 1.4 miles in 25 min.	1. 3.8-3.9 miles in 60 min.
2. 1.5-1.7 miles in 30 min.	2. 4 miles in 60 min.
3. 1.8-2.0 miles in 35 min.	3. 4.1-4.5 miles in 65 min.
4. 2.0-2.3 miles in 35 min.	4. 4.6-4.7 miles in 68 min.
5. 2.4-2.7 miles in 40 min.	5. 4.8-4.9 miles in 70 min.
6. 2.8-3.0 miles in 45 min.	6. 5 miles in 75 min.
7. 3.1-3.2 miles in 45 min.	7. 5.1-5.3 miles in 78 min.
8. 3.3-3.4 miles in 50 min.	8. 5.4-5.5 miles in 80 min.
9. 3.5-3.7 miles in 55 min.	9. 5.6-5.9 miles in 85 min.

Fitness 1

See hiking program for 20 lb. pack.

Fitness 2

If you achieved a score of high average on the *Harvard Step Test* or fair on the *12 Minute Run,* start on Chart 1-Level 2. Spend one week on Chart 1-Levels 2, 5, 6, 8, and 9, and Chart 2-Levels 2, 4, 6, 8, and 9. It is recommended that you participate 4 to 5 days a week. When Chart 2-Level 9 is reached, 4 days a week is sufficient.

Fitness 3

See hiking program for 20 lb. pack.

HIPS

Practically every woman in today's society (and many men) have complained about spreading hips. Sedentary living is the culprit.

Although you require more than routine exercises to reduce the circumference of the hips, it is important to be aware of the various muscles of the hip area and the specific exercises that can be used to firm the musculature. See CALORIES, SPOT EXERCISES and WEIGHT CONTROL.

The *psoas major* and the *iliacus* muscles are often thought of as one muscle and are called the *iliopsoas*

*HILL CLIMBING PROGRAM (100 feet ascent per minute)

Chart 1	Chart 2
1. 10 minutes	1. 38 minutes
2. 15 minutes	2. 40 minutes
3. 18 minutes	3. 43 minutes
4. 20 minutes	4. 45 minutes
5. 23 minutes	5. 50 minutes
6. 25 minutes	6. 53 minutes
7. 30 minutes	7. 55 minutes
8. 33 minutes	8. 58 minutes
9. 35 minutes	9. 60 minutes

* See ENDURANCE and ENERGY COST OF ACTIVITIES for an explanation of these charts.

Fitness 1

See hiking program for 20 lb. pack.

Fitness 2

If you achieved a score of high average on the *Harvard Step Test* or fair on the *12 Minute Run,* start on Chart 1-Level 2. Spend one week on Chart 1-Levels 2, 4, 6, 7, and 9, and Chart 2-Levels 2, 4, 5, 7, and 9. It is recommended that you participate 4 to 5 days a week. When Chart 2-Level 9 is reached, 4 days a week is sufficient.

Fitness 3

See hiking program for 20 lb. pack.

muscle. The *psoas* is attached to the spinal column and the thigh bone, while the *iliacus* is attached to the hip and the thigh bone. Those muscles act together and flex the thigh, aiding it in rotating outward. If the thigh bone is locked or set, as when you touch your toes without bending your knees, the *iliopsoas* muscle aids in flexing the trunk towards the thigh.

To develop the *iliopsoas* muscle, use the regular sit-up. Lie flat on your back on the floor, with your hands behind your head. Then sit up and return. Keep your legs straight. (Placing them under a chair or bar may help.) There's another exercise that enables you to develop the iliopsoas—leg-lifting—but it's not recommended. Here's why. The *rectus femoris* and the *iliacus* are attached to the pelvis, while the *psoas* portion of the *iliopsoas* is attached to the spine. Therefore, when the legs are raised from the floor, the front of the pelvis is tipped forward and downward, and the spine is pulled forward. The only muscles that can stabilize the pelvis are the abdominal muscles. If the abdominal muscles are weak, then leg lifting may aggravate the lower back. Although it is popular as a waist-reducing exercise, the muscles primarily involved in trimming the waist line (the rectus abdominis, the transverse, and the oblique muscles) are not affected.

The Buttocks

The *gluteus maximus* is the largest and the most superficial of the three gluteal muscles. It is that muscle that forms the rounded mass of the buttocks. As the antagonist of the *iliopsoas*, it aids in your regaining an erect posture after bending over.

The *gluteus medius* and *gluteus minimus* are overlapped by the *gluteus maximus*. They abduct the thigh and rotate it inward.

Some of the other internal muscles of that area are the *pyriformis*, the *obturator internus*, the *superior gemellus*, the *inferior gemellus*, the *quadratus femoris* and the *obturator externus.*

To firm the buttock area, try this one. Lie flat on your stomach with arms behind your head. Arch your legs and chest off the floor and return.

Another buttocks firmer starts with you down on your hands and knees with your arms straight. Drop your head down, round your back, and bring your knee close to the nose. Then raise your head, and at the same time stretch your right leg back and up as high as possible. Repeat several times with the right leg, then alternate.

You can also try bench stepping to firm the buttocks. A wooden box or bench will do. Step up with your right leg, followed by your left. Then step down with your right leg followed by your left. The cadence should be step up, step down, and so on. Be certain to keep a steady rhythm. The first time you do the exercise, 24 steps in one minute is a reasonable goal. Stop if you become winded or unduly fatigued. Work up to five minutes. It is also an excellent cardiovascular exercise.

To firm the buttock area and remove excess fat is rather difficult. A prudent diet, a good posture, an active life, and the above exercises are necessary if you want to keep good tone. Exercises alone may not seem to produce desirable results, but a combination of the four will.

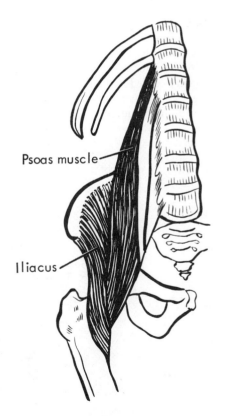

Psoas muscle

Iliacus

Iliopsoas muscle.

HORSEMANSHIP

The modern horse, consisting of many types, springs mainly from two groups—namely, the Northern or cold-blooded group, and the Southern or hot-blooded group. Crossbreeding and interbreeding have produced many kinds of horses all over the world. There are Shetland ponies, Welsh ponies, thoroughbred horses, the Norwegian pony, Icelandic ponies, Dartmoor ponies, Percheron horses, Jutland dray horses, Arabian horses, Hackney ponies, the Australian Waler, the Austrian Lippizaner, and the Appaloosa horse of the western United States.

For centuries man has depended on and used the horse as a means of transportation, an aid during war, for work, and as a hobby. Some of the uses of the horse today are pleasure riding (divided into park riding, riding in the country—called hacking—and fox hunting), show jumping and racing (flat, steeplechase and point-to-point).

Pleasure riding of all kinds is a sport for men, women and children. There are riding clubs throughout the United States specifically for boys and girls. They are taught practical care and handling of horses and tack and concepts of horsemanship. Competition is keen among districts, regions and sections, with national champions being ultimately named.

Show jumping requires coordination, good sensory perception, and a thorough knowledge of the ability and temperament of the horse. Women, men and children can participate in show jumping. There are special classes for children. Men and women, however, compete among each other. Competition is categorized into the thoroughbred jumper, the open jumper, the green hunter and the experienced hunter classes. Points are accumulated during one show and over the season resulting in a champion horse at the close of the season.

Racing consists of flat racing, har-

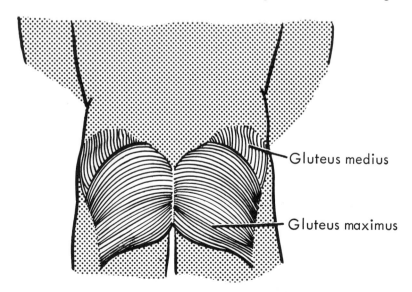

Gluteus medius

Gluteus maximus

Superficial muscles of the buttocks.

ness racing, steeplechase and point-to-point racing. All except point-to-point racing are limited to men riders. Point-to-point races are usually held in the spring season and are classified into men's and women's races. All kinds of racing require a thorough practical knowledge of riding and concepts of horsemanship, including a knowledge of the horse's ability and temperament.

No matter what the type of riding, reach an adequate state of physical fitness before participating in this exciting sport.

Contribution to Physical Fitness

Riding contributes little to circulo-respiratory endurance. However, muscle endurance and muscle strength in the arms, shoulders, back, legs and abdominals are developed through repeated riding. In addition, strength and endurance are needed for the adductor, extensor and flexor muscles of the legs. Flexibility is also needed.

The amount of physical fitness needed and developed depends on the length you will participate in the sport in a given time, the schooling of the horse, and the chosen kind of riding activity.

Conditioning Programs

Since riding develops little circulatory-respiratory endurance, you would be wise to include in the conditioning program some form of interval running. A program of isometric exercises and muscle endurance would be in order for development of arms, shoulders, back, abdominals and legs. Before participation in any form of riding you need to develop balance, coordination, strength, and endurance—especially of arm, shoulder, back and leg.

Most Common Injuries

The most common injuries are back and arm muscle strains and stiffness in those areas and in the gluteal muscles. More serious injuries may occur from falling, or being thrown from, the horse. These range from head injuries and clavicle fractures to the less serious muscle strains. That's one reason for the show jumping rider, fox hunter and race rider wearing a hard cap and bowler.—*Gloria Young*

Associations:

Professional Horsemen's Association of America, 751 Closter Dock Road, Closter, New Jersey 07624.

United States Equestrian Team, Inc. (USET), Gladstone, New Jersey 07934.

Division of Girls' and Women's Sports (DGWS). See ORGANIZATIONS.

HUNTING

The oldest of all recreational activities, hunting was once a means of survival that has turned into a major sport pursued by millions. Man has always been a hunter. But no longer does he hunt mainly for food for the household. He's found other reasons and pleasures. Our ancestors enjoyed this sport, and we inherited the passion for stalking game from them. There is the thrill of the chase and the unforgettable enjoyment in bagging an animal. There is the joy of being with companions and the story telling. There is a great opportunity to commune with nature and refresh your soul.

A hunter will endure many discomforts in cold and rainy weather, but the thrill of trying to capture his game as he takes to the hills or fields or mountains often keeps his spirits high. Each year there are more and more hunters but less and less area on which to hunt. There is better equipment produced year by year to take game, but, unfortunately, less game to stalk. Increased population has taken away many agricultural lands and reduced the natural game habitat. Game departments are greatly concerned about that situation, and have taken measures to keep hunting as an interesting recreational activity. It is up to the hunters themselves to help preserve this sport by being true sportsmen.

Physical Qualities Needed for Participation

The different methods to hunt will determine how much endurance you need. One method is taking a stand, whereby the hunter tries to blend in with the surroundings and sits or stands as quietly as possible. He waits for the animal to come walking through its natural habitat. You should have knowledge of the animal's habits and food and possess a great deal of patience and concentration. Watch the wind and keep it against you all the time.

Another method used in hunting big game is the drive. Several hunters will cover territory planned before-

hand, and a hunter or two will take stands further away in hopes that animals will be driven by the places where they are waiting. The drivers will need certain stamina, for they will have to walk through difficult terrain, heavy with underbrush or rocks.

A hunter can also track the animal he wants to hunt, but on dry, hard ground that's almost impossible. Ideal hunting conditions consist of a layer of light, dry snow from two to three inches deep on the ground with none in the trees and bushes.

A dog is a valuable accessory when you go small-game hunting. The dogs either flush out the game from its habitat or point where the hunted game is hiding. The hunter walks along with the dogs and the stamina he needs depends on how much hunting he will do in a day and what type of terrain is covered.

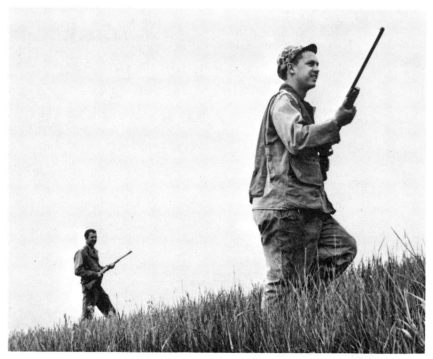

A pre-season program of physical conditioning makes the inclines seem less steep and the valleys more abundant.

Conditioning Programs

Hunters of all ages pursue the type of hunting that suits their individual likes. The conditions and environment have much to do with how a day's hunting is enjoyed. Take it easy when hunting and don't push too hard by driving continuously after the game. Since hunters can get quite winded climbing a small mountain slope because of the extra weight of equipment and clothing, get in condition before hunting season by walking as much as possible through fields and over hills.

Here are some exercises you may find valuable:

A. Isometric Exercises
   1. any general leg exercise
   2. any general arm exercise
   3. abdominal strength-tone exercise
   4. chest strength-tone exercise
B. General Exercises
   1. running (jogging and sprinting)
   2. running in place
   3. rope-jumping
   4. walking at a fast pace for a distance
   5. sit-ups
   6. chin-ups
   7. push-ups
   8. ½ knee bends
   9. squat thrusts
C. Other—see WALKING and HIKING for programs that will enable you to develop good physical condition for hiking.

Importance of Gun-Handling Knowledge

The most important physical attribute to possess is good eyesight with proper knowledge of handling guns and bow and arrows. Your gun should be fitted to your physique and should not be too heavy but comfortable, easy to handle and adequately balanced. Practice your marksmanship before the hunting season and become well ac-

quainted with your equipment. Safety measures cannot be stressed too much or too strongly, and it is your duty to take heed of all precautions. Never handle firearms carelessly, and always carry the gun with the safety on. Don't point the muzzle of the gun toward a companion or a dog and never fire across a companion. Always observe courtesy in the field.

When you know how to handle your firearms adequately, choose a method of hunting described previously and condition yourself accordingly. The better condition you are in and the more you know about your firearms and the habitats of the game, the more you will enjoy hunting.—*Jean A. Hecht*

HYPOKINETIC DISEASE

Hypokinetic disease, a term coined by Drs. Hans Kraus and Wilhelm Raab, refers to the insufficient motion of man. The basic concept is that over a biologically short period of time man has progressed from a primitive state to a highly civilized, domesticated being. He has moved from a highly vigorous and strenuous life that exposed him to the elements, to a life that is similar to the inactivity of an animal, in an extremely well-protected cage. With changes such as those there must be major reactions to the human organism. Granted, the human body has the ability to adapt to new circumstances—an outstanding trait of the organism—but the adaptation can occur only within certain limits. Outside of those limits the organism may be thrown off balance.

That is what has happened with the human body. The striated musculature constitutes a major portion of our body weight and has a far greater function than merely providing for locomotion. The action of the striated muscles influences circulation, metabolism and the endocrine balance of the body. Furthermore, the bones, posture and the position of the body are influenced by those muscles. Finally, and very importantly, the striated muscles serve as an outlet for our emotions and nervous responses, for those muscles allow us to react and respond to the various stimuli that bombard us.

Urban man, today, is an overrested, overfed, overstimulated, overprotected, underexercised, underreleased, underdisciplined person. A few thousand years ago, man and his wife and children were involved in a life-and-death struggle with their environment. The body was prepared for action. In an instant that body could fight or flee. In either case physical action was involved—fight or flight.

Civilization as a Cause of Hypokinetic Disease

Because of our current mechanized society civilized man can do neither—fight nor flee. He must contain his release. By suppressing his biological response he builds up stress—stress that affects his physical and emotional states. If continued and not checked or controlled, physical and/or emotional disease will result. Typical physical diseases are endocrine malfunctions, cardiovascular disorders, metabolic ailments (overweight), gastrointestinal upsets and malfunctions, and musculoskeletal dysfunction. The emotional diseases are neurosis, anxiety, depression, compulsion and maladjustment. Each of these diseases, whether they are emotional or physical, can cause a tension state that results in further ailments which may be either physical or emotional. What compounds the problem even further is that a physical disease may cause the person to exercise less, which in turn causes more suppression.

In spite of modern conveniences, better nutrition, and modern medical advances, many people in western society, particularly the United States, suffer from a variety of diseases which are mainly a result of inadequate adjustment to the society. Such diseases as psychosomatic disorders, chronic backache, diabetes, peptic ulcers, cardiovascular disease, obesity and tension ailments are associated with the hypokinetic disease syndrome.

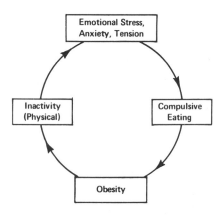

At least one out of four adults carries undesirable excess poundage, a factor predisposing to coronary heart disease. As the diagram shows, tension and stress lead to compulsive eating, which shows up as fat, which leads to further indolence, which closes the gate on tension release. Vigorous exercise not only sheds pounds (and the first to go are excess fat) but provides an outlet for tension. Moreover, it steps up the basal body metabolism and actually curbs the appetite for more calories than are necessary to maintain a "steady state" of desirable weight.

Importance of Exercise

It is apparent that our culture is going to become more mechanized in the future, causing man to do less physical work. It is imperative that each person select an activity program and *follow it for life.* Parents must encourage their children to develop adequate activity patterns and learn to want to exercise. Instead of hypokinetics the direction should aim toward kinetics (movement). Movement will allow the human organism to release its pent-up emotions through socially acceptable responses. Because of the release of the tension the chain of events is broken in the development of the syndrome. See DEGENERATIVE CARDIOVASCULAR DISEASE, DIGESTIVE SYSTEM, ENDOCRINE SYSTEM, HEART DISEASE, LOAFER'S HEART, LOW BACK PAIN and STRESS.

ICE SKATING

Ice skating is enjoyed by people all over the world, especially in countries that have very cold winter weather. In fact, in many areas skaters have moved to indoor arenas to prolong the skating season.

People of all ages enjoy skating. Children, soon after they learn to walk may be introduced to skating. Senior citizens, 70 years of age or more, may also enjoy it. You may play many recreational games such as tag, follow the leader, crack the whip, and hockey on the ice, or you may merely skate for the sheer enjoyment and/or exercise.

Contribution to Fitness

Ice skating is an excellent means of exercise. The major muscle groups of the body, such as the legs and arms, get an excellent workout because of their vigorous movements. The lungs and heart also get a good workout if the skating is strenuous enough. If the skating is done vigorously, you'll burn the calories and increase circulo-respiratory endurance.

Misconceptions About Skating

Many people shy away from ice skating because they claim to have "weak ankles." That reasoning is not valid. Most so-called weak ankles are the result of improperly fitting skates. Skates should always be at least one size smaller than shoe size and should always be fitted. It is particularly important that the heel fit properly to avoid early fatigue or the feeling of weak ankles. Another misconception is the belief that you must wear a heavy sock when skating. Heavy socks stop circulation, so that it is best to wear

light wool stretch socks. If your feet get cold, you can make covers for outside of the skates by taking a pair of men's woolen socks, splitting them at the bottom for the blades, and then pinning them alongside the skates.

Proper lacing is also important in avoiding fatigued ankles. Skates should be laced loosely at the toe and very tight up the ankles, then looser again for the remainder of the shoe.

Since ice skating is a high-energy-cost activity it may be used to help improve your fitness level, especially your circulo-respiratory and muscle endurance. Below is an ice skating program that takes into account the important principles of training.

If you desire to improve your strength and power for this activity see WEIGHT TRAINING and ISOMETRICS. The weight training and isometrics exercises may also be used to prepare your body for athletic competition.

Figure Skating

Figure skating is a highly competitive sport of grace and perfection. Experience and success in figure skating require dedication and superior physical coordination and condition.

Classes of Competitive Skating

Competitive figure skating is divided into three general classifications: 1. Singles, in which men and women execute school figures and free skating programs. 2. Pairs, in which men and women free skate together in unison. 3. Ice dance, in which a man and a woman perform compulsory dance patterns and free dance routines.

Singles ability for men and women is measured by a series of nine figure tests of increasing difficulty. There are 69 compulsory figures, consisting of a series of two- and three-lobe circles, called figure eights and serpentines, respectively. The compulsory figures to be skated in competition remain unknown to the contestant until just a few minutes before the meet. Com-

*ICE SKATING PROGRAM (Vigorous)**

Chart 1	Chart 2
1. 5 minutes	1. 21 minutes
2. 8 minutes	2. 23 minutes
3. 10 minutes	3. 25 minutes
4. 12 minutes	4. 26 minutes
5. 15 minutes	5. 28 minutes
6. 16 minutes	6. 30 minutes
7. 17 minutes	7. 32 minutes
8. 18 minutes	8. 35 minutes
9. 20 minutes	9. 36 minutes

* See ENDURANCE and ENERGY COST OF ACTIVITIES for an explanation of these charts.
** Doesn't include rest periods, times out, etc.

Fitness 1

If you achieved a score of poor or low average on the *Harvard Step Test* or a score of very poor or poor on the *12 Minute Run,* start on Chart 1-Level 1 and spend one week at each level until Chart 2-Level 9 is reached. It is recommended that you participate 4 to 5 days a week. When Chart 2-Level 9 is reached, 4 days a week is sufficient.

Fitness 2

If you achieved a score of high average on the *Harvard Step Test* or fair on the *12 Minute Run,* start on Chart 1-Level 4. Spend one week on Chart 1-Levels 1, 3, 5, 7, and 9, and Chart 2-Level 9 is reached, 4 days a week is sufficient.

Fitness 3

If you achieved a score of good or excellent on either the *Harvard Step Test* or *12 Minute Run,* continue your current program or select Chart 2-Level 9 as your level of participation. Four days a week is sufficient.

pulsory figures are designed to demonstrate a skater's ability at restricted and prescribed movements. They provide the basic moves for all of ice skating and as a result, they count 60% toward the overall title. Free skating counts for 40%. In free skating the skater is permitted to use his originality in creating a program of jumps, skims and footwork, presenting it in an interpretive manner to music.

In pair skating a man and woman perform in such a harmonious manner that they give the impression of being molded together. Pair skating is often the most spectacular figure skating event because it features all the free-skating movements of single skating, plus the daring risks in which a man raises his partner into the air and lowers her to the ice again. Acrobatics are not permitted, and the movements must be continuous.

In ice dance there are compulsory dance patterns, just as single skating requires compulsory figures. Also, compulsory dances count 60% toward the overall title as against 40% for free dance. There are 20 ice dances of set and optional patterns that have been arranged into six tests. The compulsory dance patterns include such areas as the Dutch Waltz, the Fox Trot, the American Waltz, and so on.

In contrast to compulsory dancing, free dance does not have a required sequence of steps but consists of a non-repetitious combination of new or known ice-dance movements, displayed according to the dancer's own ideas and arrangement.

Contribution to Fitness

Because of the duration of the activity, skating develops leg muscle endurance and circulo-respiratory endurance. In pairs and ice dance, muscle strength and endurance of the upper body are also developed. Figure skating also contributes to agility, balance, coordination and flexibility.

Conditioning

Training for figure skating is very demanding. You must spend hours on the ice practicing both school figures and the basic routine. You must perfect the fundamental skating stroke and the stopping motion which best suits you. Then you learn to skate in a backward motion and more progressively to the turns, jumps and spins.

To accomplish a high degree of performance requires a great many hours on the ice. Without question, figure skating is one of the most exacting of sports. The school figures require precise and accurate movement, while the free skating routines and dance movements require constant practice so that the moves are perfectly timed.

Figure skating, however, can be enjoyed as an excellent means of daily recreation. (Because it is a high-energy-cost activity, it is a noteworthy activity for developing circulo-respiratory endurance.)

Although competitive years usually range between teen-age years and the early 20's, figure skating can be enjoyed by people of all ages. In Europe, especially those countries behind the Iron Curtain, people may engage in the sport until their late 20's and early 30's. The reason for the difference in the countries is largely a result of the lack of true definition between an amateur and a professional. In the United States most of the top competitive skaters learn to skate before they are 10 years old.

Injuries

Most common injuries associated with figure skating are from falls on the ice which cause contusions and abrasions. Occasionally fractures of the ribs, clavicle, wrists, or humerus may

result. Jump turns, which are currently very popular and are executed in a very spectacular style, have increased the number of sprains and strains to the knee and ankle. In pair skating, contusions pose a hazard, not only from contact and falls but from being caught on the sharp skate edges. When several other people are skating on the ice, the incidence of injury increases as a result of collision.

Association:

United States Figure Skating Association, 575 Boylston Street, Boston, Massachusetts 02116.

INDIAN CLUBS

If you're an "oldtimer," chances are you have some memories of an exercise device which has now passed almost completely from the scene—the Indian club. Back in the late 1800's and early 1900's, Indian club exercises were as popular as weight training is today. In fact, club swinging was the forerunner of weight training and was practiced for largely the same motives—the building of impressive and powerful upper-body muscles. Although the barbell has pushed Indian clubs out of the muscle-building picture, there's no reason why the swinging way to fitness shouldn't stage a comeback. Club swinging does have the very important advantage of improving the range of motion and strength of the wrists, hands and arms. It also teaches agility, coordination and concentration.

Origin

Indian clubs, contrary to what some people believe, were not adapted from clubs used by American Indians. They were brought to this country from India by way of British soldiers who saw them being used by the strong men and gymnasts of that country. One of the earliest promoters of Indian club exercises in America was Simon D. Kehoe. Back in the 1860's, he sold rosewood clubs ranging in weight from

1 to 12 pounds each for as little as $1.50 a pair. General U. S. Grant was a Kehoe customer and said that his clubs were "of the nicest workmanship." Kehoe awarded medals to champion club swingers and explained a wide variety of club techniques in his beautifully printed book *The Indian Club Exercise*, published in 1866.

Shaped like a skimpy, elongated bowling pin, the club is grasped around its neck and moved in various patterns ranging from simple warm-up exercises to intricate rotations that take many hours of practice to learn. One reason that the Indian club has passed out of fashion is that its use can be discouraging in the early stages. Although the less complex club exercises can be done by anyone, mastering exhibition swinging requires perseverance.

Contribution to Fitness

But a good club swinging exhibition can be a moving sight. Walter A. Johnson, a professor of physical education at the University of Wisconsin, has stated that club swinging is made to order for a high school student who has a leg handicap yet wants to contribute to a physical education program. "I remember doing just that sort of thing when teaching in high school, and I shall always recall the feeling of personal gratification when watching that particular boy perform his solo. Girls do very nicely swinging clubs, as many of them start baton twirling at an early age and adapt quickly to clubs."

Club swinging is also very useful for rehabilitation of certain types of arm and shoulder injuries. Professor Johnson says that club swinging can also be used in adaptive physical education where particular restrictions of activity are imposed because of physical handicaps. "Anyone having swung clubs will vouch for improvements of muscular endurance of the arm, grip strength and joint mobility," he says.

"The prime movements of club swinging involve the shoulder joint, elbow joint, wrist joint and a rotation inward and outward of the arm. It is possible to have both clubs doing exactly the same movement or, if one desires a greater challenge, have each club doing something different."

Method of Holding the Clubs

There are different methods of holding the clubs. Kehoe's 102-year-old book advocates this method: "Take good care to grasp the handle firmly, close to the ball, extending the thumb along the shank, which you will find enables you to control its movement and prevent it from wandering out of the direction you desire it to go. This is the general hold, where the thumb can be used to guide the movements." He notes that in the more intricate twirling movements it is necessary to relax the grasp, "holding the club entirely between the thumb and forefinger during a part of the movement, but regaining a complete hold again on the finish."

A more modern book, *Gymnastics in Education*, advises holding the index finger instead of the thumb in a straight line with the club when extending it at arm's length. It says that the club should "slide between the thumb and index finger" when doing circles behind the shoulder and similar complex movements. "In a circle high or low in front, the knob of the club should be grasped by the thumb and first two fingers."

Elementary Club Swinging

"One picture is worth ten thousand words." That phrase was probably first coined by someone trying to learn how to swing Indian clubs by following only a set of written instructions. Here is a sample of the turgid prose an enthusiastic 19th century club swinger had to deal with if he were to master Simon D. Kehoe's mail-order approach to club swinging: "Execute the Outer Front with the left hand, carrying the Club outwardly to the left, and describing a reverse sweep from that of the Inner Front, with the left hand." Fortunately, Kehoe had access to the talents of a fine wood engraver, so that his students who couldn't figure out the words could see what they were supposed to learn to do.

If you are interested in adding club swinging to your own exercise repertoire, you should seek the personal tutoring of a physical education instructor who has learned the rudiments of the technique in college. You will probably have difficulty finding an expert, because many colleges have eliminated club swinging completely.

Springfield College in Springfield, Massachusetts, is one of the few physical education schools still requiring all students to master that art. Dr. Ervin R. Schmid of the College's physical education department stated that, "We keep club swinging in our program because we believe it still has value for several areas in physical education, as well as to present another form of exercise. Indian club swinging is a healthful and most pleasing form of exercise when accompanied by good music."

Some club exercises are simple and easily learned. If you can't find a competent instructor, you can at least get the feel of swinging by trying the simpler movements. Whether you succeed in progressing to more elaborate exercises will depend on your own physical potential and perseverance.

Most Indian clubs sold today are light in weight. A typical modern club is 16 inches long and weighs one pound. A club of that relatively light weight is primarily useful for exhibition swinging but also can help to loosen joints and increase flexibility. All leading sporting goods stores still carry clubs or can order them for you.
—*Robert Rodale*

INDIVIDUAL RATES OF RESPONSE

Individual rates of response apply to one of the physiological principles of training. Each person has his own level of response to a training program. In athletic participation, some individuals seem to arrive at a high level of condition long before others. The reason why this different attainment occurs is not clear, although it is probably dependent upon many variables, which may be physical, mental, environmental and heredity. A few of these specific variables are (1) present physical condition, (2) age, (3) body type, (4) weight, (5) rest, sleep and relaxation, (6) nutrition, (7) freedom from disease, (8) proneness to injury, (9) motivation, and (10) ability to learn new skills. See HEREDITY and TRAINING.

INFECTION

An apparent misconception among many people is that the physically fit or athletic person tends to possess a greater resistance to infection than does the sedentary person. Almost all research done in that area indicates that the physically fit enjoy no more resistance to infection than do their inactive counterparts. A portion of that misconception can be traced to the active, physically fit person's apparent vitality and vibrance. He looks like the "picture of health." And he probably is healthy, but available evidence suggests that his resistance to infection is no greater than that of the inactive person. History has shown numerous times that "strong" men are affected by infection and epidemics to the same degree as ordinary men.

In his book *Physiology of Exercise*, Ernst Jokl tells of the results of his Kentucky Physical Fitness Experiment conducted in 1958-59. He found that there was no significant difference in the number of school days missed between trained and untrained children. During the experimental period an influenza epidemic struck, and while absenteeism increased markedly, no change could be found in the ratio of trained and untrained children.

An attempt has been made to show that the physically fit are more resistant to upper respiratory tract infections than the unfit. Peter Karpovich offers two explanations:

1. The physically fit person produces enough body heat during exercise to prevent chilling.

2. It is possible that the physically fit individual can become better adapted to temperature changes than the person who is not accustomed to being exposed to adverse weather conditions.

Infection and Fatigue

Some medical authorities believe that infections and illness are more likely to affect you during periods of fatigue when the body's resistance is said to be "down." One effect of training is that it helps you to ward off fatigue. Remember that athletes frequently work themselves so hard that they approach fatigue or near fatigue. For an athlete to postpone fatigue he must approach fatigue frequently. His body must become accustomed to working in a state of near fatigue. In effect, he pushes his fatigue level back. For that reason athletes actually tend to lower their resistance, at least temporarily, following strenuous exercise.

Infection and Exercise

Another popular fallacy concerning illness and infection is that you can "sweat out" a cold. There is little evidence to support that contention, and in certain instances where severe infection is evident, continued exercise may aggravate the infection. Laboratory demonstrations have shown that animals injected with that bacterial infection before or after exercise were more affected by the bacteria than animals that did not exercise preced-

ing or following the injection. Consequently bed rest is recommended for certain severe infections.

Exercises may indirectly aid the spread of certain types of infection. Actually strenuous exercise may use up so much energy that hardly enough is left for the body to use to mobilize its defenses against the infection. During rest the body can concentrate its energies against illnesses and infections.

Frequently, fitness seekers are required to workout in poor weather conditions. Some physically fit persons develop a false sense of immunity with respect to bad weather conditions. A disdain for good health habits (dressing warmly, avoiding getting wet, drying adequately following shower, etc.) can make one more susceptible to infection, whether physically fit or not.

It is true that a higher degree of physical fitness does permit you to withstand greater physical stress, but there seems to be little correlation between your ability to withstand physical stress and your ability to resist infection.

Resistance to infection is largely an individual matter and depends on several factors, of which your level of physical fitness is only one consideration. A few very significant factors are eating habits, resting habits, cleanliness and other health habits. Numerous variables exist when trying to trace or compare the abilities of various groups to resist infectious diseases. For this reason studies of this nature are often complex and inconclusive.

Dr. Ernst Jokl has explored exhaustively the problem of physical fitness and immunity and states: "Physical fitness does not bestow an improved capacity to resist infectious diseases."

INJURIES[*]

The treatment of athletic injuries is a branch of sports medicine, the study

[*] This chapter was critically reviewed by O. W. Dayton.

of man's endeavor to improve his physical performance. See SPORTS MEDICINE. The prime impact of the treatment of athletic injuries is to prevent permanent loss of function as a result of these injuries, to prevent injuries when possible, and to speed the recovery.

This particular branch of sports medicine has received a considerable amount of attention in recent years because of professional sports and the need to return the top-notch athletes to regular form after an injury. The treatment of injuries, however, should not be limited to professional athletes. A quick recovery and the prevention of a permanent loss of function are extremely important for the college or high school athlete, the intramural or sandlot athlete, or for any person who engages in many of the various forms of exercise and sports. For a more exhaustive and technical presentation concerning the medical care of athletic injuries, consult the following texts. O'Donoghue, D. H. *Treatment of Injuries to Athletes*, Philadelphia; W. B. Saunders Co., 1962; Klafs, Carl E. and Daniel D. Arnheim. *Modern Principle of Athletic Training*. St. Louis: The C. V. Mosby, Co., 1963. Dayton, William O. *Athletic Training and Conditioning*. New York: The Ronald Press Company, 1960. Morehouse, Laurence E., and Philip J. Rasch. *Sports Medicine for Trainers*. Philadelphia: W. B. Saunders Co., 1964.

Classification of Injuries

One of the simplest and clearest techniques of classifying injuries is to separate them into two specific groups: *exposed* and *unexposed*. An exposed injury refers to any condition which is external and results in the exposure of superficial and underlying tissue, such as a cut. An unexposed injury, however, is internal like a bruise, although it may be initiated by some external force.

Exposed Wounds

There are four specific types of exposed wounds.

1. Abrasion—Abrasions are the tearing of the upper layers of the skin. They may or may not bleed, and weeping may also be present. That type of wound should be carefully cleaned with soap and water and treated with an antiseptic. Apply a dressing coated with a bland ointment.

2. Laceration—A laceration is a tear in the skin that leaves an interruption of normal continuity. The wound may or may not be a jagged-edged cavity. The degree of separation of the skin will establish the necessity for sutures. Sutured wounds heal faster and usually have less scarring—a physician must make that decision. Treat the lacerated wound the same way as an abrasion.

3. Puncture Wound—Puncture wounds may occur during many physical activities. A puncture wound is usually a deep penetration of the tissues by some pointed object such as a track-shoe spike. It is particularly dangerous because the individual may be subjected to lockjaw if tetanus bacilli are introduced to the blood stream. Although most puncture wounds are small on the surface, they should be examined carefully to establish the degree of underlying tissue injury. Keep the wound dry and report to a physician immediately.

4. Incised Wound—Incised wounds appear when a person receives a blow over a sharp bone or over a bone that is not properly padded. That type of injury is not as serious as the other three types of exposed injuries.

Unexposed Wounds

Unexposed or closed wounds are those internal injuries which do not break the skin. They include contusions (bruises), strains, sprains, dislocations and fractures. Occasionally, however, fractures may be exposed if a part of the broken bone breaks through the skin.

1. Fractures—A fracture is the breaking of a bone. The break can range from a partial to a complete separation of the bony parts. Generally, they are divided into two types: *simple* and *compound*. A simple fracture is a break in a bone without puncturing the skin. A compound fracture is one in which the bone punctures the outer skin, thereby making the injury an exposed wound. To treat a fracture, immobilize the affected bone before moving the person. If an extremity is fractured, it must be splinted. If the fracture is severe, the person may have to be treated for shock. Great care should be taken in handling any fracture, and you must consult a doctor immediately.

2. Dislocations—A dislocation is the separating of the articulating surfaces of the joint as a result of forces that cause the joint to go beyond the normal anatomical limits. Dislocations are divided into two classes: *subluxations* and *luxations*. Subluxations are partial dislocations in which there is an incomplete separation between the articulating bones. A luxation is a complete separation between the articulating bones. In both types of dislocations, deformity, swelling and tenderness are present.

After reduction, treat a dislocation with ice and apply a compression bandage to the affected area. The cold and compression will reduce or retard the swelling as a result of internal hemorrhaging and the clot will be kept smaller. Keep the compression bandage and ice on the area for an hour on smaller joints and up to 24 hours for larger joints. Give support and immobilization to the affected joint for a period of two days to three weeks, depending upon the extent of the injury.

3. Contusions—Contusions or bruises are a result of a blow to the body. The blow, depending upon its severity, may cause an injury ranging from a superficial bruise to a deep tissue tear and hemorrhage. In a contusion there is a flow of blood and lymph into the surrounding tissues. Since all this blood congregates at one spot, a hematoma forms (the hematoma is a soft, spongy mass that is absorbed very slowly). After a few days the blood clots, making drainage of the blood very slow. The hematoma must remain in a liquid state if it is to be reduced rather quickly. To reduce hemorrhaging, a pressure bandage and an ice pack should be applied during the first 24 hours. After that period, apply heat to keep the affected area in a liquid state, and thus provide better absorption. A contusion may affect the bones, thus causing a bone bruise.

4. Strains—A strain is an overstretching or tearing of a muscle or, in a few instances, a tendon. The tear is usually a result of an abnormal muscular contraction. The strain may range from a small separation of connective tissues and muscle fibers to a complete muscle rupture or tissue tear.

After the rupture or tear of the blood vessel or capillaries, hemorrhage is present, and shortly a hematoma is organized. The hematoma is then absorbed, and clotting takes place. To prevent too much hemorrhaging, a compression bandage and ice pack should be applied for at least 30 minutes. Overnight, keep ice on the affected muscles. Elevate the affected area when possible.

5. Sprains—A sprain is one of the most common injuries occurring in physical activity. Usually it is a result of a violent joint twist that produces a stretching or tearing of one or more ligaments surrounding the affected joint. Other tissues such as the tendons and nerves may be affected.

INTELLIGENCE

Intelligence is the capacity for reasoning and understanding. It is an aptitude for grasping truths, facts and meanings. So conceived, intelligence is an innate quality. Contrastedly, physical fitness refers to the level of physical condition that an individual attains and, as such, is an acquired quality.

Relationship Between Intelligence and Physical Fitness

Are intelligence and physical fitness strongly related? Terman, a pioneer in intelligence testing, noted three decades ago that physical weakness was found nearly 30 per cent fewer times in children of higher intelligence than in those of lower intelligence. However, other studies do not support that position. While some evidence is more favorable than others, the valid generalization from available findings is that, although there appears to be a slight positive correlation, no appreciable relationship has been established between intelligence and physical fitness.

That lack of a strong correlation between intelligence and physical fitness becomes more understandable upon examination of the relationships involving another factor—academic achievement or performance. First, the correlation between intelligence and academic achievement (which may be regarded as the application of intelligence) is not as strong as might be expected. This apparent discrepancy is attributed to achievement-motivation, which in essence determines the amount of application to a task. A person who possesses average intelligence and a high level of achievement-motivation can equal if not surpass in academic performance an intellectually gifted person who operates at a low level of achievement-motivation.

Relationship Between Academic Achievement and Fitness

A second consideration is academic achievement and physical fitness, for academic achievement is regarded as a function of intelligence. Although studies vary in their findings, there is evidence that academic achievement and physical fitness appear to be somewhat related. Careful analysis will reveal that a common denominator—achievement-motivation—seemingly exists between academic performance and physical fitness. Apparently, individuals who strive to attain a high level of physical fitness tend to apply themselves similarly to achieve a high academic level, and vice versa. Consequently, people who aspire to achieve or perform well tend to apply themselves diligently to whatever task is at hand. Related to this, it is interesting to note that some studies have disclosed that students improved their academic performance when working toward improvement in physical fitness and motor ability. They apparently transferred desire to achieve from one characteristic to another.

Although physical fitness evidently is not related to intelligence, it does appear to have some relationship with how well a person applies this innate quality—intelligence—to academic matters.—*Carlton R. Meyers.*

INTENSITY OF EXERCISE

How much should you exercise? What activities should you select? Those are questions that occur to all of us as we plan our exercise program. To help determine the length of your workout, the degree of your exercise period, and the type of physical routines, there are three important considerations. They are time, calories consumed and pulse rate.

Time

The minimum time that you should exercise is 30 minutes 3 to 4 days a week. Of course, 5 to 6 days a week would be most desirable. The intensity of exercise in the 30-minute period is described below.

Calories

You should burn off 300 to 500 calories during a thirty-minute period, and preferably around 400 to 500. Under ENERGY COST OF ACTIVITIES good illustrations of what activities meet that requirement are presented. Those people who prefer to utilize specific exercises, can note the number of calories burned off per minute for various exercises. Remember, you need not be a slave to those figures. They are to serve merely as a guide so that you can make a realistic appraisal in selecting activities and exercises. Remember that your height and weight will cause some discrepancy in the number of calories consumed in the various activities and exercises. See WEIGHT CONTROL for a more detailed explanation. It's better to consume 400 to 500 calories in one-half hour than to burn 450 in one hour, for a greater stress is placed on the body. Naturally, however, the consumption of 450 calories in one hour of exercise is better than using up no calories at all because of little exercise. You won't be able to consume 400 to 450 calories in a half hour immediately. It may take you weeks or months to achieve the required exercise level in a one-half hour period. Your initial physical condition will play a critical role in the amount of exercise you can perform in the beginning. Give careful consideration to your current physical condition before you begin any exercise program.

Pulse Rate

Pulse rate is a second factor to consider in intensity of exercise. Dr. M. F. Graham states that the heart rate of an individual should "reach a peak of at least 60 per cent of its capable range for 'several minutes'." If you have a resting rate of 72 beats per minute and a peak rate of 180, subtract 72 from 180 or 108. Sixty per cent of 108 is 65. Sixty-five added to 72 is 137. A satisfactory workout, therefore, should raise your pulse to 137 and maintain it for several minutes. See PULSE RATE for the range of your age group and a more detailed discussion. Usually an exercise level that requires 400 to 500 calories to be burned in a half hour will produce a pulse of 60 per cent of your range.

Dr. Kenneth Cooper in his book *Aerobics* goes a long way in helping a person select activities that will be of sufficient intensity for improving a person's circulo-respiratory endurance. See PROGRAMS. Also see EXCESSIVE EXERCISE for a related discussion on intensity of exercise.

INTERVAL TRAINING

Interval training is a sophisticated training technique developed by Wol-

ENERGY COST OF SELECTED EXERCISES

Exercise	Rate No. of Completed Exercise Sequences Done Per Minute	Energy Cost In Calories
Side Bends	14	1.2
Alternate Toe Touch—Sitting	14	1.4
Side Arm Fling	28	1.8
Alternate Leg Raises, Supine Position	10	2.5
Alternate Side Bends, Shoulder Touches	14	2.8
Knee Raises, Supine Position	14	3.3
Sit-ups, Hands Behind Head	20	4.0
Sprinter's Stretch	14	4.7
Push-ups	28	6.5
Burpees (4-count)	14	9.3

demar Gerschler in the 1930's. His technique first bore fruit when one of his pupils, Rudolph Harbig, astonished the track world by running the 400 meters in 46.0 seconds and the 800 meters in 1:46.6—unbelievable times in those days. Despite the outstanding success of Harbig, the interval training technique did not become popular until another of Gerschler's pupils won an Olympic gold medal for the 1,500-meter run in the 1952 Games. Since that time, most middle- and long-distance runners in the world use the system in total or in part.

Guidelines

Gerschler's concept was that for training to be successful, it was necessary to carefully control the distance, interval, repetition and time of the runner. His idea was to run a series of repeat efforts at a given distance with a controlled amount of rest. Gerschler established several guidelines for the technique, often called the *Gerschler-Reindell Law.*

1. Before the performer begins his series of repeat efforts, such as 10 to 20 440-yard runs, he should get his pulse to 120 beats per minute by a preliminary warm-up.

2. The next step is to run the first series of repeat efforts in a certain period of time so that the heart rate reaches the 170-180 beats per minute range.

3. After step two, the runner walks or jogs until his heart returns to 120-140 beats per minute. When he reaches that point, he starts the next series of efforts to get his pulse up to the 170-180 range. Then he repeats the entire process. The time that it takes for the pulse to drop from 170-180 to 120-140 is not to exceed one minute and 30 seconds. As the performer improves, the recovery time should shorten. Gerschler felt that cardiovascular training occurs during the recovery phase of the work, when the pulse is being reduced from the 170-180 range to the 120-140 range.

Interval training has evolved until today there are two basic forms of the training technique—slow and fast.

Slow Interval Training—Here the performer works, runs, or swims at a speed slower than race speed with a short rest interval and an incomplete recovery of the heart rate. The rest must always be shorter than the work interval. Slow interval training develops circulo-respiratory reserve, but it does not contribute to speed.

Fast Interval Training—This permits longer rest intervals, but the work effort is more intense. The emphasis is on speed. That type of training is beneficial to both the heart and skeletal muscles.

Objections to Interval Training

Many teachers and coaches of sport originally jumped on the interval training bandwagon. They were not cautious, however, and excluded many other effective training techniques. Today, some experts are very anti-interval training. Percy Cerutty of Australia, for example, is one who is very much opposed to interval training. Here are his objections:

1. The monotony of the daily training breeds boredom and a loss of interest because of little or no variation in the program.

2. No allowance is made for the practice of speed acceleration or variation of pace as is found in actual running.

3. No allowance is made for human fallibility and inconsistency. Great athletes, usually being emotional and temperamental, soon rebel against the regularity and regimentation.

4. The system allows little if any race practice and no personal originality.

5. When a program proves to be beyond a runner's capacity, physical breakdown and/or mental discouragement follow.

6. When a program does not equate an athlete's progressive possibilities, then it tends to produce an athlete

who seldom works to his full capacity, or even to the point of exhaustion.

7. The athlete instinctively yearns for a freer, less inhibited expression of himself, and sooner or later dislikes the system.

8. The progress, or repetitive rate, is largely governed by the pulse rate or the stop watch. Little or nothing of the human element of individual differences is considered.

9. At first, interval training did not pay attention to upper body strengthening or the techniques of breathing and movement.—*Percy Cerutty*

Most experts feel, however, that interval training can be used quite effectively as one method of training for the athlete and as a part of the training program for the noncompetitor who wants to get into condition. It is an extremely efficient conditioner of the heart and muscles.

Interval training is not the only training method, although there is no better training technique to enlarge the heart volume. But the increase diminishes quickly. Other techniques (Over Training and Fartlek) are more effective in maintaining the enlarged heart volume. The advantage of interval training, however, is the increasing of endurance in a short period of time.

Typical Interval-Training Program

Below is a typical interval-training program or schedule for the mile run, designed by Percy Cerutty.

After a slow warm-up, such as calisthenics, to elevate the pulse to 120, the following procedure and steps are advocated:

1. Run 440 yards in 70 seconds to elevate the pulse to the 170 to 180 range. Rest for a period of time until the pulse drops to 120-140. Repeat the 440 yards at the 70-second pace. Run 10 to 20, 440-yard runs of 70 seconds with rest intervals in between.

2. As your condition improves, then run the 440 yards in 68 seconds following the same procedure as above.

3. Continually drop your time until you run 10 to 20, 440 yards at 60 seconds or even faster. Also shorten the rest interval.

That program is an example of slow interval training with a gradual progression toward fast training designed specifically for an athlete. You can modify the above program for your own needs. The guideline is your pulse. You may reduce the distance or the speed depending upon your physical condition.

There is a considerable amount of overlapping in training techniques, and it is difficult to differentiate one from the other. Today there is no one pure system used, for many coaches, teachers, trainers, and athletes will borrow from other techniques to attain peak performance and condition. For a discussion of other techniques and related articles see FARTLEK, JOGGING, LYDIARD, OVER TRAINING and REPETITION TRAINING.

ISCHEMIC HEART DISEASE

Certainly nobody can deny that ischemic heart disease (IHD) is a disease with many causes. And under no pretense would I dare to claim that physical exercise is a panacea for this jig-saw puzzle of a problem. Take a look at the list of recommended ways to deter heart disease:

1. Reduce if overweight.

2. Decrease saturated fats in the diet.

3. Stop smoking cigarettes.

4. Control high blood pressure.

5. Exercise regularly.

6. Shun needless tensions.

What Can You Do?

After eliminating predisposing hereditary factors, about which you can do nothing, you are left with a number of acquired factors about which you can do much.

Start your attack by concentrating on three major fronts—dietary, anti-

THE FIGHT OR FLIGHT (ADRENERGIC) RESPONSE

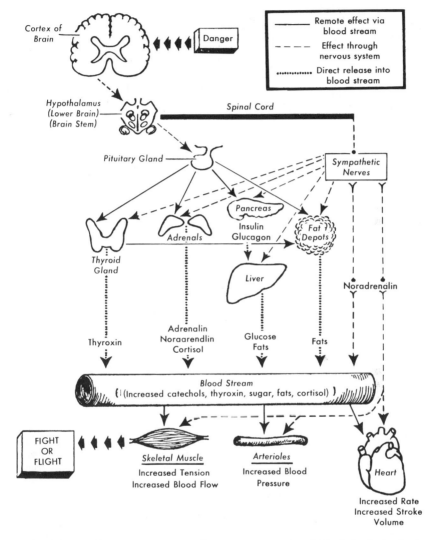

The fight-or-flight response is a complex, primitive one in which the body is physiologically prepared to do battle with, or to flee, an imminent danger. Under the influence of the brain, the endocrine glands release the necessary materials into the blood stream, with a resultant increase in blood pressure, heart rate, muscle tension, and flow of blood to the skeletal muscles in particular. The normal means of releasing the stored-up tension resulting from this "adrenergic" response is through the skeletal muscles i.e., through exercise. When such release is not available to the body, heart and blood-vessel disease is aggravated (see text). Modern-day tensions of living produce the same overall effect as external dangers, but modern civilization denies man the fight-or-flight release, except through exercise.

tension and physical exercise. Those items I have termed the Big Three. Exercise is the common denominator. Physical activity exerts both a dieting and tension release effect in itself, whereas dieting and passive anti-tension measures do not in themselves exert an exercise effect.

Dieting

Few researchers can deny the quantitative dieting effect of exercise—specifically, its calorie-spending effect. Frequently, a vicious cycle is broken.

Much remains to be proved about the qualitative dietary effect of exercise. Epidemiologic studies, however, tend to indicate that vigorous physical life to some extent nullifies high fat, high cholesterol intake. In all fairness, however, it remains to be conclusively shown that physical exercise can, in a population susceptible to IHD, completely nullify the effect of a diet high in saturated fats. Perhaps it is a matter of exercise intensity and duration.

Exercise vs. Tension

The effect of exercise on tension is a favorable one, although the distinction must be made between tension of the anxiety type and tension associated with hypertension—a medical problem of chronic, sustained elevations in blood pressure.

The exercise-tension relationship is complicated and is based on the fight or flight theory. There are many pathways and effects of fear stimuli on the neurohumoral system. These pathways were originally designed to prepare the organism in danger for fight or flight. In modern, competitive societies like our own, the fear stimulus is often triggered in the subliminal areas of the brain. The end-effects of such stimuli are the humoral buildup of blood fats, blood sugar and catechols. The effect of the neurohumoral response on the cardiovascular system is increased heart rate, cardiac output, blood pressure and muscle tension. All those factors are seen in the chronically fear-

ful, tense, or anxious individual, and all are common to coronary-proneness. In the primitive situation for which that mechanism was originally designed, man could either fight or flee his fear stimulus and thus utilize the wonderful body responses which prepared him to do so. In so doing, he used up his circulating fats and fat stores, his catechols, and thus his tensions. But modern man, often insecure and anxious, striving to keep up with the Joneses, and harboring a repressed desire to punch his boss in the nose, cannot fight or run. To do so would be to admit defeat, to let his family down, to lose face. So he is caught in a vicious cycle.

Accentuate the Positive

Exercise, the common denominator of the "Big Three" factors in a coronary-control program, is the only one of the three which accentuates the positive and plays down the negative. Dieting is full of don'ts. Shunning tension is full of don'ts. But *exercise is full of do's.* It fosters the positive approach to a program otherwise full of prohibitions.

Vigorous exercise also breeds confidence, confidence that you can still use your entire body. So powerful is its effect that dieting, if necessary at all, comes with utter ease, and tensions melt like butter on a hot plate. So forceful is its psychologic impact that confidence alone may well explain the subjective improvement exercise produces in many coronary patients when objective studies in such patients remain unaltered.

But if exercise is indeed the foundation for anti-coronary programs, it must fulfill certain requirements. It cannot be just any old exercise. To promote cardiovascular fitness, exercises should be done with clocklike regularity, should force you to reach certain minimal pulse rates—considerably higher than accepted as adequate not too many years ago—and should result in the expenditure of certain minimal amounts of calories per session. Programs should lend themselves to gradation, versatility, economy of time and money, and "agelessness"— adaptability to any age and physical condition.

And as Dr. Warren Guild and others have pointed out, exercise must, over the long haul, be fun. Otherwise motivation will lag, and dropout rates will soar. For a part of each week, you must be willing to "work at play" to become a kid again and to play games to escape the confines of ritual and the pressures of circumstance. We all know, aging may be in large measure an unwillingness to return to the freedoms of childhood. For who can play and be old at one and the same time?

At best, it is difficult to teach an old dog new tricks—or an old heart to rise to new demands. It can be done. But the best time to start is in childhood because ischemic heart disease is, pathogenetically, a pediatric disease. As a pediatrician, whose main interest in any disease process lies in prevention, I must conclude that exercise must be ingrained in the child, becoming a part of his habit pattern, like brushing teeth. And there must be some for everyone—not just the gifted 10 per cent. So if you can conceive, as I do, that a good program of lifelong physical exercise can be life-extending and happiness-producing, a common denominator in the battle against ischemic heart disease, then take the concept first to the child, next to the young adult, and lastly (but not least) to the middle-aged and the aged. For in just that order will it serve its ultimate purpose—to halt the onslaught of the great white plague that is IHD.— M. F. Graham

ISOMETRICS

Faddism versus Fact

Great popular emphasis has recently been placed on the use of isometric exercises for the development of strength.

Because of either commercialism or an attempt to get on the publicity bandwagon, many companies have produced methods, gadgets, and exercises to extol the huge benefits of isometrics. Unfortunately, many of these methods are based more on fantasy than on fact. But with an understanding of some basic facts you can capitalize on isometric exercises. Remember that no exercise or exercise method can be a panacea for all exercise problems.

Exploitation of Research

Sales promotions have extoled the usefulness of the isometric contraction. That usefulness has been supported unquestionably by fundamental research in isometrics. However, the commercial literature usually fails to note the following:

1. When researchers conduct a scientific study, they normally isolate muscle groups as much as possible so that little or no substitution of other muscles can take place.

2. The force being exerted is often, almost always, measured. (Any device or exercise program using isometrics which is not based upon the above two principles is not thoroughly valid.)

3. Summaries from textbooks describing the physiological effects of exercises are often taken out of their proper context. The original scientific investigators have frequently published material which was based upon isotonic work, but the new copied summaries claim that isometrics will develop the same physical capacities or produce the same physiological effects. That is nothing more than an assumption.

Conditioning Needs

In both physical education and fitness programs there are four distinct types of conditioning needs.

1. *Cardiovascular efficiency*—or the adaptive response of the heart to exercise.

2. *Muscular strength*—the ability to accomplish an activity at peak per-

formance without injury. Strength is the ability to work against a specified resistance.

3. *Muscular endurance*—the ability of the muscle to respond repetitively for a relatively long period of time.

4. *Flexibility*—defined both as the elasticity of a muscle group and the effective use of the muscle group throughout its maximum range of motion. The maximum effective range of motion will vary among individuals. Flexibility is closely allied to strength.

You should develop each of those four areas of response according to your needs. Some activities stress one or two areas more than they do the others. It has long been recognized that participation in sports, for example, does not necessarily produce the optimal fitness benefit. Thus, special conditioning programs have arisen to make you more proficient in your chosen activity.

Values and Limitations of Isometrics

Isometrics can develop strength and, if used properly, can offer a great deal to any physical education or athletic program. The studies using practical application of isometrics, which were undertaken at the Southern Illinois University Laboratory of Applied Physiology and Laboratory of Physical Education (Men), thus take on a timely and special significance. These studies have led to the following conclusions:

1. *The greatest value found so far in the use of isometrics has been to evaluate the strength of various movements surrounding joints.* That method of strength evaluation is extremely effective after injury because medical authorities can determine the exact area or areas of weakness and apply the proper rehabilitation technique. Moreover, the testing allows evaluation of the effectiveness of the applied corrective method or of any applied conditioning program.

2. *An isometric contraction can develop muscular strength at any point of stimulation throughout a range of motion.* Electromyographic studies have indicated that certain muscles act only in parts of the range whereas other muscles act only in parts of the movement. For example, in knee extension, which is mainly an act of the *quadriceps femoris* muscle, the *rectus femoris* and *vastus intermedius* are primarily responsible for the movement beginning with full flexion and ending at approximately 125° extension. The *rectus femoris* and *vastus intermedius* then gradually reduce their action, and the *vastus lateralis* and *vastus medialis* take over and become responsible for the action to full extension.

There is available a multiple-angle testing method which readily measures the strength of muscle groups at various points in the range of movement. That method of testing has permitted the conduction of isometric strength studies which point up the necessity of strengthening more than one point in a range of motion.

3. *The isometric contraction must be highly controlled to achieve proper strength development.* In various strength studies, scientists have found that when a weakness exists in muscles ordinarily used in normal movement, other muscles adaptively take over to a varying extent. The strong muscles get stronger because of overuse, and the weak muscles get weaker because of disuse. Therefore, it is especially important that the weakened areas be properly stimulated. That can be effectively accomplished with isometric exercises if the athlete is positioned to allow only a minimum of compensatory accommodation.

4. *Evaluation of the effect of isometric exercises is necessary if strength gains are to be realized.* No external work takes place during an isometric contraction. Therefore, unless some form of measurement is handy, there is no way to know whether or not you

are actually exerting the force necessary to build strength. Studies have indicated that many people will not exert pressure to develop strength. That may be because of (a) lack of motivation, (b) lack of belief in the benefit of isometrics, (c) lack of kinesthetic sense to exert full power, and (d) malingering or other psychologic complications.

5. *Isometric exercises are not the whole answer to the conditioning needs of most people.* Isometric exercises are extremely effective for the development of strength, but their effectiveness is increased if they are used with proper adjunctive isotonic and stretching exercises.

6. *An isometric conditioning program using gross exercises is often more detrimental than beneficial.* That would include exercise programs such as pressing the whole body against a bar or applying gross resistance with rope or straps and without the benefit of measurement. Such programs may develop the wrong muscles, partly through unwanted muscular substitution and partly because of failure to use the full ranges of motion about joints.

Recommendations for Isometrics

In Physical Education Classes

1. Isometric testing and strengthening can be beneficially applied to children and adults who need a corrective program, as well as to those who have insufficient strength to handle their body weight in such activities as chinning, dipping and push-ups.

2. Isometric testing and strengthening can be used appropriately in activities such as postural work, sports and dance if the students cannot properly perform the activity.

3. In general, isometric exercises can be used in the development of strength.

4. An isometric exercise program

should be individual rather than general.

In Athletics

1. All members and prospective members of a team should be tested by isometric methods to determine what muscle groups of their body need strengthening.

2. A muscle-strengthening program should be designed for each athlete on the basis of the testing. That program should include isometric, isotonic and stretching exercises.

3. Muscle testing may be necessary after athletic injury to determine the optimal time when the athlete can return to competition. An athlete with a severe knee injury one season will start the next season with the same injury unless specific remedial exercises have been applied to the injured areas.

A Definition and a Distinction

An isometric contraction is a muscular contraction in which you exert force against a resistance that does not move. It is like trying to push a stalled automobile.

An isotonic contraction is one in which you exert muscular force against a resistance that does move. If the stalled automobile actually moves, then the contraction is isotonic.

The muscular tension built up in the isometric contraction is converted in the isotonic contraction to actual work (that is, force moved through distance).—*Jay A. Bender, Harold M. Kaplan and Alex J. Johnson* from the *Journal of Health, Physical Education and Recreation,* May 1963.

You can effectively use isometrics to develop strength for a particular movement. That is, a golfer can position his body and club in such a manner that will simulate contact with the ball. By exerting his body maximally in that position, the muscles being used in a golf swing will develop maximum strength—an important attribute in many sport activities. Remember, strength and power are not synonymous. Strength will improve performance, but power will add a further dimension in performance. For a discussion on how to improve power see POWER and WEIGHT TRAINING.

Below are a series of isometric exercises for general body development. Do not perform these exercises without following the preceding guidelines and discussion on isometrics.

Isometric Exercises

1. *Neck Press*—From a standing position, place the palm of the left hand against the left side of the head. Press with the *head against the hand.* Repeat on the right-hand side, front, and back of the head.

2. *Doorway Press* (1)—Stand in the center of a doorway, feet comfortably apart. Place the hands against the doorway jambs so that the arms are extended upward above the head with the palms against the jambs. Press with both hands against the edges of the doorway. Be certain to keep the body straight. The doorway press develops the muscles of the shoulder and of the chest under the arms.

3. *Doorway Press* (2)—Stand in the center of a doorway, feet comfortably apart. Place the hands against the sides of the doorway, while the arms are extended downward. The back of the palms are touching the door jamb. Press outward with both hands. This variation develops the muscles of the shoulders, upper arms and upper back.

4. *Doorway Press* (3)—Stand in the center of a doorway, feet comfortably spread. Place the hands against the sides of the doorway so that they are at shoulder height. The arms will be bent. The palms are touching the sides of the door jamb. Press against the sides. That press develops muscles of the front of the chest.

5. *Doorway Press* (4)—Stand in the center of a doorway, feet comfortably apart. Place the hands against the sides of the doorway so that they are at thigh height. The back of the palms are touching the door jamb. Press against the sides. That version develops the muscles of the shoulders and upper arms.

6, 7, 8—*Doorway Push*—Sit or stand in a doorway. Place the arms at the side of the body so that the hands are at hip height. The palms are placed on the outer borders of the doorway. Press forward as though you were attempting to bring the arms forward so that the hands would meet in front of your body. Repeat the same exercise with the hands at shoulder height and extended above the body. The muscles affected are the chest (*pectoralis major and minor*), the deltoid, and the muscles of the chest under the arms (*serratus anterior*).

9. *Backward Press*—Stand about 12 to 18 inches away from a smooth wall with the back facing the wall. With your arms alongside the body, place the palms against the wall. Keeping your arms straight, exert a pressure against the wall as though attempting to push the wall over. That press develops the muscles of the upper back and arms.

10. *Floor Press*—Lie flat on your back with the upper arms at shoulder height and your elbows bent so that your forearms are bent over the upper arms. Make an effort to push the elbows against the floor as hard as possible. The floor press develops the muscles of the upper back.

11. *Reclining Press*—Assume a supine position on a floor or mat with your arms along side the body, palms facing downward. Exert pressure downward with your hands and make an effort to raise your pelvis from the floor. The heels of the feet, the hands and the back of the head should be the only parts of your body touching the floor. That version develops most of

the posterior muscles of the body, including the shoulders and upper arms.

Upper Arms (Back): Triceps

12. *Triceps Press*—Grasp a towel or rope in both hands. The right hand is just above the right shoulder. Your left arm is alongside the left side of your body, and the arm is flexed so that your left hand is near the small of your back. Attempt to extend both arms by trying to raise your right hand and lowering your left. Repeat, reversing the above. That exercise develops the muscles of the back of the upper arm.

13. *Arm Push*—Flex the arms and position the hands directly in front of the chest. Place the fist of one of the hands in the palm of the other. Push both hands against each other. The arm push develops the muscles of the back of the upper arm. This exercise can be performed at abdomen or face height.

14. *Bar Press* (Horizontal)—Assume a horizontal position underneath an immovable bar (door-bar). The bar should be directly in line with the armpits and approximately 24 inches high. Grasp the bar with a regular grip and press upward as hard as possible. The bar press develops the muscles of the back of the upper arm and the chest.

Upper Arm (Front): Biceps Brachialis

15. *Arm Curl*—Assume a standing position with the feet on top of the loop of a rope, hold the other end of the rope by the hands. Keep the upper arms perpendicular, and the lower arms parallel to the floor. With rope pulled taut, exert a pull and hold. That curl develops the muscles of the front of the upper arms.

16. *Reverse Push-up* — Assume a prone position on the floor. Place the palms of the hands on the floor at hip height with the fingers pointing down toward the toes. Force the hands downward, keeping the body in con-

tact with the floor. The push-up develops the muscles of the front of the upper arm and chest.

17. *Forearm Press*—In a sitting or standing position, hold the right forearm across the body, bend your arm at the elbow, so that the palm is facing upward. Place the left hand on the wrist of the right hand. Press upward with the right forearm—resist with the left. That exercise develops the muscles of the front of the upper arm.

Forearms and Wrist

18. *Wrist Grip*—Grasp the handle of a baseball bat or some other similar object, and squeeze it as hard as possible. If you can't find a suitable object, clenching the fist together as tightly as possible may be just as beneficial. The wrist grip develops the muscles of the forearm and hand.

19. *Wrist Turn*—Take the handle of a baseball bat and hold it with both hands at arm's length, directly in front of the chest with the hands about five inches apart. Attempt first to turn the handle inward resisting with the other hand. Then try to turn the handle outward, resisting with the other hand. Repeat with the other arm. That turn develops the pronator and supinator muscles of the forearm.

Lower Back

20. *Body Arch*—Assume a prone position with the arms crossed in front of the chest so that the upper body is resting on the elbows. With the pelvic area and toes touching the floor and the heels under a heavy object (bed) try to lift the object. Keep the legs straight and lift from the hips. The body arch develops the muscles of the lower back, including the *gluteus maximus* (buttocks area).

21. *Dead Lift*—Stand on a rope with the feet spread at hip width. Bend the trunk forward slightly and bend the legs so that the thighs are parallel with the floor. Hold the arms straight at the sides of the body, grasping the rope.

Attempt to straighten the trunk and legs. That lift develops the muscle of the lower back and *gluteus maximus*.

Abdomen

22. *Sit-Up*—With the feet placed under a chair or held by a partner, place the upper body at a 45-degree angle from the floor. Extend arms in front of the body. Hold the position for 10-20 seconds. If you cannot maintain the position, then it may be necessary to move the upper body to reduce the stress. To make the exercise more difficult, lock the hands in back of the head.

23. *Stomach Pull*—Assume a standing, sitting, or lying position. Exhale and then contract the abdominal muscles as though attempting to push the muscles to the back bone.

24. *Abdominal Curl*—Assume a supine position with the arms at the sides. Attempt to curl upward and forward, while keeping the lower back on the floor.

Legs

25. *One-Leg Squat*—Assume a standing position next to a wall and extend the left leg forward. Squat with the right leg until the right upper leg and lower leg form a 90-degree angle. Place your hand against a wall, if necessary, to maintain balance. Hold this position without bending the trunk. Reverse with the other leg.

26. *Leg Tensor*—Sit in a chair or assume a standing position and extend the right leg. Tense the leg muscles as much as possible and hold for ten seconds. Repeat with the other leg. Both the squat and the leg tensor develops the muscles of the front of the upper leg (Quadriceps).

27. *Leg Push and Pull*—Assume a supine position with the knees raised to a position above the hips. Place the lower legs parallel to the floor, crossed at the ankles. Force the ankles against each other, pulling down with the top ankle and pushing up with the bottom ankle. Repeat with the ankles crossed in the opposite direction. The muscles of the front and back of the upper leg are exercised.

28. *Leg Wall Push*—Stand with the back toward the wall with one foot about 12-18 inches from the wall and the heel of the other foot against the wall. Push backward with the heel that is against the wall. Repeat with the other leg. That exercise develops the muscles of the back of the upper leg.

29. *Thigh Abductor*—Assume a supine position with the ankles crossed. Attempt to force the feet away from each other, keeping the legs straight.

30. *Thigh Abductor*—Assume a supine position. Force the legs against each other.

Lower Legs

31. *Foot Push*—Assume a sitting position and raise the right thigh toward the chest. Loop a towel around the ball of the right foot. Attempt to push the right foot downward making the movement at the ankle joint. This is a good exercise to develop the muscles of the back of the lower leg.

32. *Ankle Flex*—Assume a sitting or standing position and attempt to flex the foot upward from the ankle joint. Exert resistance with the hands or some other object to give a workout to the muscles of the front of the lower legs.

ISOTONICS

The term isotonics refer to exercises that produce movement. The opposite of isotonic exercises are isometric exercises, which involve no movement. Isotonics are superior to isometrics because they allow for movement of the muscles and, therefore, exercise the muscles over their full range of motion —an important ingredient in maintaining flexibility. When any muscle moves, it is said to have moved isotonically, for the fibers of the muscle must either shorten or lengthen for movement. The most popular forms of isotonic exercises are calisthenics and weight training. For a discussion of related subjects see EXERCISES, ISOMETRICS, MUSCLE SYSTEM and WEIGHT TRAINING.

JOGGING

A number of medical authorities believe that a regular program of jogging improves the function of heart, blood vessels and lungs. A program of jogging will increase the amount of oxygen that can be carried to the tissues of the body. There is also evidence that additional blood vessels are formed in skeletal and heart muscle as a response to exercise programs such as jogging. In some areas of the country, postcoronary patients are being placed in supervised programs of jogging and walking in order to facilitate their recovery.

Jogging requires a large expenditure of energy. It is, therefore, an excellent supplement to a weight-reducing or weight-control program. However, in order for a person to lose weight by jogging, he must also reduce his intake of calories. Contrary to popular belief, exercise such as jogging does not intensify appetite.

Jogging is best defined as slow-pace running. The distance and speed vary among individuals, but they are closely related to the person's level of fitness, age and sex. A younger person is usually capable of jogging at a greater speed for a longer distance than an older individual. Women usually jog at a slower rate and for shorter distances than men of the same age. There is no general agreement among professional educators on the optimum speed and distance required to maintain fitness. One of the advantages of jogging is that it allows each person, regardless of his condition, age, or sex,

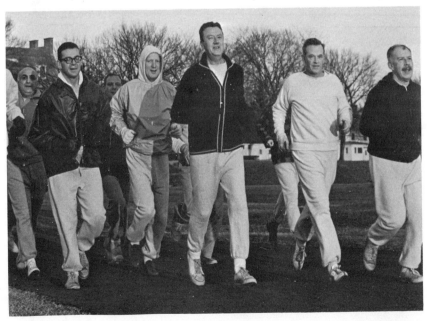

Because jogging is informal and non-competitive, many people have found it an enjoyable way to exercise in a group.

to determine the speed and distance of his workout. If he feels tired after jogging a distance, he may stop and walk for a while and then continue jogging. If he feels strong and is not out of breath, he can increase both the pace and the distance of the workout. Following this procedure makes it difficult for the jogger to overexert himself. This type of program is well suited to those who enjoy complete freedom from formal, competitive activities—*Douglas W. King*

How to Jog

Make sure you jog relaxed and natural. Choose a style easiest for you:

(a) *Heel-to-toe-technique*—Land first on the heel of your foot and then rock your body forward to take off on the ball of the foot. This detailed action is used by most long distance runners, since it's not tiring.

(b) *Flat-footed*—Instead of hitting first with the heel, the entire foot lands on the surface at the same time. This method distributes pressure over the entire foot, and often eliminates potential bruising when running overland or on a hard surface.

(c) *Ball-heel technique*—Land on the ball of your foot and then settle to the heel before taking the next step. This form of jogging is often instinctive with former track sprinters who are used to running on their toes. Women too are inclined toward that technique, perhaps because they are used to wearing high heel shoes. The ball-heel movement produces a strain for many joggers and you may not find it as comfortable as other techniques.

A Jogging Program

Start slowly by alternately walking and jogging a quarter mile the first week. For example, alternate jogging and walking 110 yard distances to complete the quarter mile. (Quarter mile equals 440 yards.)

Continue using the jogging/walking sequence and gradually build up to one mile by the end of week five. The sixth week jog 330 yards and walk 110 yards. The seventh week, start jogging a mile at a speed which would permit you to talk easily with a running companion.

You should be able to complete the mile in 8 to 10 minutes. By the end of 10 weeks, you should be working up to 1½ mile distances. See chart:

Jogging to Stop Smoking

A doctor who smoked for 41 years gave up smoking and hasn't smoked in nearly a year. A salesman who smoked for 20 years also quit and hasn't smoked for 18 months. Both have beat the smoking habit and both credit jogging for making them give up cigarettes.

The experience of those California jogging enthusiasts is not unique. Others are discovering that jogging is one of the easiest and best ways to quit smoking. The heavy smoker who has tried every possible way to give up smoking and failed will be happy to know that jogging takes only a few minutes a day. You're jogging when you cover a mile in seven minutes or more—you're running when you do it in less.

Weeks	Distance Miles	Walk or Jog		Weeks	Distance Miles	Walk or Jog
1	up to ¼	Walk/Jog		6	1	Jog 330 Yds. Walk 110 Yds.
2	¼	Walk/Jog				
3	¼	Walk/Jog—Begin to Emphasize Jogging		7	1	Jog
				8	1¼	Jog
4	½	Jog/Walk		9	1¼	Jog
5	1	Jog/Walk		10	1½	Jog

"I used to smoke two packs of cigarettes a day and I smoked for 41 years," commented Dr. Delmar Mitchelson, an Encino, Calif., obstetrician. He weighs 180, stands 5 feet-11 and has a 33-inch waistline. He's 59 years old.

Two years ago before he started jogging, Dr. Mitchelson said he was a "prime candidate for a heart attack." He was overweight (he had a 37-inch waistline), didn't exercise enough, had high blood pressure and smoked excessively. "Jogging motivated me to quit," he says. "I ran for about a year while smoking and didn't do too well. I knew smoking was holding me back from increasing my distance. It affected my wind. I had read medical articles on the subject. One day I decided to quit smoking altogether. And I did. After only 24 hours, I didn't have any trouble with the urge to smoke. I was too busy jogging. I haven't smoked for 43 weeks and never get the urge."

Ten miles a day of running is my average now and I run seven days a week, the doctor added. He ran 3,000 miles last year and already has run 1,000 miles this year. A few months ago he was the only one of four jogging enthusiasts who was able to complete a 26-mile run from Encino to the city of San Fernando, even though he was the oldest. Besides getting his weight down, trimming his waist and quitting smoking, he said his blood pressure is now normal.

Gene Neumeier, a 42-year-old medical supply salesman, is another jogging enthusiast who credits a running program to aiding him in giving up smoking.

"I tried hard to quit smoking for 10 years. I smoked a pack a day for 20 years. I was in bad physical condition. I was overweight, got short of breath with the slightest exercise. When I first started jogging, my heart would pound and my chest would hurt. I knew my chest hurt from all the years of smoking. That's when I decided to quit smoking. It was real tough at first. It bothered me for 45 days, left me quite nervous, but members of the jogging club—particularly the doctors—told me to run more . . . that the jogging would help cure me of my nervous tension. And it did, particularly

as I increased my distance. I haven't smoked for 18 months."

"I like to golf and I used to feel real tired and short-winded around the 13th or 14th hole. Now, after nearly three years of jogging, I play as much as 36 holes without getting tired. I feel more alert and I've lost 14 pounds and reduced two inches at the waist. I've heard of quite a few of our club members who quit smoking after they started jogging. They all saw how it affected their wind and felt pain in their chest."

Can't Smoke and Run

Dr. Richard Steiner, a pathologist at Long Beach Community Hospital, commented on why so many joggers had quit smoking. "I think it goes hand in hand—it's incompatible to smoke and run. Joggers see how smoking cuts their wind and affects their cardiovascular system, so they cut down on smoking and finally quit. Any jogger who smokes will find it difficult to run more than a mile. I preach to joggers not to smoke, but if they can't give up smoking and want to quit running, I tell them it's better to run and smoke than not run at all."

Commented Dr. Steiner: "Tension leaves you when you jog, even for only a half hour . . . that relaxed feeling alone helps you to cut down on smoking. That tired feeling at the end of a day is mostly a frame of mind. If you jog, you won't have to lay down in front of the TV and fall asleep. You'll have more pep in the afternoon and evening."—*Jack Scagnetti*

Wintertime Jogging

Your winter months should provide as much outdoor pleasure as your summers, which means that you need a carry-over sport for wintry weather. Skiing and sledding are ideal. So are skating and paddle tennis. Wintertime jogging maintains your summertime endurance and increases your enjoyment of whatever sport you choose.

Most men and women do their most resultful work between Labor Day and July Fourth. During that period, they need their full strength, energy and resourcefulness. As the tensions mount, they must be able to relax. As work piles up, they must change priorities without hitting the panic button. That ability stems only from a profound feeling of competence, calm, and excellence which, in turn, is the product of a regular exercise program.

Special Preparations for Winter Jogging

Feet. Tennis shoes or sneakers are out. I wear heavy socks and my regular running shoes except for wet and very cold weather. When it's really cold, I pull on two pairs of socks, the inner pair of silk or thin cotton, the outer pair of wool. In snow or slush I wear a pair of lined hiking shoes. They are heavy, but their extra weight gives me an extra workout.

Legs. The legs have fewer nerve endings close to the surface than the torso, so they are less influenced by cold. Two layers usually suffice—a pair of thin underdrawers and a pair of heavy army pants, sweat pants, ski pants, or Levis.

Torso. Keeping the chest and rib cage warm is the secret of outdoor running. I experimented until I discovered the proper number of layers of clothing needed. Thick and furry materials are a drag. A lot of thin layers, permitting air to flow between, are best. For cold days, I wear a long-sleeve undershirt, woolen sport shirt, pullover sweater and a windbreaker. On a very blustery day, I leave off the windbreaker and add a heavy, thigh-length coat or mackinaw which hugs my hips.

Warm-up. The winter warm-up should be extended. My usual summer warm-up is a 15-minute walk. Winters, I add a second 5 minutes at an ever faster walk. In general, the older you are, the more time you should devote to warming up.

Road Conditions. Expect your footing to be treacherous, both rougher and more slippery. Adjust your pace accordingly. These extra stresses on your ankles, which stretch and strain

the tendons, increase your agility and ankle strength and contribute to your skills on the ski trail or on the paddle tennis court.

When It's Too Cold to Jog. Experience has taught me that my lungs don't enjoy air colder than 20 degrees above zero. Your own experience will indicate your own tolerance. Dr. Acors Thompson of Falls Church, Virginia, says, "Most of us who take up jogging are 'insiders' who breathe warm air most of the time. Such people will have difficulty running in cold air. I'm one of them. When the temperature gets below 30 degrees, I start coughing badly. Under such circumstances, you must find an indoor track (school or YMCA) or run in place in your own home while listening to music or watching TV."

When Illness Strikes. Even joggers get colds. Then they must face the question of whether or not to abandon their daily workouts. Doctors say, "If you have any infection, don't run. Your body has suffered an insult. Help it to recover before you add any extra stresses."

What is happening is that white corpuscles in your blood stream are busy surrounding and disarming the attacking viruses. That takes time. You can help best by living normally, eating nutritionally balanced meals, and getting a full night's sleep. A recovery program also includes a mild exercise designed to keep blood circulating. If you're on your back, raise your legs over your head and "pedal" for a bit each morning and night. If ambulatory, walk slowly up and down flights of stairs.

Admittedly, jogging is more complicated during the winter than during the summer. But the increased energy and good feeling that it spawns enables most men to do it without a second thought. If a person has adopted jogging as a way of life, then he absorbs its extra requirements with the same equanimity with which he orders

°JOGGING PROGRAM

Chart 1	Chart 2
1. Jog 55 yds./walk 55 yds.— ½ mile in 7-8 min.	1. Jog 110 yds./walk 110 yds.— 2 miles in 21-22 min.
2. Jog 55 yds./walk 55 yds.— ¾ mile in 11-12 min.	2. Jog 110 yds./walk 110 yds.— 2 miles in 20 min. 1 Day jog 220 yds./walk 110 yds.
3. Jog 55 yds./walk 55 yds.— 1 mile in 15-16 min.	3. 2 Days jog 110 yds./walk 110 yds.— 2¼ miles in 25 min. 2 Days jog 220 yds./walk 110 yds.—2¼ miles in 24 min.
4. Jog 110 yds./walk 110 yds. 1 mile in 12-14 min.	4. Jog 220 yds./walk 110 yds.— 2½ miles in 27 min.
5. Jog 110 yds./walk 110 yds. 1¼ miles in 15-16 min.	5. Jog 220 yds./walk 110 yds.— 2½ miles in 26 min.
6. Jog 110 yds./walk 110 yds. 1¼ miles in 13-14 min.	6. 2 Day jog 220 yds./walk 110 yds.— 2¾ miles in 29 min. 2 Day jog 330 yds./walk 110 yds.—2¾ miles in 28 min.
7. Jog 110 yds./walk 110 yds. 1½ miles in 15-16 min.	7. Jog 330 yds./walk 110 yds.— 3 miles in 33 min.
8. Jog 110 yds./walk 110 yds. 1½ miles in 14 min.	8. Jog 330 yds./walk 110 yds.— 3 miles in 31-32 min.
9. Jog 110 yds./walk 110 yds. 1¾ miles in 18 min.	9. Jog 440 yds./walk 110 yds.— 3 miles in 30 min.

° See ENDURANCE and ENERGY COST OF ACTIVITIES for an explanation of these charts.

Fitness 1

If you achieved a score of poor or low average on the *Harvard Step Test* or a score of very poor or poor on the *12 Minute Run*, start on Chart 1-Level 1 and spend one week at each level until Chart 2-Level 9 is reached. It is recommended that you participate 4 to 5 days a week. When Chart 2-Level 9 is reached, 4 days a week is sufficient.

Fitness 2

If you achieved a score of high average on the *Harvard Step Test* or fair on the *12 Minute Run*, start on Chart 1-Level 2. Spend one week on Chart 1-Levels 2, 4, 6, 7, and 9, and Chart 2-Levels 1, 3, 5, 6, 7, and 9. It is recommended that you participate 4 to 5 days a week. When Chart 2-Level 9 is reached, 4 days a week is sufficient.

Fitness 3

If you achieved a score of good or excellent on either the *Harvard Step Test* or *12 Minute Run*, continue your current program or select Chart 2-Level 9 as your level of participation. Four days a week is sufficient.

the furnace cleaned, arranges for snow removal, and changes to snow tires.— *Curtis Mitchell*

Since jogging is a high-energy-cost activity, it may be used to help improve your fitness level, especially your circulo-respiratory and muscle endurance. Below is a jogging program that takes into account the important principles of training.

JUDO

Judo was developed in 1882 by Japanese educator Jigoro Kano, as a synthesis of various styles of *jujutsu* welded to improve the mental and physical health, of the Japanese national public.

Judo differs from *jujutsu* as a defensive system because it operates entirely without weapons as an "empty-hand" combative. *Jujutsu* often permitted the operator to employ a weapon. Physical training centers on the development of throwing techniques and grappling skills. Judo also makes full use of exercises, employed toward the development of a wholly harmonious self. Modern Judo tends to employ more calisthenics as preparatory exercises, many of which can be said to be isolated exercise.

Training methods vary greatly. Preparatory exercises "warm up" and "cool down" the body prior to and immediately after training sessions, respectively. Supplementary exercises place emphasis on form and speed in throwing techniques by the use of hundreds of repetitions of a technique performed daily against a training partner who cooperates in a set way. Sometimes the throws are completed and sometimes they are withheld. Compound exercises are used to develop skills in critical grappling situations by drills in bridging, twisting, evasive actions, and the concentration of body forces while lying down. Auxiliary exercises include the use of resistance exercises to increase body muscle-contraction power. By the use of falling exercises, upon a matted surface, trainees develop skills which enable them to withstand the powerful forces developed by throwing techniques applied against them.

Judo contributes to improvements in cardiovascular efficiency, flexibility, muscular strength, endurance, balance/agility, coordination (timing and right use of muscles) in everyday living by giving the body a sense of relaxation and acute awareness of kinesthetic values. Muscle groups stimulated are those of all major areas.

Athletic objectives in spite of their disciplinary effect can be detrimental if overemphasis is placed on "winning." Judo training must not consider the contest as its end point, and all training must not produce functional disturbances in trainees. Only through the strict adherence to a performance of a technically uniform body motion, as required in Judo techniques, will harmony of mind and body be developed.—*Donn Draeger*

Associations:

United States Judo Federation, 4367 Bishop Road, Detroit, Michigan 48224.

KARATE

Karate is a collective name used to identify about one hundred styles of deliberately designed physical/mental disciplines. Their basis is that the study and practice of "empty-hand" combative tactics will result in the improvement of personal character and health.

All styles of karate are composed of tactics employing the natural parts of the body as defensive "weapons" to respond to an attack provoked by an adversary. A wide range of anatomical parts of the human body serve as these "weapons," but either the arm, leg or head is used most often. They are ideally employed in striking, thrusting, kicking, blocking, covering, parrying, or evading actions against the weaknesses of the adversary, generally trying to injure or even kill him. Physical training for all styles centers on the development of technical skills. That development is achieved by the means of prescribed drills which concentrate on stance, movement, balance, breathing, speed and timing.

Preparatory exercises are used to strengthen and limber the joints as well as the muscles. Most of those exercises bear some relation to technique and are not entirely isolated exercises. Supplementary exercises place emphasis on efficient form in the delivery of the "weapons" both as a self-practice and a partner-practice method. Hundreds of repetitions of each particular strike, thrust, kick, block, parry, or covering action are practiced daily. Compound exercises depart from the general definition in that they deal largely with standing positions rather than recumbent ones. They include special drills for hardening of the "weapons" by means of repeated pounding against specific materials such as wood or stone to produce immunity from impact shock and pain. Speed drills are used to develop rapidity in striking, thrusting and kicking precise target areas and utilize lighted candles to focus the energy of the action on snuffing out the flame by means of the shock wave. Karate students often evaluate the efficiency of their "weapons" by attempting to break materials like wood and stone.

The actual practice of karate techniques employs three main methods: formal practice fighting, prearranged form and free fighting. Formal practicing involves both "empty-hand" tactics and use of an actual weapon. In using the "three-step style," training partners square off, one taking the role of attacker, the other a defender. The attacker, using the same technique, attacks three times. The defender blocks all three attacks using the same technique, then adds a counterattack. After sufficient skill in that method, the "one-step style" is employed. That method is more subtle and develops instantaneous response to an attack.

Prearranged form practice is always a self-practice method designed to temper the body through the disciplines of perfection of technique. Prearranged movement (specially chosen tactics in a prescribed order) are executed as a series of actions promoting the essence of karate. Each particular system has its own formal arrangement of this practice method.

The third main training method,

free fighting, is free only to the extent permitted by common sense rules of safety. That method must be attempted only after the trainee has some well-established knowledge of an experience in formal practice fighting and prearranged forms. To enter free fighting without sufficient practice and training results in "clout fighting" and the degeneration of technique by which no true karate tactics can develop. Karate training places heavy emphasis on spiritual discipline. A high degree of patience and enterprise fostered through applied spiritual discipline, the concentration of one's energies, becomes the backbone of karate—rationale. Meditation in the Zen style is the form by which the suggested spiritual discipline is accelerated.

All forms of karate are splendid developers of physical fitness, though they do not necessarily agree on the precise methods of training and the intricacies of technique.

The development of karate as a sport has been the major source of inspiration for the majority of karate devotees in the Western world. This emphasis has resulted in a narrowing of technical style, an almost complete loss of combative reality and a serious decline in spiritual discipline.

But the fact remains that in spite of these difficulties karate produces healthful exercise which contributes to improvements in cardiovascular efficiency, flexibility, muscular strength, endurance, balance/agility and coordination. In everyday living it gives the body a sense of relaxation and acute awareness to kinesthetic values. All major muscle groups are adequately stimulated.—*Donn Draeger*

KINESIOLOGY

Kinesiology is the study of human movement. It encompasses those aspects of anatomy, physics (or mechanics) and physiology that apply to human motion. Anatomically, kinesiology is concerned with the skeletal and muscular systems of man. This subject includes some physical and mechanical factors that affect human movement such as gravity, balance, motion and force. Some body movements can be considered controlled conditions of imbalance—for example, in walking or running, the individual initiates movement by leaning forward until balance is lost; he maintains forward momentum by repeatedly placing one foot in front of the other at such a rate as to avoid falling. See BALANCE.

Causes of Body Movement

Movements are the result of force. All movements initiated by the body result from nerve stimulation to the muscles which causes them to contract. The contraction of muscle tissue exerts a pulling force on the bones, changing the angles of the joints, and motion occurs. Aside from the forces created within the body, the body is capable of exerting forces against external objects, resulting in their motion. Every individual exerts force against external objects in everyday activities like throwing, pushing and lifting. The simple act of walking involves applying force against the ground to achieve forward motion. The maintenance of erect posture necessitates the application of force against the downward pull of gravity.

Besides the physical and mechanical factors, movement depends upon individual characteristics including body build, height, weight, flexibility, nerve function, age, perceptual ability and strength. Because individuals vary widely in these characteristics, some are better suited for efficient and graceful movement than others.

Contribution of Kinesiology to Fitness

A knowledge of kinesiology benefits doctors, physical therapists, physical educators, coaches, athletic trainers, and others. Doctors and physical therapists utilize kinesiological information in correcting movement problems. Those problems may be only postural, or they may be the result of a serious accident in which a person has lost the use of part (or parts) of his body. Kinesiological information is useful in establishing rehabilitative programs so that victims of serious accidents may become active members of society. Physical educators and coaches apply that information to teach students how to move and how to improve their movements from simple everyday motion to the complicated movements involved in many sports activities. Athletic trainers utilize this information to determine how sports injuries have occurred, how to treat the injury and aid recovery, and how to help the athletes avoid future similar injuries.

Every person should know the most efficient way to stand, sit, lift, walk, run, throw an object, utilize force and momentum, and apply mechanical principles to the use of tools and implements. For almost everyone, those everyday functions, efficiently performed, will have an effect on their overall fitness. The performance of movement in an efficient manner helps one to conserve energy and prolong endurance. Disregard or ignorance of the factors governing movements can result in inefficiency, wasted effort, fatigue and possible injury.

KINESTHESIA (Kinesthesis)

One of the important functions of the human body's nervous system is to provide a sensory feedback process by means of receptor organs located throughout the body. Those organs transmit sensory nerve impulses back to the central nervous system (spinal cord and brain). It is through certain specialized receptor organs that a skilled performer will be able to experience the "feel" of a movement. In fact, at times, he may be able to indicate success or failure in a physical skill through a kinesthetic perception of the sensations that his nervous system has recorded.

Kinesthesis by definition refers to your awareness of (1) the position and movement of your limbs and body space and (2) the pressures that are acting on or within your limbs and body.

In order to record position, movement, and pressure, different sensory organs are found in the tissues of the body. Earlier beliefs considered that stretch receptors, found in muscles (muscle spindles) and at the junction of the skeletal muscle and tendon (Golgi Tendon Organs), provided the necessary kinesthetic information. Mountcastle and Powell have shown that the stretch receptors *do not* provide important information in the perception of joint position. Recent evidence has identified other sensory endings as the sensory feedback receptors involved in kinesthesis. *Ruffin Endings,* the most common type of receptors in moveable joints, are concerned with the sensations of position and movement in joints. It is thought that the receptors are constantly active and have a certain discharging pattern for each position produced by the joint. *Pacinian Corpuscles* have a wide distribution throughout the body in subcutaneous tissue, joints and periosteum of bone. According to F. Hellebrant, they are sensitive to pressure and supposedly respond with a burst of impulses during joint movement but stop discharging once a new joint position has been reached. Additional sensory nerve endings associated with cutaneous and visceral sensations should be considered as playing a role in this perception process.

The sense of the body balance and space orientation are functionally integrated with kinesthesis. This is primarily the responsibility of the vestibular system located in the inner ear. The two main receptors involved, labyrinths and otolithic structures, become stimulated by accelerations, vibrations and changes in the head position.

At the present time, there is not a complete understanding of the importance of each sensory feedback receptor or maybe even the identification of all the receptors that are involved. However, it is apparent that an integration of the various receptor sensations is needed along with an interpretation of these sensations, to enable a person to develop "kinesthetic perception."

An individual through achieving a high physical fitness level does not necessarily improve his kinesthetic awareness. It depends primarily on the types of experiences that were employed in developing that fitness level.

In summarizing the previous research in this area, it appears that there is no general kinesthesia; that kinesthetic specificity exists in (a) the recording sensory feedbacks, (b) the area of the body involved and (c) the type of task being performed. From the limited evidence available, it appears that a general physical fitness level is of minor importance, whereas, selected motor experiences which have been repeated, play an important role in the sensory discriminating capacity and the perceptionality needed in kinesthesia.—*H. H. Merrifield*

KNEE

The knee, the largest and most complicated joint in the body, is a true hinge joint. The two main bones of the joint are the femur and the tibia. The lower end of the femur provides the upper articulating surface of the joint, while the head of the tibia provides the other surface. Those two surfaces are complementary to each other. That is, the convex surfaces of the lower end of the femur, the condyles, fit into the concave surfaces of the head of the tibia. The fibula serves as an attachment for muscles and ligaments which are essential to efficient movement and support of the joint.

Thirteen separate ligaments and tendons provide most of the support for the knee. Lateral stability is afforded by the *internal* and *external lateral ligaments.*

The *cruciate* ligaments keep the femur from sliding forward and backward on the tibia.

The entire joint is enclosed in a membranous sac forming the joint capsule. This sac contains bursae which secrete a lubricating fluid during joint motion. Situated on the head of the tibia are the *semilunar cartilages,* or *menisci.* They are constructed of a slightly flexible, tough, fibrous tissue. Their function is to cushion and absorb shock and aid in holding the condyles of the femur in approximation with the head of the tibia.

Functions

The knee performs two principal functions, flexion and extension. Rotation inward and outward is possible but only to a very limited extent. The flexion of the knee occurs because of the contraction of the muscles on the back of the upper leg, called the hamstrings. The extension is caused by the muscles on the front of the upper leg, called the *quadriceps femoris.*

Susceptibility to Injury

The knee, although the largest joint of the body is most vulnerable to injuries, largely because of a poor bony arrangement. The main support of the joint is from tissue, and it has very little defense against a force from the side. Injuries to the knee joint are very incapacitating, and in some instances, keep people from participating in athletics, especially contact sports.

The muscles located above and below the knee aid in stability; therefore, it is advisable to condition them properly so that the knee will be protected against injury. Many exercises can do the job well. Those mentioned under EXERCISES, ISOMETRICS and WEIGHT TRAINING are excellent.

Traditionally deep-knee bends, full squats, and duck walks were used to

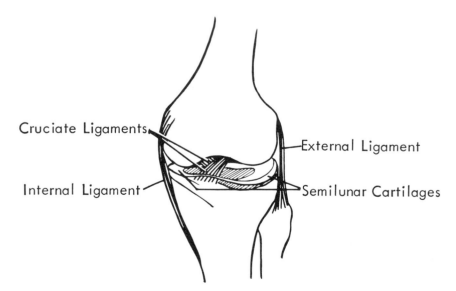

Cruciate Ligaments

External Ligament

Internal Ligament

Semilunar Cartilages

LIGAMENTS OF THE KNEE

condition the muscles of the leg. Recent investigations, however, have revealed that those exercises do more harm than good. In fact, they may cause people to be predisposed to knee injuries because they are potentially dangerous to the internal and supporting structures of the knee joint, and place great stress on the ligaments and cartilages. See EXCESSIVE EXERCISE.

Reconditioning after Injury

Once the knee has been injured, proper reconditioning should take place immediately. Many orthopedic surgeons have the injured person perform simple isometric exercises—such as contracting the extensor and flexor muscles—even when the knee is in a cast. For some unknown reason the quadrices muscles degenerate very quickly when kept in an immobile state. In fact, the atrophy is significant 24 hours after immobilization. Although it is very important that reconditioning be started immediately, at no time should the knee joint be moved until the pain has subsided and the initial stages of healing have taken place. When healing has occurred, passive exercises may be attempted.

Return to active competition or exercise should not begin until a 30-pound weight can be held a full extension of 30 seconds or until the quadriceps of both legs, injured and uninjured measure the same in circumference within ¼ inch. Take each measurement 3 inches and 8 inches above the knee cap; only after these conditions are met is the knee strong enough for vigorous participation in sports and exercises.

LA SIERRA PROGRAM

The LaSierra Program is a physical fitness program developed by Stan LeProtti for high school students in LaSierra High School, Carmichael, California. It grew out of the need for a vigorous physical-fitness program

in the high school physical education curriculum.

Ability Groups

The program is based upon three ability groups. Students are classified in the ability groups by performance in fitness tests which measure strength endurance, power, flexibility, agility and balance. The groups are color coded with members wearing the appropriate color shorts for easy identification.

Testing

When a student begins as a freshman, he is placed in the white or beginner group. He is then tested in the fall of this first year according to the items in Test Battery #1. There are three levels of performance in this battery (minimum, median and ceiling). Those levels are common in the other two test batteries, only higher. If he achieves the first two levels in Battery #1, the student remains in the white group. If he performs at the ceiling level in *all* test items, he advances to the second, or red group.

The passing of several weeks brings another testing session. If a student is still in the white group, he is given Test Battery #1. If he is in the red group, he performs Test Battery #2. Again, he must achieve the ceiling level to advance to the next group or maintain the minimum level to remain in the red group. For example, if he attains the ceiling performance of *all* the red tests, he is advanced to the third, or blue group. If he slips below the minimum performance of the red, he returns to the white group. A student who is in the white group and does not maintain the minimum white level remains in the white group since there are no lower groups.

A student must attain *all* ceiling performance standards and gain semester grade of "B" or above to move up to the next highest color group. In addition, he must present himself

PHYSICAL FITNESS TESTS
PHYSICAL FITNESS TEST BATTERY NO. 1—WHITE TEAM

	Minimum Performance	Median Performance	Ceiling Performance
PULL-UPS	2	6	10
PUSH-UPS	16	24	32
BAR-DIPS	4	8	12
SIT-UP (2 min.)	30	45	60
BURPEE (4 Count-20 sec.)	9	11	13
SHUTTLE RUN (200 Yards) ..	38 sec.	36 sec.	34 sec.
ROPE CLIMB (18′ Stand Start)	Hands/Feet w/Foot Clamp	Hands/Feet	Hands
AGILITY RUN	21 sec.	20.5 sec.	20 sec.
880 YARD RUN	3:30	3:15	3:00
MAN LIFT AND CARRY	440 Yards	660 Yards	880 Yards
PEGBOARD (Vertical)	3 holes	6 holes	1 trip
SWIM (Free)	40 sec.	38 sec.	36 sec.

with a short-trim haircut prior to color group movement.

A student must achieve *all* minimum standards of performance to remain in Red Group.

A student must achieve *all* ceiling standards of performance and gain a semester grade of "B" or above to move up to the next highest color group. In addition, he must present himself with a short-trim haircut prior to color group movement.

The tests are administered to every student during the fall and spring of the school year. Through this testing he is assigned a group. Because the testing period lasts nine weeks, it serves as a conditioner.

During the 12-week period between the testing sessions, the students who appear to be having difficulty are given intense training in specific activities to improve their performance.

In this interim, the class periods are divided into three phases. First, all three groups follow exercise routines. The white and red groups follow 12-minute strength-endurance exercises conducted at the beginning of the physical-education period. Upon completing that routine, they enter sports activity units such as flag football,

PHYSICAL FITNESS TEST BATTERY NO. 2—RED TEAM

	Minimum Performance	Median Performance	Ceiling Performance
PULL-UPS	10	12	14
PUSH-UPS	32	40	48
BAR-DIPS	12	15	18
BURPEE (4 Count—30 sec.)	19	20	21
HANGING LEG LIFTS (30 sec.)..	20	22	24
SHUTTLE RUN (300 Yards)	55 sec.	53 sec.	51 sec.
ROPE CLIMB (18′ Stand Start) ...	Hands	9 sec.	7 sec.
AGILITY RUN	20 sec.	19.5 sec.	19 sec.
1320 YARD RUN	4:40	4:30	4:20
MAN LIFT AND CARRY	880 Yards	1000 Yards	1320 Yards
PEGBOARD (Vertical)	1 trip	1 trip	1 trip
EXTENSION PRESS-UP	1	3	5
TWO MILE RUN	Complete	Complete	Complete
SWIM (100 Yards)	Complete	Complete	Complete

PHYSICAL FITNESS TEST BATTERY NO. 3—BLUE TEAM

	Minimum (Blues) Performance	Median (Purples) Performance	Ceiling (Golds) Performance
PULL-UPS	14	18	22
BAR-DIPS	18	28	32
HANDSTAND PUSH-UPS	12	14	16
*PUSH-UPS	48	62	68
EXTENSION PRESS-UP	10	15	25
PERBOARD—Vertical	1 trip	2 trips	3 trips
TWO ARM HAND HANG	1:30	2:00	3:00
BURPEE—30 Sec. Alt. 1 arm	20	21	22
ROPE CLIMB—20′ Sit Start	Hands/Feet	Hands	7.5 sec.
SHUTTLE RUN—300 Yards	51 sec.	49 sec.	48 sec.
MILE RUN	6:15	6:00	5:45
3 MILE JOG	Finish	Finish	Finish
MAN LIFT AND CARRY	1320 Yards	1 Mile	1¼ Miles
AGILITY RUN	19 sec.	18:5 sec.	18 sec.
DODGE RUN—120 Yards	26 sec.	25 sec.	24 sec.
HANGING SIT-UPS	15	20	25

* Minor test item—eliminated from test battery in 1964.

basketball, volleyball, softball, speedball, soccer, push ball, and track and field.

The blues also have exercise routines to follow before the sport activity. A typical routine includes jumping jacks —10 sets of 8; alternate toe touches— 10 sets of 8; push-ups—5 sets of 8; full

THE LA SIERRA NAVY BLUE PROGRAM
(Revised Fall 1963)

Physical Fitness Test Item	Number, Time or Distance Required
1. Bar-Dips (Parallel Bar)	50
2. Pull-Ups (Horizontal Bar)	32
3. Push-Ups	150
4. Alt. 1 Arm Burpee—30 sec.	26
5. 120 Yd. Dodge Run	24 seconds
6. 300 Yd. Shuttle Run	46 seconds
7. Rope Climb—20 feet	2 cmp. trips
8. Agility Run	17 seconds
9. Extension Press-Up—8 inches	100
10. Vertical Pegboard	5 trips
11. Handstand	45 seconds
12. Man Lift and Carry	5 miles
13. Mile Run	5 min. 15 sec.
14. Five-Mile Jog	Finish
15. Obstacle Course	Complete
16. Swim—Front Prone Position	1 mile
17. Swim—Underwater	50 yards
18. Swim—Any Combination of Strokes	2 miles
19. Execute Front Hanging Float w/arms and ankles tied— deep water	6 minutes
20. Stay afloat in deep water in vertical position—use of arms or legs permitted within 8 foot circle	2 hours

bends—10 sets of 8; push-ups—5 sets of 8; burpee—10 sets of 8; push-ups— 5 sets of 8; sit-ups—10 sets of 8; leg lifts—5 sets of 8; push-ups—5 sets of 8; extension press-ups—10; 200 stride hops; 200 straddle hops; 75 hops on each toe; 200 toe hops. After this vigorous workout, the blues also participate in the sports activities mentioned earlier.

When they complete the exercise routines and the sports activity, the students are required to run through an outdoor apparatus course which includes bar dips, pull-ups, hand walks across parallel bars, over head horizontal cables, and vertical pegboard climb.

Contribution to Fitness

The entire program is quite vigorous because of the demands of the test batteries. The maximum level of physical fitness is achieved through attainment of the "Navy Blue Test Battery." The test is quite gruelling and demands an extremely high level of physical fitness. See "Navy Blue" Test Battery.

LEGS

Thigh Muscles

The muscles of the thigh are grouped into three areas: (1) front muscles of the thigh; (2) inside muscles of the thigh; and (3) the back muscles of the thigh.

The muscles usually associated with the front of the thigh are the *sartorius* and the *quadriceps femoris.*

The *quadriceps* (four-headed) *femoris* is a very large muscle on the front of the upper leg. There are four parts of that muscle, the *rectus femoris,* the *vastus lateralis,* the *vastus medialis,* and the *vastus intermedius.* That powerful group of muscles is located on the front of the leg. They are extensors of the leg and are the muscle group that provides most of

the power in kicking a football or performing the leg-kick in swimming. The *rectus femoris* also flexes the thigh on the pelvis. Another flexor of the thigh is the *sartorius.* It is the longest muscle of the body and runs diagonally across the *quadriceps femoris* from the inside of the knee to the outside of the hip.

An exercise that will develop the extensor muscles of the legs, the *quadriceps femoris,* is the three-quarter knee bend. In that exercise, spread your feet comfortably with the back straight. To perform that correctly, you bend your knees so that your thighs are at a right angle to the floor. Your hands may be held on your hips or out in front of you. Be certain your back is kept straight. Then return to your standing position. This is a good exercise for people who have thin thighs and want them to become fuller.

To develop the flexor muscles of the thigh (the *rectus femoris,* and the *sartorius*) place your foot against a desk or a bar and push for 10 seconds. Repeat with the other leg.

The muscles associated with the inside of the thigh are the *adductor longus, adductor brevis* and *adductor magnus.* As their names imply, those muscles are the adductors of the leg. You can firm up the adductor muscles of the leg by standing in a doorway and placing the inside of your foot against the wall. Then try to draw your leg inward, keeping an erect position. Exert a pull for 10 seconds, and then repeat with the other leg.

The muscles of the back of the thigh, often called the hamstring muscles, are the *biceps femoris,* the *semitendinosus,* and the *semimembranosus.* They act as flexors of the leg and rotate the leg laterally.

To stretch those muscles, sit on the floor with your legs outstretched in front of you. Your upper body should be in an upright position. That is your starting position. Start the exercise by bending from the hips until your upper body is parallel to the legs and floor.

At first you may find this quite difficult—so work into the exercise gradually.

The thigh area, like the hip area, is a problem for many people because it is a place for fat deposits, especially for women. If you desire to slim the thighs, a prudent diet and an active life with a great deal of walking are necessary. See DIET.

Women who are interested in acquiring an attractive curve of the calf must give shape to the lower leg by developing the muscle there. Con-

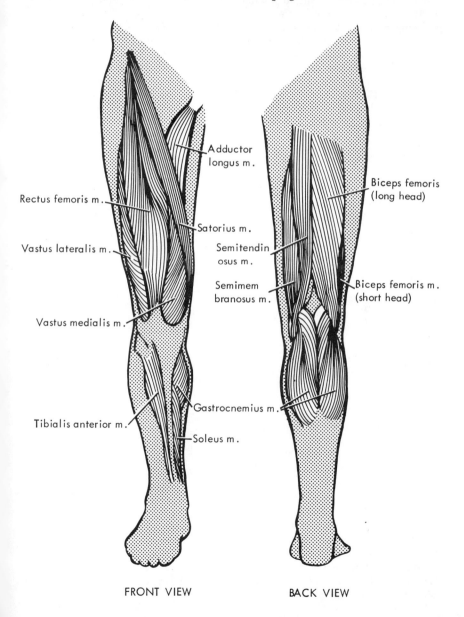

Rectus femoris m.

Adductor longus m.

Biceps femoris (long head)

Vastus lateralis m.

Satorius m.

Semitendinosus m.

Semimembranosus m.

Biceps femoris m. (short head)

Vastus medialis m.

Tibialis anterior m.

Gastrocnemius m.

Soleus m.

FRONT VIEW   BACK VIEW

trasted with the thigh and the buttocks, there is little fat on the calves. The way to emphasize the curve is to provide more muscle bulk. If you rise on your toes and look back at your calf, you'll see how the muscle becomes pleasantly rounded. This movement is almost totally dependent on the muscles of the calf, and it is a movement which you can do often. To accelerate the effort, add extra pounds to the body weight by carrying dumbbells. (An adequate set of 2 hand dumbbells with weights can be bought for about $15.00.)

To start, hold heavy dumbbells at your side with your feet comfortably balanced an inch or two apart. Then rise high on your toes as many times as you can. Before you desert this exercise, you should be able to do three sets of 12 repetitions. Next stand on one leg with the free leg raised behind and keep your balance by lightly touching the wall or a chair with your fingertips. Hold a heavy dumbbell on the side of the supporting leg and rise up and down as high and as many times as you can on your toes. You can accelerate your progress by remembering, everytime you go upstairs, to stand with the ball of one foot on the stair and the heel well out so that it can drop lower than the toes. With the calf muscles doing all the work (the handrail only there for support) lift the lower heel as high and as low as possible until your muscles ache. You can do this in your room if you step on a thick book in place of stairs. However, the best exercise of all for the legs is walking or running. If walking is selected, it must not be just a leisurely walk around the house or block, but rather a brisk, vigorous walk of thirty minutes or more. The activity will involve a great many of the muscles of the legs, and absolutely no equipment is needed except your willingness to walk. See EXERCISES, ISOMETRICS and WEIGHT TRAINING.

LIFETIME SPORTS

Charles B. Wilkinson, President of the *Lifetime Sports Foundation,* has defined lifetime sports in the following manner: "A true lifetime sport should meet the following criteria: (1) it is a game which can be played and enjoyed throughout one's life; (2) both men and women can participate; (3) no team organization is required; and (4) facilities for play are readily available." Many times carry-over sports have been used to describe activities that can be included throughout life, but often team sports were included. Lifetime sports, however, refer to many of those activities listed under carry-over sports but delete those that require team organization.

Activities included under lifetime sports are

Archery
Badminton
Bicycling
Billiards
Boating
Bowling
Camping
Canoeing
Croquet
Curling
Dance
Deck Tennis
Fencing
Fishing
Gardening
Golf
Hiking (Backpacking)
Handball
Horseback Riding
Hunting
Ice Boating
Ice Skating
Jukskei
Mountain Climbing
Mountaineering
Orienteering (No competition)
Rowing
Roller Skating
Quoits

Sailing
Skiing
Shooting
Pistol and Rifle
Sledding
Squash
Surfing
Swimming
Table Tennis
Tennis
Tobogganing
Water Skiing
Weight Lifting

Depending upon the local environment and facilities, some of those activities may be impossible to pursue, but many of them may be played in any climate with just a minimum of adaptation. It is important that the children of a community be given an opportunity to learn those activities. Parents, schools, Y's, clubs, and other recreational operations are to be aware of the need for teaching children lifetime sports. Too often the emphasis is on team sports that cannot be used in later life.

Offered in Schools

The American Association of Health, Physical Education and Recreation (AAHPER) conducted a survey of lifetime sports offered in secondary schools. In their report the AAHPER revealed that relatively little is being done in this area. The sports investigated were badminton, bowling, golf and tennis—supposedly popular activities.

Some 60 per cent of the schools provided instruction to boys and 52 per cent to girls, with 75 per cent of the students participating in half of the schools. Only 18 per cent of the schools provided bowling instruction to boys and 22 per cent to girls, with less than 25 per cent of the students participating in one-third of the schools and less than 50 per cent in two-thirds. About 26 per cent of the schools provided golf instruction to

boys and about 17 per cent to the girls, with less than 25 per cent of the students participating. Thirty-eight per cent of the schools provided tennis instruction to boys and 39 per cent to the girls, with less than 25 per cent of the students participating in one-third of the schools and less than 50 per cent in two-thirds.

Improvement Attempts

What can be done about it? The Lifetime Sports Foundation founded by Brunswick and American Machine and Foundry, two companies that admittedly have a vested interest, have placed a great emphasis on the need for lifetime sports. The companies issued a grant to the AAHPER in 1965 and initiated the *Lifetime Sports Foundation Project*, whose objectives are to have the director and his staff work with local and state authorities to improve and broaden their physical education programs. The project seeks to (1) conduct and stimulate in-service and pre-service clinics for teachers and recreation leaders, (2) identify and spread ideas about effective methods of organizing and teaching groups, use of limited space and equipment, and other improvisations and innovations, (3) investigate the nature and extent of lifetime sports instruction in schools of the nation, (4) study the psychological and physical benefits of regular participation in sports, and (5) contribute to the support of the AAHPER Outdoor Education Project.

The Lifetime Sports Education Project conducted four national clinics in badminton, tennis, golf and bowling. These clinics were designed to train master clinicians, who were then committed to assist at state-level clinics. Persons trained at the state level were then committed to serve at the local level, the goal being to develop a large number of physical educators qualified to teach tennis, badminton, golf and bowling. It appears that a

FITNESS BENEFITS OF RECREATIONAL ACTIVITIES

H–High M–Medium L–Low M-H–Depends whether recreation (M) or vigorous (H)

Sport	C-R Endurance	Muscle Strength				Muscle Endurance				Flexibility			
		Arms	Legs	Abdomen	Back	Arms	Legs	Abdomen	Back	Shoulder	Hip	Elbow	Knee
Archery	L	M-H	L	M	H	L	L	M	M	H	L	L	L
Badminton	M-H	M	H	M	M	M	H	M	M	H	M	H	H
Bicycling	M-H	L	H	L-M	M	L	H	L-M	L-M	L	H	L	H
Billiards	L	L	L	L	L	L	L	L	L	M	L	L	L
Boating	L	L	L	L	L	L	L	L	L	M	L	L	L
Bobsledding	L	M	L	L	L	L	L	L	L	L	L	L	L
Bowling	L	L-M	L-M	L-M	L-M	L	L	L	L	M	M	M	M
Canoeing	L-M-H	H	M	M	H	M-H	M	M	M	H	H	H	L
Croquet	L	L	L	L	L	L	L	L	L	L	L	L	L
Curling	L	L	M	L-M	M	L	L-M	L	L-M	M	L	M	L
Deck Tennis	L	L-M	M	M	M	L	M	L	M	H	H	H	H
Diving (Springboard)	L	L	M	M	M	L	L	L	L	M	H	L	L
Fencing	M-H	M-H	M-H	M	M	M	M-H	M	M	M	H	H	H
Fishing													
a. Deep Sea	L	M-H	L	L	M	H	L	L	M	L	L	M	L
b. Fresh	L	L-M	L	L	M	L	L	L	L	L	L	M	L
c. Surf	L	M-H	L	L	M	M	L	L	M	L	L	L	L
Gliding	L	L	L	L	L-M	L	L	L	L	M	M	L	M
Golf	L	L	M	L	M	L	M	L	L	M	M	H	M
Handball	M-H	M	H	M	M	H	M	M-H	M	M	M	H	H
Horseback Riding	L-M	M	M-H	L	M	L	M	M	L	L	M	H	M
Horseshoe Pitching	L	M	L	L	L-M	L-M	L	L	L	M	L	L	L
Hunting	M	M	M-H	M	M	M	L	M	M	L-M	M	M	M
Ice Skating	M-H	M-H	H	H	M	M-H	M-H	H	M	L-M	H	L	H
Judo	H	H	H	H	H	H	H	H	H	M	H	H	H
Jukskei	L	L-M	L	L	L	L	L	L	L	M	L	L	L
Karate	H	H	H	H	H	H	H	H	H	M	H	M	H

FITNESS BENEFITS OF RECREATIONAL ACTIVITIES

H—High   M—Medium   L—Low   M-H—Depends whether recreation (M) or vigorous (H)

Sport	C-R Endurance	Muscle Strength				Muscle Endurance				Flexibility			
		Arms	Legs	Abdomen	Back	Arms	Legs	Abdomen	Back	Shoulder	Hip	Elbow	Knee
Mt. Climbing	H	M-H	H	H	H	H	H	H	H	M	H	M	H
Motor Sports	L	L	L	L	L	M	L	L	L	L	L	L	L
Netball	M-H	L	H	L	L	M	H	M	M	M	M	M	H
Orienteering	H	M	L	M	M	M	H	L	L	M	M	M	H
Quoits	L	L-M	L	L	L	L	L	L	M	L-M	H	L	M
Rollerskating	M-H	M	H	M	M	M	M-H	M	M	L-M	L	L	H
Rowing	L-M-H	H	H	H	H	H	H	H	H	H	L	H	H
Sailing	L	M-H	M	M	M-H	M-H	M-H	M	M-H	M	M	M	M
Scuba Diving	L-M	M	M	L	M	M	M	M	M	H	M	M	M
Sculling	H	H	H	H	H	H	M-H	H	H	H	L	H	H
Shooting													
a. Pistol	L	M	L	L	M	M	M	M	M	L	L	L	L
b. Rifle	L	M-H	L	L	M	M	M	M	M	L	L	L	L
Shuffleboard	L	L	L	L	L	L	L	L	L	L	L	L	L
Skiing													
a. Down hill	M-H	M	H	M	M	M	H	M	M	M	H	M	H
b. Cross country	H	M	H	M	H	H	H	M	M	L	H	L	H
Skin Diving	M	M	M	L	M	M-H	M	M	H	M	M	M	M
Sledding	L-M	L	L	L	L	L	L	L	M	L	L	L	L
Squash	M-H	H	H	M	M	M	M-H	M	M	H	H	H	H
Surfing	L	L	H	L	L	L	L	L	L	L	L	L	L
Swimming	H	H	M-H	M	H	H	H	M	M	M	H	H	H
Table Tennis	L-M	L-M	L-M	L	L	L-M	L-M	L	L	L	L	L	L
Tennis	H-M	M	H	M	M	M	M-H	M	M	H	M	H	H
Volleyball	M-H	M-H	M-H	L-M	M	M-H	M-H	M	M	M	M	M	M
Water Skiing	M	H	M-H	L-M	M	H	H	M	M-H	L	M	L	M

good start has been made in that direction.

That National Recreation and Park Association, NRPA, realizing the need for lifetime sports instruction, undertook a *Lifetime Sports Recreation Project* in cooperation with the Lifetime Sports Foundation. The purpose of the project is to (1) encourage planned park and recreation programs of instruction and (2) promote increased participation in lifetime sports after instruction. The NRPA directed its efforts toward badminton, bowling, tennis and golf.

The efforts of the Lifetime Sports Foundation and the resulting projects have been commendable and deserve full credit for the planning and direction. But they will go only as far as the population will let them. It is necessary that all citizens recognize the necessity of such instruction, education and emphasis.

Duties of School, Parents, Community

Schools must realize that physical education instruction with participation by every student is the only goal. They must also be aware that physical education be given the same status as the other subjects in the academic curriculum. Physical educators have contributed greatly to the current state of affairs, because they have often relied on the traditional 3 or 4 sports, not analyzing why they offer certain sports, what benefits the children are receiving, and what type of instruction they have been giving. If they had been meeting those requirements, the need for the Lifetime Sports Foundation would be dubious.

School administrators are also contributors to the current state of affairs. Effective sports instruction cannot take place in a class where 60 or more pupils are present with only one teacher. Nor will one or two periods a week alleviate the problem. Three one-hour class periods a week is the minimum.

Parents must demand that their children be given proper instruction in lifetime activities. They should not judge their physical education program on the football or basketball team, but rather on the participation of the children in physical education, the type of activities they are learning, the fitness of the children, the degree of vigor in the intramural program, and the interest the children take in lifetime sports.

The community plays an important role too. It must provide facilities for recreation. Tennis courts, golf ranges, bowling lanes, playgrounds, parks and bikeways are a few of the necessary items.

Related topics and discussions are COMMUNITY, FAMILY, GOVERNMENT and SCHOOLS.

LOAFER'S HEART

Loafer's heart, a term coined by Drs. Hans Kraus and Wilhelm Raab, is characterized by its inadequate energy economy, rapid rate at rest, slow deceleration of the heart rate after exercise to the resting rate, and small stroke volume during exercise (indicating less blood flow with each beat). The loafer's heart, as its name implies, is a condition that occurs with a decrease in exercise. The opposite of the detrained heart is the trained heart or the athlete's heart. See ATHLETE'S HEART.

Kraus and Raab cite some typical cases of the loafer's heart. They have noted that one elderly woman spent 30 years in bed without interruption. Her pulse rate was over 140 beats per minute despite medication. They compared her with an extremely active aged alpinist, 87 years of age. He demonstrated no signs of cardiac failure and had a resting heart rate between 48 and 60. A concert conductor who led an extremely hectic life, traveled incessantly from concert to concert and smoked one cigarette after another. The only exercise he got was conducting. He succumbed after his fourth myocardial infarction at the age of 60. He claimed to have a normal heart by self evaluation. But Dr. Raab found that his pulse rate was around 116 per minute.

The loafer's heart in many instances can be reversed. A gradual, progressive exercise program that is geared to the individual needs of the person can improve the condition and make a more efficient organ.

See HYPOKINETIC DISEASE.

LONGEVITY

Mankind has always been interested in finding out how people can live longer. Modern advances in science and medicine have extended your life span and have enabled you to retain youth as long as possible. It is evident that the average length of life has been considerably extended over the last decade. The struggle for a better life has brought about many improvements in the living conditions of mankind. There are now better working conditions, improved nutrition, and also advances in medicine to cope with the past and present diseases. As a result of our advanced technology, today's society is softening.

Review of Literature

One of the first studies on the effects of exercise on aging by Mark B. Wakefield compared the age at death of the men who played in the Indiana state high school basketball tournament from 1911-1935 with those among men in the general population. The results favor the basketball players, because their rate of mortality was 30% less than the average for the general high school graduate in Indiana.

In a 1954 study by Dr. Thomas K. Cureton, results indicated that if the blood pressure and pulse rates are lowered as much as they are in any subject who undergoes consistent physical training, health is improved. In another study by Cureton, reported

in 1952, there was no indication that former champions show relatively greater strain or deterioration, but instead they have significantly stronger circulation and vagus tone.

In 1954, Dr. Ernst Jokl recorded his findings when the German Gymnastic Union held its annual festival for men and women gymnasts. Participants competed on the horizontal bar, the parallel bars, the vaulting horse, running, broad jumping, shot put and swimming. Training was more effective in determining physical efficiency than was chronological age because training had obliterated whatever deteriorating effect could be ascribed to aging.

Jokl also stated that there is a tendency for the decline due to aging to be retarded. Today, men and women of 60 look younger than men and women of 60 half a century ago. Regular physical exercise tends to accentuate that trend. At least one aspect of aging, the decline of efficiency, can be inhibited by 25 years and more, provided there is systematic and lasting application of suitable forms of physical training.

A third investigation by Dr. Cureton (1957) involving normal aging of adults revealed that the efficiency of the body for labor, love and life, in general, may be greatly extended by unusual care and physical conditioning in the middle-aged period.

In 1957, Dr. Etta Walters stated that the psychomotor skills developed early and kept in training can be retained by the aged to such a high degree that the older person can surpass a much younger age group in that skill.

In 1957, Dr. Henry J. Montoye wrote that regular exercise of the proper intensities and duration can do much to postpone the deterioration which commonly occurs as the individual gets older.

The effect of muscular activity on longevity was discussed by Dr. Lawrence C. Rarick who stated, "While the evidence is not clear concerning the effects of exercise on longevity there is strong support for the belief that the person will have a healthier, happy and more productive span of years late in life, by including a regular program of physical activity in his regimen of living.

In 1959, Dr. A. L. Chapman stated that muscular activity is needed in order to keep the smooth muscle linings of the blood vessels from becoming atrophic. The statement implies that exercise is important as a means of maintaining good, efficient circulation while aging.

In 1960, Dr. Fred Hein and Allan Ryan pointed out from their research that heredity is an important factor in the appearance of the evidences of aging as well as in longevity. Other studies also indicated that in middle age and beyond, exercise can be a useful means of preserving more youthful body contours, retaining functional organic reserves, and maintaining the general resiliency of the body.

Exercise Preserves Youth

Regular exercise assists in preserving the physical characteristics of youth and delaying the onset of the stigmata of aging and probably exerts a favorable influence upon longevity.

A study conducted by Drs. Elsworth Buskirk and James Counsilman revealed that the psychological and social benefits accrued during middle age through participation in exercise and recreational endeavors may be equally as important and more easily documented than physiological benefits. Since it is probable the synergism of psychological, social and physiological factors produce "gains," a wisely selected exercise program may contribute measurably toward productive life in middle age.

Dr. Henry Montoye stated that a pilot study taking into account a variety of factors indicates that although there appear to be rather distinct differences between athletes as a group and non-athlete controls as to physical capacity and other characteristics while in college; by middle age or before, those differences are not nearly so marked. Apparently few training habits carry over into later life. Mode of life and amount of physical activity at various periods of life rather than sports participation in youth may well be the important question in relation to longevity.

In 1961 Dr. Martti Karvonen pointed out that the phenomena of aging appear as opposite to those caused by training. Thus, in some populations, a decrease in the amount of habitual exercise may accentuate several age changes, whereas in other populations with life-long exercise the state of training may delay them.

Karvonen also listed the areas of needed research in regard to exercise and aging. It included reinvestigation of several gerontological problems on physically active as against sedentary subjects; statistical analysis of the interdependence of growth and physical fitness in different geographic, racial and social groups; and training studies on elderly subjects, in order to build a scientific background for the physical rehabilitation of the aged. Karvonen stated that long-term exercise may have a positive effect on health even if it does not prolong life. Such an effect would be manifested by a lower frequency of illness in such a way that subjective interpretation will not cause bias.

Dr. Dragomir stated that a correct combination of mental activity and physical exercise and sports is, at present, the best method of preserving for as long as possible the activity of the brain cells on a high level with respect to their extremely important regulating and trophic function in the organism. If activity of the brain is maintained on a high level, especially as regards their regulating and trophic function, the whole organism and all its functions will be in good health.

Physical exercises, therefore, are the best physiological means of controlling the phenomena of senescence. It should be emphasized, that the control of the phenomena of senescence—the fight for longevity—should begin as early as possible, before man has completed his development.

The results of research by Drs. J. H. Currens and P. D. White show that strenuous physical effort can be maintained for a prolonged period in a person who is well trained without the accumulation of excess lactic acid in the blood. That seems to be the most important aspect of training so far as ability for sustained physical muscular effort is concerned.

In 1964, Mateeff stated that, according to Arshavski, the new forms of intensive muscular activity which man has acquired in the course of his phylogenetic development, and which have led to increase in the vagus tonus and slowing of heart activity and respiration, have been the cause of the increased span of human life three- to four-fold as compared with the lower ape.

In 1965, Davis, Logan, and McKinney stated that although the scientific evidence is scarce and opinions vary, it can be shown that exercise is beneficial to the aging process. Dr. White states the following:

Exercise has positive effects on health. In the first place, there is the benefit of establishing or maintaining a general muscular tone throughout the body, including the heart.

A second benefit from exercise is its effect on the psyche. For many of us, exercise is a delightful antidote for nervous tension and strains.

A third benefit of exercise at any age and therefore, applicable to the "aging" is its favorable effect in helping to control obesity, a condition widely regarded as inimical to the best of health and longevity.

Recommendations and Implications

Why not exercise if the quality of your health is improved? As a result of exercise, the digestive system will be better able to function; respiration will be aided; circulation will be improved; and general muscle tone throughout the body will be better. Another benefit of exercise at any age is that it helps to control obesity.

Also, exercise has a favorable effect on mental health. For many people exercise is a delightful antidote for nervous tension, and strains, anxiety and mental concentration.

Regular exercise assists in preserving the physical characteristics of youth and delaying the onset of the stigmata of aging. Furthermore, training helps to obliterate the deteriorating effect of aging, and a decline in efficiency can be postponed until an indefinite time.

The exact reasons for aging are not known, but the process of aging and training appear to be opposites. Exercise seems to inhibit the decline of efficiency provided the body is kept in some form of training. Therefore, physical exercise is the best physiological means of controlling the phenomena of senescence and should begin as early as possible.—*Sheldon A. Chamberlain, Jr.*

A Further Note on Longevity

There are many factors that are related to longevity. H. B. Jones compiled a chart noting the magnitude of environment and heredity factors in longevity. The chart, presented below, demonstrates the life-span differences of individuals. The plus (+) before the number indicates the average number of years that are added to the normal life span, while the minus (−) indicates the number of years subtracted from the normal life span.

Notice the column labeled reversible, especially those concerned with overweight and atherosclerosis. Those are factors that can be improved through regular, moderate exercise.

Dr. Jean Meyer, Professor of Nutrition at Harvard University, has noted that a person who exercises regularly and properly will add 5 years to his

PHYSIOLOGICAL AGE AND LIFE-SPAN DIFFERENCES

Reversible Comparison	Years	Permanent Comparison	Years
Country versus city dwelling	+ 5	Female versus male sex	+ 3
Married status versus single,		Familial constitutions	
widowed, divorced	+ 5	2 grandparents lived to 80	
Overweight		years	+ 2
25 per cent overweight group	− 3.6	4 grandparents lived to 80	
35 per cent overweight group	− 4.3	years	+ 4
45 per cent overweight group	− 6.6	Mother lived to age 90 yrs.	+ 3
55 per cent overweight group	− 11.4	Father lived to age 90 yrs.	+ 4.4
67 per cent overweight	− 15.1	Both mother and father lived	
Or: an average effect of 1 per		to age 90 years	+ 7.4
cent overweight	− 0.17	Mother lived to age 80 yrs.	+ 1.5
Smoking		Father lived to age 80 yrs.	+ 2.2
1 package cigarettes per day	− 7	Brother, mother and father	
2 packages cigarettes per day	− 12	lived to age 80 years	+ 3.7
Atherosclerosis		Mother died at 60 years	− 0.7
Fat metabolism		Father died at 60 years	− 1.1
In 25th percentile of popu-		Brother, mother and father	
lation having "ideal" lipo-		died at age 60 years	− 1.8
protein concentrations	+ 10	Recession of childhood and	
Having average lipoprotein		infectious disease over past	
concentrations	0	century in Western countries	+ 15
In 25th percentile of popu-		Life Insurance Impairment Study	
lation having elevated		Rheumatic heart disease,	
lipoproteins	− 7	evidenced by:	
In 5th percentile of popula-		Heart murmur	− 11
tion having highest ele-		Heart murmur + tonsillitis	− 18
vation of lipoproteins	− 15	Heart murmur + strepto-	
Diabetes		coccal infection	− 13
Uncontrolled, before insulin,		Rapid pulse	− 3.5
1900	− 35	Phlebitis	− 3.5
Controlled with insulin		Varicose veins	− 0.2
1920 Joslin Clinic record	− 20	Epilepsy	− 20.0
1940 Joslin Clinic record	− 15	Skull fracture	− 2.9
1950 Joslin Clinic record	− 10	Tuberculosis	− 1.8
		Nephrectomy	− 2.0
		Moderate albumin in urine	− 5.0
		Moderate albumin in urine	− 13.5

life span. It is possible, therefore, to include a further entry on the list, that of exercise or the lack of it.

LOW BACK PAIN

Lumbago, lordosis, disc lesion, slipped disc—call it what you may—it's still a big pain in the back.

If you are one of the millions of Americans who recoils with lower back pain after any kind of exertion—and medical authorities estimate that one of every two Americans eventually has the problem—the time is at hand to review your postural habits and respect for proper exercise. As Dr. Hans Kraus, consultant to the late President John F. Kennedy, put it at an Industrial Medical Association convention in New York City

—More than 80 per cent of pain in the lower back is muscular in origin.

—Muscular imbalance producing pain is usually general, or postural, rather than due to local defects of the bones or joints.

—Muscular imbalances producing lower back pain are principally due to lack of exercise. Every general medical examination should include testing of the mobility and strength of muscles supporting the spine.

Dr. Kraus, associate professor of physical medicine at New York University's School of Medicine, has said that the first episode of relatively mild low back pain is an excellent opportunity for the doctor to persuade his patient to take more active exercise.

George R. Bruce, weight-training director of the Mid Valley YMCA in Van Nuys, California, also reminds back sufferers that every movement of the body is dependent upon its muscles. "It is the function of the muscles to hold the body and its contents in proper shape and in proper place." Bruce emphasizes, "The stronger the muscles the more easily they can carry on their designated functions."

Causes and Treatment

In other words, lower back pain means lack of exercise, weak muscles, lack of proper body shape, deterioration or lordosis, resultant strain on the spine, disc lesions or pressure on the nerve-crammed spinal cord. Any of those factors, alone or in combination, can cause the excruciating experience known as lower back pain. Most of them, according to Dr. Miland E. Knapp of the University of Minnesota's Medical School in Minneapolis, are curable. Treatments prescribed by Dr. Knapp include (in the acute state) bed rest, support by taping or traction, hot packs, whirlpool baths, the Hubbard tank, aspirin, codeine, selected sedatives and manipulation.

"Probably the most important procedure for relieving low back pain during the acute stage is bed rest on a firm mattress over a bed board that covers the entire surface of the spring," Dr. Knapp writes. "A firm felt mattress

is preferable, but a sponge rubber mattress with a compression ratio of 34 pounds per square inch is satisfactory and may be a little more comfortable."

Pelvic belts, corsets, and heat have proved of value in relieving pain. Moist heat appears to be most useful when muscle spasm accompanies the pain. Traction is important, too, because muscle contractures often cause prolonged disability.

Exercise as Treatment

During subacute and chronic stages, exercises may be used to strengthen weak muscles. Writes Dr. Knapp, "We usually start with postural exercises, stressing back-flattening if lordosis is present and adapting the program to fit the presenting symptoms. If weakness is severe, the best method of producing hypertrophy is progressive resistance exercises." The physician stresses that early surgical treatment is often indicated if conservative treatment fails to provide enough relief so that the patient can return to work or live in reasonable comfort.

Probably more than 90 per cent of workers return to their jobs following back injury, and only a small percentage require surgical treatment. "Work Hardening Units," similar to one developed at the Minneapolis Curative Workshop, are often helpful in preparing patients and tender backs for the rigors of an eight-hour factory or office routine again.

Under the direction of the occupational therapist, a work program is set up which simulates as closely as possible the expected work situation, and may involve shoveling sand, lifting bricks or cement blocks, pushing a wheelbarrow, sawing, or running a lathe. The patient visits the unit daily, working within his physical capacities until he can work through a six-hour-day. He is then discharged, presumably sufficiently rehabilitated to assume normal responsibilities.

Among key "Rules to Live By—From Now On," published by McNeil

Laboratories of Fort Washington, Pennsylvania, are

1. Never bend from the waist only. Bend the hips and knees.

2. Never lift a heavy object higher than your waist.

3. Always face the object you wish to lift.

4. Avoid carrying unbalanced loads. Hold heavy objects close to your body.

5. Never carry anything heavier than you can manage with ease.

6. Never move or lift heavy furni-ture. Wait for someone who knows the principles of leverage.

7. Avoid sudden movements, sudden "overloading" of muscles. Learn to move deliberately, swinging the legs from the hips.

8. Learn to keep the head in line with the spine when standing, sitting, or lying in bed.

9. Put soft chairs and deep couches on your "don't sit" list. During prolonged sitting, cross legs to rest your back.

10. Before beginning to attempt

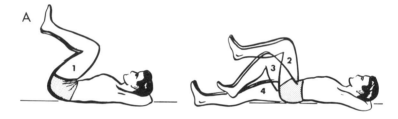

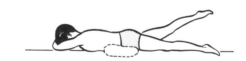

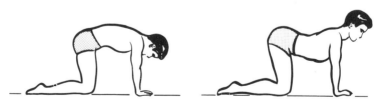

These exercises may be used to strengthen the low back area. In (A), lie on your back with knees flexed and pull them toward your chest. Then lower the legs gradually, being certain to keep the low back on the floor. Repeat. In (B), lie on your stomach with a pillow under your waist. Raise one leg at a time, lower and rest. Repeat. Assume a kneeling position as in (C) and arch your back like a cat, dropping your head at the same time. Then reverse the position by dropping your back and raising your head. Repeat several times.

physical exercises for physical fitness, consult your physician. He can then determine if the low back pain is due to faulty posture. When you commence, omit any exercise which arches or overstrains the lower back—backward or forward bends, or touching the toes with the knees straight.—*John Haberern*

Why Low Back Pain Occurs

Body mechanics, or posture, refers to the relationship of the various body parts to each other and their degree of efficiency. Many factors affect posture. Some are muscle strength, muscle tone and muscle balance. Deficiencies concerned with these factors result in varying degrees of misalignment, inefficiency, fatigue, and, not too infrequently, pain and usually manifest themselves as misalignments between adjacent body parts. Nowhere are postural complications more evident than in the low back region, and many Americans suffer from a too common malady referred to as low back ache or low back pain. The precipitator of most low back problems in the United States is lack of exercise. With adequate regular exercise, the muscles of the back are kept in good condition with respect to muscle strength, tone and balance. Barring poor postural habits, alignment can be maintained and low back problems avoided.

Muscle Strength, Balance and Flexibility

A healthy low back depends upon muscle strength and balance, flexibility, and good postural habits. Most low back problems stem from misalignment which has been caused by one or usually a combination of those factors. In some cases, misalignment can be traced to hereditary factors concerned with bone formation. Poor postural practices and a lack of exercise during the formative adolescent years may precipitate poor bone formation which can lead to permanent misalign-ment. Misalignment, regardless of its cause, puts unaccustomed strain on muscles, ligaments and other tissues.

Although muscle strength is the mechanical means by which the body is aligned, muscle flexibility is also extremely important. Flexibility is often overlooked as a source of low back problems. Muscles which are not continually stretched through exercise to maintain a functional range of motion, tend to shorten from lack of use. That is, flexibility decreases. In this situation, the ligamentous and muscular tissues are more susceptible to being overstretched during sudden exertion. The overstretching is usually followed by pain, muscle spasm, and, sometimes, loss of function. Those same symptoms frequently occur after a bout of hard physical work. Witness the number of individuals who return to work the day after a heavy snow storm complaining about a myriad of pains in the legs, back and arms. The same complaints are often registered by the weekend gardener.

Importance of Pelvis

At the pelvis, the weight of the upper body is transferred to the lower limbs. The pelvis, or pelvic girdle, is balanced on the rounded heads of the femurs (thigh bones), affords attachments for numerous muscles, and depends upon these muscles for its alignment and balance. Some of the muscles involved in the balance and alignment of the pelvis are the abdominals, hamstrings, gluteals and hip flexors. Any imbalance or weakness in those muscles can lead to pelvic misalignment, which usually manifests itself as a forward or backward tilt of the pelvis. Lateral tilts also occur and frequently result from compensation to offset a condition in which one leg is shorter than the other.

There are other causes of lateral tilts, for any situation in which a pelvic tilt exists necessarily puts abnormal tension on muscles and ligaments in the low back area. As an example, the abdominal muscles attach to the front of the pelvis and hold it up. In the case of weak abdominal muscles, the pelvis is allowed to tilt forward. The sacrum is also tilted forward, putting increased tension on the sacroiliac joint and the ligaments located on the front of the lumbar vertebrae. Forward tilt of the pelvis leads to lordosis, or sway back. It is in that situation that the "slipped disc" injury most often occurs. The fronts of the lumbar vertebrae are further apart in the lordosis condition, and the intervertebral discs tend to slide forward because of the uneven pressure exerted upon them. In addition to anterior (forward) dislocations of the intervertebral discs, posterior and lateral dislocations also occur depending on the nature of the vertebral misalignment. While vertebral misalignment sets up the disc injury, its occurrence is often the result of inefficient movement. Lifting heavy objects and loss of balance are several situations in which disc injuries frequently occur. Disc injuries usually necessitate surgical repair.

In addition to abdominal weakness, a lack of strength in the gluteals and/or hamstrings can also lead to forward pelvic tilt. While the abdominals stabilize the pelvis by pulling upward on the front, the gluteals and hamstrings contribute to stabilization by pulling down on the rear of the pelvis. If the strength of the hip stabilizers (abdominals, gluteals and hamstrings) is not sufficient to offset the action of the major hip flexor muscle, the psoas forward tilt of the pelvis can occur. The psoas originates (attaches) on the front and side of the last thoracic vertebrae and the five lumbar vertebrae, passes over the front brim of the pelvis, and attaches to the upper part of the thigh bone (femur). During contraction, this muscle lifts the leg forward. At the same time, it exerts a forward pull on the lumbar vertebrae and a downward pull on the front brim

of the pelvis. If the tendency is not adequately compensated for by the pelvis stabilizers, a forward tilt of the pelvis can result. To demonstrate the action of the psoas, lie on your back with your hands placed under the hollow of the back. With the knees kept straight, raise the feet off the floor and feel the increase in the low back curve —that is caused by the forward pull of the psoas on the lumbar vertebrae.

Another complication associated with an increased low back curve is the decrease in the size of the openings between the vertebrae in the lumbar region through which nerve fibers leave the spinal cord. That can result in pressure being put on those nerves. The pressure may be evidenced by pain in the low back area. The pain, and sometimes numbness, may also be recognized in the lower limbs since some of these nerves serve the extremities. Displaced or ruptured intervertebral discs can also put pressure on spinal nerves.

Flatback, or a decrease in the lumbar curve, is a condition resulting from a muscular imbalance in which the pelvis, or hip stabilizers, are shorter than normal. That imbalance is often accompanied by a weakness in the hip flexors. The hip stabilizers, in that situation, tilt the pelvis to the rear, and a flattening of the lumbar curve occurs. The effects of flatback are a decrease in overall body flexibility, a decrease in the shock-absorbing ability of the vertebral column, and changes in the support of the internal organs (viscera). Also a stretch is placed upon the erector muscles of the spine which leads to fatigue, spasm and pain. Pain associated with the erector muscles is usually located in the low back region where these muscles originate.

Low back misalignments sometimes give rise to upper or mid-back deviations. As an example, a kyphosis condition (abnormal backward curvature of the spine) may develop in the thoracic region to offset a swayback condition in the low back, or if a scoliosis (lateral curve) exists in the low back in one direction, a lateral curve in the opposite direction may develop in another region of the spine to compensate. Those compensatory curves are an attempt by the body to restore balance and efficiency.

Improper Lifting

The muscularly weak back is more susceptible to low back problems, but a healthy, strong back can be injured by poor postural and mechanical habits as well as trauma. Sudden violent movements and improper lifting have caused painful backs. Those injuries usually involve the straining of ligaments and muscles and, sometimes, disc complications. Lifting should be done with the powerful leg muscles, not with the back. The back muscles are responsible primarily for the maintenance of erect posture. Lifting should never be done in an off-balance position, and during the lifting of heavy objects, both feet should be in contact with the floor and the back should be kept erect.

Posture

Improper sitting posture can lead to low back problems. As in lifting, the back should be kept erect. To sit slouched in a chair puts unnecessary tension on the back muscles. Poorly designed furniture, which is constructed without regard for body structure, can cause strain, fatigue and pain in muscles. Sitting for prolonged periods of time causes shortening of certain postural muscles, particularly the hamstring muscles. If you are involved in an occupation which necessitates sitting for prolonged periods, you must exercise regularly to maintain the hamstring muscles at their proper length. Without that regular exercise, low back problems may develop as a result of the hamstring shortening.

A bed that is too soft or sags in the middle is the worst enemy of any back.

No matter what position you assume on such a bed, muscles are placed in unaccustomed and constant tension. At a time when the muscles are supposed to be completely relaxed, many of them are placed under stress throughout the night. It is no wonder that these muscles, the spinal erectors being the ones most often affected, are sore in the morning. Many medical men suggest the use of a board under the mattress to alleviate the condition.

Diet and Other Influences

In addition to muscular inadequacies and poor mechanical practices, postural misalignments and posture-based complications have several other causes. A poor diet can lead to malnutrition and obesity. Malnutrition adversely affects bone growth and development. Obesity adds stress to the structural components (bones, muscles and other tissues) of the body. Poor-fitting shoes and, particularly, high-heeled shoes can lead to foot and leg deviations which can end in pelvic misalignment. The most common foot deviation is pronation, or turning out of the foot, which frequently causes a forward tilt of the pelvis. Other possible causes of low back pain are certain diseases, psychological problems, and endocrine disturbances.

Contribution of Exercise

Many low back problems could be avoided through regular exercise. Exercise must be looked upon as a biological necessity. The body was made to move. Without adequate exercise, it is impossible to maintain the strength, tone and flexibility of the muscles concerned with the low back region. Posture is a good habit which must be instilled in each individual early in life and be accompanied by good nutrition, adequate rest and sleep, and regular exercise. In adolescents and adults who have already developed postural misalignments, re-education is necessary. The postural muscles must be improved through exercise. At the same time, the advantages of good posture must be emphasized because advanced or persistent bad backs necessitate support, physical therapy and rehabilitation.

Exercises recommended for the low back contribute to strength and flexibility of the muscles involved. Although strength is one aim, the exercises are not strenuous in themselves. Most low back exercises are performed in a sitting or lying position. In these positions, the back is well supported during the exercises.

For more information, see EXCESSIVE EXERCISE, FATIGUE, HYPOKINETIC DISEASE, INJURIES, LOW FITNESS and OBESITY.

LOW FITNESS

The first prerequisite in correcting low fitness is motivation to exercise. You must see a real need to improve your fitness level for both immediate and long-range effects. See MOTIVATION for a discussion on how to increase motivation. Also see MOTIVATION OF THE LOW FITNESS PERSON.

The second step is to determine what basic fitness components you need to correct. The four prime fitness components are muscle strength, muscle endurance, circulo-respiratory endurance and flexibility. Flexibility is important to avoid injury, muscle strength is essential for good posture, muscle endurance is a necessity in maintaining good posture and in continuing activities throughout the day, and circulo-respiratory endurance is necessary because of its relationship to reducing degenerative cardiovascular disease, in providing stamina for a day's work. Those components are also important so that you have adequate reserve to meet any emergency without placing undo stress on the body or endangering it. See FLEXIBILITY, MUSCLE ENDURANCE, CIRCULO-RESPIRATORY ENDURANCE and STRENGTH

for a complete discussion. Other fitness components become important as you engage in various sports and activities.

In achieving an adequate level of fitness, don't take a haphazard approach, for it will probably be ineffective and neglect the necessary principles of training. (See TRAINING.) Simply following a running or cycling program will not develop all the fitness components—you must search for a better program. Dr. Cureton's continuous rhythmical exercise program (see CONTINUOUS RHYTHMICAL EXERCISE), or the systematic program outlined below are sound approaches. The following program allows a progressive development of each of the various vital components of fitness. The weeks allotted for each step of the program are merely arbitrary but you can use them as a guide for establishing your routine.

Low Fitness Program

Step 1. Step 1 of the program should last 6 to 8 weeks. In some cases, it will last longer or shorter, depending upon the fitness level. The first step is to measure the flexibility of your various joints. To do so, see the series of flexibility tests listed under TESTS. You ought to take all tests included under that section and pass them all before progressing to Step 2.

To improve your flexibility, perform those exercises listed under EXERCISES for flexibility and gradually try to extend your range of movement in the exercise. Do not use forceful movements but rather slow stretching movements. The neck, shoulder, back, hips, knees, ankles and wrists should all be exercised. That phase of the program requires only 10 to 15 minutes. Continually check on your progress to see if you have achieved a passing grade in each of the flexibility items. The first phase of the program should take you 6 to 8 weeks. Once you have passed all the test items, you are ready to progress to the second phase of the program.

Step 2. Step 2 of the exercise program, emphasizes strength development, which begins with a strength test. The tests as described under TESTS are excellent. However, it will require weight-training equipment. Once you have established your strength level, you are ready to progress to the strength-building phase of the program with weight training exercises a major part. Attempt to develop specific parts of the body—neck, arm and shoulder, back, abdomen and legs. Ten to twelve lifts are selected and the objective is to do three sets of 8 repetitions maximum for each lift. See WEIGHT TRAINING for a discussion on how to build strength and STRENGTH. Calisthenics can also be used to build strength, but care must be taken that the emphasis is on muscle strength and not muscle endurance. For that reason, the approach outlined under EXERCISES must be followed. Isometrics can also be used as a means of developing strength. But because of their limitations, it is a technique to follow only as a last resort or when equipment is not available. See ISOMETRICS.

That phase of the program should last 6 to 8 weeks. It may take quite a bit longer, especially if you have a very low strength level. It is also important to note that flexibility exercises are continued in this program but that they make up only about 10 minutes of the routine and gradually decrease each week until they consume only five minutes of the daily workout.

Step 3. Emphasis in Step 3 is on muscle endurance. To test your muscle endurance, a series of tests are provided under TESTS. Prime emphasis is placed on the upper body. Use weight training and calisthenics and emphasize the various body parts—neck, arms and shoulders, abdomen, back and legs. If weight training is used, concentrate on 3/8 maximum load and lift it 1½ to 2 minutes. Do 3 sets. See

MUSCLE ENDURANCE for a discussion on how to build that particular component of fitness. You can also use calisthenics along with exercises on apparatus. See EXERCISES. As with the strength exercises, include flexibility exercises at the outset of the program. They should take up about five minutes and can be used quite effectively as a warm-up. As the end of 8 weeks, retest your muscle endurance to see what kind of progress you have made. If you have demonstrated a significant improvement, you are ready to progress to Step 4.

Step 4. You now progress into building the most important component of fitness—circulo-respiratory endurance. Here emphasis is placed on developing cardiovascular function. Activities including cycling, swimming, running, walking, hiking, skating, squash, handball, tennis, and the like can be used to improve cardiovascular function, provided that you adopt a progressive program. To measure your circulo-respiratory endurance, take one of the tests described under TESTS. One of the best is the *Harvard Step Test.* If you score below 50, you are classified in poor physical condition. If you score between 50 and 80, you are in average physical condition. If you score above 80, you are in good physical condition. Another test is *Cooper's Twelve Minute Run/Walk.* Again there are various classifications indicating your fitness category. On the basis of your test scores on either the *Cooper Twelve-Minute Run* or the *Harvard Step Test,* you are able to select an exercise program. Refer to the particular entries of the book that develop circulo-respiratory endurance where you will find a progressive program that will allow you to develop circulo-respiratory endurance.

If you are classed at poor physical condition, you should remain at least 2 to 3 weeks at each level. If you are classed in fair physical condition, spend 1 to 2 weeks at each level. On the other hand, if you show a fitness level of good or above, you may start on the second chart and spend one week at each level. To maintain flexibility, it would be an excellent idea to warm up before each activity with five minutes of flexibility exercises. You might also try to perform several isometrics to maintain a reasonable degree of muscle strength. At six-week intervals, retest yourself with the battery of the *Cooper Twelve-Minute Run* or the *Harvard Step Tests* depending upon the one you selected first. Once you demonstrate a good or excellent fitness category, you can then progress into Step 5. You should spend an average of 8 to 20 weeks in Step 4.

Step 5. Up to this point, you probably have exercised five days a week. Now that you have achieved a high level of physical fitness, you can cut back your efforts to only three or four days a week. Be sure to select an endurance activity that will continue to keep you fit throughout the year, including both indoor and outdoor activities such as running, cycling, running in place, swimming, rope skipping, skating, basketball and squash. Start off the workout by 5 to 10 minutes of flexibility exercises, followed by 30 to 45 minutes of the selected endurance activity, and then 5 minutes of cooling off. Include flexibility exercises in the cooling off. You can maintain muscle endurance and circulo-respiratory endurance by the endurance activity and flexibility with the flexibility exercises which precede and conclude the exercise program. To maintain muscle strength, include some spot isometric exercises or perform occasional weight-training exercises or some calisthenics directed toward developing strength.

Once you reach that phase of the program constantly reevaluate your fitness status. A fitness test every two to three months is not unreasonable. Merely repeat those tests which you used initially. If at any time you notice

that you are slipping in one of the four fitness categories, it is time to reestablish the desired level of fitness for that particular component. Follow the same general principles set forth above and under TRAINING.

LYDIARD TRAINING SYSTEM

The Lydiard system of training was developed by Arthur Lydiard of New Zealand, who trained both Peter Snell, the 1960 Olympic 800 and 1,500 meters champion, and Murray Halberg, the 1960 Olympic 5,000 meters champion. The system is often incorrectly called "marathon training" but, in effect, is much more. Dr. J. Kenneth Doherty describes the Lydiard Training System as a wise balance between stamina and speed training, between training and competition and between utilizing the many systems of training.

This long-range running program covers 52 weeks a year, 7 days a week, and involves extensive distance running that requires up to 100 miles per week. A great emphasis is placed on being quite judicious in the selection of the meets and recovery period after the meet, not on overcompeting. Some meets are run as developmental races, which are in effect part of the training for the one major performance.

Elements of the Program

The basic elements of the program are time running (3 to 4 weeks), cross-country running (12 to 14 weeks), marathon training (8 to 10 weeks), speed-hill training (6 to 8 weeks), track training (12 to 14 weeks), and the training off period (3 to 6 weeks).

Time Running

At the outset of the training program, you begin by running steadily at an easy pace. Disregard pace and mileage. Gradually increase the time until you can run two hours steadily without stress.

Cross Country

Lydiard divides the cross-country training into two six-week periods. The first six weeks includes running against time and later mileage running up to 100 miles per week. The second six-week period includes faster running and time trials of various distances, paces and efforts. Delay actual competition until it is needed for motivating and aiding your development.

The cross-country big race.

If you have trained for a year, the system allows for 10 days of easier effort. Running takes place, but it is not nearly so strenuous. The workout is a steady, even pace.

Marathon Training

One hundred miles a week is the key to the Lydiard system. The running is done 7 days a week, which averages out to 14 miles a day. Usually the week is divided into 3 days of 20 miles and 4 days of 10 miles. The marathon training is continued until 18 weeks prior to the start of the important track competition.

Speed-Hill-Training

The most demanding and strenuous element of the Lydiard System is the speed-hill-training. Consequently, six weeks are devoted to this phase of the training program. After warming up with a two-mile jog, choose a fairly steep hill about ½ mile long. You run up the hill lifting the knees high. Emphasis is on the springing motion rather than the speed. After reaching the top, sprint down the hill with relaxed strides. When you reach the bottom, you then do a series of sprints such as 3-220's and 6-50's, on alternating runs. Do the hill run and sprints four times.

Track Training

The track training, like the cross-country running, is divided into two six-week periods. The first six-week period simply stated is a combination of interval and repetition training. See INTERVAL TRAINING and REPETITION TRAINING.

The second six-week period is a continuation of that training except that it includes developmental races. Lydiard urges you to race twice a week during the last phase. However, those races are mainly under and over distance races, for the main focus of attention is on future big track races. But these races are stressed because Lydiard advocates that to become fit for racing you must race, not just run.

Big Track Race

The big track race refers to the actual race—the goal of your training program.

Training Off Period

The training off period will vary with the length of training for the program and is about 3 to 6 weeks. The running is usually around 45 to 60 minutes of light jogging over varied terrain. Once a week, there is a long run of about 20 miles.

Lydiard System and Fitness

The Lydiard System is primarily a system for the training of cross-country and middle or long distance track men. It is a long-range training program that is extremely demanding and allows you to train at your own rate without undue emphasis on continual competition. The system places a great deal of stress on the training but avoids overcompetition—a normal pitfall in the United States.

You can follow this technique if you are interested in conditioning your body for physical fitness, for it is an excellent body training technique. It is necessary, however, that you be physically strong enough to train by this technique, for it is quite demanding on the human body. Lydiard, himself, did not let Halberg engage in the program completely until he felt he had adequate strength and stamina for such rigorous training. See FARTLEK INTERVAL TRAINING, JOGGING, OVERTRAINING, REPETITION TRAINING and TRAINING.

MASSAGE

Massage is an ancient method of injury treatment. As far back as Classical Greece, and possibly earlier, massage was recognized as a useful means

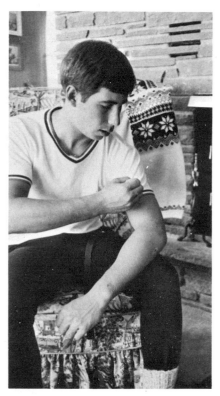

By cupping your hands and beating lightly against the skin, you can easily produce an invigorating and stimulating sensation. Move up and down with the cupping movement and continue only until the skin develops a slight coloration.

in aiding recovery from injuries. According to Dayton, "Massage is the scientific and systematic manipulation of tissues for therapeutic purposes."

Techniques

There are four techniques generally used in massage. 1. Stroking or effleurage, consists of firm, even stroking with the palms of the hands. 2. Compression, or petrissage, is a kneading motion in which the muscles are gently rolled, lifted and squeezed with varying amounts of pressure. 3. The friction technique is applied with the tips of the fingers or the heels of the palms and is administered in a circular pattern with gentle pressure. 4. Percussion is probably the least popular massage technique and consists of light blows delivered alternately by each hand. Gentle stretching, although not actually considered one of the techniques, definitely has a place in the art of massage.

Massage and Injuries

The intelligent application of massage to injuries facilitates their recovery. However, massage should never be applied to a new injury. It is important that the healing process be underway before massage is used. Unwise and early use of massage may actually hamper recovery. Generally, massage should not be used for at least 48 hours after the occurrence of the injury. Massage is also not advisable when a person is suffering from a skin irritation or rash. When less friction is desired use a powder, oil, or a liniment. Massage for therapeutic purposes should be employed only by someone experienced in its application.

The process of recovery from injuries involves the removal of excess fluids that have collected, the actual repair of the damaged tissue, and the breakdown and removal of adhesions and destroyed tissue substances. Massage increases circulation in the area of the injury. The blood brought into the area by the increased local circulation provides nutritive, rebuilding materials, and facilitates the removal of the excess fluids and tissue debris from the injury. Massage is also a useful means of helping to relieve pain and stiffness resulting from spasms and unaccustomed work.

Massage and Exercise

Massage is most beneficial when it is accompanied by a carefully planned exercise program. The exercise should be light at first and should increase as tolerance increases. While massage aids in the breakdown of the adhesions which form as part of the healing process, exercise aids the removal of the adhesions through absorption. Without exercise, the adhesions, which are nonelastic, will remain and interfere with the elasticity of the healed tissues. Massage accompanied by exercise following injuries assures the return of the preinjury range of motion to the injured tissues. Exercise also aids the rebuilding of muscular strength in the area of the injury.

MECHANICAL DEVICES

With the tremendous upsurge in interest for physical fitness, there has been a corresponding upswing in the manufacture of mechanical devices that purport to dramatically increase your level of physical fitness. Those devices have been flooding the American and European markets as panaceas for achieving optimum fitness; some can be purchased for a few dollars, while others cost $100 or more. Many of them claim to insure immediate, effortless fitness.

To review all the pieces of equipment that are available at the present time is unthinkable—the list is too lengthy. Furthermore, since new gadgets and gimmicks are flooding the markets weekly, a résumé of the present ones would be quickly outdated. There are, however, several guidelines to follow in evaluating the

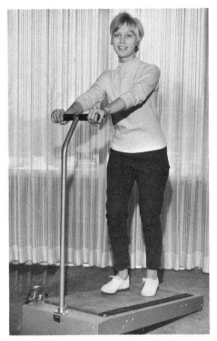

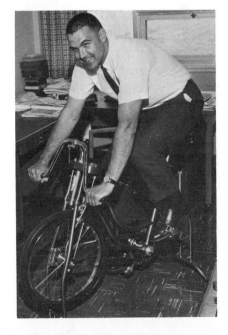

Two of the most popular mechanical devices are the inclined treadmill (top) and the stationary bicycle (below). Both make important contributions to the improvement of cardiovascular fitness.

exercise device before you consider a purchase.

Every exercise device must be measured in relation to the specific fitness components. That is, does the exercise device cause the body to be exercised properly to develop those vital factors of physical fitness? Below are a series of questions and statements that should be weighed in relation to each exercise device in order to evaluate the equipment.

1. Does the equipment or device do what it claims to do? Too often the advertising is geared to merely sell a product. For example, *if the device claims to* improve circulo-respiratory endurance, it must allow the heart rate to be increased to 140 beats per minute or more for *a sustained period of time.* The accelerated pulse must last for several minutes, not just a few seconds.

If the exercise device claims to improve muscle strength, be certain that it causes the muscles exercised to exert at least 2/3 maximum effort. If you can lift 100 pounds over your head as a maximum effort, you will not improve arm and shoulder strength unless the device allows you to lift 2/3, or 67 pounds, above your head several times every other day. To build strength, isometric (no movement) or isotonic (movement) exercises may be used. Best results for strength improvement by the isometric method involves maximally contracting the muscle for 5 seconds, 5 to 10 times or more a day. For weight training exercises (isotonic), 3 sets of 6 repetitions maximum is required to improve muscle strength.

If the exercise device claims to improve muscle endurance, it must force the muscle(s) being exercised to become fatigued to the point where continued exertion is practically impossible. The work load, however, is not to be so great that after a few contractions you can no longer continue, for then strength rather than endurance is

involved. You should be able to do at least 15 to 35 repetitions before you cannot continue. Weight training is an illustration of building muscle endurance. Suitable weight can be lifted 30 to 35 times without stopping; several sets of those repetitions complete the routine.

If a device claims to increase flexibility, emphasis must be foremost on allowing the muscles to go through their full range of motion. That is, there should be a complete contraction and extension of the muscle group(s). An isometric exercise will not improve flexibility; for to improve flexibility requires movement. Remember you improve flexibility at a specific joint. There is no such thing as a flexible person—he just has flexible joints.

2. Some devices are popular as an effortless way to get fit. The fact is there is no simple way to become physically fit other than hard work. Fitness does not come easily. From the above discussion, it is apparent that an activity will have to last from 30 to 60 minutes to qualify as a complete fitness device and as a means of developing the vital aspects of physical fitness. Major offenders of the easy way to get fit are the isometric-fitness and the spot-exercise people.

3. Do the advertisers use nebulous terms to describe their product? For example, a favorite expression is, "Improves muscle tone." Exactly what is muscle tone? Muscle tone is the state of contraction of the muscle even while you are at rest. The degree of contraction is dependent upon the response of the muscle to the nervous system; and the tone will vary depending upon the stimulation that it receives from the nervous system whether you are lying down or standing up. Evidence in research has been conflicting on whether muscle tone is improved with exercise or not; in fact, muscle tone is a controversial term in itself. See MUSCLE TONE.

Another favorite claim is that the

device improves circulation. The only kind of circulation that really counts in physical fitness is that of the efficiency of the heart and the blood vessels. To improve that efficiency, the pulse rate must rise to 140 beats per minute as a result of the exercise for a sustained period of time.

A third popular advertising method is to say that the device redistributes the fat of the body. Fat accumulates as a result of inactivity and overeating. The only way to reverse that condition is to cut down on the food intake and increase the activity level. The calorie outgo must exceed the calorie intake if you expect to lose weight. Merely exercising one limb or a certain muscle group is not very efficient. It may firm up the muscle behind the fat; but it will not generally remove the fat unless it is an extremely hard, long term exercise. The fat must be removed with activity that is of sufficient intensity to burn up more calories than consumed. Studies have shown that mechanical vibrators or massage devices do not take off or redistribute fat; one authority claims that if you use them for 15 minutes a day for a year, you'll lose only *one pound* according to the caloric cost calculations. See MYTHS OF EXERCISE.

4. Personal testimonies are another dangerous technique in promoting an exercise device. For example, a certain university used a dynamic tension machine to help condition their athletes and is now placed first in the league. The inference is that the piece of equipment must be good because of such success. Remember it takes talent, hard work, good coaching, and desire to make a champion, not just one exercise device.

5. A final approach used by some is that the piece of equipment gives you all the benefits that you would derive from swimming a mile or walking four miles. That comparison is erroneous, unless the piece of equipment allows you to get your pulse rate up as high as it would in the compared event, burn as many calories (see ENERGY COST OF ACTIVITIES) or involve similar or as many muscle groups.

Remember, there are a good many exercise devices that are being overlooked because of the worthless items so prevalent on the market. Exercise devices can be used in helping you attain physical fitness—perhaps not all of the components of fitness, but some of them. If you are fully aware of the limitations of the exercise device and the derived benefits, you will be a satisfied customer. Remember: you must do the work; the device can only improve your efficiency of doing it.

There is no easy, effortless way to get fit. To attain a reasonable degree of physical fitness that will be healthful for your body requires hard work, dedication and enjoyment. See EQUIPMENT.

MEDICINE BALL

Introduction

Medicine ball activities are used by those who want to strengthen arm, shoulder and trunk muscles. Generally, you need a partner to catch the heavy (6 to 8 lbs.) medicine ball.

Basic Positions and Throws

1. Basic Position—For each of the following throws, the starting or basic position is always the same. You hold the ball next to the chest with your hands behind and under the center of the ball. One foot is slightly ahead of the other.

2. Chest Pass—Assume the basic position. Then step in the direction of the throw as you push the ball from your chest by extending the arms.

3. Underhand Throw—Assume a basic position and bend from the waist. Then swing the ball backward and between your legs, keeping the arms straight. Once the back swing is

complete, swing the ball forward and upward, releasing it for the throw.

4. One-arm Throw—Assume the basic position and then turn slightly to the right (if you are right-handed). Place your right hand on the back of the ball and your left hand underneath it. Bring the ball past your right hip and then up to shoulder height. At that point, step forward on your left foot and throw the ball by moving the right arm forward in an arc.

5. Overhead Throw—Assume a basic position and raise the ball overhead, dropping it down slightly behind the head. Then step forward and swing both arms forward, releasing the ball. Many calisthenics, informal games, or guerrilla drills can be adapted for use with a medicine ball.

Individual Exercises

1. Running with Ball—Assume a basic position and, while holding the ball directly in front of your body, run forward or in place.

2. Squat Thrust with Ball—Assume a basic position, then perform a squat and place the ball on the ground between your legs. Hug the ball as you extend your legs backward and then return them to the squat position. Keeping the ball directly in front of you, return to the standing position.

3. Trunk Rotation—Assume the basic position and then raise the ball overhead as you would in an overhead throw. Keeping that position, execute a series of trunk twists (rotating to the left and right).

4. Chest Raise—Assume a prone position and place the medicine ball behind your neck, holding it with both hands. Then raise your head and chest off the floor.

Dual Exercises

1. Bend and Throw—Stand 10 feet apart, facing your partner. Holding the ball in an overhead position, bend forward swinging the ball between your legs and release it with an under-hand throw to your partner. He catches it and repeats the action.

2. Distance Throws—Stand far apart and attempt one of the four basic throws (chest, underhand, overhand and one-arm). Try for distance. The partner marks where the ball landed and, standing on that spot, returns the ball, throwing it in the same maneuver.

3. Dual Run with Ball—Both partners face each other about five to 10 feet apart. One has the ball. As you start to run (one forward and the other backward), execute chest passes between each other. Also try running laterally.

4. Dual Sit-Ups—Both partners sit on the floor with legs interlocked. One partner holds the ball overhead and reclines on the floor. He then performs a sit-up, passing the ball to you. Catch it above your head (the throw is only a matter of inches), sit up, and return the throw. The sit-ups may be executed as rapidly or as slowly as you wish.

MENSTRUATION

During the first two days of menstrual flow, strenuous activity should usually be curtailed. Mild exercise should be substituted and may be helpful in alleviating pain or the feeling of congestion. Of course, many women still continue strenuous training despite menstrual flow with both good and bad effects. Dr. P. O. Astrand and his associate conducted an experiment in which he found 1/3 of the girls reporting lower abdominal pain as a result of swimming training. Another study conducted by the American Amateur Athletic Union revealed that 85 per cent of the women could compete normally, whereas 15 per cent had increased pain and flow. Since women vary considerably in experiencing discomfort during menstrual flow, participation in demanding physical activity becomes a personal preference. To prohibit or encourage such participation by anyone other than the woman herself is impractical.

Another point that has received considerable attention is what effect the menstrual cycle has on performance. Again, research reveals conflicting results. Some findings show that performance is improved during menstrual flow, others have found no change or a decrease in performance, and still others indicate that performance is best after the menstrual flow. Again it is apparent that each woman is to be her own judge on what effect menstrual flow has on her performance.

Dysmenorrhea (painful flow) is a problem that plagues some women, and ranges from a few slight twinges in the abdominal and low back region to violent cramps, nausea and headaches. Gynecologists estimate that 20 to 30 per cent of the dysmenorrhea cases are due to organic causes such as ovaries, cysts, endocrine imbalance, or infection. Seventy to 80 per cent of the cases are functional, caused by poor posture, insufficient exercise, fatigue (lack of sleep), weak abdominal musculature, and malnutrition from poor eating habits or dieting.

Many of the basic causes of painful flow can be alleviated through proper exercise, exercise that strengthens the muscles of the abdominal area and relieves tension. It has not been conclusively proved whether the benefits are physiological or psychological. Probably it is a combination of the two.

A study conducted by Ruth Harris and Etta C. Walters at the University of Michigan pointed out the contributions of exercise in relieving dysmenorrhea. Eighty-seven per cent of a group of freshmen who suffered from moderate or severe cases of dysmenorrhea and then performed prescribed abdominal exercises for a minimum of 8 weeks showed a decrease in the severity of dysmenorrhea.

Exercises for Reduction of Dysmenorrhea

Here are a series of exercises that can be effective in reducing dysmenorrhea. They are used for relieving the congestion in the abdominal area caused by poor posture, poor circulation, or poor muscle tone, and for relieving back and leg pain.

1. Mosher Exercise—Lie on your back with your knees bent, feet flat on the floor, and right or left hand resting lightly on the lower abdomen. Slowly force your abdominal wall up against the hand as far as possible. Slowly contract the abdominal wall and relax. Repeat 10 times. Breathe normally throughout the movement.

2. Cat Exercise—Kneel on your hands and knees. Raise your back as high as possible while tucking your pelvic girdle under and contracting the abdomen. Relax completely and allow the back to sag. Repeat 8 to 10 times, maintaining rhythm throughout.

3. Knee-Chest—Kneel with your knees approximately 12 inches apart, hips directly over the knees, and your chest as close to the floor as comfortable. Hold the position for 3 to 5 minutes. Slide into prone position.

4. Thigh-Chest—Kneel with your knees about 12 inches apart. Your chest and abdomen are resting on your thighs, and the hands are back by the heels. Take 3 or 4 deep breaths. Keeping at same position, move your arms out in front of your head. Breathe 3 or 4 times and stretch your fingertips forward, pushing the hips backward with each inhalation. Release on each exhalation.

5. Billig's Exercise—Stand sideways with your shoes off, 18 inches from a wall. Place your forearm on the wall with your shoulder and elbow in line. Place the opposite hand on hips. Now tilt the pelvis backward, contract the abdominal and gluteal muscles; and flattening the lower back.

Hold the chest high. Now stretch the hips forward and sideward toward the wall. Do not twist the hips. See PREGNANCY, FEMININITY and WOMEN.

MENTAL HEALTH

Despite the use of tranquilizers and other chemical therapy, mental illness or emotional disturbances continue to be the foremost health problem in the United States. In recent years, various authorities have stated that more hospital beds are occupied by the mentally ill than by the physically ill. In addition, millions at home are incapacitated to various degrees by less severe forms of mental illness.

The person who possesses sound mental health is flexible, not rigid, in his behavior and responses. He maintains contact with reality, and he usually deals effectively with his environment. The desirability of possessing sound mental health, defined by Dr. Gladys Scott as "being comfortable with one's self and with others," is unquestioned. An individual is willing to strive toward that goal if he believes that positive results can be expected.

Physical Fitness and Mental Health

Because the possession of a desirable level of physical fitness produces many direct benefits, any possible benefits to the maintenance of good mental health (or emotional health) might best be considered a dividend.

Man is an entity—a united organism that cannot be divided. What happens to him physically affects him mentally, and vice versa. His nervous system, for example, serves equally these two components. That relationship is the basis for the belief that a release of physical tension through physical exercise causes an accompanying release of mental tension, or "nervous strain," since the opportunity is provided to express tension through action in a socially approved manner. The mental and physical unity of man is emphasized by Dr. Emma Layman, a psychologist, who points out, "Although we give lip-service to the idea of mind-body unit and have done so for many years, we continue to speak of physical health and mental health as if they were developed independently and constitute two separate entities." She emphasizes that the two are intimately related and that each affects the other.

Physical educators, recreators, health officials, medical doctors, physiologists, psychologists, and even philosophers have long maintained that the possession and maintenance of physical fitness benefits the human organism in a number of ways, including the gaining of satisfactions, the releasing of tensions, and the promoting of adequate patterns of adjustment to sound mental health. Indeed, some of the important objectives of physical education are based on that premise. In addition, a limited amount of substantiated research findings exists affirming that the possession of physical fitness and favorable mental health go together or are related.

Athletics and Personality Traits

In most of the studies reviewed, investigators have attempted to study various groups in which measured, personality traits (a crude indication of mental health) have been compared for subgroups who have been classified according to participation or nonparticipation in athletics or other vigorous physical activity. Although a common finding is that an athletic group possesses a higher degree of one or more favorable personality traits than a nonathletic group, that conclusion does not actually prove that participation in athletic-type activity causes favorable personality traits to be developed. Perhaps the possession of those traits causes one to participate in sports. Also, other factors not studied could be involved. Regardless of these shortcomings, the studies to be reviewed represent the most authoritative attack yet made in the scientific investigation of mental health and physical fitness.

A series of studies have yielded findings that mentally retarded children when placed in an intensive physical conditioning program for several weeks sometimes gained several I. Q. points as compared to a non-participating control group who remained essentially constant in their I. Q. Although the possibility exists that the extra attention given to the children in the physical-conditioning program may explain the increase in functional intelligence, another explanation is that their improved physical fitness enabled them to function mentally with increased efficiency, which would probably be accompanied by an associated improvement in self-satisfaction and mental health. Several investigators have concluded that (1) participation in athletics and the development of the physique and motor skills result in an improvement in social adjustment; and (2) engaging in play and athletics enhances social development.

Lula C. Lion conducted a study involving 200 freshmen college women. He found a significant relationship between self-concept and body concept in most of the five dimensions measured, which suggests that body security is related to personal security for facing one's self and the world. That fact, then, reinforces a need for physical fitness as it relates to mental health.

Drs. C. C. Cowell and A. H. Ismail studied the relationship between the degree of personal acceptance, motor fitness, and athletic aptitude of 83 ten- to twelve-year-old boys. They found that boys who score high on physical measures are likely to have leadership potentialities, to be accepted at close personal contact by their friends, and to be well adjusted socially.

The California Psychological Inventory was administered to 334 team sport athletes and nonparticipants by Jack Schendel. Based on his findings, he concluded that psychological differences existed between athletes and nonparticipants. Ninth-grade athletes possessed more desirable personal characteristics than nonparticipants. Twelfth-grade athletes generally possessed desirable personal-social-psychological differences when compared to nonparticipants, but that finding was reversed when college athletes and nonparticipants were compared.

In a study of 100 nonathletes and 400 high school athletes classified by sport, Dr. Howard Slusher compared personality traits with athletic participation. He found intelligence to be significantly lower and hypochondria (morbid anxiety about health) to be higher for all athletic groups than for the nonathletes. The football and wrestling groups had strong neurotic profiles, but the swimmers displayed little of those characteristics.

The California Psychological Inventory and the Phillips JCR Test (a vertical jump, a 100-yard shuttle run, and chinning) were administered to 818 high school boys by J. Burton Merriman. He concluded that motor ability is related to personality traits. The upper motor ability group (which possessed the highest level of physical fitness) scored significantly higher on intellectual and interest measurements than the lower motor ability group. Few significant differences were found on personality traits when athletes and nonathletes were matched on motor ability.

Stress

The findings of two studies perhaps clarify somewhat a small part of the relationship between physical fitness and mental health. Ernst D. Michael reviewed studies on stress and exercise and found apparent evidence that the stress-adaptation mechanism was conditioned through exercise. A lack of activity was thought to reduce the ability to withstand stress. The evidence indicated that adaptation to exercise gave a slight degree of protection against emotional stress. On the basis of his findings, Michael theorized that regular daily exercise improves the ability to withstand emotional stress through the effects of hormones on the nervous system. Dr. Celeste Ulrich measured the stress exhibited by college women when in competitive situations. She conjectured that "exercise while imposing a stress may also act as a homeostatic regulator of the body with regard to the resolution of physiological reactions elicited by emotional stressors," thus perhaps, resulting in an improvement in emotional health.

When considered in total, the findings of the studies reported above give some indication that regular participation in sports or exercise in general, develops a few personality traits that are considered favorable. However, in some instances, the findings contradict this conclusion. Also, for most personality traits, no distinguishable differences were found. A claim can perhaps be made that well-adjusted individuals tend to participate in physical activity. The findings reported indicated that physical fitness or participation in sports or exercise does not appear to make much of a positive contribution to the personality traits indicative of a well-adjusted person. In all the studies reviewed, personality traits and other variables were measured only once. No attempts were made to do long-term studies on the effects on personality or mental health of participation in regular physical activity for several months or longer. That type of approach would provide more substantial evidence than any of the studies yet attempted. Based on the findings of the research completed to date, it must be concluded that many gaps exist and that at this time little in the way of definitive conclusions can be made.

Why Recreation Contributes to Mental Health

In her book *Mental Health through Physical Education and Recreation,* Emma McCloy Layman, who has served as head psychologist at a children's hospital and a mental health institution, expresses the opinion that programs of physical education, recreation, and athletics "especially lend themselves to the possibility of realizing mental health valves" for the following reasons:

(a) They are concerned with the development of physical fitness, an important requisite for mental health.

(b) They contribute exceptionally well to the satisfaction of certain basic physiological and psychological needs.

(c) They "provide opportunities for spontaneous emotional expression (a characteristic of a well-adjusted or mentally-healthy person) and release from strain."

(d) They "provide acceptable channels for satisfaction of fundamental needs and desires in which emotions find a healthy outlet."

(e) They "provide release from strain, which relaxes and refreshes the participant, who may be physically tired but who experiences a reduction in his tensions and worries. That release is especially important for the adult who has few socially approved outlets from strain and tension."

(f) "Attitudes and habits developed in the physical education class, on the athletic field, and in the recreation group transfer readily to real-life situations for children and adults, because of the similarity between the social interaction involved in activities in these situations and those found outside the school and supervised group. Many of these benefits should also come to physically fit adults who engage in carry-over types of physical activity."

Dr. William Menninger, founder and director of the Menninger Clinic in Topeka, Kansas, for many years, made the following conclusion on the basis of clinical experience and research findings with his patients: "There are many outside the professions of play leadership who doubt that there is any necessity or value other than a fun value for the adult in his play activities.

"Mentally healthy people participate in some form of volitional activity to supplement their required daily work. This is not merely because they wish something to do in their leisure time, for many persons with little leisure make time for play. Their satisfaction from these activities meets deep-seated psychological demands quite beyond the superficial rationalization of enjoyment.

"Too many people do not know how to play. Others limit their recreation to being merely passive observers of the activity of others. There is considerable scientific evidence that the healthy personality is one who not only plays, but who takes his play seriously. Furthermore, there is also evidence that the inability and unwillingness to play reveals an insecure or disordered aspect of personality.

"Good mental health is directly related to the capacity and willingness of an individual to play. Regardless of his objections, resistance, or past practice, any individual will make a wise investment for himself if he does plan time for his play and take it seriously."

Some authorities, who have had years of observation and first-hand experiences with mental health and physical fitness, strongly believe that the two are intertwined and that one is important to the other. That position is reported by Ernst Michael, the head of a college physical education department, who has written, "Because of the fact that all illness and all healthiness are psychosomatic in nature, physical fitness and mental health are inseparable. Of course, the level of one will not always match the level of the other, but eventually an impairment in one area will have a detrimental effect on the other." Therefore, unless contrary evidence is uncovered by better designed, more sophisticated, long-term scientific research, the belief that physical fitness and mental health are related seems to have some justification.—*Donald R. Casady.* See PERSONALITY and SOCIAL CONTEXT.

METABOLISM

Metabolism the sum of many complex biochemical reactions, is the conversion of the body's organic material into useful energy for use in physiological processes. Resting or basal metabolism is the collective metabolism of the body while at rest.

Measurement of Metabolism

Metabolism may be measured by either direct or indirect methods. The former refers to the amount of heat produced per unit of time, while the latter refers to the oxygen consumed by the body in a stipulated period of time. The measurement of heat production involves the use of elaborate equipment and, for that reason, is seldom used. As a result, metabolism is most often measured by determining the oxygen consumed (direct method). Heat production can be determined from the oxygen consumed and is expressed as kilocalories (calories). The consumption of 1 liter of oxygen is equal to approximately 5 calories.

The amount of oxygen consumed by the body (metabolism) depends on several factors, including temperature, skill, nutrition, fitness level and body weight. The most important is body weight. If you compare the metabolism of large and small people, the difference will be striking. In such a case, metabolism is often expressed as the amount of oxygen consumed, or heat produced, per kilogram of body weight, or per square of body surface. Since fat does not consume oxygen and varies considerably from person to person, metabolism is sometimes expressed in terms of the "fat-free weight." See OXYGEN INTAKE.

The standard resting or basal metabolism rate for the typical person, weight around 150 to 160 pounds, is approximately 1.17 calories per minute, or 70 calories per hour. Based on the statistics presented above, the average person consumes slightly less than one-quarter of a quart of oxygen per minute, or about 14 quarts of oxygen per hour.

ing muscles and the skin. In a variety of ways, the entire body is affected by the metabolic process which provides the energy for exercise. It is on those adjustments that the numerous activities in this book have been classified.

Research has demonstrated that for exercise to be truly beneficial, especially to the circulatory-respiratory system, the pulse rate must be raised sufficiently, enough calories must be burned up, and that the oxygen consumed must be sufficient. The figure below illustrates that the three properties of beneficial exercise are directly related.

Classification of Work	Oxygen Consumed Per Minute	Calories Burned Per Minute	Pulse Rate Per Minute
Low	¼- ½ Quart	1.17- 2.49	
Mild	½-1 Quart	2.5 - 4.99	Less than 100
Moderate	1 -1½ Quarts	5.0 - 7.49	Less than 120
Moderate High	1½-2 Quarts	7.5 - 9.99	Less than 140
High	2 -2½ Quarts	10.0 -12.49	Less than 160
Very High	2½ Quarts +	12.5 +	170 and above

Effect of Exercise

Exercise requires an increase in metabolic reactions that supply energy for the varied activities of the living cells. There is an increased requirement for the transport of oxygen to muscles and the removal of waste products from the muscles which requires an adjustment in respiration and circulation. See OXYGEN REQUIREMENT. Those adjustments involve stepped-up breathing and circulation and diversion of blood to the work-

A great many sports and activities are classified on work-intensity basis: as high-energy cost to low-energy-cost activities.

Because various activities vary in intensity, you are able to sustain those routines for longer periods of time— an important implication for establishing workout periods and guidelines for work.

Another important aspect of metabolism is oxygen debt. Simply stated, oxygen debt occurs during certain

GUIDELINES FOR WORK

Classification of Work	Length of Time that Work Can Be Maintained
Low	Indefinite
Mild	Eight hours a day
Moderate	Eight hours a day for a few weeks
Moderate High	Eight hours a day for a few weeks
High	Four hours—two or three times a week
Very High	One to two hours. A pulse rate of 180 or more— only a few minutes.

levels of exercise when the muscles demand more oxygen than they can receive. For example, you may be able to take in only 3 quarts of oxygen per minute but exercise at a rate that requires 4 quarts of oxygen. You, therefore, incur a debt of 1 quart of oxygen for each minute of exercise. At rest, your oxygen intake will remain above your normal resting level, which may be ½ quart, until the debt has been repaid. During the period of exercise, therefore, ¾ of the necessary energy was obtained by aerobic metabolism and ¼ by anaerobic metabolism. See OXYGEN DEBT for a more complete discussion. See also ENERGY COST OF ACTIVITIES.

MIDDLE AGE

Can a middle-aged person still engage in vigorous exercise? After 30 should he start tapering off his activities and direct his efforts toward less strenuous activities? What really happens in middle age? Those are all questions that concern the person who is approaching that age bracket.

What Is Middle Age?

The process of aging varies considerably from one person to another, making it difficult to classify a certain group of people as middle-aged. Ideally, physiological age should be used as a classification, but most often middle age is used to refer to people between 30 and 60.

Many changes occur to the body during middle age. Often, people assume that those transformations occur because they are merely getting older and the body is slowly wearing out. But the fact is some of these modifications occur or are speeded up because of sedentary living and resultant obesity.

From early adulthood to old age, numerous changes take place in the cardiovascular, kidney, respiratory, muscular and endocrinological functions. Some cardiovascular changes recorded are a slow but steady increase in resting blood pressure, especially after age of 40, and a higher systolic blood pressure during exercise with a slower recovery. There is also an apparent rise in cholesterol levels. Research has demonstrated, furthermore, that there is a decrease in the maximum heart rate experienced during exercise and that cardio-output at rest decreases with age, with the most significant drop occurring between the ages of 35 and 45 and a steady decline thereafter.

Kidney function changes appreciably during middle age. The standard glomerular filtration rate increases until around 45 to 48 years of age, after which there is a steady decline. Kidney plasma flow also decreases.

With increasing age the respiratory system shows a decrease in vital capacity, maximal breathing capacity, and maximum oxygen intake.

Other significant changes are a decrease in basal metabolism rate, in nerve conduction velocity (affect reaction time), in work rate, and in muscular strength, muscle endurance and circulo-respiratory endurance. It appears that during middle age a person's tolerance to heat decreases, thereby inhibiting activity in hot, humid climate. Sexual activity or vigor decreases with age. Moreover, there is a very gradual increase in weight, that may go unnoticed for quite sometime. This process is often called "creeping obesity." See also AGING.

Why Age Brings Changes

One theory advanced by Dr. Nathan Shock is that aging is really "the progressive changes that take place in a cell, tissue, or organism with the passage of time. The end result of those changes is an increase in mortality rate with increasing age."

Although those adjustments are inevitable owing to aging of cells and tissues, that aging, at least during the middle years, may be the result of dis-use. Much of the decline may result from cessation of work. It becomes apparent, therefore, that inevitably you will age, but that you need not age as fast. Exercise and diet can go a long way in helping you avoid the pitfall of disuse and the resulting complications. See DEGENERATIVE CARDIO-VASCULAR DISEASE.

Research tends to indicate that exercise can aid significantly in slowing down the aging process during middle age, for exercise can be helpful in reducing cholesterol and blood pressure. See CHOLESTEROL and BLOOD PRESSURE. It can also positively affect oxygen intake, muscular strength, muscle endurance, circulo-respiratory endurance and weight. See MUSCULAR ENDURANCE, OXYGEN INTAKE, OBESITY, STRENGTH, CIRCULO-RESPIRATORY ENDURANCE and WEIGHT CONTROL.

Although many of those changes are associated primarily with physical performance, improvement, or maintenance, of the functions can go a long way in slowing down the aging process at least by giving you greater stamina for the day's work and providing you with a desirable hobby. Improvement in several of those areas can also help you to reduce the possibility of developing degenerating cardiovascular diseases that may be a great plague now and in later life.

How Much Exercise?

It is becoming quite evident that during middle age a person need not taper-off his training as previously believed. The traditional concept was that a middle-aged person should concentrate on activities that were not demanding. Today, however, vigorous exercise is becoming a prerequisite for a healthy organism. In fact, the exercise level must be sufficient to get the pulse rate up to at least 140 and burn up to 300 to 500 calories in ½ hour. See INTENSITY OF EXERCISE. Of course, the program for making that goal will be slower than in earlier

years. It will also be imperative to warm-up and taper-off, because the circulatory system will not be as flexible. See WARM-UP and TAPERING OFF.

Provided the person has the medical approval and follows the previously described principles, there is no danger in vigorous exercise. In fact, it will be quite helpful to most middle-aged people. See EXCESSIVE EXERCISE.

MOTIVATION

There are thousands of people who have inspired themselves to make action a part of their daily lives. Some have gotten in the habit of doing only a few mild calisthenics each day, while others have become long-distance runners. But regardless of what levels of physical achievement those successful fitness-seekers have sought to achieve, they have made use of the same basic psychological principles to break out of their sedentary ruts. No matter how many "fitness failures" you have experienced in the past, there is no reason why you, too, can't use these successful ideas that help make exercise an automatic part of everyday life.

First thing to realize is that everyone is different. If you would set out to try to find two people with the same combination of height, weight, body build, physical skills and mental outlook you would soon see that you have an impossible task. Yet all those qualities are ingredients in the fitness equation. Each has a profound influence on how well a person can go through a certain set of exercises and keep following a particular routine from day to day. And add to those strictly personal differences the variations in the way we live and work, the different facilities for exercise we have available and also the variation in fitness goals we are trying to achieve.

Most people who make up their minds to try to correct their flabby shape, pick up a pamphlet outlining a specific exercise program. Two of the most popular are the Canadian Air Force 5-BX program and the booklet *Adult Physical Fitness* put out by the U.S. government. Hundreds of thousands of those exercise plans have been distributed. They give an exact set of exercises which have been engineered by experts, and there is no doubt that they constitute an effective fitness program. Differences in individual strength and fitness potential are accommodated by the listing of levels of achievement which call for different numbers of repetitions of exercises and some changes in the program. But all newcomers are given one set of exercises to do, and as they get proficient at those they graduate to level two, and on up.

While many people have made good use of these standard exercise programs, and in fact some have made them a permanent part of their lives, the number of dropouts far exceeds those who remain faithful to the exact program in the manual. It is really too much to expect that one specific set of calisthenics, even though they are most carefully thought out by experts, will please everybody all the time. So if you have tried one of the standard programs and eventually given it up, don't consider that you are a permanent fitness failure. There is more than one route to fitness. In fact there are probably as many ways to become fit as there are people. You simply have not yet found the best way for you. If you keep looking, sooner than you think you will find a way to exercise that you will enjoy, and which will help you toward the fitness you are hoping for.

Choosing A Fitness Type

There are three broad types of fitness which appeal to average people:
1. Circulo-respiratory fitness, the conditioning of the heart and lungs to improve your "wind" and provide protection against heart attacks. Continuous movement that will increase your heartbeat promotes cardiovascular fitness. Fast walking, jogging, bicycling, climbing, swimming and many other sports are the exercises widely used.

2. Building strength. Young people go for body power improvement in a big way, but it also appeals to middle-aged men and women who are looking for greater ability at sports and health benefits like prevention of low back pain. Calisthenics, isometrics, and mild weight training are the most popular strength-building exercises.

3. Improving body contours. Streamlining waists and hips, trimming down thighs, filling out the arms—those are typical goals of many people. Calisthenics will help, but so will cardiovascular exercises like jogging and swimming. A variety of exercises is best for achieving that goal.

Do some thinking now and decide what kind of fitness you personally want to achieve. Maybe you are after several kinds of fitness. If so, it might help to list them in the order you consider important.

Start your search for action by deciding which activities appeal to you most. Make it a point to sample them, even if you don't think at the outset that you will make them permanent parts of your exercise plan. Jogging doesn't appeal to you, you think? Well, run around the block anyway just to see whether you might like it. You are not a potential cyclist? How do you know until you try? Make a quick study of your home town or neighborhood for fitness opportunities, and possibly make a list of things you might do close to home. Put down every activity that occurs to you, whether you think you will like to do it or not. Decide after you try how you rate these activities for personal appeal.

Ignore Your Inhibitions

Right here you are going to run into the biggest stumbling block to fitness—the fear that you will look funny doing something different, or that your lack of skill at a sport or game will expose you to ridicule. You may be afraid to try tennis because you think you'll look stupid handling a racket, or you won't want to try jogging because you think people will make jokes.

Being concerned about how you'll look jogging down the street or riding a bicycle is even more ridiculous. The fact is that most experienced exercisers get to like demonstrating that they are not just one of the pack of human sheep who don't have the drive or imagination to do things that are unusual. Their view of the world is not limited to what they can see from their automobile windows or on their television screens. Exercisers get to sense nature directly, in all its moods, and enjoy the experience fully.

Slash Away at Excuses

Most intelligent people realize that they should exercise to be healthy and to feel vigorous, but their failures to follow a regular program have created feelings of guilt. Gradually, they cease trying to fight off the vice of sluggishness, and make a mental list of excuses for doing nothing. "If I walk, my feet will hurt." "If I run, I will perspire and my clothes will get messy." "Whenever I exercise I get hungrier, eat more and gain weight." All excuses of that type are basically fraudulent, for there are safe, sane and pleasurable ways for everyone to exercise, even those who have had heart attacks, hernias, and many other real health problems. If you are going to break out of your sedentary rut for good, you will have to slash away at the excuses for not exercising that have plagued you—but it must be done carefully and thoughtfully. Enthusiasm should be directed at the goal of moving closer to fitness every day, not to setting records or becoming a strong man overnight.

Aching feet can be one of the most crippling of disabilities. Few people want to exercise when their feet hurt. If you have that problem, look carefully at your shoes. Do they provide plenty of room, ample cushioning for the pounding of constant walking, and the proper support for the complex bone and muscle structure of the foot? Try different shoes or get advice from a foot specialist until your feet are healthy. Then go on to exercise pleasurably.

Don't let your initial enthusiasm trick you into exceeding your capacity. Starting a walking program with a 10-mile hike is foolish. So is rushing through a calisthenic program, or constantly testing yourself by probing the outer limits of your strength. Mature people should do most exercises gently, being careful not to put too much leverage on joints or to stretch the body unthinkingly.

Sure, sooner or later you will get aches and pains, but your enthusiasm for exercise will last longer if you try to prevent them. And you can help yourself greatly by learning which kinds of pains to ignore and which to heed. Most simple pains from exertion should be ignored, because more exercise will help iron them out. If in doubt, rest for a few days until they go away. Then resume your program with the same vigor as before. Being able to understand and cope with minor exercise injuries is extremely important to maintaining interest in a fitness program.

Picking a time for exercise is a problem for some people. Many of the exercise books say that you should set aside a definite time each day for exercise, a practice which probably suits some people but not necessarily all. The nonexerciser may get hung up at the outset of his plan on the decision when to start. He may think he is too groggy in the morning before breakfast, too rushed after breakfast, too busy to exercise at work, and too tired in the evening. Actually, he is just putting into action the excuse process, especially if he is telling himself that at certain times of the day he is too lethargic to get moving. Experienced exercisers know that there is nothing like a little movement to spin the cobwebs out of the head and perk up flagging spirits, especially if the exercise is something you enjoy doing. But you have to make a start sometime—anytime—to know that a fitness program can really be fun. Just start, seek out the fun of fitness, and you'll be darn sure to start making time for exercise—because almost everyone can make time for fun.

Keys to Motivation

Personal associations and relations with other people are extremely important to exercise motivation. Like it or not, we naturally give weight to what other people are doing, and what they think of us. Because most of us live in a society of unfit people, we must exert unusual personal effort to inspire ourselves to move. People with leadership qualities are best able to muster the magnitude of will power needed.

A good example of a civilian group effort for fitness was the recent National YMCA Marathon, a "race" where teams of 25 joggers from different local Y's sought to cover the simulated distance from New York to San Francisco in the shortest time. Canton, Ohio's, Y won the 1967 championship in the record time of 6½ days, through a tremendous group assault on the distance by business and professional men who logged an average of 18 miles of jogging each day. One man ran 42 miles in one day, for high individual honors.

Here are some comments from the runners themselves: "The spirit of this race is spreading. Even guys not in the race are running more after seeing that everyone is running." "A man can do so much more than he ever thought physically possible," said another man.

Yes, it is possible to break out of a sedentary rut. First start your mind working in the right direction. Your muscles will follow right along.—*Robert Rodale*

MOTIVATION OF THE LOW FITNESS PERSON

Motivation is difficult to define and describe in specific terms. We may know when a person has it and when he does not. But, many times, it is difficult to tell why one person is and another is not motivated. A part of this very complex general phenomenon is the difficulty to determine how a person becomes motivated. Motivation is very individual. The solutions required to motivate a low-fitness person are about as variable as the many sizes and shapes of people. In fact, the size and shape of a person might give some hints for the solution of the puzzle.

Importance of Goals

An important concept underlying the motivation of anyone is that he must establish a goal or an aim which is sufficiently attractive to give him the necessary perseverance. That requires emotional as well as intellectual involvement, and it may be necessary if the person has developed a defeated attitude to encourage him to choose a long-term goal. Getting a person to consciously or sub-consciously select a goal is ordinarily not too difficult, however, because most low-fitness individuals would prefer to be in a higher fitness category.

Self-discipline and Sub-goals

To help a person develop the quality of discipline necessary to stay with a physical conditioning program long enough to make physiological changes is a much more difficult problem than it is to get him to select a goal. That requires specific sub-goals (progressions) with some type of reinforcement for each evidence. It would be motivating to experience some improvement in those characteristics. Some measurements must be recorded that will reflect changes accurately. The experience of some success or sincere encouragement from the supervisor with a personal interest may be sufficient to carry the person through the "I want to quit stage." After a period of time self-evaluation, test performances and the personal feeling of well being should be sufficient to help the individual develop a positive attitude toward his physical condition.

The motivation to undertake and continue a conditioning program must come from within the individual rather than from another person. That really means that he must develop an attitude that will require him to keep on the conditioning program. Frequently, when a person begins a conditioning program, he is highly motivated and has a good attitude. The enthusiasm often fades rapidly, however. Our sedentary habits and pressure-society tend to destroy enthusiasts. One of the things that is strategic in keeping an individual on the program is the realization of some success toward reaching the major objectives of the program. If one objective is to lose weight, even a small weight loss will be encouraging.

Recently I visited the United States Marine Corps basic training center at Parris Island, where I saw some almost unbelievable perseverance and consequent results accomplished with extremely low-fitness young men. They were part of the special training battalion which is composed of men selected for a program of intensive physical conditioning because of their low-fitness level. The beginning level of many of these poorly conditioned men was as low as I have ever observed. Yet, in an average time of about 14 days, a large percentage of those men were able to progress from

the special training battalion back to regular marine basic training. The average weight loss of the overweight marines was 1.1 pounds per day even though their caloric intake was approximately 2,400 calories. Of course, the motivation and time devoted were much greater than that allotted by the average individual for training, but the results clearly showed the possibilities of changes in physical status with very hard effort. The reason for the intensive motivation of that group seemed to be one of peer status since the big desire was to get back with their regular training group. A major reason why a boy of that type enlists in the Marine Corps is that he believes the Corps can *make men* and he is not satisfied with his present status. Thus, he has internal motivation.

Factors Involved in Low Physical Fitness

In order to motivate a low-fitness person, you must gain some background as to why that person is in his present condition. The reasons for low physical fitness, like the solutions to the motivation problem, are many and varied. The low-fitness individual may have an adverse reaction to physical conditioning because of his early experience in playing games. He may simply have not had early experience in physical activity, or he may have been somewhat slower in picking up the various skills, thus being chided or teased so that he avoided almost all physical activity. Consequently, he slowly but steadily fell behind in years of physical development, all in all a very vicious cycle.

Many times the reason for low fitness is simply the individual's body build. Individuals with certain body health (somatotypes) find it very difficult to participate successfully in some activities. After a series of failures, it is easy to develop a "defeated" attitude.

Low fitness status may be related

to maturity since the individual may not be able to make a realistic self-appraisal of himself. If he does not realize his poor physical condition or if he honestly believes that he is doing the "best he can do," it is quite easy to fall farther behind.

General Principles

The low-fitness individual needs to realize that fitness is important enough so that he wants to make a change. That importance generally hinges on the aspects of the physiological benefits of physical health or possible peer status rewards which can be expected with increases in strength, endurance and general physical skill. According to Hein and others, the contributions of physical activity to physical health are: (1) assisting in weight control, (2) preventing cardiovascular disease, (3) decreasing aging and increasing longevity, and (4) helping to prepare one to meet emergencies. Orientation to those benefits may impress some. In fact, if the serious nature of the low fitness condition is not sufficient to motivate the person, then the possible benefits that can be gained through exercise may provide useful motivation. In that sense, the benefits could serve a "reward function." If the person gets involved enough to realize that someone really wants to help him and the desire to improve his physical health becomes important enough so that he is motivated, he still may be missing one link before he will begin to "involve" himself. He needs to realize that a reasonable solution to his dilemma exists, i.e., that it is possible for "him" to actually gain some of the benefits of exercise. The young men in the special training battalion of the Marine Corps have shown that satisfactory results are possible even if the beginning status is tremendously low.

If you attempt to motivate a low-fitness person, demonstrate to that person that you have a genuine desire to *help him*. If the low-fitness person can get the "feeling" that you are really interested in his physical well-being, the prerequisite to motivation participation is frequently satisfied.

Specific Techniques for Motivation

In addition to the general principles of motivation to be considered for the low-fitness individual, the following specific principles related to the conditioning program should be considered by physical educators, medical doctors, parents, Y directors, and anyone else who is vitally interested in improving another person's low fitness level.

1. Show a sincere interest in the person.
2. Be enthusiastic in your guidance.
3. Develop rapport and get to know the individual.
4. Be aware of differences in philosophy and personality and try to understand the thinking of the person in consideration.
5. Approach strong points and assist in developing a positive attitude.
6. Find out the reasons for the poor physical condition—one of the better ways is to get the person to write an autobiography after rapport is gained.

In addition to those principles mentioned above:

1. Determine the current status of the individual.
2. Design a good measurement program that will be motivational and also assess the subject in terms of his objectives. (Fatty tissue and cardiovascular measurements are of interest to adult men, strength and endurance are important to young boys and men, and body measurements and personal appearance are important considerations for girls.)
3. Develop a good program designed for the individual.
4. Remove fears of the individual and then subtly lead him into successes in those areas. For example, if

the person is fat, it is not a good idea to ask him to support his body with his arms or work on high apparatus because it is easy for him to get hurt in trying to do a simple dismount off the equipment.

5. Guide him toward interesting articles on fitness techniques and values.

6. If at all possible, get a partner of similar ability to work with him.

7. Develop progress reports and go over them with the person at intervals.

8. Make the program fun and exciting so the person is eager to come back for more.

9. Let the individual help you plan his program and try to teach him how to do it so that he can plan his own conditioning program after a period of time. In other words, make certain that there is some "education" in the physical "training" program.

The motivation of a low-fitness individual in physical activity is very difficult. The individual case study approach is generally recommended, including utilizing the advice of a multidisciplinary group. It is important to consider the medical, health, academic and personal-social aspects of an individual. That means that the medical profession, nurses, teachers, counselors, parents, and peers of an individual may have important information that you can use in motivating the low-fitness person to reach his objectives. In fact, if you are going to be successful in working with low-fitness individuals the most important underlying attitude is to want to *help* each individual rather than just outlining a program and telling him to get on with it.—*Arne L. Olson.* Adapted from *The Pennsylvania Journal of Health, Physical Education and Recreation*, July 1967.

MOTOR ABILITY

Dr. Thomas K. Cureton, notes that motor ability is the ability to execute any motor skills—athletic or not. Type-

writing, washing dishes, driving a car, hitting a golf ball, kicking a soccer ball and running are all examples of motor skills.

Performance Levels

Everyone has a different performance level in the many motor skills. Cureton recognized these differences and indicated that a motor genius is a person who learns many motor skills quickly and excels in several. Athletically, a good example of that type of person is the decathlon champion. At the opposite end is the motor moron. He is the person who has difficulty in learning and performing many motor skills. Most people fall somewhere between these extremes, for motor ability for the majority of the population is specific rather than general. That is, you may excell in one sport or activity but perform poorly at another.

Components of Motor Ability

There are many separate components involved in motor ability. The major ones are speed, power, agility, balance, muscle strength, muscle endurance, circulo-respiratory endurance, flexibility, kinesthesia, reaction and movement time, motor educability, motor fitness and physique or body type. (For a discussion of these particular components, see the individual entry.) Other vital components are hand-eye coordination, foot-eye coordination, rhythm, vision, and arm and hand steadiness. Further refinements of hand-eye coordination are aiming and dexterity.

Hand-eye and foot-eye coordination—Those two components indicate the relationship between the eyes and hands and the eyes and legs regarding timing and the extent to which the eyes and limbs act together in performing a skill. It is the manner in which the limbs respond to the visual stimuli that a person receives. The movement may be large such as in shoveling snow or more refined as in typewriting.

Rhythm—Somewhat related to kinesthesia, rhythm is the movement or force experienced in muscle action. The muscle action is controlled, thereby giving you a smooth movement rather than a "spastic" or uneven movement.

Vision—That component refers to what you perceive with your eyes. It includes peripheral vision, depth perception, and the ability to estimate the location of a moving object.

Arm and hand steadiness—Arm and hand steadiness is, as its name implies, the steadiness with which arm and hand movements can be made, such as putting a thread through the eye of a needle and pistol shooting.

Aiming—Aiming is a limited form of eye-hand coordination, such as skeet shooting or adjusting a microscope.

Dexterity—Dexterity, a further refinement of eye-hand coordination, is the ability to make coordinated arm, hand and/or finger movements in a rapid response. Cradling a lacrosse stick or seeing how rapidly you can put a series of blocks in corresponding holes are examples.

Motor ability is really the ability to put all these separate components into a coordinated pattern for a certain skill. Many people call that ability *coordination*. You usually learn how to coordinate those components by actually practicing the skill. (See MOTOR LEARNING.)

Importance of Practice

The practicing of a skill, according to Dr. Franklin Henry at the University of California, helps you store the coordinated pattern in the brain in what might be called a memory drum. Whenever you need to perform that skill you call upon that memory drum to "play back" that skill, and the movement is made somewhat automatically depending upon how well it was learned previously.

For example, when you were first learning to drive a standard-shift car you may have thought it was practically impossible to coordinate all the necessary skills needed for driving. Yet after regular practice, the actions became automatic. You no longer had to "think" about putting in the clutch and releasing the pressure on the gas pedal before moving the gear shift. You learn to react to various stimuli without even consciously thinking about it. The same is true when you learn to walk, eat, run, throw a ball, or ride a bike. When you are riding your bicycle and start to lose your balance, you adjust automatically by turning your wheel in the direction in which you are falling.

There is some carry-over from the learning of one skill to another, although not as much as traditionally assumed. For example, a person who has learned to play tennis and plays it quite well will probably learn the game of badminton more quickly than a person who has never held a tennis or badminton racket. Both skills involve hitting an object with a racket, and both may involve some similar strategy. The transfer or carry-over is usually in the initial stages of learning a new skill because of the similarity to skills previously learned. The actual stroking of the object, however, is different. In tennis, the movement requires the entire arm with the main action at the elbow and shoulder, while in badminton wrist action is the most important. Therefore, if all things are equal, after a period of practice, the non-tennis player may match or surpass the tennis player in badminton skill. The skills that carry over to another skill and the skills that interfere with the learning process are not well established. Generally, the parts that are identical transfer easily, but similar parts of a skill seem to conflict for some performers and make the new skill more difficult.

It is apparent that motor ability is

dependent upon the exposure to various activities and skills. The more exposure generally, the greater the skill level. The degree to which you can learn a skill, however, is limited by heredity. (See HEREDITY). A child must, therefore, be exposed to many activities in order to develop his motor abilities to his capable level. Participation in one sport or activity will certainly not make him a well-rounded individual for participation in a variety of activities. See ATHLETIC PARTICIPATION FOR YOUNGSTERS.

Some of you may wonder about the person who seems to learn everything well, such as the motor genius that Dr. Cureton talked about. An individual may be born with a high degree of motor educability (see MOTOR EDUCABILITY). He may have been genetically endowed with a higher degree of muscle strength, speed, or kinesthesia than the average person, thereby permitting him to excell in many activities. Or he may have been that fortunate individual who was exposed to a wide range of activities as a child, therefore giving him a large "memory bank" to draw on. The major portion of the population, however, does not fall in that fortunate category.

A series of motor ability tests (see TESTS) have been devised to measure motor ability. The results of the tests, however, should be interpreted as a measurement of your experiences in motor activities rather than your total coordination. See MOTOR FITNESS and PHYSICAL FITNESS.

MOTOR BEHAVIOR

Motor behavior is a general term used to refer to movements which are used in skilled performances. The movements must be observable. They are not the movements of the heart rate, blood circulation, nervous impulses and the like. The movements need not be goal directed or voluntary.

MOTOR EDUCABILITY

Motor educability is the ease with which you learn new physical skills. It is related to such terms as coordination and general athletic ability and is determined by the speed with which you learn a new skill even though you had never seen the game played or were not aware of the skills involved.

Some researchers believe that motor educability is not being valid since the learning of a skill is specific to the task being learned, not the overall ability of the person. The fact remains, however, that some people learn faster than others when attempting a motor skill. Dr. Bryant Cratty states that those quick learners of a motor skill are highly motivated, possess above average strength, are able to analyze quickly and correctly the mechanics of the task, and are free of excess tension in learning the task. That is, they do not demonstrate an over amount of inhibitions in learning the skill. Too much inhibition can cause you to refuse to learn a new skill for fear of being embarrassed or ridiculed.

The entire area of motor educability and whether there is such a component is a fertile field for investigation by researchers. See MOTOR ABILITY, MOTOR FITNESS, PHYSICAL FITNESS and TESTS.

MOTOR FITNESS

According to Dr. H. H. Clarke, the term "motor fitness" originated during World War II, but its exact definition is a subject of controversy. Clarke suggested that motor fitness has a wider connotation than physical fitness and has more dimensions or factors involved. For the purposes of this discussion, motor fitness will be taken to mean the fitness of the motor apparatus of the body which enables it to initiate and sustain or repeat the development of force in a variety of situations.

First, it must be recognized that man is a unity, a complex integrated being. The division of mind and body is outdated. The physical and mental functions in man are interrelated in such a way that one cannot isolate the physical from the mental processes involved in the performance of a motor task. And yet we must look at the different aspects of the complex processes involved in motor performance in order to determine their precise make-up.

In considering the composition of motor fitness, there would appear to be few clearly defined, readily identifiable factors. In their place are found loosely defined, often interchangeable terms, such as strength, power, endurance, stamina, balance, speed, agility, flexibility and mobility. Those terms are used to describe extremely complicated areas which indicate some of the many physical abilities which man possesses. It is believed that motor fitness, as defined above, can be considered to depend upon exertion of force, speed of movement, range of movement and work capacity.

The performance of a motor task would also inevitably involve some mechanism to control the motor apparatus of the body because of the information supplied by the perceptual apparatus of the body utilizing the senses of hearing, sight, touch and kinesthesis. That mechanism would control, for a specific motor task, the amount of force required, the speed, direction, and extent of the movement, and the supply of energy. However, the controlling mechanism and the perceptual apparatus of the body are not included in this concept of motor fitness—the state of preparation of the motor apparatus—and will not be discussed further.

Exertion of Force

The ability to exert force is related to the size of the muscle fibers and, consequently, to the total cross-section of the muscles involved. The strength of a muscle or group of muscles is the maximum force that can be exerted in a single effort. The amount of force that can be exerted by muscles varies in different situations because different variables are involved, such as the position of the body. The expression of strength is highly specific to the situation and needs differentiating into the following three types:

Isometric or Static Strength

That type of strength is demonstrated when force is exerted against an immovable object. It is measured by means of a dynamometer or cable tensiometer in situations where force is exerted until a maximum is reached. The amount of movement in the testing instrument is minimal and nonexistent at the time the maximum force is exerted.

Isotonic Strength

That type of strength is demonstrated when movement occurs while force is applied. The magnitude of the strength is represented by the maximum resistance that can be moved in a given direction from a particular position. Isotonic strength is involved in two types of muscular contraction:

a. a concentric contraction which occurs when the muscle shortens while developing sufficient tension to overcome the resistance, e.g., flexing the elbow joint with a weight in the hand.

b. an eccentric contraction which occurs when the muscle lengthens while under the control of the individual but exhibits tension throughout the range of movement, e.g., extending the elbow joint to slowly lower a weight in the hand.

Explosive Strength

Sometimes referred to as power or energy mobilization, it involves the ability to exert maximum force or energy in an explosive act. The distinguishing feature is the speed of the movement—the speed with which one can exert maximum force. It is demonstrated when you are required to throw yourself or an external object as far or as high as possible.

Speed of Movement

This is the ability of all or part of the human body to cover a given distance in the shortest possible time. It is related to the explosive strength of the muscles, and to a large extent, speed of movement and explosive strength are probably dependent upon the speed of muscle contraction. The structure of the muscle has implications for the speed of movements. In many muscles, there are both red and white fibers which have different characteristics. White muscle fibers are capable of contracting more quickly, reaching maximum tension more rapidly, and returning to their normal resting length in a shorter time than red muscle fibers, which are able to sustain a given contraction for a longer period of time.

The structure of man is basically a lever system utilizing bones as levers and joints as hinges, with the muscles supplying the motive force, aided by gravitational force in some situations. The majority of the levers in the human body are third class levers which favor speed and range of movement. If two levers of differing lengths move through the same angle in the same time, the moving end of the longer lever will travel a greater absolute distance than the moving end of the shorter lever. Because the time of movement is the same for both levers, the rate of movement (or speed) of the end of the longer lever is greater than that of the short lever. The majority of the motor tasks performed by man involve a series of levers working together, resulting in the required speed of the movement being achieved with the greatest economy of effort.

That phenomenon is revealed in situations demanding rapid body or limb movement, such as fast running, quick change of direction, and rapid movements of the arms and the legs.

Range of Movement

The ability to move the body parts through a wide range is dependent upon the freedom of movement in the joints of the body. The movement possibilities in joints, in terms of direction and extent, depend upon the shape of the bone surfaces of the joint, and the placement of muscles, ligaments, and other soft tissues such as the joint capsule and cartilage. That ability is ideally measured in terms of the number of degrees through which a given part of the body can be moved in a given direction. For a more detailed discussion, see FLEXIBILITY.

Work Capacity

The ability to continue performing an activity or the capacity to continue working involves either sustaining or repeating a sub-maximal effort. There are three types of work capacity.

Static Work Capacity (or Static Endurance)—the ability to maintain a sub-maximal static or isometric contraction. It can be expressed in terms of the length of time for which a given force of contraction can be maintained (that is, the holding time). Müller has pointed out that the capacity depends solely on strength, and that strength and holding time cannot be trained separately. The holding time is the same for all subjects and all muscle groups in any state of training. For example, according to Müller, 50 per cent of the maximal isometric strength for any subject and any muscle group could be held for approximately one minute.

Muscular Work Capacity (or Muscular Endurance)—the ability to repeat a sub-maximal effort as many times as possible. It appears to be related to the isotonic strength of the muscles and, to some extent, the blood supply to the muscles. The types of activity in which it is most often demonstrated are pull-ups, push-ups, leg lifts, and sit-ups. There appears to be an extremely wide range of ability in those test situations. For example, the number of sit-ups recorded varies from none to over 500.

For most people, the effort required is usually close to the maximum possible either by approximately the maximum strength of the person, in which case only a very few repetitions are made, or by approximating the maximum rate of working, in which case a time limit is used, for example, sit-ups in two minutes.

Circulo-Respiratory Work Capacity (or Circulo-Respiratory Endurance)— the ability to repeat a sub-maximal effort for as long as possible. That capacity is demonstrated particularly when the individual works in "steady state." The oxygen requirements of the activity are met largely by the oxygen supply during work. It reflects the aerobic capacity of a person—his ability to supply oxygen while working. It is dependent, to a large extent, upon the capacity of the heart and also upon the metabolic reserves. The intensity of the work is lower than that required in muscular work-capacity situations. The heart is called upon to pump vast quantities of blood to supply the oxygen needed by the working muscles. For low intensity work of long duration, the metabolic reserves of glycogen and fatty acids appear to be the limiting factor rather than the capacity of the circulo-respiratory system to supply oxygen.

The maximum attainable oxygen intake serves as the most significant criterion of the circulo-respiratory work capacity. It varies according to type of activity, state of training age and the extent of the musculature used at the time. Studies with highly trained athletes have shown that the amount of muscle mass involved in the performance of the activity is an important factor, because higher capacities are found if the test involves running, whereas smaller maximum capacities are found when the arms are used. At rest, the average oxygen intake for an adult male is approximately 0.25 liters per minute. The maximum oxygen intake recorded with some athletes is over 5.6 liters per minute.

Conclusion

The level of motor fitness achieved is primarily a function of the type and amount of activity to which a person is exposed. All of the force areas discussed above respond remarkably to training if designed and carried out in accordance with the fundamental principles of training. See MOTOR ABILITY and PHYSICAL FITNESS.—*E. R. Sandstrom*

MOTOR LEARNING

The efficiency with which you learn a motor skill is important not only for the time it saves but for the positive attitude which you develop when you learn the activity rapidly and easily. Greater enthusiasm and, consequently, greater participation are evident in those activities in which you experience early success. Conversely, you are likely to avoid those activities which have proved frustrating in early attempts. Therefore, for physical fitness values, as well as other benefits which result from frequent participation, it is important that the learning of physical activities be as efficient and pleasant as possible.

Efficiency in Learning and Teaching

The development of efficiency in the learning or teaching of skills must begin with some understanding of the learning process itself. Motor learning refers to the acquisition of skills involving bodily movement. Careful analysis reveals that acquiring most recreational or sports skills is an active, thoughtful process. Blind trial-and-error efforts are not only frustrating but largely ineffective. In learning a new skill, a thoughtful person may observe someone else perform the task, mentally put himself through the activity, and then attempt to duplicate the performance. After analyzing his performance and receiving advice from other persons, he may try again, making those adjustments which seem appropriate to him. Certain motor skills are learned slowly by some persons because of their inability to see the relationship between the response and the results. Action, feedback, evaluation and repeated action are major factors in the successful development of a motor skill. Learning a motor skill, therefore, is both a physical and a mental process. As such, it requires the total involvement of the learner in order to insure effectiveness.

Importance of Reinforcement

The most important single ingredient in the learning of skills is *reinforcement*. That concept, which had its roots in Thorndike's *Law of Effect*, refers to any condition which increases the probability that a given response will recur on subsequent occasions when similar conditions exist. Reinforcement is usually some type of pleasant occurrence such as the realization of success in the particular task, or being praised by the teacher. For example, the young baseball pitcher who makes the proper finger-wrist snap in his delivery may notice that the ball curves in the desired manner. As a result of this pleasant experience (success in curving the ball), he will most likely remember the particular finger-wrist action and, therefore, repeat it on future occasions.

The process of teaching motor skills involves guidance into appropriate responses and the reinforcement of these responses. It is true, however, that a great deal of learning takes place without formalized teaching. For example, the young pitcher may accidentally discover the wrist snap-curve ball relationship. But if he has no guidance, he wastes much time through the exploration of many inappropriate responses. On the other hand, when the learner is guided in his efforts, the process is usually speeded, and there is less waste of time. The first important function of the teacher, therefore, is to reduce the amount of irrelevant effort.

A second function of the teacher is to praise or, in some other way, reinforce appropriate action, especially when the activity does not produce results which are immediately obvious. For example, the bowler may exhibit an improved delivery but with no sudden improvement in score. In such a case, the teacher must reinforce his form, thus reinforcing that part of the performance. The role of the teacher in providing reinforcement is especially true in activities such as dance, swimming and gymnastics, where correct or incorrect responses are not always apparent. A valuable aid in the learning of any activity is to analyze the skills so that any small degree of improvement can be noticed. Recognition of any small amount of progress is most stimulating and the best assurance that it will be retained.

Mental Practice

The learning of motor skills may be greatly improved by the use of *mental practice* along with the regular physical practice. Mental practice refers to the imaginary or hidden experience which mentally duplicates the physical performance of the task. Research has shown that such thought when used in combination with regular practice can result in as much improvement as if the total practice time were spent in physical practice.

Mental practice can, in effect, serve to lengthen the practice session or provide more trials during a particular work period. Very often a person who is learning a sport skill will have a limited number of trials because he has to wait his turn or does not have ready access to the facilities or equipment. Use of appropriate mental practice during those sessions can provide for the learning of skills during such periods.

Mental activity in relation to the learning and performance of motor skills may take several forms. Those include (1) review which immediately precedes, follows, or coincides with performance; (2) formal or informal rehearsal which takes place between work periods; and (3) decision-making which relates to the strategy or planning of the activity. Review is most frequently noted when the gymnast, diver, bowler, or high jumper pauses briefly prior to beginning his performance to mentally go through a perfect execution of the task so that, during the actual performance which follows, the sequence of movements will be most vivid in his mind. The person who is upset because of a prior failure, the person who is unable to concentrate because of certain distracting factors, or the person who rushes into the performance without such deliberation most often commits common errors. Some performers review the performance immediately after it is completed, apparently in an effort to firmly establish a good routine. Occasionally a golfer, bowler, or some other performer will orally remind himself of a particular point during the performance in order to avoid a certain fault.

Situational decision-making has traditionally been encouraged by athletic coaches. For example, a baseball coach will say to each of his fielders "assume that every ball will be hit to you and plan ahead so that you'll know what to do with it." In most other team activities, performers are similarly encouraged to prepare ahead for any eventuality.

A sound habit is to review or mentally rehearse each skill prior to its performance at a practice session. Then time can be saved by reducing the usual amount of routine physical practice. Although the value of that technique is most obvious with new skills, it can also be helpful in preventing faults with familiar activities and insuring that the level of performance is as high as possible.

Distribution of Practices

Wise *distribution of practices* is one of the most critical factors in the learning of skills. It has long been established that individuals do not learn simply because they practice. Still there is the widely held assumption that learning is simply a factor of time spent in practice. The more you practice, the more you learn. A great deal of research has been conducted in recent years in regard to the massing or distribution of practice. Such investigation has involved verbal and novel motor tasks as well as regular sports skills and has established the following generalizations:

1. Distributed practices are generally more efficient for learning and performance than are massed practices.

2. Relatively short practices (in time or in number of repetitions) make for more efficient learning than do longer practices.

3. Progressively decreasing the concentration of practice periods during the learning period seems advantageous.

4. Progressively decreasing the length of practice periods during the learning period appears to make learning more effective.

5. Proficiency which has been gained over a long period of time is retained better than that which is developed within a short period.

6. Individuals or groups who are more competent in a particular activity can effectively practice that activity for longer periods than can persons or groups who are less competent.

Similarly, older children are able to practice longer than younger ones.

7. In physical education or sports activities, the number of repetitions or trials (shots, throws, dives, etc.) should be considered as the unit of practice rather than the time spent at the work session.

Those recommendations may be applied in a single practice period, or they may be put to use equally well on a seasonal basis. For example, during a unit of basketball, the instructor may attempt to teach dribbling, lay-up shots (with the right and left hand), jump shots, free throws, pivoting, passing (different types), faking, guarding, fast breaking and many other fundamentals of individual and team play. Some teachers might take a full period to try to do a thorough job in teaching one or two of these skills. Consequently a rather long practice (especially in number of repetitions) for the one or two skills will result. On the other hand, the teacher who makes effective use of short, distributed practices would have the students move more rapidly through a greater number of the skills during the class period. Each player may receive only three trials at a particular pivoting maneuver during the early part of the class. However, the teacher might well take the class through more than one round of the skills during a single period. It is probably better that the student practice two rounds of 5 left-handed lay-ups rather than one round of 10 trials of the same shot. The technique of going through the circuit of skills more than once, or covering a greater number of skills during a class period, seems to be an effective use of short and distributed practices.

The use of short work sessions on each skill demands that the skill be practiced on several occasions in order to develop adequate competency. For example, in the discussion of daily basketball practice, it was mentioned that several fundamental skills should be included each day. During the first few days of practice, it seems desirable to spend a relatively long period on each skill as it is introduced. On the following days, after some degree of success has been attained, a shorter period of time is devoted to the specific skill. Other new skills should be introduced on successive days and handled in a similar manner, with relatively long practices immediately after the skill is introduced. In this manner, several activities are included within each class period with the possibility of devoting different amounts of time to each. Group activity, whether in a lead-up drill or the total game, also can be conducted in this manner. One way of achieving distribution is to include game play (with other activites) only for a short period during the class time. Another way is to devote the total class time to the game but to introduce sufficient rest periods for the purpose of instruction, whether in fundamentals or in team strategy.

Transfer of Skill

The learning process becomes more efficient if the teacher and learner take full advantage of opportunities for transfer of skills. Being aware of these opportunities and planning for transfer can make the learning and performance of many skills easier. Many different activities have movements which are almost identical. Therefore, once the basic movement has been learned, it can be used in many activities. However, when the individual does not recognize that some particular movement is applicable, much time is lost in attempting to learn a new response. In popular skills, it is assumed that transfer would take place from rebound tumbling to diving, from the overhand throw in baseball to the overhead smash in tennis, from the soccer kick to the soccer-type field goal kick in football, and from the forehand and backhand strokes from tennis to squash. An analysis of common sports activities will reveal numerous other possibilities for transfer.

In addition to specific movements, certain general principles or concepts can be transferred to different activities. Those include such components as footwork, body positioning, and general strategy from tennis to squash, the general use of the follow-through technique in throwing or striking skills, and the strategy of double teaming (2 on 1, 3 on 2, etc.) in team sports.

In order to accomplish maximum transfer, it is important that new activities be analyzed for (1) specific skills, (2) general movement principles, and (3) strategy (where applicable) so that maximum carry-over from previously learned activities can be brought into use.

Retention

All skill learning will be more valuable if you are able to remember it for a reasonably long time. If skills cannot be remembered and therefore performed on the appropriate occasion, the time spent in practice will be largely wasted. In fact, there can be no improvement from trial to trial without some retention, because the learning of advanced concepts or skills depends upon an understanding and retention of certain prerequisites. Despite the obvious importance of remembering what has been learned, both teachers and students have been primarily concerned with immediate performance, often to the neglect of techniques which might improve long-term retention.

The retention of an unpracticed skill follows a decelerating curve. That is, most rapid forgetting takes place soon after the completion of practice. As time passes, less and less is forgotten, so that after a time practically no more forgetting occurs. Theoretically, a skill once learned is never completely forgotten. That is true despite the fact that an older person may not have the physical capability to perform a task that he learned in his youth.

The retention of motor skills may be improved by several techniques. Perhaps the most important of these is to initially learn the skill to a high level of competency. Overlearning, or the continuance of practice after the skill has been learned, is extremely helpful in promoting long-term retention. Research has shown that a certain amount of drill, following the first successful performance of the activity, is a sound investment. Such practice tends to "set," or reinforce, the learning so that it will be remembered longer.

Another technique which tends to promote retention is to learn the skill on a distributed practice schedule, i.e., work sessions that are spread out. Several studies have shown that most skills learned over a long period of time will be retained longer than those which are learned on a "crammed" practice schedule.

Skills which are meaningful to the learner are remembered better than those which are less well understood. Activities which are well organized, which are related to the individual's previous skills, and which seem appropriate will be learned and remembered best. Most people remember learning skills in which the required action was just the opposite of what seemed to be the right way to perform. Such a situation slows down learning and hinders retention. Therefore, it is a wise idea to clearly organize and understand the task before the beginning of practice.

You should avoid the learning of skills which are similar to the one which is to be retained. Such similar skills tend to be confusing when you attempt to perform the originally learned task. Therefore, the boy who is in the process of learning a proper baseball swing should not practice golf during that period. Though there are some similarities, the golf stroke is so different that it would interfere with the retention of the baseball swing. A second activity which is similar to the first should be delayed until the first one is well learned.

Reviewing is of great importance in the retention of skills. To be most effective the reviews, or brief practices, should be done reasonably soon after the conclusion of the learning period.

Interest

Skills which are of great interest to the person will be learned better and therefore remembered longer. The person will have a tendency to think about the skill (mentally practice) more frequently if his motivation is high. In general, an interesting task, well organized and practiced under desirable conditions, leads to good learning. Good learning, in turn, leads to good retention.—*Joseph B. Oxendine*

MOTOR PERFORMANCE

Motor performance is a voluntary, goal-directed movement and is an aspect of motor behavior. A typical example of motor performance is attempting to kick an extra point in football. Motor performance can be affected by a series of factors including skill level, personality, and anxiety or tension. See MOTOR BEHAVIOR and MOTOR SKILLS.

MOTOR SKILL

Motor skill is a reasonably complex motor performance for the individual, and the skill may be more complex for one person than another. The term "skill" indicates that some learning has taken place and that the movement is done in a coordinated manner. The speed and accuracy of movement are increased, and there is a decrease in the number of errors. To perform a motor skill requires learning. It cannot be done as a reflex or learned in a

single trial. See MOTOR BEHAVIOR and MOTOR PERFORMANCE.

MOUNTAIN CLIMBING (MOUNTAINEERING or ALPINISM)

Mountain climbing, a sport that has flourished since the 1800's, requires careful planning, adequate equipment, physical skill, endurance and daring.

Proper equipment includes packsacks containing first-aid supplies, food, additional clothing, and, if necessary, sleeping bags, cooking gear and a tent or shelter. Boots that are made of leather with rubber soles will be necessary. In some instances, rubber soles with lugs and/or leather soles with nails are desirable. An ice axe may also aid the mountaineer in cutting steps in ice and snow, keeping his balance, and stopping himself from falling. A mountaineer should also know how to use a compass and maps, because trails may be nonexistent or difficult to find.

If a day trip is planned, a climber usually begins at dawn so that adequate time is allowed for ascent and return. A good climber can expect to cover a mile of vertical height a day on low, easy mountains. On more difficult peaks, the mountaineer may cover only a few hundred feet a day. Furthermore, on high altitude climbs, the climber will be slowed by a lack of oxygen. See ENVIRONMENT (Altitude). Because of the lack of oxygen the climber will have to decrease the pace or use special oxygen equipment.

In treacherous climbing areas, climbers will rope themselves together in groups of two, three, or more so that one climber may act as a base or a hold if another slips or gets into trouble.

There are three phases of mountain climbing—hiking, rock climbing and climbing on ice and snow.

Famous climbing areas throughout

the world are United States—the Rocky Mountains, the Cascade Range, and the Sierra Madre Mountains; Canada—the Rocky Mountains; South America—the Andes Mountains; Asia—the Himalaya Mountains and the Karakoram Range; and Europe—the Alps.

Benefits

Regular participation in mountaineering will result in an improvement in circulo-respiratory endurance, for it is classified as a high-energy-consumption activity. Muscle endurance and strength will also be developed because it is quite demanding upon the major muscle groups, especially the leg muscles which get a good workout in walking, climbing, chimneying and rapelling.

Conditioning Programs

The two most important qualities to develop for mountaineering are leg-muscle endurance and circulo-respiratory endurance. Without those factors, you will soon falter and fail. The best way to condition for mountaineering is to get out on the trail and hike—the more strenuous the region the better. If there are any rocky cliffs available, use them regularly. When hiking, you should be able to cover 20 miles comfortably. Furthermore, as you are hiking, try to pace your breathing and breathe deeply. Traditionally, mountaineers train by inhaling for 6 to 8 paces, holding for two, and then exhaling for 6 to 8 paces.

There are also specific indoor exercises for further preparation: gradual, progressive *toe touching* (standing and sitting); *three-quarter knee bends* with weights and *walking squats* for developing the leg musculature; and stepping up and down on a chair for conditioning the legs and circulo-respiratory system. Start the exercise by standing in front of a chair and stepping up and down with both feet at 24 to 30 steps a minute. At the beginning, one minute is sufficient; you

should work up to 5 minutes of bench stepping. An alternate technique is to stand beside the chair and step up with only one leg for 25 steps, repeating with the other leg. Running or jogging are also important.

* MOUNTAIN CLIMBING PROGRAM

Chart 1	Chart 2
1. 10 minutes	1. 38 minutes
2. 15 minutes	2. 40 minutes
3. 18 minutes	3. 43 minutes
4. 20 minutes	4. 45 minutes
5. 23 minutes	5. 50 minutes
6. 25 minutes	6. 53 minutes
7. 30 minutes	7. 55 minutes
8. 33 minutes	8. 58 minutes
9. 35 minutes	9. 60 minutes

* See ENDURANCE and ENERGY COST OF ACTIVITIES for an explanation of these charts.

Fitness 1

If you achieved a score of poor or low average in the *Harvard Step Test* or a score of very poor or poor on the *12 Minute Run*, start on Chart 1-Level 1 and spend 1 week at each level until Chart 2-Level 9 is reached. It is recommended that you participate 4 to 5 days a week. When Chart 2-Level 9 is reached, 4 days a week is sufficient.

Fitness 2

If you achieved a score of high average on the *Harvard Step Test* or fair on the *12 Minute Run*, start on Chart 1-Level 2. Spend one week on Chart 1-Levels 2, 4, 6, 7, and 9, and Chart 2-Levels 2, 4, 5, 7, and 9. It is recommended that you participate 4 to 5 days a week. When Chart 2-Level 9 is reached 4 days a week is sufficient.

Fitness 3

If you achieved a score of good or excellent on either the *Harvard Step Test* or *12 Minute Run*, continue your current program or select Chart 2-Level 9 as your level of participation. Four days a week is sufficient.

Since mountain climbing is a high energy-cost-activity, it may be used to help improve your fitness level, especially your circulo-respiratory and muscle endurance. This mountaineering program takes into account the important principles of training.

Although mountain climbing takes a great deal more time than one hour, the program will give you an idea of the essentials for developing fitness.

Mountain Clubs

1. American Alpine Club, 113 East 90th Street, New York, N.Y. 10028.

2. Appalachian Mountain Club, 5 Joy Street, Boston, Massachusetts 02108.

3. Appalachian Trail Conference, Inc., 1916 Sunderland Place, N.W., Washington, D.C. 20036.

4. Colorado Mountain Club, 1400 Josephine Street, Denver, Colorado 80206.

5. Dartmouth Mountaineering Club 23 Robinson Hall, Hanover, New Hampshire 03755.

6. Denver University Alpine Club, 2050 E. Evans, Denver, Colorado 80210.

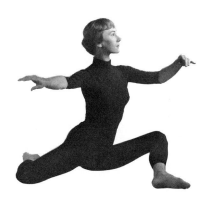

Movement education makes a person aware of his body and its efficient use.

7. Iowa Mountaineers, P.O. Box 163, Iowa City, Iowa 52242.

8. M.I.T. Outing Club, Massachusetts Institute of Technology, Cambridge, Massachusetts 02139.

9. Mountaineers. Mailing address: P.O. Box 122, Seattle, Washington 98111. Main Clubroom location: 719½ Pike Street, Seattle, Washington 98111.

10. Sierra Club, 1050 Mills Tower, San Francisco, California 94104.

MOVEMENT EDUCATION

Movement education is a relatively new idea in physical education. The program, developed in Germany and England, is in use in some American schools and, with exposure, should become more popular. Movement education, sometimes referred to as educational gymnastics, is directed toward young children and early adolescents. It deals with a student's awareness of his body, and the factors which determine movement, such as time, weight, space and flow. The program allows each child to have a physical movement experience all his own. Since each child is allowed to progress at his own rate and level, frustration is less likely to occur. Emphasis is placed on conscious control of the body.

The children are provided with problems that make physiological demands. No instructions are given as to how to solve the problem. There is no right or wrong way to solve the problem. Each child attacks the problem in a series of conscious movements which he himself determines. The child is made to be aware of the movements he is using, because actions learned in this way are more likely to be retained as reflex movements. In movement education the objective is to have each child develop an awareness of his ability to use his body efficiently. The child will acquire a repertoire of *basic movements* (running, jumping, leaping, hopping, rolling, pushing, pulling and others) which he can recall and use when necessary.

One advantage of educational gymnastics is that it recognizes individual differences in children. It is not concerned with competition. In a competitive situation where winning is the desired outcome, it is difficult for a child to concentrate on the movement he is going through. Many children who are slow learners may become frustrated in a competitive program. Educational gymnastics, or movement education, will better prepare individuals for later competition as well as giving them an appreciation of their bodies and bodily movements.

MUSCLE

There are three types of muscle tissue: *cardiac* or heart muscle, *smooth* or *nonstriated* (involuntary), and *skeletal* or *striated* (voluntary).

Cardiac Muscle

The heart muscle, or *myocardium*, is an involuntary muscle that contracts in a rhythmical manner. It is controlled by the involuntary nervous system. The cardiac muscle is similar to both the smooth muscles (both are involuntary) and the skeletal muscles (both are striated). Yet it is different from those two other types of muscles because the fibers of its muscle are not entirely separate. The cardiac muscle requires an uninterrupted supply of oxygen, and failure to receive adequate blood containing the invaluable oxygen will result in tissue damage. To reduce that possibility, the heart maintains an especially rich blood sup-

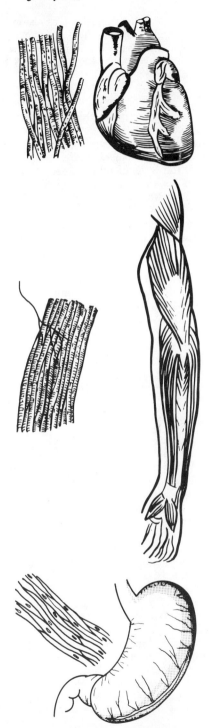

These drawings show the three types of muscle tissue—cardiac muscle, which makes up the heart (top); skeletal muscle, which moves bones and joints (middle), and smooth muscle, which makes up the walls of various organs like the stomach.

ply. Since the coronary vessels and the capillaries literally bathe every fiber of the heart, the heart is able to perform with a great capacity. See CIRCULATORY SYSTEM.

Smooth Muscle

Smooth, or involuntary, muscle tissue composes the walls of the various organs associated with digestion—the esophagus, stomach, intestines, and also the walls of other visceral organs such as the bladder, ureters, uterus and partitions of the organs. Blood vessels are also lined with smooth muscles. The involuntary muscles are those over which we do not have any control and have no sarcolemma (covering membrane).

The involuntary muscle contracts very slowly, and the contraction is quite long. There is very little expenditure of energy with the contraction so that the muscles are not subject to fatigue. The smooth muscles are able to stretch considerably to enlarge such hollow organs as the stomach, bladder and intestines. See CIRCULATORY SYSTEM and DIGESTIVE SYSTEM.

Skeletal Muscle

The skeletal, or striated, muscles are those muscles that primarily protect the vital parts of the body, help maintain circulation of the blood, assist in body balance and posture, and are responsible for movement of the body. There are over 600 such muscles of the body.

Skeletal muscles are made up of long cylindrical fibers or cells that are arranged parallel to one another. Those tiny fibers range from a hundredth of an inch to almost two inches in length and are enclosed in a thin elastic membrane. Units of 100 to 150 fibers are bound into bundles which are held together in larger bundles. The large bundles are then incased in a membrane or sheath to form the muscles. The sheaths merge at the ends of the muscle and form the ten-

dons that attach the muscle to the bone. See MUSCLES, SKELETAL.

MUSCLE-BOUNDNESS

For decades, people have claimed that if you lift weights you will become muscle-bound. Why that opinion about weight training arose is not clear. Because it is very likely that since the earliest lifters were exceptionally strong men and were poorly coordinated, people assumed that weight lifting and muscle-boundness went together. Muscle-boundness is a term used to describe that person who is heavily muscled, slow, and awkward in his movements. He is characterized by the gorilla walk and a poor degree of flexibility. Even athletic coaches have been afraid of encouraging their athletes to lift weights and feel that boys who are exceptionally well developed do not have the flexibility or the grace of movement that the non-weight training athletes have. Fortunately that concept of weight training is changing. A considerable number of research studies have been conducted in the past 20 years to determine whether weight training does result in a muscle-bound individual. The results reveal:

1. There is no such phenomenon as muscle-boundness, at least in the sense that heavy or large muscles produce an awkward or inflexible person.

2. People who have trained with weights are stronger and faster and have quicker movement time than the person who does not train with weights.

3. People who train with weights have as much, if not more, flexibility than those who do not train with weights.

4. Some studies have revealed that people who train with weights are better coordinated than the average person.

If all those findings are true, why do some weight-training people seem to have poor flexibility and coordination, and why do they appear so awkward? The key to the entire phenomenon is to train with weights properly. If weight training is performed in a correct manner, the participant can expect to improve strength, physique, flexibility, coordination and movement time. But if he rejects the proper principles and guidelines, he can expect to reduce his flexibility and coordination and develop an improper physique.

Principles of Proper Weight Training

1. Be certain that you allow the muscle being exercised to go through its full range of motion. For example, if you are performing a barbell curl, be certain that you start the motion with the weight resting against the thighs and then bring the barbell all the way to the chest. The muscles are then contracted and extended through their full range of motion. That movement must occur at every joint. The joints are not to be exercised in only one direction.

2. Exercise muscles on both sides of the joint. Some lifters develop one group of muscles and completely ignore the antagonist muscles (the opposite muscles). For example, if you perform only pull-ups to develop the flexor muscles of the arms and do nothing for the extensors (hips), you will develop powerful flexors and weak extensors. That condition will result in your having arms partially flexed at the elbows because the flexors draw the arm upward. The same situation may occur at the other parts of the body.

3. Engage in stretching exercises for the joints which will help increase your flexibility. See EXERCISES.

4. In lifting for a sport you will find it advantageous to engage in the sport or activity on the days that you do not lift. For example, to improve your golf swing, you must practice that separate skill. Just performing with the weights will not improve the swing.

Following those principles when performing weight-training exercises will help you achieve those benefits mentioned above. See WEIGHT TRAINING.

Furthermore, you should also realize that isometric exercises can contribute to inflexibility. Isometric exercises do not allow the muscles and the joints to be exercised through their full range of motion. It is imperative, therefore, that isometrics be only one small part of your conditioning program. Isometrics are fine for developing strength, but they have some very serious limitations. See ISOMETRICS.

MUSCLE CRAMPS

When one of your muscles contracts powerfully and painfully, you have a muscle cramp. The contraction may occur at any time—at rest as well as during activity. Cramps usually occur without warning. Occasionally, however, you may be able to feel one "building up."

The cause of the cramp is unknown. Dr. Peter Karpovich has several ideas concerning the causative factors. First, a cramp may be the result of "a lowered threshold or irritability of motor nerves, resulting in a sudden increase in the frequency of nerve impulses going to the muscle." Second, the threshold of irritability of motor units may be lowered, thereby contracting the units beyond their limits. In that instance, since the muscle fiber has contracted too much, it may remain shortened for a long period of time, unless stretched. Third, the chemical acetylcholine, produced by the nerve endings for muscle contractions, may not be destroyed quickly enough by cholisesterase.

When a cramp occurs, the best remedy is stretching the affected muscle and firmly kneading it. If the leg muscle is affected, walking for a few minutes usually eases the pain. However, if you sit down (as natural impulses dictate), the cramp will probably continue.

If you get cramps frequently, it is best to avoid vigorous movements until you have warmed up properly. It's a good idea to take a look at your diet, too. A deficiency in calcium, sodium, and vitamin B may help to cause a muscle cramp. See MUSCLE SORENESS AND STIFFNESS.

MUSCLE ENDURANCE

Muscle endurance is the ability of the muscle or groups of muscles to persist in an activity or movement. The number of push-ups you can do is a typical measure of arm and shoulder muscle endurance. When the muscles become fatigued, you are forced to stop because the muscles of the arms and shoulders become fatigued, not because you become breathless as you would in a circulo-respiratory exercise or activity.

Muscle Endurance versus Muscle Strength

Muscle endurance is often confused with muscle strength, and vice versa. Many people perform push-ups under the assumption that they are demonstrating muscle strength. Muscle strength is the maximum effort made with one contraction. So the push-ups, done many times, demonstrate the muscle endurance of the arm and shoulder, not strength.

The strength of the exercising muscles, however, is a limiting factor in muscle or local endurance. If the work load is easy or light for strong muscles, only relatively few muscle fibers are needed to be brought into play. As these fibers become more fatigued, their threshold of irritability is raised, and they fail to respond to the stimuli. See ALL-OR-NONE LAW. As a result of the increased stimuli, fresh fibers are stimulated or aroused, and they take over while the fatigued fibers rest. When rested, those fibers can later be stimulated if necessary. On the other hand, when the muscle is relatively weak, many fibers will have to come into play to perform the same function that the strong muscles did. When those fibers become fatigued, there are fewer fibers to take over the already fatigued fibers. As a result, the muscles are no longer able to continue.

Consequently, strength and muscle endurance are very closely related. The strength of the muscle will complement the muscle's endurance by allowing for more efficient contraction during exercise.

Types of Muscle Endurance

There are two types of muscle endurance. (1) Dynamic endurance (isotonic) is the ability of the muscles to raise and lower a submaximal load. An example is pull-ups. The muscles are forced to contract and extend during the movement. (2) Static endurance (isometric) is the ability of the muscles to maintain a static contraction without movement. An example would be carrying a heavy box for a considerable distance. The muscles are stimulated, even though there is no actual movement, for as long as possible. If it is a maximum contraction, all the muscle fibers of that muscle come into play.

Factors that Affect Muscular Endurance

There are several factors that influence endurance.

Age

Although there is little evidence on what effect age has on muscle endurance, it is apparent that there are some differences between the various age groups. Research has demonstrated that young children do not tire as quickly as high school children. It is traditionally assumed that as you get older, muscle endurance decreases. But that assumption has not been thoroughly investigated by research. Perhaps the local endurance decreases because you become less active.

Sex

If the strength factor is eliminated, there is no difference between the sexes concerning muscular endurance. Since the male is stronger biologically, he can persist in an activity over a longer period because the task is actually easier for him, for fewer fibers are needed for him to perform the task. If, on the other hand, the strength factor is negated, women probably have the same amount of muscular endurance as men.

Motivation

One of the most important factors in local endurance is motivation. That is the ability to persist in the activity despite the pain and discomfort encountered. Motivation varies considerably from person to person. It will also vary within an individual. If you are interested in what you are doing, you may not even notice the onset of fatigue or may be more willing to persist in the activity. On the other hand, if you are bored, you may just quit at the first sign of fatigue or become mentally tired before the actual physical fatigue sets in. Motivation is a highly personal phenomenon, that often varies greatly in each person.

Skill

The higher the skill level, the slower the onset of fatigue. Many of the unnecessary movements are eliminated, allowing more efficient motion and causing fewer muscle fibers to come into play. Training will improve the skill level considerably.

Temperature

The temperature and humidity have a great deal to do with local endur-

ance. Extreme heat or cold will result in poorer performance. There seems to exist an optimal muscle temperature. See ENVIRONMENT.

Fat

Fat is excess weight composed of non-contracting material. Since weight increases the amount of work, even for a simple movement, fat cuts down on your endurance. The excess fat can be likened to placing an extra weight, such as a book, on the arm and then attempting to do a series of barbell curls. The book makes the arms tire before they normally would because of the extra work needed to complete the movement.

Circulation

Since the blood carries oxygen to the muscles, it is vital that the circulation of the muscle be sufficient to prolong the activity. The rate at which the oxygen is delivered to the muscles is dependent upon the rate of circulation, and the rate of circulation is dependent upon the stroke volume of the heart.

Training and Muscle Endurance

To develop dynamic muscle endurance you must follow the overload principle, which means that the muscles are repeatedly and regularly stimulated by a greater-than-normal exercise load or rate. The overload principle also is used in building strength, but in muscle endurance training, the emphasis is placed on high repetition-low resistance training. The exercise is performed many times, and the resistance or work load is relatively light. The resistance, however, cannot be so low that there is no appreciable overload. Specifically the guidelines to follow for building muscle endurance is this: The exercises should be repeated at the rate of 30 per minute. You should reach voluntary exhaustion in about 1½ to 2½ minutes. If you are exhausted before that point, the load is too heavy, and you are developing more strength than endurance. If, on the other hand, you are able to exercise longer than the 1½ to 2½ time period, the work load is too easy, and you are not really overloading the muscle(s). It appears that to work at the above rate for the stipulated time requires that the muscle(s) must work against three-eighths maximum load. Following those guidelines weight training is an excellent means of developing dynamic muscle endurance. Four sets for each exercise should be sufficient.

To develop static muscle endurance requires that you exert a maximum contraction until you are voluntarily exhausted. The length of time will vary considerably from person to person. One word of caution, however, at the outset of static muscle endurance training, do not present a maximum effort for two weeks. A typical training method of developing static muscle endurance of the arm and shoulder girdle and the flexors of the forearm is to assume a flexed arm position for as long as possible several times a day, each day during the training period. See STRENGTH, TRAINING and WEIGHT TRAINING.

MUSCLE SORENESS AND STIFFNESS

Muscle soreness and stiffness are the logical aftereffects of strenuous physical activity. They may occur immediately following the activity, or after some delay, which is usually the next day. Often the soreness and stiffness lasts for only a few days, although after periods of severe exercise, they may last for a week.

Medical authorities have been unable to conclusively prove what causes soreness and stiffness, but there are two commonly accepted theories. One is that metabolic waste (lactic acid) remains in the muscle for a few hours after exercise and thereby initiates pain in the muscle receptors. That theory would account for the fact that the untrained person takes longer to recover from exercise stress than the trained individual; for the latter, having an improved circulatory system, is better able to supply the muscle with nutrients and remove lactic acid.

The other theory is that muscle soreness may be the result of tiny muscle fiber tears that occur during severe muscular activity. That minor injury would probably result in the soreness or stiffness that appears a day after the activity.

To avoid a great deal of muscle soreness or stiffness, plan your conditioning program to progress gradually, especially during the beginning stages. That approach will allow the muscles of the body to acclimate themselves to the work placed upon them. Of course, the muscles can easily slip back into inefficiency. Therefore when you have reached a high plateau of fitness, make every effort to sustain it.

If you do become sore or stiff from physical activity, light exercises or general activity will often provide temporary relief, although the pain usually occurs upon cessation of exercise. Tapering off will also help to avoid such undesirable aftereffects. See TAPERING OFF.

MUSCLE TONE

Muscle tone or tonus is a common term among fitness-minded people. It is commercial companies, physical educators and even doctors who use it to describe the physical benefits from using their products or programs. Yet there is a great deal of controversy over what muscle tonus actually is and whether it can even be improved.

Traditionally, muscle tone has been described as a mild state of contraction or firmness evident in the muscles even when they are relaxed. It has also been used to describe the health of a person, the feeling being that poor health habits and lack of exercise will result in poor muscle tone. Other observations have noted that muscles which are used more, such as the anti-gravity muscles (those which hold the body upright—calf, front of thigh, buttocks, abdominal wall, and back) have a greater muscle tone than the other muscles of the body.

Cause of Muscle Tone

The popular thinking has been that muscles demonstrated their tone as a result of random stimuli from the nervous system to the muscles, a result of heredity or exercise, good health habits and general well-being. At present, neurophysiologists agree that electromyography (study of muscle activity by electrical impulses) shows that in the normal human being there is complete relaxation of the skeletal muscle while at rest. Although a person is able to completely relax all neuromuscular activity in the muscle, that does not mean there is no tone or tonus in the muscle—it simply means that the term needs to be redefined. Dr. J. V. Basmajian in his book *Muscles Alive* states that the general tone of a muscle is determined by the natural fullness and pressure of the muscle and the connective tissue. That fullness and pressure, called the passive component, is continuous throughout life. It is also determined by the active contraction of the muscle in response to the stimuli of the nervous system. The active component is due to the neuromuscular system and is not always present.

Some muscles of the body contain only the active component, whereas others contain only the passive component. Those muscles that are involved in posture, the anti-gravity muscles, contain both active and passive components and, therefore, demonstrate better muscle tone.

The feel of good muscle tone is the result of the fullness and pressure of the muscles and the response of the muscles to the stimuli of being touched. If the muscle is not stimulated, then the active component will be missing.

MUSCLES, SKELETAL

The skeletal or striated muscles are those muscles that primarily protect the vital parts of the body, help maintain normal circulation of the blood, assist in body balance and posture and are responsible for locomotion of movement. There are over 600 skeletal muscles which work in pairs (prime movers and their antagonists).

The Structure of Skeletal Muscle

A muscle is made up of many tiny fibers, each fiber being a cell, varying in length from a hundredth of an inch to almost two inches in length and ten to 100 plus microns in width (a micron is 1/1000 mm.). The thickness of the muscle depends upon the animal and the muscle, not on the length of the fiber. Those muscle fibers do not run the entire length of most muscles.

The muscle fiber, which is composed of *sarcoplasm*, is encased in a thin elastic membrane called the *sarcolemma*. The sarcolemma, in turn, is covered with the *endomysium*, a substance which separates the muscle fiber from its neighbors. Although the endomysium separates each single fiber, it connects them into a bundle, somewhat like the mortar between bricks. Fifteen to 150 fibers may be connected in that manner to form a primary bundle.

The primary bundle is covered with a membrane called the *perimysium* which separates the primary bundles from one another but yet, like the endomysium, connects the bundles together. The series of bundles connected by the perimysium are called secondary and tertiary bundles. The bundles are covered by the *epimysium* —the outer covering of the muscle.

The latter unit, that surrounded by the epimysium, forms the muscle. The sheaths merge at the ends of the muscle and form the tendons that attach the muscle to the bone.

The muscle fiber is the basic unit of the muscle. Each fiber is a mass of protoplasm, called sarcoplasm, and contains a series of nuclei and striations. The striations are called myofibrils or fibrils—meaning smaller fibers. Each myofibril has a number of light and dark bands that run parallel to one another across the fibers. They are what give the muscle its striated appearance. The light bands are called I bands, and the dark bands, A bands.

Both of the myofibrils are composed of two kinds of protein. The A band is made up of actin and myosin; while the I band is made up of only actin.

How the Muscle Contracts

The most widely accepted theory for muscle contraction is the Huxley sliding filament theory which proposes that the filaments, actin and myoxin, merely slide by one another when they are stimulated. Activated either electrically or chemically, the sliding causes the sacromere (material that makes up a muscle fiber) to shorten. Then the fiber and the entire muscle shorten. The shortening is a contraction, and contraction of the muscle is necessary for movement.

Why the myosin and actin filaments slide over one another has not been completely determined. It appears that there are protein bridges coming from the myosin filaments toward the actin filaments, and they are slightly slanted. When the impulse for contraction is received by the muscle fiber, a chemical is released and causes the bridges to grasp, pull and regrasp the actin filaments. Since the actin filaments are attached to the outer borders of the sacromere, they are brought toward each other, forcing the muscle to shorten. That contraction usually results in movement

of a bone at one end of the muscle, while the bone at the other end is usually stabilized by other muscles.

All-or-None Law

A single muscle fiber will contract to its fullest extent when stimulated, provided that the impulse is strong enough to excite the fiber. If the impulse is not strong enough, on the other hand, the fiber will not contract. That is the all-or-none principle.

The strength of the contraction, however, depends upon the number of fibers excited. For example, when you lift a light object, less strength is needed than when you lift a heavy object. The force of the contraction, therefore, is dependent upon the number of fibers excited by the impulse. A strong impulse will excite more fibers to contract (maximally, according to the all-or-none principle) than a weak impulse. See ALL-OR-NONE LAW.

Chemical Constitution of Muscle

Striated muscle consists of 75 per cent water, 20 per cent protein, and 5 per cent mineral and various organic substances. The primary mineral of the muscle fiber is potassium. The principal non-protein nitrogenous substances are adenosine triphosphate, creatine, phosphocreatine and urea. The main proteins are myosin and actin.

The Chemistry of Muscular Contraction

The energy of contraction takes place through chemical reactions. Those reactions may be explained through a series of cycles. The energy for contraction is obtained from a breakdown of adenosine triphosphate (ATP) to adenosine diphosphate (ADP) and free phosphate (P). The reaction is the first to occur when the muscle fiber contracts. The conversion of ATP to ADP is the immediate source of energy for the contraction of the muscle.

Since the supply of ATP in a muscle is very limited, the length of time a muscle could contract would be very short if it were not for a quick method of replenishing the ATP. The chemical process that is described above, ATP converted to ADP + P, is reversible; and ADP and phosphate can be resynthesized to replenish the supply of ATP. The process of breaking down ATP to ADP plus phosphate and the resynthesizing of ADP plus phosphate to ATP is called the *ATP Cycle*. The cycle provides most of the energy necessary for muscular contraction. Since energy is required for resynthesizing ATP, however, another source of energy is needed.

The second source of energy is the *phosphocreatine cycle*. Phosphocreatine (PC) exists in the muscle and can be broken down into creatine and phosphoric acid. The energy released during the cycle provides the energy to resynthesize ATP. As in the ATP cycle, it is also reversible; and therefore, if a third source of energy were not available, the process also would soon deplete the available sources of energy.

The *glycogen-lactic acid cycle* provides the third source of energy. During digestion, carbohydrates are broken down into several substances, one being glucose (sugar); glucose is converted to glycogen and is stored in the liver and the muscles. The glycogen remains in the liver until the glycogen stored in the muscles is depleted. When the depletion occurs, muscle glycogen, in a complicated process, breaks down into lactic acid. The energy released in the breakdown is used for the resynthesis of phosphocreatine. One-fifth of the lactic acid is oxidized to form carbon dioxide and water. The combination with oxygen yields enough energy to resynthesize the remaining four-fifths of the lactic acid into glycogen. The water and carbon dioxide are considered waste products and are removed from the body.

The latter cycle, with glycogen converted into lactic acid, is different from the ATP and phosphocreatine cycles in that it depends upon material (oxygen) from outside the body.

Below is a summary outline of the chemistry of contraction.

When a muscle is exercised at a moderate rate, the oxygen supply is

SUMMARY OF CHEMICAL CHANGES IN MUSCLE CONTRACTION

1. Adenosine Triphosphate (ATP)	breaks down to:	Releases energy for contraction
Adenosine Diphosphate and free phosphate (ADP) (P) (Reversible)		
2. Phosphocreatine (PC)	breaks down to:	Releases energy for resynthesis of ATP
Creatine & Phosphoric acid (C) (P) (Reversible)		
3. Glycogen (G)	breaks down to:	Releases energy for resynthesis of phosphocreatine
Lactic Acid (LA)		
4. Lactic Acid (one-fifth) Oxidized		Releases energy for resynthesis of glycogen from remaining (four-fifths) Lactic Acid

adequate; and the waste products can be removed. In that case, there is no buildup of lactic acid, and the muscle can be exercised or "worked" for a long period of time. However, when a muscle is exercised vigorously, the oxygen supply may not be adequate; and there is a consequent buildup of lactic acid. When the lactic acid level concentration reaches 0.3 per cent, contraction becomes very difficult; and at 0.4 per cent, the muscle is not able to contract.

Muscle Relaxation

Why a muscle relaxes when it is no longer stimulated is not fully understood. One very chemically complex theory proposes that there is a relaxing agent called the Marsh-Bendall factor, which inhibits the breakdown of ATP for muscle contraction. Simply stated, the process of relaxation is as follows: there are two chemical elements involved—magnesium and calcium. The magnesium is bound to the relaxing agent (the Marsh-Bendall factor) and the calcium to the actomyosin. When the muscle is stimulated, the magnesium transfers to the actomyosin and the calcium to the Marsh-Bendall factor. That transfer inhibits the Marsh-Bendall factor and allows the ATP to be broken down for muscle contraction. When the stimulation ceases, the Marsh-Bendall factor again inhibits the breakdown of ATP and the muscle relaxes.

Muscular Fatigue

When a muscle is stimulated repeatedly over a period of time, the contraction and relaxation of the muscle decreases; and if continued, the muscle will fail to contract at all. The loss of capacity to contract is called fatigue.

It has been postulated that the site of fatigue is in one of three places: (a) the nerve, (b) the muscle-nerve junction (motor end plate) and (c) the muscle itself.

Skeletal Muscle System

The skeletal muscle system's responsibilities are to produce movement of the body and/or any of its parts and to maintain the body in an upright position. The muscular system is very complex and performs its tasks by moving the bones of the body. The muscles span the bones and joints and act as cables by pulling the bone in the direction desired.

Most of the muscles work in pairs; when one contracts to pull the bone, the other stretches. If you bend your arm to "make a muscle," the biceps contracts and the triceps stretches. When the arm is straightened, the reverse occurs. An *agonist* is the name given to a muscle responsible for a particular movement, while an *antagonist* has a primary responsibility of causing a movement exactly opposite to that of an agonist.

That pairing of muscles enables you to perform movements without a jerking motion; for as rapidly as one muscle contracts, the other stretches, thereby acting as a break.

Terms

There is a certain nomenclature that is used to determine the direction in which a muscle moves.

Extension indicates that the limb is being extended; while *flexion* indicates that the limb is being bent. An extensor muscle extends a joint; while a flexor muscle flexes or bends a joint. Two other important terms are abduction and adduction.

Abduction is a lateral movement away from the midline of the body; while *adduction* is a medial movement toward the midline of the body. An abductor muscle, therefore, moves a limb away from the body, and an adductor muscle moves the limb toward the body. For further information on skeletal muscles, see: EFFECTS OF EXERCISES, FLEXIBILITY, MUSCLE ENDURANCE, STRENGTH, MUSCLE SYS-
Continued on p. 332

SKELETAL MUSCLES

Name	Origin	Insertion	Action
MUSCLES OF HEAD & FACE			
Frontalis	Skin of eyebrow	Epicranial Aponeurosis	Elevates eyebrow, wrinkles forehead
Occipitalis	Occipital bone	Epicranial Aponeurosis	Draws scalp backward
Orbicularis oculi	Frontal bone and maxilla	Lateral & medial palpebral ligaments	Closes eyelids, causes squinting
Corrugator	Frontal Bone	Skin of Eyebrow	Wrinkles forehead and causes frowning
Orbicularis Oris	Various muscles running to lip	Fibers around oral opening (Sphincter)	Draws lips together
Zygomaticus	Zygomatic bone	Obicularis oris muscle	Results in smiling, mirth & kindly disposition
Buccinator	Maxilla and mandible	Sides of mouth	Pulls lip and cheek against teeth
Masseter	Zygomatic arch	Lateral surface of Ramus	Enables mastication
Temporal	Temporal fossa	Coronoid process of mandible	Enables mastication
Pterygoids	Upper aspects of skull	Medial surface of mandible	Causes mastication & opening of mouth
MUSCLES OF THE NECK			
Platysma	Subcutaneous tissue of neck	Mandible, skin of cheek	Wrinkles skin of neck, lowers corners of mouth
Sternocleidomastoideus	Upper border of sternum, clavicle	Mastoid process of temporal bone	Turns head toward shoulder, rotates head
Longus Cervicis	Cervical and thoracic vertebrae	Base of occipital bone	Flexes head forward
Longus Capitis	Cervical and thoracic vertebrae	Base of occipital bone	Flexes head forward
Rectus Capitis Anterior	Cervical and thoracic vertebrae	Base of occipital bone	Flexes head forward
Rectus Capitis Lateralis	Cervical and thoracic vertebrae	Base of occipital bone	Rotates the head
Scalenus anterior	Cervical Vertebrae	Ribs	Aids respiration and bends vertebral column
Scalenus medius	Cervical Vertebrae	Ribs	Aids respiration and bends vertebral column

SKELETAL MUSCLES—*Continued*

Name	Origin	Insertion	Action
Scalenus posterior	Cervical Vertebrae	Ribs	Aids respiration and bends vertebral column
MUSCLES OF TRUNK			
DEEP MUSCLES OF THE BACK			
Splenius capitis	Lower half of ligamentum nuchae	Mastoid process of the temporal bone and occipital bone	Straighten back, aids in bending backwards
Splenius cervicis	Spines 3rd to 6th cervical vertebrae	Transverse process upper two or three cervical vertebrae	Straighten back, aids in bending backwards
Sacrospinalis iliocostalis longissimus spinalis	Saerum, spines of lumbar & 11th & 12th thoracic vert.	Lumbar, thoracic & cervical vert. Posterior part of ribs.	Straighten back, aids in bending backwards
SUPERFICIAL MUSCLES OF THE BACK			
Trapezius	Occipital bone 7th cervical vert. & all thoracic vert.	Clavicle, acromion & spine of scapula	Raise and shrug shoulder, extend head, turn head side to side. Brace back shoulders
Latissimus dorsi	Spines of last 6 thoracic & upper lumbar vert., iliac crest	Anterior surface upper part of humerus	Adducts arm, rotates inward, depresses shoulder
Rhomboideus major	Upper four thoracic vert.	Medial border of scapula	Steadies the scapula
Rhomboideus minor	Occipital bone, 7th cervical, 1st thoracic vert.	Medial border of scapula	Steadies the scapula
Levator Scapulae	Transverse process atlas, axis	Upper part of medial border of scapula	Draws scapula upwards
DIAPHRAM MUSCLES OF ABDOMINAL WALL			
Diaphram	Between thoracic and abdominal cavities	Linea alba	Is necessary for inspiration and expiration
External oblique	Lower eight ribs	Aponeurosis to pubis, iliac crest, linea alba	1. Raise pressure in abdomen 2. Aid vomiting 3. Aid defecation 4. Cause expulsion of child at parturition 5. Aid expiration of air

Muscle	Origin	Insertion	Action
Internal oblique	Anterior part of iliac crest & inguinal ligament	Lower three ribs & linea alba	Same as above
Transverse abdominis	Iliac crest, 12th rib, cartilage of lower ribs	Aponeurosis, linea alba, pubis	Same as External oblique
Rectus abdominis	Pubis & pubic symphysis	Cartilages of 5th, 6th, 7th ribs	Same as above
MUSCLES OF THE CHEST			
Pectoralis major	Clavicle, sternum, aponeurosis of external oblique	Outer lip of bicipital groove of humerus	Adducts and medially rotates arm, draws forward or medially when arm is extended
Pectoralis minor	3rd, 4th, 5th ribs	Coracoid process of scapula	Pulls scapula forward
Serratus anterior	Lateral surface of 1st to 8th rib	Medial border of scapula	Draws scapula forward and laterally
Subclavis	1st rib	Lower surface of clavicle	Depresses scapula and shoulder
External intercostal	Lower border of a rib	Upper border of rib below	Elevates ribs as in inspiration
Internal intercostal	Ridge of the inner surface of a rib	Upper border of the rib below	Depress ribs as in expiration
MUSCLES OF SHOULDER & UPPER LIMB			
SHOULDER			
Deltoid	Spine of scapula and acromion	Deltoid tuberosity	Abducts arm, rotates it laterally & medially
Subscapularis	Subscapular fossa of scapula	Lesser tuberosity of humerus	Rotates arm medially. Holds humerus in cavity
Supraspinatus	Subscapular fossa of scapula	Lesser tuberosity of humerus	Rotates arm medially. Holds humerus in cavity
Infraspinatus	Subscapular fossa of scapula	Lesser tuberosity of humerus	Same as above
Teres minor	Subscapular fossa of scapula	Lesser tuberosity of humerus	Same as above
Teres major	Axillary border scapula	Anterior surface upper half of humerus	Adducts, extends & rotates arm medially
THE ARM (HUMERUS)			
Coracobrachialis	Coracoid process of scapula	Middle third of humerus	Adducts and flexes arm
Biceps brachii	Short head: Coracoid process of scapula / Long head: Scapula above glenoid cavity	Posterior part of tuberosity of radius	Flexes elbow & is a strong supinator of forearm

SKELETAL MUSCLES—*Continued*

Name	Origin	Insertion	Action
Brachialis	Lower half of humerus	Tuberosity and coronoid process	Flexes elbow joint
Triceps brachii	Long head: Below glenoid cavity; Medial head: Lower half of humerus; Lateral head: Upper half of humerus	Olecranon process of ulna	Extends forearm, long head; extends and adducts arm
MUSCLES OF THE FOREARM			
Flexor carpi radialis	Medial epicondyle of humerus	2nd and 3rd metacarpal	Flexes wrist, and abducting
Palmaris longus	Medial epicondyle of humerus	Palmar aponeurosis	Aids in flexing the wrist
Flexor carpi ulnaris	Medial epicondyle of humerus; Olecranon process	5th metacarpal pisiform, and hamate bone	Flexes wrist, adducts hand
Flexor digitorum sublimis	Medial epicondyle of humerus	Medial epicondyle of humerus	Flexes the fingers and possibly wrist
Brachioradialis	Lateral epicondyle of humerus	Lateral styloid process	Flexes the elbow joint
Extensor carpi radialis longus	Lateral epicondyle of humerus	Base of 2nd metacarpal	Is an antagonist of flexor muscles of fingers
Extensor carpi radialis brevis	Lateral epicondyle of humerus	Base of 2nd and 3rd metacarpal	Is an antagonist of flexor muscles of fingers
Extensor digitorum	Lateral epicondyle of humerus	Base, middle, distal phalanx of four digits	Extends fingers & opens hands
Extensor digiti minimi	Lateral epicondyle of humerus	Base of metacarpal	Extends little finger and wrist
Extensor carpi ulnaris	Lateral epicondyle of humerus	Base of metacarpal	Steadies the wrist during flexion of fingers
Anconeus	Lateral epicondyle of humerus	Tendons and muscles to bones of wrist, hand and fingers	Assists the triceps in extending elbow
Supinator	Lateral epicondyle of humerus, lateral side of ulna	Upper one third lateral side radius	Supinates forearm
Pronator teres	Humeral head: Medial epicondyle of humerus; Ulnar head: Coronoid process of ulna	Middle one third of lateral surface of radius	Pronates and flexes forearm

MUSCLES OF THE LOWER LIMB
MUSCLES OF THE ILIAC (HIP) REGION

Muscle	Origin	Insertion	Action
Psoas major	Bodies of 12th thoracic to 5th lumbar vert.	Lesser trochanter of femur	Adducts, flexes thigh; rotates it medially
Iliacus	Iliac fossa of ilium	On fibers of psoas major	Adducts, flexes thigh, rotates it medially; Assists weakly in flexing trunk
Psoas minor	12th thoracic, 1st lumbar vert.	Into the pubis	Extends thigh, rotates it laterally
Gluteus maximus	Iliac crest, side of coccyx & sacrum	Gluteal tuberosity of femur & linea aspera	Abducts the thigh, rotates it inward
Gluteus medius	Outer aspect of ilium	Greater trochanter of femur	Same as above
Gluteus minimus	Outer aspect of ilium	Greater trochanter of femur	Rotates thigh laterally
Pyriformis	Inside pelvis, surface of sacrum	Greater trochanter	Rotates thigh outward
Obturator internus	Pelvis	Greater trochanter	Same as above
Superior gemellus	Spine of ischium	Same as above	Same as above
Inferior gemellus	Tuberosity of ischium	Same as above	Same as above
Quadratus femoris	Same as above	Femur	Same as above
Obturator externus	Margin of obturator forearm	Medial side of greater trochanter	Rotates thigh outward

MUSCLES OF THE THIGH

Muscle	Origin	Insertion	Action
Tensor fasciae latae	Iliac crest and anterior superior spine of the ilium	Iliotibial tract	Extends knees
Sartorius	Iliac spine	Medial upper side of the tibia	Flexes the thigh, is an abductor & lateral rotator of thigh
Quadriceps femories	Two tendons from ilium	Insets rectur femoris into patella	Extends the leg at knee, flexes the thigh on pelvis
Rectus femoris			
Vastus lateralis	Greater trochanter of femur	Same as above	Same as above
Vastus medialis	Lower part of the trochanteric line	Same as above	Same as above
Vastus intermedius	Upper two thirds of femur	Same as above	Same as above
Gracilis	Pubic symphysis pubic arch	Shaft of tibia below condyle	Adducts & flexes thigh
Adductor longus	Pubis and pubic arch	Middle one third of linea aspera	Are powerful adductors of the femur
Adductor brevis	Outer surface of pubis	Upper part of linea aspera	Same as above
Adductor magnus	Pubis & ischium	Full length of linea aspera	Same as above

SKELETAL MUSCLES—Continued

Name	Origin	Insertion	Action
Biceps femoris	Two heads: tuberosity of ischium & linea aspera	Lateral side of head of fibula & lateral condyle of tibia	Flexors of leg & rotates leg laterally
Semitendinosus	Tuberosity of the ischium	Medial surface of shaft of tibia	Same as above
Semimembranosus	Tuberosity of the ischium	Medial condyle of tibia	Same as above
MUSCLES OF THE LOWER LEG			
Tibialis anterior	Lateral condyle & shaft of tibia	Base of 1st metatarsal bone & median cuneiform	Flexes and inverts foot
Extensor hallucis longus	Middle anterior of fibula	Upper surface of base of distal phalanx	Dorsally flexes ankle, foot; & extends toe
Extensor digitorum longus	Lateral condyle of tibia & upper surface of fibula	Four outer toes	Flexes ankle & foot, extends 4 outer toes & abduction of foot
Peroneus longus	Upper ⅔ of lateral & shaft of fibula	Tendon at ankle	Steadies the tibia & arch of foot
Peroneus brevis	Lower lateral part of shaft of fibula	5th metatarsal bone	Everts the foot and prevents inversion
Gastrocnemius	Two heads from the medial & lateral condyle of femur	Calcaneus	Flexes leg, adducts & inverts the foot
Soleus	Head of fibula, and medial side of the tibia	Calcaneus	Same as above
Popliteus	Lateral condyle of femur & posterior ligament of knee	Upper surface of tibia	Flexes the knee joint
Flexor hallucis longus	Posterior surface of lower ⅔ fibula	Plantar surface of base of distal phalanx of toe	Flexes the toes & steadies metatarsal bones
Flexor digitorum longus	Posterior surface of tibia	Medial malleolus	Same as above
Tibialis posterior	Tibia and fibula & aponeurosis	Navicular bone	Inverts foot & longitudinal arch
MUSCLES OF THE HAND			
Abductor pollicis brevis	Ligament in front of wrist joint	Proximal phalanx of the thumb	Moves thumb forward & rotates it inward
Opponens pollicis	Ligament in front of wrist	Metacarpal bone of thumb	Flexes metacarpal bone of thumb
Flexor pollicis brevis	Same as above	Proximal phalanx of thumb	Flexes proximal phalanx of thumb

Adductor pollicis	Oblique head: Capitate & trapezium bone; Transverse head: 3rd metacarpal bone	Same as above	Draws thumb into palm of hand
Palmaris brevis	Ligament in front of wrist	Skin of hand	Wrinkles skin of palm
Abductor digiti minimi	Pisiform bone	Proximal phalanx of little finger	Abducts little finger
Flexor digiti minimi	Hamate bone	Same as above	Flexes the proximal phalanx of little finger

MUSCLES OF THE FOOT

Extensor digitorum brevis	Outer & upper surfaces of calcaneum	Tendon to big 1, 2, 3, 4 toes	Extends toes
Abductor hallucis	Medial surface of the calcaneum	Proximal phalanx of big toe	Abducts great toe
Flexor digitorum brevis	Calcaneum plantor surface	Tendons	Flexes toes
Abductor digiti minimi	Calcaneum plantor surface	Proximal phalanx of little toe	Abducts little toe
Flexor hallucis brevis	Cuboid bone	Proximal phalanx of great toe	Flexes big toe
Adductor hallucis	2, 3, 4, 5th metatarsal bones	Proximal phalanx of great toe	Adducts great toe
Flexor digiti minimi brevis	5th metatarsal bone	Proximal phalanx of little toe	Flexes little toe

NOTE: The most important functions of the foot muscles are to steady the toes and hold them for support. The muscles also maintain the arches of the foot.

TEM, MUSCLE TONE and STITCH IN THE SIDE.

MYTHS OF EXERCISE

Exercise and the results it brings to the human body are too often grossly misunderstood. Here are five of the modern myths about exercise.

1. Exercise increases your appetite, resulting in increased weight.

No! Exercise, especially continuous rhythmical activities such as jogging, swimming, cycling, rowing and skiing, will actually depress the appetite. Tests on college students indicate that after an hour or so of physical activity in the late afternoon, they are unable to eat more than a small portion of their dinners. Dr. H. L. Taylor and his colleagues have shown that adult men who increase their exercise level above that of the very sedentary did not experience an accompanying increase in food intake.

Dr. Jean Mayer's studies of dietary histories and activity schedules in obese and normal-weight high school girls show that although caloric intakes were generally larger in the non-obese group, the obese girls gained more weight. Reason? The overweight group spent only half the time in sports or in exercise of any sort. Similar results have been reported by many other investigators.

Dr. Mayer is convinced that inactivity is the most important cause of "creeping" overweight in modern Western societies. It is wrong to think that you can maintain your weight by only regulating your food intake. To live in our modern, sedentary world without becoming obese means that you either will have to step up your activity or be mildly or acutely hungry all your life! See APPETITE.

2. Exercise is unrealistic because it requires so much work to burn up the calories in only one piece of pie.

No! You frequently read that the caloric equivalent of a pound of fat can be burned only by walking 36 hours, playing volleyball for 11 hours or splitting wood for 7 hours. That's true. But what most people don't realize is that exercise doesn't have to be continuous to burn up the calories. You lose as much weight in walking for 36 hours straight, as you do in walking for 18 hours on two different occasions, or for 12 hours at 3 different times or for 9 hours on any 4 outings. Any exercise has a cumulative effect even if it is done for only 20 to 30 minutes each day. For instance, a half hour of handball or squash daily would enable you to lose 16 pounds a year.

Dr. L. H. Newburgh states that the more overweight a person is the more calories he uses in exercising. Consequently, any increase in caloric intake of a physically active person causes only a slight increase in weight because of the energy cost of moving the extra poundage. On the other side of the coin, in a sedentary, obese individual, less energy is expended moving the extra weight and therefore weight gain is much more rapid. A sedentary person is exposed to the danger of overweight to a much greater extent than one who makes a practice of daily, or at least frequent, exercise.

Dr. Mayer reports some interesting results of an experiment conducted in the Nutrition Department at Harvard. Undergraduates were made to double their food intake—already in the vicinity of 3,000 calories—without increasing their weight. They had to work hard to achieve that result, especially as classes limited the time they could devote to exercise. But, by exercising they did manage to lose an extra 3,000 calories per day. See CALORIES.

3. Using vibrating belts and tables, massage, rubber sweat suits and steam baths will make you lose fat.

No! You cannot pummel, vibrate, massage, or steam fat away. Excluding surgical removal, there are only two effective methods for reduction of body fat. The first involves modification of the diet to reduce caloric intake. The second is increasing energy expenditure through physical activity. In addition, exercise increases the proportion of muscle to fat. Muscles become less infiltrated with fat and hence stronger and more efficient. Naturally, a combination of proper diet and exercise is the most effective way to reduce body fat.

Trying to reduce by steam baths and rubber sweat suits results in a temporary loss of body fluid. After a few glasses of water, the weight is quickly replaced. The physiological phenomenon called water balance is a very delicate adjustment that should be left to your natural desire for water. To withhold fluid in order to show a weight loss results in dehydration and eventual lack of proper bodily functions.

Perspiration is a natural mechanism which helps keep your temperature at normal levels. Evaporation of perspiration has a cooling effect. To prevent or retard that process by wearing a rubber suit, often results in sluggishness or a slow down in your physical activity schedule. If you drive yourself to a point of discomfort by continuing the activity, heat exhaustion may result. See MECHANICAL DEVICES.

4. Running will cause "athlete's heart" (an abnormal and dangerous condition).

No! That misconception still persists despite years of study showing that a continuous program of running or jogging will develop a stronger, more efficient heart. The heart is a muscle as well as an organ. If it can pump a greater volume of blood with each beat, it will not have to beat as many times. After a program of jogging, the heart rate per minute at rest decreases. The heart also recuperates faster after exercise in the trained individual, indicating good circulatory efficiency.

If the heart is already diseased, violent and strenuous exercise could result in more damage. But exercise has never been proven to be the direct cause of a coronary death in a person with a normal, non-diseased heart. The noted physiologist, Dr. Arthur Steinhaus states that autopsy records show that a healthy heart has never been damaged by exercise, no matter how strenuous. Even the rare cases of acute cardiac dilatation recover perfectly.

Athletes, such as long distance runners, may develop a larger and stronger heart than the average person for his size, but this is not the pathologically enlarged heart seen in certain kinds of heart disease. The larger heart of the endurance athlete appears to be a perfectly normal and functional adaptation to the demands placed on it.

The trained heart is superior in every way. With each beat it pumps twice as much blood as does the untrained heart. Consequently, the frequency of beats is reduced. The heart of Donald Lash, world's champion in the two-mile race, pumped so much blood that he was able to absorb over 5 quarts of oxygen per minute. The untrained person does well to absorb about half that amount.

A sudden break in training has never been shown to be harmful in spite of claims made by some so-called authorities. The enlarged heart of a highly trained athlete becomes smaller after the training season. See ATHLETE'S HEART.

5. Once you pass forty years of age, you are too old to engage in strenuous exercise.

No! Aging can best be described as loss of cardiovascular, respiratory, renal and even endocrinological function. Physical training through exercise and sport helps prevent such deterioration and thus keeps you younger longer. Chronological age is far different from physiological age. Some men at 30 years of age have the heart and arteries of a 60-year-old and vice versa.

Dr. Ernst Jokl studied older gymnasts in Germany and found that those who were continuously active maintained exceptional athletic performance well into their sixties. He concludes that regular exercise acts as "preventive medicine," that it prevents degenerative disease and slows down the physical deterioration associated with aging.

Dr. Shock has described in careful scientific detail all the various physiological functions that degenerate as a result of aging. The next important task is to show, in the same careful detail, how an exercise program can retard that deterioration. In addition, exercise criteria should be set up in accord with age and normal activity. Excessive muscle power is not particularly essential for older citizens. Kinetic exercises such as walking, jogging, swimming and cycling as opposed to static exercise such as push-ups, weight lifting and sedentary routines should be recommended. Excessive muscle mass and contraction may impede rather than speed up venous return to the heart. See AGING and MIDDLE AGE.—*Sidney B. Sward*

NECK

Muscles and Exercises

The *platysma* is a broad, thin muscle that covers the side of the neck from the second rib to the chin. It is a weak muscle that wrinkles the skin of the neck and lowers the corners of the mouth and also serves to decrease the hollow between the jaw and neck.

The *sternocleidomastoid* is a second neck muscle that turns the head downward to one side, depending upon whether the right or the left sternocleidomastoid muscle contracts. The muscle is a very prominent one of the neck and can be easily seen or felt by turning the head to the side.

One of the best exercises you can do for strengthening the neck muscles, especially the *sternocleidomastoid* and the *platysma*, is to lie flat on your back with your head and neck hanging over the side of a bench or bed. Allow your head to hang and turn it to the side. Then raise your head 10 times. Perform the exercise 10 times. Then turn your head to the opposite side and repeat. Another exercise that aids in strengthening the platysma, thereby helping to prevent a sagging appearance in the neck, involves clenching your teeth and raising the head slightly. You should feel tension in the entire area. Hold the position for a count of 10. Turning the head in a circle is a simple but helpful exercise. Begin by tilting the head backward and turn it to the side, front, side and back again. Make an attempt to turn the head as far as possible to each side. A series of 5 turns to the right and 5 to the left is a good beginning level. Another exercise is to place the hand along the side of the head and exert pressure against the hand. Be certain to push with the head and to resist with the hand. (Since the arm muscles are stronger, some injuries have occurred by pushing with the hand rather than the head.) Hold for a count of 10, and then repeat on the other side. That exercise is particularly good for strengthening the sternocleidomastoid muscle. For more exercises see WEIGHT TRAINING, ISOMETRICS and EXERCISES.

NEUROMUSCULAR SYSTEM

The neuromuscular system is the integration of the muscular and the nervous systems. For a complete understanding of the neuromuscular system, review MUSCLES, SKELETAL.

The human body is comprised of hundreds of muscles which allow it to move. Those muscles, however, would be incapable of movement if it were not for the impulses they receive from the nervous system. The nervous system consists of the brain and spinal cord (central nervous system) and the network of nerves (peripheral nervous system) and is divided in two ways: the *somatic* and *autonomic* systems. You have no control over the autonomic system, such as the heart rate and the smooth muscles of the digestive system. The somatic system consists of both the central and peripheral nervous systems; that is, the brain, the spinal cord and the peripheral nerves.

Somatic System

Here the discussion of the neuromuscular system is confined to the somatic system. That system is concerned with the reception of an impulse from the environment. The *sensory* nerves pick up the impulse and carry it to the spinal cord and/or the brain. A motor pattern is organized either in the brain or in the spinal column, and the impulse from the spinal cord and/or brain is then sent via the *motor* nerve to the muscles so that the response can be made. The simplest movement is made in a *reflex arc*, often called an involuntary movement. No thinking takes place—the impulse merely travels from the sensory nerve to the spinal cord. There the motor nerve picks up the impulse, and the message is sent back to the muscles telling them to move. Other movements are much more complicated and may cause the impulse to go up to various heights of the spinal cord before descending with the motor pattern. On the other hand, the movement may require interpretation by the brain so the sensory impulse will have to go to the brain, and then sent back down to the spinal column to the appropriate level where the motor nerve carries the impulse to the muscles for a response or movement.

The strength of the contraction of a muscle, the endurance of muscle, the posture and muscle tonus, balance and movements are all dependent upon the neuromuscular system.

Strength of a Muscle Contraction

Obviously, it takes less strength to lift a pencil than it takes to lift a metal pipe, despite the fact that similar muscles are used. The lifting of a heavy object requires a more powerful contraction than does the lifting of a light weight. The number of muscle fibers of a specific muscle determines the strength of the contraction. If a few fibers are stimulated, the contraction will be weak. If many of the fibers are stimulated, the contraction will be strong. See ALL-OR-NONE LAW.

Muscle Endurance

Muscle endurance is controlled by the neuromuscular system since the general physiological site of fatigue is the *motor end plate*. The motor end plate is the junction between the nerve ending and the muscle fiber. The gap between the nerve and the muscle fiber is called a synapse. To allow the impulse to travel across this gap, acetylcholine is released and then destroyed by an enzyme. Fatigue occurs at the gap or synapse because the enzyme does not work efficiently when it must quickly and repeatedly destroy the acetylcholine. To recover, the synapse must have a short period of rest which allows time for the enzyme to function.

Posture

The basic element of posture is the *stretch reflex*, which is very important in the maintenance of posture. It is best developed in the extensor muscles, which are usually involved in maintaining the posture of the body against gravity. Those muscles help to keep the body from flexing at the hip and knee as a result of gravity. Although the maintenance is primarily reflex, the involvement of the brain is necessary to maintain the posture. A loss of consciousness also involves a loss of maintaining the upright posture. See POSTURE.

Muscle Tonus

Muscle tone is the mild state of contraction or firmness of the muscle that is evident even when the person is relaxed. The tone or tonus is the result of the natural fullness and pressure of the muscle and the connective tissue and the contraction of the muscle in response to the various impulses it receives from the nervous system. See MUSCLE TONE.

Balance

Closely allied to posture is balance, or the ability of the person to maintain equilibrium in various positions. When a complex or simple motor skill is performed, it is essential that you be in the correct position so that the necessary movements can be made. The positioning of the body is considered to be complex reflex patterns which are the result of various stimuli you receive through the various sense organs—touch, smell, sight, hearing. For example, when running, you suddenly trip and start to fall. You do not think the correct response out; you automatically react to the situation and compensate by running faster until you have reestablished the correct running posture. See BALANCE. Closely allied to that phenomenon is KINESTHESIA.

Body Movements

There are two types of body movement—reflex and voluntary. The typical reflex movement occurs when you place your hand on a hot stove and pull it away quickly. That response was not learned but, instead, inborn. Here one of the sense receptors is stimulated and you respond accordingly.

Voluntary movements are much more complex. The impulses for voluntary movement originate in the cerebral cortex of the brain, and the various parts of the brain control the voluntary movements. There is a specific motor area of the brain which allows movement of the different parts of the body.

Besides all those functions, the neuromuscular system is also responsible for coordinating the movements of the body. Without that coordination, the body would move in a purposeless manner. Smooth, coordinated movements depend upon smooth, coordinated muscle action. Thus, the nervous system must stimulate the motor units at the proper time. In effect, it synchronizes the motor units. The synchronizing is done by having the nervous system decide the number of units to be stimulated and the number of times they are to be stimulated and to coordinate when the various units are to be fired.

Training and the Neuromuscular System

Training for a specific activity or skill will result in an improvement in that activity or skill, provided the correct skills are practiced. Repeatedly practicing an activity or skill will result in actual storage of the coordinated pattern in the brain in a memory drum. Whenever you need to perform that skill, you simply call upon the memory drum to "play back" the skill, and the movement is made automatically. See MOTOR ABILITY for a related discussion and reference. Training will also result in training the synapses (the joint at which a nervous impulse passes from one cell to another). At the synapse, there may be several other nerve fibers. To provide the correct response, the proper fiber must be chosen. If you practice the skill, the actions will become habitual.

For related articles see COORDINATION, MOTOR EDUCABILITY, MOTOR FITNESS, MOTOR LEARNING and REACTION TIME.

NUTRITION

"Nutrition is the science of food and its relation to health," says the National Research Council. Nutrition deals with food and how the body makes use of food and is concerned with the ingredients in foods and their chemical reactions within the body. Knowledge and application of the principles of nutrition are necessary as an aid in developing strong bodies and good health through a proper diet. Your diet, or your food intake, directly affects your growth, development and ability to live an energetic life. "You are what you eat" is an often-referred-to statement that summarizes the value of good nutrition. The study of nutrition tells you which foods are necessary and how to determine and prepare a balanced diet. A basic knowledge of nutrition is essential in preparing food, whether it be for yourself, a small family, an institution, patrons of a public eating place, or an athletic team.

Dietary Problems

Advances in nutrition accompanied by new discoveries in medicine in the United States have led to such beneficial developments as greater size and weight and longer life expectancy. But, while the U.S. has the most abundant supply and variety of foods of all the nations of the world, it does not necessarily follow that all U.S. citizens are well nourished. Many middle-aged Americans suffer from chronic conditions which can be attributed to inadequate nutrition. It is possible to get enough to eat to satisfy hunger and yet not fulfill the nutritive requirements of the body. What kinds of foods are eaten is more important than the quantity of food eaten. Studies have shown that one out of every five American school children has an inadequate diet. The foods most often lacking are dairy products, vegetables and fresh fruits, particularly citrus fruits.

In many nations of the world, starvation and malnutrition are commonplace. Starvation simply means not getting enough food to carry on life processes efficiently. Malnutrition means not getting enough of specific necessary foods. Starving and malnourished individuals suffer from a myriad of afflictions, including poor physical and mental condition, problems with teeth and gums, poor complexions, nutritional anemia, night blindness and many others.

Another dietary problem, particularly prevalent in the United States, is overnutrition. Far too many Americans are overweight. The excess weight causes not only physical problems but may lead to psychological problems as well.

The most common reasons for inadequate diets are ignorance of nutritional facts, taste preferences, cultural customs, habit, poverty, fad foods and combinations of those. Eating is largely habitual. People become accustomed to certain foods that they enjoy and are hesitant to make changes. Too often the selection of foods is done on a taste basis with little regard for their nutritional value. Overeating is also habitual. Poor eating habits centering on the choice of foods usually begin early in life and are difficult to change. Teenagers, because they are in their major growth and development years, should have the best possible diet. Instead, many survive on hamburgers, french fries and soda, a diet that cannot possibly provide all the ingredients necessary to build a strong, healthy, attractive body.

Nutrition education can play an influential role in correcting the poor eating habits of many people. Through education, people can be made aware of the benefits of good nutritional practices. Education is also helpful in teaching those from low-income groups how to get the most nutrition from their food dollar. Other things being equal, good nutritional practices will favorably affect vitality and longevity. Aside from appearance and a feeling of well being, a well-nourished person is usually well adjusted emotionally.

Metabolism

The body is the sum of many chemical reactions. Every bodily function is the result of chemical combinations within the body. Those reactions are grouped under the heading of *metabolism,* the body's utilization of foods. The ingredients involved in those reactions are provided by the breakdown of foods in the process of digestion. Digestion results in the formation of numerous chemical substances that the body can use to carry out its many functions. As in any chemical reaction, human metabolism depends on a delicate balance of substances involved. Following digestion, the usable substances are absorbed into the blood stream and transported to the various body tissues, where they take part in the many phases of metabolism. The unusable substances are not absorbed and are eventually eliminated from the body.

Food consists of six different classes called nutrients: (1) carbohydrates, (2) proteins, (3) fats, (4) vitamins, (5) minerals and (6) water. Those nutrients are used by the body as fuel to accomplish work, to build and repair body tissues and to regulate body processes. If the body is to operate at an optimum level, those nutrients must be supplied in sufficient amounts. Where there is an inadequate supply of particular nutrients, the function in which they participate must necessarily suffer. After a time the nutritional deficiencies are reflected in your overall health.

Whether active or resting, the body continually expends energy. Even when the body is at rest, energy must be supplied for the beating of the heart, respiration, and many other forms of cell activity. The basal metabolic need (energy needed during rest) for a 24-hour period is approximately 11 calories per pound of body weight. A calorie is a measure of heat and is expressed as the amount of heat necessary to raise the temperature of one pound of water 4 degrees on the Fahrenheit scale. For example, the basal metabolic requirement for a 150-pound man for a 24-hour period would be 11 x 150, 1,650 calories. The energy requirement for each individual is dependent upon a number of factors, the most influential of which is the amount of physical activity engaged in. It is not uncommon for a person engaged in strenuous physical activity to expend as many as 4,000 calories in a day. See CALORIES.

Body weight is an excellent barometer for determining the adequacy of diet. Underweight is an indication that the energy supply (food intake) is not sufficient to meet energy needs, while overweight indicates a more than adequate intake of calories. The maintenance of ideal weight is an indication that the energy intake is balanced with energy output.

Nutrients

An interesting, and necessary, biological relationship exists between plants and animals. Animals cannot make their own nutrients. They must get them from plants. In plants, the combination of carbon dioxide, oxygen, water and nitrogen-containing substances takes place as a result of sunlight acting upon the chlorophyll of the plants. That combination results in the formation of organic chemical compounds called carbohydrates, fats and proteins. Organic compounds consist of three basic elements, carbon, hydrogen and oxygen, and when combined with oxygen (oxidation), they release energy. They differ from each other according to the relative amounts of the three basic elements.

After ingestion by animals, the substances are broken down into simpler chemical substances that the body can use to build and repair its own tissues and to provide energy. The plants in turn utilize animal wastes. The animal waste products are broken down by bacteria in the process of decay into substances which plants can use to carry on their own life functions. The relationship between the plant and animal kingdoms is called the "nitrogen cycle." Neither plants nor animals could exist without the other.

Carbohydrates

Carbohydrates are either simple sugars or a complex combination of several sugars. The sources of carbohydrates are fruits and vegetables. Some vegetables rich in sugars include beets, carrots, onions, turnips and sweet potatoes. The sugars that the plants do not use for their own functions are stored as starch for future energy needs. *Starches* are formed by the combination of several sugars and are found in the seeds and roots of plants. Animals can easily digest starches into their simple sugar components for quick energy fuel. The primary sources of starches are grain and grain products, including breakfast cereals, noodles, pastries, as well as certain vegetables.

Cellulose is a form of carbohydrate found in the leaves, roots, seeds and skins of fruits and vegetables and is practically indigestible by man and other animals. Its value is that it gives bulk to the food wastes and, thereby, facilitates their removal from the body.

Glycogen is the carbohydrate product that can be stored in limited amounts in certain animal tissues (liver and muscles). For that reason, it is often referred to as animal starch. When needed, it can easily be converted into simple sugar units (glu-

cose) and oxidized to meet energy needs.

Carbohydrates have been labeled the "body's most preferred foods," since they are the easiest nutrients for the body to digest and use. Aside from providing quick energy, they also furnish some important proteins, minerals and vitamins. In addition, they are generally pleasing to the taste. When the carbohydrate stores in the body become inadequate, as in prolonged, strenuous muscular activity or starvation, the body can make adjustments that will allow it to oxidize, burn fats and, infrequently, proteins to fulfill energy needs. Unfortunately, the utilization of fats and proteins in place of carbohydrates is less efficient and chemically more complex and can go on for only a limited amount of time before other body functions begin to suffer.

The single most important indicator of carbohydrate need is the amount of physical activity engaged in. If, for any reason, the body is not supplied with enough carbohydrate fuel to meet energy needs, a condition called hypoglycemia (lack of sugar) exists. That condition produces a feeling of extreme fatigue.

The average American diet consists of 40-50 per cent carbohydrates, 10-15 per cent proteins, and 30-40 per cent fats. The percentages differ throughout the world. In many of the poorer nations, carbohydrates make up a considerably larger percentage of the diet.

Fats

Fats are a class of nutrients made up of fatty acids and glycerin, an organic alcohol. Fatty acids contain large amounts of carbon and hydrogen and small amounts of oxygen. Most fat nutrients are supplied by animals, including animal products such as butter, fatty meats, fish, egg yolks, poultry and other dairy products, salad and cooking oils, margarine, chocolate, nuts and peanut butter. Pound for pound, fats provide more usable energy fuel than either carbohydrates or proteins. They also take longer to digest and, therefore, have a longer-lasting satisfying effect on appetite and hunger.

The body can store fats. Aside from being energy stores, fat deposits in the body serve another useful purpose. Moderate amounts of fatty (adipose) tissue provide support, protection and insulation for the internal organs. When more fatty foods are ingested than the body can use or store efficiently, complications develop. Excess fat cannot be used, and its storage becomes obvious and unattractive. Not only does it serve no useful function, but excess fatty tissue can present numerous health problems for the body. An increased burden is placed on the heart and other internal organs. Movement becomes less efficient and less desirable and leads to laziness. Many overweight people suffer from postural problems caused by the additional load placed on the skeletal and muscular systems. Insurance statistics have shown that overweight individuals have a shorter life expectancy than those who maintain normal weight.

Proteins

Proteins are present in all living tissues. They make up vital parts of cells and are the main constituents of muscles, nerves, glands, and many hormones. In addition to carbon, hydrogen and oxygen, proteins also contain nitrogen. Protein molecules are large and are composed of many nitrogen-containing compounds called *amino acids*. Individual protein molecules may consist of several different amino acids. Before the body can utilize proteins, they must be broken down into their component amino acids by the digestive system. Then they can be absorbed by the blood and carried to the tissues, where they are selectively removed by cells in need of specific amino acids. The cells combine the

amino acids they have selected to form their own characteristic proteins. Those new proteins are used by the cells to carry out their own life functions.

The body uses proteins to build and repair body tissues and, in emergency situations, can oxidize proteins to meet energy needs. The use of proteins for energy can go on for only a limited time because while proteins are being oxidized for energy, the building and repairing of body cells and tissues must necessarily be affected. Though the body can use carbohydrates or fats to meet energy needs, it cannot substitute either of those components to perform the function of proteins, since neither can supply the necessary amino acids. The process of life is a rigorous experience for body cells and tissues. In the process, many millions of cells are destroyed daily. If the protein supply is not sufficient to offset the daily destruction of cells, the body will actually begin to waste away since the destroyed cells cannot be replaced. Therefore, a diet lacking in proteins must have a detrimental effect on growth and development.

Although proteins are necessary if life is to continue, they are not required in large amounts. Foods which are rich in proteins include meats, fish, eggs and nuts. Other foods which contribute lesser amounts of proteins are dry cereals, breads and most fruits and vegetables. Many of the foods that are rich in proteins also provide some minerals and vitamins. A wide range of protein ingestion is conducive to health and necessary during periods of rapid growth, or cell formation, as in adolescence, pregnancy and convalescence. It is a common practice among doctors to prescribe high-protein diets for pregnant women and individuals with diseases, in whom there is a high degree of cell destruction or damage.

Vitamins

Vitamins are organic substances that occur in small amounts in natural foods. They provide for chemical control of numerous body functions and play an important role in energy production, normal growth and development, reproduction, resistance to infection and general health. Most vitamins act as catalysts, substances which initiate, or change the speed of chemical reactions. Almost all the body's many chemical reactions require the presence of catalysts if they are to occur. Without those substances, many reactions and life itself could not continue. Catalysts that promote reactions in living tissues are called "organic enzymes."

Most plants can manufacture the vitamins they need, but you must get your vitamins from the foods you eat. The major sources of vitamins are meats, particularly liver and kidneys, fruits, vegetables, milk, eggs, fish and certain cereals. Deficiencies in the various essential vitamins can hinder the normal functioning of the body. Those deficiencies are evidenced by such afflictions as night blindness, poor bone and tooth formation, scurvy, stunted growth, lack of vitality, poor condition of skin and mucous membranes, and a loss of appetite and weight.

The vitamins considered most important when dealing with human nutrition include vitamin A, three members of the B complex group, C, D, E, K, B$_{12}$.

Vitamin A promotes normal growth, increases resistance to infections and contributes to the general condition of the epithelial tissues, those that line the passageways of the body. A lack of vitamin A leads to night blindness and poor condition of the skin and mucous membranes. The best sources of vitamin A are fish liver oils, milk, milk products, egg yolk, vegetables (spinach, broccoli, lettuce, carrots, green beans) and fruits (apricots and peaches).

Vitamin B Complex is actually a group of about ten vitamins needed by the body in small amounts. The most important members of the B complex group are thiamin, niacin and riboflavin. *Thiamin* facilitates energy production from carbohydrates and influences nervous function. A lack of thiamin may lead to nervous irritability, growth impairment and loss of appetite and weight. *Niacin* plays an important role in cell respiration and carbohydrate oxidation and contributes to good digestion. Niacin deficiency leads to a disease called pellagra. *Riboflavin* aids the utilization of protein and is important to growth and general health. A diet deficient in riboflavin is evidenced by poor skin condition and itching eyes. Foods that are rich in B vitamins include milk, yeast, liver, kidneys, fish, eggs, vegetables, lean meats and fresh fruits.

Vitamin C, or ascorbic acid, prevents scurvy, a disease characterized by weakness, bleeding gums, loss of teeth, and swelling in various parts of the body. The primary source of vitamin C is citrus fruits.

Vitamin D, the "sunshine vitamin," promotes the formation of strong bones and teeth, prevents rickets, and aids the absorption of important minerals by the body. An inadequate intake of vitamin D leads to bone deformities, protruding abdomen and restlessness. The body can manufacture vitamin D if sufficiently exposed to sunlight. Food sources include fish liver oils and milk fortified with vitamin D.

Other important vitamins are vitamin B$_{12}$ (blood formation), vitamin E (neuromuscular function) and vitamin K (normal blood clotting).

Minerals

Minerals are inorganic chemical substances which, like vitamins, play an important part in regulating body functions. In addition, they are essential to the structure of bones and other body tissues. The proper functioning of numerous organs depends upon a constant supply of several important minerals. Some of the essential minerals, and the most clearly understood from the standpoint of function, include calcium, phosphorus, iron, copper, iodine, sodium and potassium.

Calcium and *phosphorus* are necessary for the formation of strong bones and teeth. Calcium is also important in the regulation of the irritability of the nervous system. The major source of those important minerals is milk. Other foods rich in these minerals are cheese, green leafy vegetables and nuts. The need for calcium and phosphorus exists throughout life but is greatest during times of rapid growth and development.

Iron is a major component of the hemoglobin of the blood. Since the amount of oxygen that the blood can carry is dependent upon the amount of hemoglobin in the blood, the importance of iron is evident. A lack of iron in the diet will affect the ability of the blood to carry oxygen, since not enough hemoglobin can be formed. Deficiencies of iron can be avoided if the diet includes sufficient amounts of meat (particularly liver), eggs, green leafy vegetables, bread, cereals and certain other foods.

Copper aids the body's utilization of iron. The need for copper is small, and a well-planned diet will supply the necessary amount.

Iodine, another mineral that the body requires in small amounts, affects thyroid gland function. A lack of the mineral in the diet can lead to an enlargement of the gland, a condition known as "simple goiter." The chief sources of iodine are sea foods, marine plants and iodized salt.

Sodium and *potassium* salts are essential to the maintenance of water balance in the body and the functioning of nerves and muscles. The amount of water retained by the body is regulated by, among other things, the amounts of the salts present in the body tissues. Following periods of intense physical exertion, particularly during warm weather when the body loses more water and salt than normal, it is important that the replacement of water also be accompanied by replacement of the salt. If the salt is not replaced, the body will not be able to retain the water. In athletics, that situation is met by the administration of salt tablets or liquids that contain those salts. Normally, there need be no concern about sodium and potassium intake if a well-balanced diet is followed. See SALT TABLETS.

Other minerals that are considered important for normal body function are chlorine, fluorine, cobalt, magnesium, manganese, molybdenum, selenium, sulphur and zinc.

Water in Nutrition

Water accounts for about 70 per cent of the body weight. All of the body fluids are basically watery solutions. The three main fluid compartments of the body are:

1. Intracellular fluid, which exists within the cells.

2. Extracellular fluid, which exists between the cells and provides the environment in which they exist and perform their respective functions.

3. Plasma, a fluid, which consists of 92 per cent water.

Those fluids are made up of water and dissolved inorganic mineral substances. The chemistry of animal life involves exchanges between these fluids and combinations of the various solutions.

Historical incidents have shown that you can exist for as long as three or four weeks without food, but if deprived of water, you will die within a few days.

Water is acquired in three ways, water taken as drink, water contained in ingested foods, and water formed within the body as a result of the oxidation process. Water is lost from the body through urination, defecation, perspiration and evaporation. In the average adult, the daily water loss amounts to about three quarts, the amount which must be replaced daily. Two quarts of that requirement are provided by the food ingested. The other quart, approximately six glasses, must be taken daily as drink. Normally the thirst mechanism is sufficient to induce you take enough water. The fluid requirement varies from day to day depending on certain factors, the most important of which are perspiration, temperature and the amount of exercise or strenuous work in which you engage. Under conditions of extreme exertion, heat and excessive perspiration, a special effort is necessary to meet the water loss.

Exercise and Nutrition

At the present time, there is no scientific evidence to indicate that physical performance or fitness can be improved by modifying a basically sound diet. There is no doubt, however, that a less than adequate diet can impair the attainment of a high degree of physical fitness and maximum physical performance.

You cannot achieve physical fitness by merely paying close attention to obtaining an adequate diet. Likewise, you cannot achieve it by merely directing your efforts toward exercise. Adequate nutrition, exercise, rest, relaxation and other good health habits are all essential to obtain a desirable physique, organic health, and motor capacity physical fitness. Other important considerations for obtaining physical fitness are a healthy outlook on life and good motivation.

Diet Considerations

Calorie Intake—Normally, if you are not overweight, it is necessary to consume enough food daily to meet the energy demands of your training or exercise program. If you do not eat a sufficient number of calories, you will find it difficult to achieve maximum fitness. There is a strong possibility that you will also experience a decline in physical performance if that practice is continued too long. Sometimes the decline is referred to as staleness. See STALENESS. However, you should not consume more food than you need, or that will result in an increase in body weight despite the additional activity.

Proportion of Foodstuffs—There are many opinions of what constitutes a proper proportion of carbohydrates, fats and proteins, and there is little evidence to really support any of them. The chart shows approximate percentages, and these will vary from one person to another. The percentage of protein consumption, higher than is traditionally considered necessary, reflects what is needed by a person on a training program strenuous enough to result in increased muscle mass, thereby increasing the demands of protein. The fat consumption is considerably lower than that in the typical diet consumed in America, for many current diets contain a proportion of almost 50 per cent. Many authorities on degenerative cardiovascular disease feel that the 45 to 50 per cent proportions of fat is much too high, and that 30 to 35 per cent is much more desirable. Some have recommended that the percentage be reduced to 20 per cent, particularly for those who do not intend to exercise.

Carbohydrates—Carbohydrates are used primarily in muscular work. But if the exercise is long and the carbohydrate reserves diminish, fat is metabolized. When the carbohydrate stores can be refilled or maintained, endurance will be improved. A small amount of muscular efficiency is increased if carbohydrates rather than fat are consumed. If you intend to engage in endurance activities, be certain to have a diet rich in carbohydrates prior to the event. That recommendation should not be misinterpreted to mean that "extra-energy" food right before all activities is bene-

SUGGESTED PERCENTAGES OF BASIC FOODSTUFFS°

Foodstuffs	Calories		Percentage
	Men	Women	
Carbohydrates	1350-1650	1080-1320	45-55
Fat	900-1050	720-840	30-35
Protein	300-750	240-600	10-25

° Based on 3,000 calories for men and 2,400 calories for women.

ficial. The activities involved are of an endurance type. The taking of additional carbohydrates *during* an endurance activity, such as cross country skiing or very long distance running, will enable you to persist in the activity for a longer period of time.

Fat—Fat provides the fuel for muscular work when the carbohydrate reserves are lowered. There is some indication, moreover, that fat may be utilized even when the carbohydrate reserves are not lowered. It has been demonstrated, however, that the burning of fat is about 10 per cent less economical than the consuming of carbohydrates. Because of the reduced economy, a greater strain is placed on the respiratory system, for more oxygen is needed to burn up the fat.

Protein—Several research studies have shown that protein is not metabolized during exercise in the well-nourished person. Traditionally, a great deal of meat has been used at training tables in an effort to get the athletes the necessary protein for the upcoming athletic event. The benefit of the steak or other meat is largely psychological rather than physiological, however. The requirement for protein is not increased when performing exercise unless there is an increase in muscle mass.

Vitamins—Vitamins in the normal diet are essential for good performance. Where vitamins are lacking in diet, taking additional vitamins may improve performance.

There is one additional aspect regarding nutrition and exercise. Try to eliminate, as much as possible, those foods that furnish only calories without contributing to their share of vitamins and minerals. For example, substitute fruit and fruit juices for dessert, candy, soda and the like. See DIET.

OBESITY

Historically, obesity was considered a sign of success and well being. Fatness in men was thought a sign of prosperity, while plumpness was thought to enhance a woman's charm. Many fat individuals were admired because of their jolly personalities, and it was generally felt that fat people were happier and more carefree than the average person. Today, fat people come in second. Medical science tells us that obese people are not well nourished and strongly suggests greater risks for obese persons to such major disorders as heart disease, high blood pressure, diabetes and respiratory difficulties. The danger of developing other diseases also increases with fatness as does the possible damage to various normal body functions. Furthermore, obesity is a hazard for pregnant women and may produce infertility in men who possess rolls of fat on the thighs.

The association between obesity and mortality is real, even though the present cause and effect relationship is slim and obscure. However, insurance companies seem to feel the relationship is genuine and, consequently, are charging higher premiums for those who are fat. Economically the fat person is also penalized when buying clothing and furniture, securing transportation, and paying for the excessive quantities of appetizing foods. The concerned fat person also spends a great deal of money on potential cures or weight-reducing remedies.

Regardless of the health and monetary implications, obesity is also an esthetic problem and can lead to adverse psychological reactions. In our society, fat people are regarded as unattractive and unwanted and hence may develop feelings of insecurity, loneliness, tension, anxiety, defeat and neglect. Along with those numerous emotional disturbances, are associated physical discomfort of walking and the obvious discrimination encountered when competing for certain jobs.

Obesity Defined and Assessed

The two terms *obesity* and *overweight* are not synonymous. Obesity is a bodily condition marked by excessive, generalized deposition of fatty (adipose) tissue. The term "overweight" simply implies overheaviness, with no direct implication with regard to fatness. As discussed here, overweight may be entirely within a normal range of fatness. A person may be overweight because he is muscular (muscle tissue weighs more than fatty tissue), has a high degree of bony development, or has a condition marked by excessive accumulation of fluid in the tissues, which again is not directly related to the accumulation of fatty tissue.

The implication here concerns the use of standard height-weight tables to assess obesity. The practice of using the tables can be extremely misleading. A person should not be considered obese and restricted to a demanding diet solely because he is labeled overweight by standard height-weight tables. Certainly a fullback on a professional football team would be classified as overweight, but seldom is he obese.

How then can you tell if you are fat? There are numerous scientific techniques that could provide the answer. However, the best single method of assessment appears to be the utilization of skinfold calipers.

From a practical point of view, general fatness can be determined by simply looking in a mirror. In reality, the appraisal of the nude body is quite often a more reliable guide for estimating obesity than body weight. If the appearance test fails to give the answer, pinching the back of the upper arm (triceps area) can offer a realistic assessment. The U. S. Department of Health, Education and Welfare reports that a skinfold held between the thumb and forefinger thicker than one inch is an indication of body fatness.

Causes

The many causes of obesity fall into the following categories: environmental, genetic, psychological and physiological.

Environmental factors have made available all types and amounts of food while stifling the lack of opportunity and desire to exercise. Food habits, regardless of their inadequacies, continue to be practiced among various cultural groups, and food and drink are still the ultimate expression of hospitality at all social functions. Young mothers now consider large weight gains in early infancy as highly desirable, and comparing the eating habits of their infants to those of other infants leads them to introduce table foods too early. That usually results in the forcing of large quantities of food. Often parents allow those infants to eat as frequently as they want while minimizing physical activity.

Genetically, reports from studies of human populations strongly suggests the existence of a hereditary factor. For example, a study of M. L. Johnson and others showed that 8 to 9 per cent of children of normal-weight parents were classified as obese. When one parent was obese, the prevalence of obesity increased to 40 per cent. When both parents were obese, it rose to 80 per cent. Studies of twins and other groups support the genetic theory as a cause of obesity.

Studies of obese persons have also made it clear that overeating is frequently associated with emotional trauma. The onset of obesity in a number of subjects can be identified with some particular stress period. Bruch suggests that overeating may be a balancing factor in adjustment to life. If overeating is to be stopped, the individual must be helped to find some other form of emotional support. Failure to do so may result not only in unsuccessful weight reducing but may produce trauma far worse than the obesity it was designed to cure.

Many obese people delude themselves into believing that their fatness is caused by glandular disturbances. That is very rarely the case, although some types of obesity do result from improper functioning of the glands. The glands secrete the hormones which control metabolism, appetite and the body's utilization of fat. Less than two per cent of all obesity cases are believed to be of such origin. Those cases can often be controlled or cured by hormones given under a doctor's direction.

Although each of the above factors may have contributed to the development of obesity, the basic cause still remains the consumption of more calories than are expended, with the surplus food energy being converted into body fat. Simply stated, that means overeating and underexercising. Unable to burn all the fuel (food) it takes in and does not eliminate as waste, the body stores the surplus as fat. The fat tissue is not simply inactive stored material. Fat goes to work quickly and makes more fat.

Treatment

As always, the best treatment for obesity is prevention. During the pre-

ventative stage, you only need to concern yourself with keeping the caloric intake below your energy requirement or eating less food than the body requires for energy-producing purposes (work). When you neglect to practice prevention, you will usually become involved with treating much more than a simple balancing of energy requirements. The problem now becomes two-fold as you must overcome the original problem of energy balance as well as face the mounting social and psychological problems.

Exercise

The effectiveness of an increased level of activity in establishing caloric balance has been alternately overrated and underrated. As with dietary therapy, the area of reducing through exercise has been saturated with quackery. Miracle methods advertising instant results with little effort have been and will continue to be completely unsuccessful for the perplexed heavy person. *There simply is no method that is quick and effortless.* On the other hand, you hear that it is relatively impossible to lose weight through exercise. It has been stated that a caloric equivalent of a pound of fat can be matched only by walking 36 hours, splitting wood for 7 hours, or playing volleyball for 11 hours. However, the implied idea is that the cost of exercise depends entirely on the exercise being done at one stretch. Regarding that, Jean Mayer cites that, although splitting wood for one-half hour every day, by no means an impossible task for a healthy man, would add up to seven hours in two weeks. If it represents a regular practice, it would, by the very reasoning of the detractors of exercise, represent a caloric equivalent of 26 pounds of body fat in a year. A half hour of handball or squash a day would be equivalent to 16 pounds a year.

Moreover, most energy costs have

been quoted for an average man. Mayer feels that if the energy cost of exercise is approximately proportional to body weight (and it is), it follows that a heavy person will require more energy and, hence, burn up more body fat for the same amount of exercise as the person of desirable weight. Therefore, energy expenditure and weight loss would be greater in the case of a larger or heavier man.

Food and Exercise

Another misconception concerning food and exercise contends that exercise is usually followed by an increase in food intake. Mayer feels the increase can take place only if the individual was fairly active to start with. If he was sedentary, he can step up his activity without any such increase in appetite. Conversely, if activity is decreased below a certain point, appetite does not decrease correspondingly. In fact, it may increase somewhat. The result, of course, is an accumulation of fat.

Insufficient activity has been a more frequent finding among obese subjects than is an abnormally large food intake. In a study involving motion pictures, it was shown clearly that the average fat girl expends far less energy during scheduled exercise periods than does her nonobese counterpart. It was also found that the onset of excessive weight gain among fat children generally occurred during the winter, which suggests the possible importance of inactivity in the development of obesity. Researchers have also shown that fat girls eat less—*not more*—than normal-weight individuals but spend as much as two-thirds less time on preoccupations involving motion of the body. Fat women have also been shown to be less active than the nonobese.

However, even with the evidence in support of the values of exercise in maintaining or reducing weight, many claim they have tried exercising and have experienced very little success. That result is due to either or both of two reasons.

1. In most cases, fat people do not exercise hard enough nor with any degree of consistency. Obese people begin their exercise in poor physical condition and, thus, become discouraged immediately from sore muscles and fatigue, acquired from trying too much too soon. Properly conceived, an exercise program should build up gradually, with regularly scheduled periods of exercise at least five times per week. Results will not be immediate and fantastic, but like the program, they will come gradually and consistently. Over a period of one year, 10 to 20 pounds assuredly can be lost if proper training procedures are followed.

Psychological Deterrents

2. Most heavy people, after a month or so of physical exercise, usually become disheartened when they climb on the scales and find that their weight has remained the same or, in some cases, that it may have actually increased. It is significant to note that weight is not necessarily a good guide in fat loss because muscle tissue is heavier than fat tissue, and muscle tissue is the normal by-product of strenuous exercise. As a result of strenuous exercise, a person will probably lose a good deal of fat tissue (which should be the ultimate goal) but may gain or remain the same weight because the fat loss is usually compensated for by an increase in muscle tissue. Consequently, individuals are actually shedding ugly fat tissue and should be pleased with their progress.

The increase in muscle tissue need not be bulky and ugly, which is what most women usually fear. Exercise improves the tone of weak, sagging muscles and thereby improves the contour of specific areas of the body, such as the abdomen, chest, hips, buttocks, thighs, calves, etc. Even though the actual weight of most muscles will increase when exercised, a properly developed and supervised program can prevent a corresponding increase in bulk. That fact can easily be exemplified by the women who have participated on our Olympic gymnastic teams. They have indeed developed a toned musculature system and have still managed to keep themselves thin and attractively contoured. Dancers and ice skaters are additional examples of the same type of reasoning.

For those who choose not to exercise, fat can accumulate in most people by only a few calories a day. In fact, an excess of only 100 calories a day can produce a 10-16 pound weight gain a year. Hence, inactivity has been labeled the most important factor explaining the frequency of creeping overweight in our society. To combat the creeping weight problem, the concept of prevention cannot be overemphasized. There is no doubt that weight reduction can lead to general improvement in health and social status. However, there are still some disorders in which fatness can leave permanent health and social damage. Indeed, for these people, second place can become a permanent position on the ladder of life. See OVERWEIGHT and WEIGHT CONTROL.—*William A. Banaszewski*

ORGANIZATIONS

Several organizations have a vital concern in physical fitness. The following are just a few of those actively involved in promoting physical fitness and related areas.

AMA Committee on Exercise and Physical Fitness

The chief purpose of the Committee is the promotion of interest in physical fitness for both the medical profession and the public of all ages and sexes. The Committee is also concerned with the relationship of exercise to health and the coordination of AMA physical fitness efforts with those of other private and public agencies. Its address is 535 North Dearborn Street, Chicago, Illinois 60610.

Amateur Athletic Union

The AAU was founded in 1888 in an effort to control the unscrupulous practices that were threatening to destroy amateur athletics. Today, the AAU is divided into associations—both state and regional areas—which hold their own competition as well as national meets and tournaments. The AAU registers its amateurs and probes the country to see that its standards are maintained.

The AAU has jurisdiction over 19 sports including basketball, bobsledding, boxing, gymnastics, handball, horseshoe pitching, ice hockey, swimming, tobogganing, track and field, tug of war, volleyball, water polo and wrestling. Many of its sports assist the United States in training for Olympic competition. The AAU provides many interesting publications; its address is 231 West 58th Street, New York, New York 10019.

American Association for Health, Physical Education and Recreation

The American Association for Health, Physical Education and Recreation—a department of the National Education Association—is the voluntary professional organization which brings together teachers, administrators, leaders and students in these related fields. The AAHPER membership, now more than 50,000 is concerned with the present condition and future progress of physical education and dance, health education and school nursing, athletics, safety education, recreation, outdoor education and programs of professional preparation for leadership in these areas. The AAHPER serves members at all levels —elementary and secondary school, college and university, and community. It provides the framework through which the profession contributes to the well-being of people everywhere. While their responsibilities and interests vary, AAHPER members share a common purpose of working to strengthen and improve school and community programs. They promote public understanding of the values of these programs to children, youth and adults. And they have shown that personal and professional benefits increase as these objectives are accomplished.

The AAHPER has many publications, two of which are the *Journal of Health, Physical Education and Recreation* and the Research Quarterly. See PUBLICATIONS. The address of the AAHPER is 1201 Sixteenth Street, NW, Washington, D.C. 20036.

American College of Sports Medicine

The ACSM was established to advance and disseminate knowledge dealing with the effect of sports and other physical activities on the health of human beings at various stages of life. The organization includes physicians, physiologists, physical educators, dentists, nutritionists, psychologists, anthropologists, physical therapists, coaches, trainers and others interested in human fitness. The College is a professional organization that holds scientific meetings and workshops and publishes a newsletter, a scientific journal, and an *Encyclopedia of Sports Medicine*. There are three types of membership: Fellow, member, student member. To be a Fellow requires that you possess an earned doctorate degree, are a member of ACSM for one year, attend at least one regional or national meeting of the ACSM, and demonstrate further qualifications such as experience in publications in the area of sports medicine. To become a member, you must be sponsored by one Fellow of the College in good standing. The address of the College is: American Col-

lege of Sports Medicine, 1440 Monroe Street, Madison, Wisconsin 53706.

Athletic Institute

The Athletic Institute is concerned with the nation-wide promotion of athletics, physical education and recreation. The overall objective of this nonprofit organization is to motivate every community in America toward developing sports, physical fitness and recreation programs with adequate facilities, good leadership, programming and general participation. The Institute has produced audiovisual aids to help people become more proficient in sports. Such materials as 35 mm sound slide films, 8 mm loop films, handbooks and instructional guides are available. They have also sponsored symposiums and clinics on exercise and sports. The address of the Institute is: 805 Merchandise Mart, Chicago, Illinois 60654.

International Council of Health, Physical Education and Recreation

The ICHPER was established and developed on the concept of international cooperation. It serves to bring together teachers, administrators, leaders, national departments of physical education, and professional associations concerned with health, physical education, sports, and recreation into one organization and represents their concerns at the international level. Through the strengthening of professional ties among colleagues and departments as well as associations from all continents, the ICHPER fosters international understanding and goodwill and encourages the development and expansion of educationally sound programs in these fields in all countries.

The ICHPER collaborates at an international level with the WCOTP; with ICHPER members; with national and international organizations for health, physical education, sports and recreation; with national departments of physical education; with schools, institutes and universities; with related agencies such as Unesco, FAO, WHO, and UNICEF; and with interested colleagues and individuals throughout the world.

The address of the Council in the United States is ICHPER, 1201 Sixteenth Street, NW, Washington, D.C. 20036. Membership entitles you to receive the following publications: *ICHPER BULLETIN* (newsletter), *GYMNASIUM* (journal reporting international aspects of the profession), and Proceedings of ICHPER Congress (highlights and speeches of meetings).

Lifetime Sports Foundation

See LIFETIME SPORTS and AAHPER (under ORGANIZATIONS).

National College Physical Education Association for Men

The objectives of the NCPEAM are to advance physical education in institutions of higher learning, including: basic instruction, intercollegiate athletics, intramural athletics, research and teacher education. The College holds an annual meeting in which the subjects mentioned above are discussed. The *Proceedings* of the meetings are then published by the AAHPER. Its address is 205 Huff Gymnasium, University of Illinois, Urbana, Illinois 61822.

National College Physical Education Association for Women

The NCPEAW is the sister organization of NCPEAM. Its objectives are similar to those of the Men's College, has an annual meeting and publishes a *Proceedings* of the meeting.

Both the NCPEAM and the NCPEAW have a joint publication called *Quest*. The purpose of this journal is to publish analyses of professional practices and current thinking in the area of physical education. It is also used to provide a forum and outlet for other scholarly and aesthetic

presentations. Its address is 205 Huff Gymnasium, University of Illinois, Urbana, Illinois 61822.

National Collegiate Athletic Association

The NCAA was established in 1905 when 13 university representatives gathered in New York City to bring about reforms in football playing rules. Later 62 schools took part in a mass meeting called for by the preliminary group of 13. From that group evolved the NCAA. Today the NCAA is the governing group of over 600 colleges. It conducts championships in 13 sports, sets policies, keeps records, formulates rules, and guards against gambling and other unethical practices. Offices are located at: Suite 206, Fairfax Building, 11th and Baltimore, Kansas City, Missouri; and The National Collegiate Athletic Bureau, Box 757, Grand Central Station, New York, New York 10017.

National Federation of State High School Athletic Associations

The NFSHSAA governs the activity of 20,000+ high schools in 49 states and several Canadian provinces. It cooperates with other athletic organizations in writing the rules for a number of sports and compiling records. It also regulates traveling, equipment and other pertinent areas. Ninety-five per cent of the member schools have basketball teams, 50 per cent have football teams, and 60+ per cent have baseball and track teams.

The offices are located at 7 South Dearborn Street, Chicago, Illinois 60602.

National Foundation for Health, Physical Education and Recreation

The National Foundation for Health, Physical Education and Recreation is a private, nonprofit, tax exempt corporation formed in 1966 and sponsored by AAHPER. Its main purpose is the advancement of education through deeper understandings of the contributions of health education, physical education and recreation to the health and well being of all people.

The Foundation is constituted to receive and administer bequests, grants and special and general contributions, and to extend membership to individuals and groups. Membership in the Foundation is open to individuals and groups concerned with the advancement of health, physical education and recreation. Special invitations are extended to members of the profession, members of allied professions, sports and education writers, institutions, agencies, organizations and suppliers. A membership reply form and an information brochure will be sent on request. For more information write to: National Foundation for Health, Physical Education and Recreation, 1201 Sixteenth Street, NW, Washington, D.C. 20036.

The National Jogging Association

The National Jogging Association is a nonprofit, nationwide federation of jogging groups and individual joggers, recently incorporated to:

1. Promote healthful jogging by physically qualified people countrywide.

2. Stimulate and maintain motivation among joggers.

3. Foster the preventive maintenance concept in health preservation.

4. Increase communication among joggers through a nationally circulated Newsletter or Magazine.

5. Set standards of performance and safe guidelines for participation at various individual levels of fitness.

6. Provide understanding of the benefits of jogging—and of the precautions to be observed by the physically deconditioned.

7. Serve as a central repository for data on jogging, which can be computerized for research purposes as the years pass.

8. Serve as a clearinghouse for questions relating to jogging.

9. Sponsor research in exercise physiology and in the techniques of safely increasing total human performance and maintaining physical fitness.

10. Get the endorsement of the medical profession for the Association's objectives, standards and guidelines.

11. Mobilize the influence of jogging groups to provide jogging trails, tracks and supporting facilities.

12. Provide any desired degree of unity among jogging groups for coordinating programs and activities and attaining objectives.

For information write to: The National Jogging Association, P. O. Box 19367, Washington, D.C. 20036.

President's Council on Physical Fitness and Sports

See GOVERNMENT.

Project on Recreation and Fitness for the Mentally Retarded

See *AAHPER* under ORGANIZATIONS.

ORIENTEERING

Orienteering is a game of physical and mental challenge, for it involves a great deal of physical stamina and

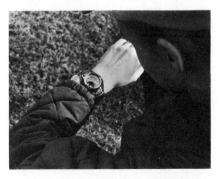

Proper use of a compass is essential in covering an orienteering course. Often the participant is asked to surmount natural obstacles in an unfamiliar terrain.

a good bit of decision-making and planning. Orienteering originated in Sweden, where it is a national, mass-participation sport. It is slowly being adopted by other countries of the world.

Orienteering involves hiking, climbing, running, jogging and walking, and adds a new dimension, mental involvement. That makes the activity all the more challenging.

Orienteering demands the use and knowledge of a detailed map and special compass. The map used is usually on a scale of about 2½ inches for every mile on the ground and presents in detail the terrain of the area, including rivers, lakes, streams, forests, roads, paths, railroads, fences, other important landmarks and land undulations (mountains, hills and valleys)— a very important aspect. The compass, helps the orienteer measure angles and distances on his map or find a bearing.

The participant is given a compass and a specially marked map of the area. The marks on the map indicate the control stations and coincides with the course to be covered. The course is established by an organizer to make the course easy or difficult depending upon the competitors' ability and experience.

The course is designed to cover all kinds of terrain, and many natural obstacles or problems are presented. Throughout the course, *control stations* are set up, which are found either in consecutive or random order, depending upon the rules of the game. The control stations on the ground coincide with the marks placed on the map. They are strategically placed so that they cannot be seen from one station to another. In fact, they are usually seen only from 20-35 yards away, the purpose being that the orienteer must use the map and compass to find his objective—the station. The control stations are marked on the ground with red and white flags about 24″ by 18″ and on the map with small red circles.

The object, therefore, is to have the orienteer begin at the starting line, progress to the various controls, mark his control card at each station, and return to the finish line. All those maneuvers are attempted in the shortest time possible. Each control station must be reached. If one is missed, a penalty is incurred.

The orienteer, from the start, plots his course to achieve the first control station. For that he reads his map, compass and protractor. The control station is marked with a red and white flag and is placed so that it may be observed from 20 to 35 yards away, which allows the orienteer to come within a few yards of the control despite very minute errors in calculations. The control is not hidden. Once at the control station, the orienteer marks his control card with a marker or has it marked by the control official. Now the contestant sets his sights on the next control. He aligns his compass on the map and then plots his objective.

To get to a control, there is a good deal of decision making. On the map, it may appear that the shortest distance between two points is a straight line—if the land is flat. But if the terrain has elevations of considerable height or other obstacles, taking another route may be more efficient physically and less time consuming. There are other techniques, which the experienced orienteer learns with practice, that will assist him greatly in reducing his time.

Conditioning Programs

Orienteering is a high-energy-cost activity and, therefore, requires that you be in excellent physical condition to (adequately participate). Since orienteering contests may last 100 minutes or more, cause you to sprint on open fields, do some hill climbing or rock climbing, you need to be in good condition.

To adequately prepare for orienteering, spend about 30 minutes every other day running. At first, you should run about 10 minutes, covering 1 mile. Each day increase by 1 or 2 minutes until you are able to run 30 minutes. If that is too demanding, start out by

* ORIENTEERING PROGRAM

Chart 1		Chart 2	
1.	10 minutes	1.	35 minutes
2.	15 minutes	2.	35 minutes
3.	15 minutes	3.	40 minutes
4.	20 minutes	4.	40 minutes
5.	20 minutes	5.	45 minutes
6.	25 minutes	6.	50 minutes
7.	25 minutes	7.	50 minutes
8.	30 minutes	8.	55 minutes
9.	30 minutes	9.	60 minutes

* See ENDURANCE and ENERGY COST OF ACTIVITIES for an explanation of these charts.

Fitness 1

If you achieved a score of poor or low average on the *Harvard Step Test* or a score of very poor or poor on the *12 Minute Run*, start on Chart 1-Level 1 and spend 1 week at each level until Chart 2-Level 9 is reached. It is recommended that you participate 4 to 5 days a week. When Chart 2-Level 9 is reached, 4 days a week is sufficient.

Fitness 2

If you achieved a score of high average on the *Harvard Step Test* or fair on the *12 Minute Run*, start on Chart 1-Level 2. Spend one week on Chart 1-Levels 2, 5, 7, 9, and Chart 2-Levels 2, 4, 5, 7, 8, and 9. It is recommended that you participate 4 to 5 days a week. When Chart 2-Level 9 is reached, 4 days a week is sufficient.

Fitness 3

If you achieved a score of good or excellent on either the *Harvard Step Test* or *12 Minute Run*, continue your current program or select Chart 2-Level 9 as your level of participation. Four days a week is sufficient.

jogging and gradually increase the speed until you are able to cover 3 miles in at least 30 minutes.

After you have adjusted to that routine, you can then progress to step 2 in the training program. Start out by jogging for about 10 minutes. Then choose one of the following forms of running.

Interval Running—Select a distance of about 220 yards. Plan to cover the distance in about 36 seconds. Run one 220 at that pace, and then rest for 2 minutes. Then run again. That should be done 6 to 30 times depending upon your condition and level of competition. Gradually reduce your rest period as your physical condition improves. See INTERVAL TRAINING.

Continuous Running—Select or mark off a course from 3 to 6 miles that covers various terrains. Run at a continuous pace.

Fartlek—Set up a similar course to what was done for continuous running. Instead of running the course at the same pace, vary your speed from all out sprinting to steady running to light jogging. See FARTLEK.

Contribution to Fitness

Since orienteering is a high-energy-cost activity, it may be used to help improve your fitness level, especially your circulo-respiratory and muscle endurance. Below is an orienteering program that takes into account the important principles of training.

OVER-DISTANCE TRAINING

Over-distance training requires the runner, cyclist, skater or swimmer to train at distances greater than the distance of his specific event. The pace, naturally, is slower than that of the intended competition event. For example, a runner training for the 440-yard dash may run a series of 880 yards or runs of two to three miles in daily preparation.

The most common reasons for using

the over-distance training technique are: (1) to develop or improve circulorespiratory and muscle endurance; (2) to give the performer an opportunity to work on the proper mechanics of running, cycling, or whatever; (3) to develop confidence so that the performer will be able to run the shorter distance in competition because of his ability to cover long distances relatively easily; (4) to break away from the monotony of training continually for speed.

Over-distance training is usually most advantageous early in the season when emphasis is placed on building endurance and stamina and on correct form. See FARTLEK.

OVERLOAD PRINCIPLE

The overload principle is basic to any program of physical conditioning. Simply stated, it means that when repeatedly and regularly stimulated by a greater-than-normal exercise load or rate, the body adjusts and increases its capacity to perform physical work. If you want to improve your physical fitness, repeatedly subject your body to an exercise routine more vigorous than normal. When the body adapts to an exercise level, the work level must be increased so that the body is stimulated by a greater than normal exercise load. You remain at that level until the body adapts further. The procedure is followed until the desired level of fitness is achieved.

Three Methods

There are three methods to increase the exercise load: (1) increase the resistance, (2) increase the length of the exercise, or (3) increase both the resistance of the exercise and duration.

You can increase the resistance by adding weight (adding weight in weight training), increasing the speed in which the exercise is performed (attempting to run a similar distance in a shorter period of time), or a com-

bination of the two. You can increase the length of exercise, by increasing the number of repetitions of exercise (more repetitions in calisthenics or weight training), by increasing the distance over which the exercise is performed (running a greater distance) or by increasing the repetitions and the distance.

Overload should be gradual to permit adaptation to take place without undue strain on the body. Although it is normal to have some muscle soreness and tiredness at the start of training, it is unnecessary, however, for such discomfort to be excessive to the point where you limit your daily activity.

Excellent examples of programs that utilize the overload principle are weight training, interval training and circuit training.

For further information, see ADAPTATION, PROGRESSION and TRAINING.

OVERTRAINING

Sometimes in an effort to attain an exceptionally high degree of fitness, you may begin to train frequently and quite intensely—a pattern that is particularly true in athletic training. At first, there is considerable improvement. But when you lose interest and your performance starts to fall, you are overtrained and begin to enter a period of staleness. The overtraining and resulting staleness are not to be confused with *retrogression*. See RETROGRESSION and TRAINING. When performance declines, you usually try even harder to improve, compounding the entire situation and only adding to that overtrained state. Shortly you become frustrated and develop feelings of inadequacy.

Signs of Overtraining

Some of the outward signs of overtraining are a feeling of tiredness, loss of weight, poor appetite, occasional headaches and failure to sleep well.

You may also notice definite behavior changes, such as lassitude and irritability. Many times those symptoms are not evident to the overtrained person but only to those around him. Dr. Wolfgang Wolf notes that there are several measurable physiological changes that accompany overtraining —increased resting heart rate and blood pressure, increased frequency of breathing, a rise in blood sugar and increased basal metabolism.

Overtraining varies from one person to another. In his study, Dr. Wolf showed that there are five basic reasons why a person may become overtrained. (1) the basic personality of the person (he is bored easily); (2) the type of sport (usually those sports that require speed, strength, and good coordination predispose the person to overtraining); (3) too early specialization on top performance by relatively young performers; (4) overexertion through occupation and participation in an activity (a sort of burning the candle at both ends); and (5) overuse of caffeine stimulants, such as coffee and colas.

A further problem is that the person may be attempting to reach a goal that is beyond his capacity or ability. As a result, he feels frustrated with too much competition. And in athletic competition, you cannot expect to give a maximum effort every few days, for the body needs time to recuperate.

Treatment

To recover, the best technique is to suspend training for a time or taper-off the training and not work as intensely as before. A checkup by the family physician might also be in order to determine if there are any serious physiological disorders causing the reduced performance. The symptoms of overtraining usually disappear after a week or so away from the work.

Preventing overtraining is a matter of recognizing the basic causes of the overtraining syndrome. Also by being aware that each person is different and has his own capacity, you will not be continually comparing your progress with that of your neighbor. Each person has his own individual rate of improvement. See INDIVIDUAL RATES OF RESPONSE.

Another vital concept is variety in the workout. Repeatedly doing the same thing, day after day, can only result in boredom. Be willing to put variety in your exercise and activity routine. Even Roger Bannister, when conscientiously training for the four-minute mile, took time off to go rock climbing. He considered it to be part of his training routine. If a world record holder considers it important to vary the workout, so can you. For more information, see STALENESS IN TRAINING AND RACING.

OVERWEIGHT

Your overall health is the product of several factors: heredity, disease, environment, stress, emotional stability, exercise and diet. For every individual, there is an optimum diet that will adequately supply the essential nutrients for growth, development and good health. Variations from that diet can lead to many complications, particularly malnutrition. Malnutrition can result from a lack of food, or even from too much food or the wrong kinds of foods.

Despite an abundance of food, many Americans are poorly fed. They choose their foods poorly with little regard for nutritional value, and they eat excessively. Many overweight people overindulge in animal fats, dairy products and sweets. Modern labor saving devices, particularly the automobile, have contributed to the overweight problem by reducing man's need to expend energy. Overweight places the body systems under a constant strain and can lead to life-shortening diseases, including heart disease and vascular problems, diabetes, kidney afflictions, digestive disorders, cancer, arteriosclerosis, high blood pressure and others.

Research and insurance statistics have shown a relationship between longevity and weight. The 1959 Build and Blood Pressure Study by the Society of Actuaries showed that a moderate degree of underweight is favorable to long life, other factors being equal. Overweight was disadvantageous and increased the mortality rate. In other words, overweight people are more susceptible to complications which might lead to early death.

When trying to determine the status of their present weight, many people refer to average weight charts. Those are a poor guide since the average includes overweights as well as underweights. Normal, or ideal weight, is generally considered to be about 20 pounds below average weight. Ideal weight charts have been developed that take into account your age, height, sex and size of frame.

Basically your weight is determined by food intake and energy expenditure. Constant weight can be maintained if food intake and food usage are balanced. When food intake becomes excessive and outstrips usage, the excess must be stored by the body as adipose tissue, or fat. The body is capable of storing a limited amount of fat efficiently. In fact, moderate amounts of fat tissue are necessary for good health, because it contributes to support, protection and insulation for various organs of the body and serves as part of the foundation for the skin. But when the excess no longer can be stored efficiently, fat presents an unattractive health hazard.

Active people have higher energy requirements than sedentary individuals. Therefore, their caloric intake must be greater to meet their needs. Compared to carbohydrates and proteins, fats are concentrated energy foods; they provide approximately twice as much energy fuel as the same

amounts of carbohydrates and proteins. High fat diets are not harmful to those who are physically active, since they burn up the fat reducing the chances of overweight. Unfortunately, people who are not physically active often indulge in high fat diets. Overweight can also be caused by a high carbohydrate diet as well, since excess carbohydrates are converted to fat for storage by the body.

Overweight can usually be traced to two factors—overeating and a lack of exercise. When weight is gained, there is more body tissue to be maintained. The skeletal and muscular systems are placed under an obvious strain to support the additional load thrust upon them. A not so obvious, but very dangerous, strain is placed on the cardiovascular system. The accumulation of fatty tissue means an increase in blood pressure, which causes the heart to work harder to overcome the increased resistance. In the overweight, or obese person, muscle tissue, which aids blood flow, is negligible or has been replaced by fatty tissue. Adipose tissue actually hampers blood flow, since it is not very vascular (i.e., not well supplied with blood vessels). In obese inactive people, the blood vessels become less elastic and lose some of their ability to aid circulatory function. In the overweight person, the heart must assume a greater degree of the responsibility for moving the blood through the body. The heart of the normal individual gets assistance from the blood vessels and muscle tissues.

Once the capacity of the body fat stores is reached, any additional fats remain in the blood and are circulated throughout the vascular system. It is possible for those fatty materials to become deposited on the inner lining of the blood vessel walls narrowing the arterial openings and leading to a hardening of the arteries, or arteriosclerosis. Arteriosclerosis results in a loss of the elasticity in the arterial walls. Aside from those complications, fatty deposits in the blood vessels pose another threat; solid parts of the deposits may break away from the vessel lining and be carried throughout the vascular system (the system of blood vessels). It is possible for one of the particles to become lodged in a vessel opening, blocking the blood flow through it. If that vessel serves a major organ (heart or brain), the blockage could be fatal.

Much interest has been directed lately to a substance called *cholesterol,* which belongs to a class of fats referred to as sterols. Cholesterol, as well as several other fatty substances, is a normal constituent of certain body tissues and aids some functions. Its source is certain foods, but it can also be formed in the body. Cholesterol level in the blood depends upon the same factors that control the levels of other food substances in the body—intake and usage. The fact that cholesterol can be formed in the body, as well, makes control of the cholesterol level in the blood of some individuals difficult. Blood cholesterol level does fluctuate in normal individuals, and some can tolerate a higher level than others without complications.

Attempts have been made, with a degree of success, to link high blood cholesterol levels to the incidence of coronary heart disease and other circulatory problems. In those diseases, cholesterol deposits form on the arterial linings and restrict blood flow.

Fat nutrients account for approximately 40 per cent of the American diet, which is considerably higher than most other countries. According to most nutritionists, the optimum fat content of the diet is about 20-25 per cent. Fat consumption, connected with the fact that many Americans tend to be sedentary, throws some light on the problem of overweight in the United States.

There is no immediate or easy method to remove excess weight. None of the reducing fads or short-cut methods has been proven effective. The answer to losing weight is simple; cut down on calorie intake and increase calorie usage. Losing weight is not pleasant; old eating habits must change, and new habits must be formed with respect to diet and exercise. The goodies and the between meal snacks must go. Those who can never find time to exercise must make time.

Aside from aiding weight control, regular vigorous exercise provides numerous physiological benefits; it leads to increased lung efficiency, more efficient transport of nutrients and oxygen, better removal of wastes, conditioning of the blood vessels and strengthening of the heart. The heart is a muscle. Like other muscles, its efficiency, strength, endurance and size increase with exercise. As the heart becomes better conditioned, it can pump more blood with less effort; it pumps more blood per stroke and reacts quickly to emergency needs. The heart of the obese person works harder at rest than does the heart of the physically fit person. It is not capable of working at the capacity of a healthy heart. In an emergency situation, that heart cannot be depended upon since it is unaccustomed to meeting the demands of intense exertion. Not only may it fail to meet the demands of a given situation, but it might fail completely, resulting in permanent damage or even death.

The greatest value of regular exercise is that it accustoms the heart and the rest of the organisms to physical stress; and survival depends, to a large degree, upon your ability to cope with stressful situations, both physical and mental. There seems to be a positive relationship between the ability to withstand physical stress and the ability to withstand mental or emotional stress.

The problem of overweight is not strictly a physical problem; but for many overweight people, it is also a very definite emotional problem. Many fat people are ashamed of their physical appearance. They are, for the most part, reluctant to get into situations where their physical excess puts them at a disadvantage (i.e., athletic situations, social events, etc.). They do not like to move because they are poor at moving. The adages "everyone loves a fat man" and "fat people are jolly" cannot be further from the truth; most fat people are miserable under their facade of jolliness; they may appear to be happy on the outside, but they are figuratively and literally dying on the inside. To some, the fat person is nothing more than an unattractive, lazy individual who is ruled by his stomach and exhibits no control over his appetites. To medical authorities, he is sick.

Why People Overeat

Why do people overeat? Some overeat from habit; some simply for the enjoyment they derive from eating, while others use eating as a means of meeting unpleasant situations. Psychologists have found that some obese people rely on food to fulfill desires which have not been met. The psychological implications of overweight is a study in itself, and a complex one. Overweight among children and adolescents can precipitate life-long physical and emotional problems. Dr. Hilde Bruch speaking on the emotional significance of the preferred weight said: "A feeling of harmony and integrity about one's self and one's body is an important, central experience for a healthy emotional development. The hapless youngster who according to his constitutional makeup is inclined to grow heavy, is continuously exposed to a negative critical attitude and derogatory comments. His concept of self, as well as his body image, is built during childhood from all sensory and psychic experiences. If there is continuous insult to a person's

physical makeup, he will be unable to develop a valid feeling of self-esteem and of unity between his psychic and physical self."

As already mentioned, there is no easy way to lose excess weight. It involves sacrifice and hard work. Some encourage the overweight person to purchase certain gadgets or miracle drugs to make weight losing easy. Some suggestions for easy weight reduction include belts, vibrating machines, corsets, soaps, reducing foods, steam baths and drugs. The only real reducing foods are those that are satisfying and provide essential nutrients but are low in calorie content. Steam baths do reduce weight; but that loss is only due to sweating, and the water is rapidly replaced. Drugs advertised for weight reduction should be regarded with suspicion and not used except under the supervision of a physician. The indiscriminant use of such products can pose a threat to your well-being.

Knowledge of the principles of nutrition is valuable in losing weight. With such knowledge, you can select foods that provide nourishment without the excess calories. Any physician can help in the planning of a weight watcher's diet by investigating your eating habits and daily energy requirements. Caloric charts and booklets have been compiled that can be used to determine the caloric value of various foods. H. Diehl estimates that, if you could reduce the daily caloric intake by 50 calories for a year, you would lose 5 pounds, other things remaining equal (exercise, etc.). A 100 calorie per day decrease would result in a 10 pound weight loss in a year. The value of exercise in a weight reducing program cannot be over-emphasized.

Underweight

Just as some individuals have an overweight problem, others have an underweight problem. While a slight degree of underweight is desirable, some people are too much below normal weight. Evidence seems to show that underweight does not pose any of the myriad problems associated with, and attributed to, overweight. Like overweight, underweight is based on the relationship between calorie intake and calorie usage; but in the latter condition, calorie intake cannot keep pace with calorie usage. Fat tissue, a moderate amount of which is necessary for good health, is negligible in the underweight person. Underweight persons tend to tire easily and usually lack strength.

The solution, in most cases of serious underweight problems, is to get the person to take in more food. Usually, the diet of the underweight person does not supply the essential requirements; they do not ingest enough food to meet energy and development needs. It is important that they choose foods carefully when trying to gain weight. Care must be taken to assure that the necessary daily vitamin and mineral needs of the body are met. Where there is a lack of appetite, an attempt should be made to select foods that are tasty. Some authorities suggest eating more frequently including a small meal or snack before bedtime. Quite often, the underweight person does not get enough sleep; extra sleep, during which time energy expenditure is at a minimum, is helpful in gaining weight. Exercise helps by increasing the demand for food fuel. Exercise also leads to the development of muscle tissue which adds bulk and weight to the body. See DIET, NUTRITION, OBESITY, WEIGHT GAINING and WEIGHT CONTROL.

OXYGEN DEBT

The human body depends on oxygen for survival. Even during the period of greatest inactivity, such as deep sleep, the requirement for oxygen, although minimal, still exists. The body's need for oxygen is directly proportional to its degree of activity. The more active the body, the greater is its need. Under normal circumstances, the body is able to supply itself with enough oxygen to meet its demands.

On occasion, the body needs more oxygen than its circulatory and respiratory systems can provide. That can happen under two different, but related, sets of conditions. In one instance you may start performing an activity, such as climbing a flight of stairs, at a fixed rate of work which requires an increased but constant expenditure of energy. To meet the increased energy expenditure, the oxygen *requirement*, likewise, is instantaneously increased to a new level. However, it takes the body from several seconds to several minutes to adjust its oxygen supply or intake to the new required level. Thus during that adjustment period, the demand or requirement exceeds the supply.

Under the second set of conditions, you are faced with a performance task, such as running a 100-yard dash, in which the level of energy expenditure needed to perform the task requires an oxygen intake greatly in excess of your maximal oxygen intake capability. See OXYGEN INTAKE. Throughout the entire performance of that task, the supply is unable to meet the demand.

In both of the above examples, you are able to climb the stairs or run the 100-yard dash even though your oxygen requirement is greater than your ability to provide oxygen, either temporarily or entirely during the performance. During those intervals where the oxygen demand or requirement exceeds the supply, you form what is termed an *oxygen debt*. It is the formation of that debt which allows you to perform successfully without having to stop as a result of an oxygen deficiency.

Recovery Period

The term *debt* implies an obligation or something owed, and that is applicable to the term *oxygen debt*. Immediately following the performance of an activity in which an oxygen debt is formed, there is a period, referred to as the recovery period, in which your heart rate, breathing rate and depth, level of oxygen intake, and other physiological parameters are all elevated above the so-called resting levels. It is during that period that the oxygen debt is repaid. The duration of the recovery period depends on the magnitude of the oxygen debt.

The physiological processes which allow the formation and repayment of the oxygen debt are not entirely understood. What is known concerning the biochemical transformations enabling the occurrence of the phenomenon are detailed and complex. In its simplest terms, however, an oxygen debt is formed because of the following chain of events. During the normal formation, expenditure and reformation of energy (energy cycle), oxygen functions in a capacity where it removes certain end products of metabolism, thus allowing the energy cycle to continue uninterrupted. In the absence of sufficient oxygen, those end products accumulate. That blocks the energy cycle, and the result is a reduction in the available energy sources, which quickly leads to a cessation of the activity. Because of the formation of lactic acid, the energy cycle can continue for a certain period of time in the absence of oxygen, because lactic acid formation functions as a temporary substitute for oxygen. The duration of that period depends primarily on the level of accumulated lactic acid. During the recovery period, the oxygen intake in excess of the "resting" level is used for the greatest part to reduce that lactic acid back to its normal level. Thus the lactic acid serves to allow the forma-

tion of an oxygen debt and remains to remind the debtor that oxygen is owed, once it becomes available in sufficient quantity.

The oxygen debt accumulated under the conditions of a 100-yard run is explained by the lactic acid mechanism. However, under the conditions of stair climbing, it is open to question as to whether lactic acid is or is not involved.

The amount of oxygen debt that you can incur seems to be an individual matter. There is some evidence which indicates that cardio-respiratory training will increase the size of the debt that can be tolerated and also that athletes can tolerate larger debts than nonathletes. The ability to sustain a larger debt would be advantageous because it would increase your performance potential. However, it has yet to be determined whether that result is from a physiological adaptation or from your being better able to withstand the discomfort associated with the accumulation of a higher debt. The latter would be associated more with a psychological adaptation.
—*Jack H. Wilmore*

OXYGEN INTAKE (UPTAKE)

One of the primary functions of the respiratory and cardiovascular systems is to provide oxygen, via the blood, to the body tissues. Oxygen is taken into the lungs from the atmosphere during the inspiration phase of the breathing cycle. From here, it diffuses through the lung tissue into the blood, where it chemically binds to the hemoglobin of the red blood cell. The oxygenated blood is then carried through a great vascular network to the microscopic capillaries which permeate the tissues at that point, diffusing from the blood across the capillary membrane to the tissue, in proportion to the needs of that particular tissue.

The amount of oxygen released by the blood and used by the body's tissues during a fixed period of time is referred to as *oxygen intake*. Oxygen *up*take and oxygen consumption are two additional terms that are used interchangeably with oxygen intake, all three terms denoting the same physiological phenomenon.

Although oxygen is not the source of energy for any general body or muscular activities, as is sometimes commonly believed, it is intimately involved with the biochemical processes which synthesize the primary energy sources. Without oxygen, those biochemical processes cannot continue, and the tissues involved would live only a matter of several minutes. Thus, even though oxygen is not the source of the body's energy, the amount of oxygen used by the body over a certain period of time (oxygen intake) is directly proportional to the energy expended by the body to perform its many tasks. It is in that sense that the term *oxygen intake* gains its physiological significance.

Connection with Cardiovascular and Respiratory Systems

Through its reflection of the organism's energy expenditure, the oxygen intake also reflects the efficiency of the cardiovascular and respiratory systems. At that point, oxygen intake can be related to cardiorespiratory fitness, the latter being one of the most important components of total body or physical fitness. See CIRCULO-RESPIRATORY ENDURANCE. The relative degree of efficiency of the cardiovascular and respiratory systems is indicative of the cardiorespiratory fitness level; the greater the efficiency, the higher the level of fitness. Thus, to evaluate cardiorespiratory fitness, that degree of efficiency must be assessed.

Oxygen intake, under certain conditions, reflects the efficiency of the cardiovascular and respiratory systems. Research has shown that you have a definable limit as to the greatest quantity of oxygen you can deliver to your tissues during an allout performance of a large muscle activity, such as running. That limit is referred to as your maximal oxygen intake. Theoretically, those people with larger maximal oxygen intakes have greater efficiencies and consequently higher cardiorespiratory fitness levels. That is due to their ability to deliver more oxygen to their tissues over a fixed

AVERAGE MAXIMAL OXYGEN INTAKE VALUES FOR SELECTED GROUPS*

Level of Conditioning	Number of Subjects	Age Group	Maximal Oxygen Intake	
		years	$ml/kg/min.$[1]	$ml/LBW/min.$[2]
Runners	5	18-29	65.8	71.2
Athletes	15	18-29	52.8	57.5
Phys. Ed. Majors	42	20-33	58.6	
	16	20-26	50.5	
Normal-Trained	50	18-25	55.4	
Normal-Average	24	17-33	50.0	
	22	18-30	49.3	54.6
	11	20-29	48.7	
	36	20-29	44.7	
	39	18-29	44.6	53.1

* Adapted from the publication Wilmore, Jack H., "The Influence of Motivation on Physical Work Capacity and Performance," *J. Appl. Physiol.* 24:459-469, 1968.
[1] milliliters of oxygen/kilogram of body weight per minute.
[2] milliters of oxygen/kilogram of lean body weight per minute.

period of time, which implies that they have a greater available energy source and thus the potential for performing more work (increased endurance).

The above theory is partially substantiated by the fact that your maximal oxygen intake will increase significantly as a result of a cardiorespiratory training or conditioning program, such as running. Additional support for that theory is given by the data presented in the accompanying chart, comparing the average maximal oxygen intake values of selected groups of individuals, each group possessing different degrees of cardiorespiratory fitness. Those values are expressed in relation to your body weight (maximal oxygen intake/body weight). Maximal oxygen intake is directly related to your muscle mass regardless of your respective level of cardiorespiratory fitness. By dividing the maximal oxygen intake by your body weight or, even better, lean body weight (body weight—weight of body fat), the influence of the muscle mass is reduced considerably, and the resulting value is more truly representative of cardiorespiratory efficiency and fitness.—*Jack H. Wilmore*

OXYGEN SUPPLEMENT

In the 1932 Olympics, the Japanese swimming team administered oxygen to its athletes in an effort to improve their performance. The incident would probably have gone unnoticed, except for the fact that the Japanese dominated the various swimming events. Ever since that time, a great many coaches around the world have used oxygen to "assist" their athletes, especially in track meets and football games.

The practice of utilizing oxygen to assist an athlete has drawn a great deal of controversy. There are those who feel that the oxygen helps a person physiologically as well as psycho-logically. Others feel the benefits are merely psychological. Still others feel that the use of oxygen has absolutely no effect upon performance.

Therapeutical Basis for Administering Oxygen

Even in the mildest physical activity, there is an increased demand for oxygen by the cells. In order to meet that demand, the entire respiratory system steps up its activity by increasing the depth and rate of breathing. The amount of increase, naturally, is dependent upon the intensity and length of the activity. At the same time, the exchange of gases in the lungs and cells is much more efficient.

During exercise, the physiological adjustments that take place are directed toward transporting more oxygen to the exercising muscles. The blood under resting conditions leaves the lungs about 95 per cent saturated with oxygen and returns to the lungs about 70 per cent saturated. The other 25 per cent has been used by the tissues of the body. But during exercise, the blood returns to the lungs only 5 per cent saturated, which indicates the body's need for more oxygen. During exercise, however, when the blood passes through the lungs, it does not remain there as long as during rest because of the increased heart rate. Actually, it is in the lungs only about one-fourth of the time that it would be if you were at rest. To compensate for that decreased time, the small vessels of the lungs dilate and provide for greater diffusion of oxygen to the blood. The compensation will take place adequately, provided the oxygen intake does not exceed 4+ quarts per minute, which is about 12 to 16 times the consumption of oxygen at rest. If the exercise is more severe, the oxygen diffusion will be incomplete, thereby reducing the oxygen saturation of the arterial blood.

At first, the popular conception was that additional oxygen could improve performance because more oxygen would be available in the lungs for diffusion, thereby increasing the hemoglobin saturation, and making available more oxygen in the blood solution. Since there are .2 cubic centimeters of oxygen present in each 100 cubic centimeters of blood, the increased oxygen intake would supposedly increase the amount of oxygen in solution to about .6 cubic centimeters per 100 cubic centimeters of blood. The problem is, however, that the above statements apply only while you are breathing the oxygen. Once the breathing of oxygen has stopped and the rebreathing of the atmospheric air begins, the entire process reverses itself and returns to the level prior to breathing the additional oxygen. Breathing of additional oxygen improves performance only when used during the actual performance.

Applied research supports the above discussion. A. T. Miller conducted an experiment in which he administered oxygen before, during and after a treadmill run. He found no changes in heart rate, blood pressure, blood lactate, or even endurance when the oxygen was administered before exercise. He also found no improvement in recovery for the measurements mentioned above as a result of breathing oxygen. His study did reveal, however, a decrease in blood lactate and an increase in running time to exhaustion *when oxygen was administered during exercise.* In the same study, he was able to demonstrate a psychological effect for breathing atmospheric air that had been marked *oxygen,* for the subjects to see. That fact may explain why some studies have indicated an improved performance after breathing oxygen.

E. R. Elbel, D. Ormond and D. Cluse found similar conclusions regarding the administering of oxygen during and after exercise. *They found that oxygen administered during exercise revealed significantly slower heart*

rates. When oxygen was administered during recovery, there were no significant changes in oxygen debt repayment, but the pulse rates were significantly slower. The pulse rates, however, were rather small—1 to 5 beats per minute.

Conclusions of Research

It may be concluded from the previously cited research and thought that:

1. The administering of oxygen does not produce a more efficient physiological function unless it is utilized during the actual exercise. The improvement of performance, if there is any, is unquestionably psychological.

2. The administering of oxygen after performance does not aid in recovery to any appreciable extent.

3. Improved performance will undoubtedly occur if oxygen is breathed during the actual event, but that, of course, is impossible in virtually all activities except mountain climbing.

OXYGEN REQUIREMENTS

The human organism, like all other living organisms, requires oxygen to survive. In all the living cells of the body, oxygen is combined with energy fuel in a constant life process called oxidation. The fuel is provided by the breakdown of foods in the digestive system. The food fuel, in the form of glycogen, is transported to the cells via the blood stream, where it is utilized. The combination that takes place in the cells is complex, but simply stated:

Glycogen + Oxygen → Carbon
dioxide + Water + Energy

The energy produced is used by the various cells to carry out their specific functions. The body is capable of storing the fuel (glycogen) in the cells as potential energy to be released during oxidation. Oxygen, on the other hand, cannot be stored by the body and must, therefore, be continually supplied to the cells. The supply function is performed by the respiratory and circulatory systems.

Exercise and Oxygen

Muscular contraction is one of the many functions that oxidation makes possible. Exercise, or physical work, is the result of muscular contraction. Since exercise can occur at varying levels of intensity, it follows that oxidation, which supplies the energy for contraction, must occur at a level proportional to that of the muscular activity. During increased physical exertion, more fuel and oxygen are used by the muscles involved. Since glycogen can be stored in the cells, it is readily available to the needy muscles. To meet the increased demand for oxygen brought on by the intensified muscular activity, certain changes occur in the respiratory and circulatory apparatus. There is an increase in the rate and depth of breathing which makes more oxygen available to the blood to carry to the area of intensified activity. There is increased cardiac activity to transport more blood to the working muscles more rapidly, and the ability of the blood itself to carry oxygen also increases. Those same adjustments also serve to facilitate the removal of waste products, particularly carbon dioxide, which result from oxidation.

Up to a certain intensity of physical exertion, the circulatory and respiratory adjustments that occur are sufficient to supply enough oxygen to continue a given activity almost indefinitely. In that situation enough oxygen is supplied, not only to allow the activity to continue at the same level, but also to assure adequate removal of the waste products. Work of such an intensity that the oxygen supply is sufficient to satisfy the oxygen demand is referred to as *aerobic* (with oxygen), or *oxidative* work. That is, the energy produced is the result of the oxidation of glycogen. When oxygen supply is sufficient to fulfill the oxygen demand for a task lasting over a few minutes, you are said to be performing in a condition of *steady state*. Steady state is a condition of equilibrium between the oxygen supply and the ability of the muscles to accept and use the oxygen while continuing the exercise. The degree of steady state varies. Obviously, a steady state exists during rest or minimal physical exertion (easy walking). For each individual there is a *maximum steady state* at which he can function. Maximum steady state is considered to be the maximum level at which you can perform sustained work, that is, the maximum rate at which you can work and maintain the equilibrium between oxygen demand and muscle use. That factor separates the physically fit person from the unfit person, for the fit person can maintain a higher maximum steady state in the performance of the same task.

Anaerobic Functions

There is for each person a limit to the ability of the muscles to receive and use oxygen efficiently. When the intensity of work, or exercise, reaches a level at which the oxygen supply cannot keep pace with the oxygen demand, chemical (metabolic) changes occur in the muscle that will allow it to continue to function *anaerobically* (without oxygen), or *nonoxidatively*. In anaerobic work, the changes make it possible for the food-fuel to be broken down without oxygen (anaerobically). The means of producing energy for muscular contraction is valuable in emergency situations but is very inefficient and wasteful and can continue for only a short period of time. When compared to aerobic metabolism, which results in the complete breakdown of glycogen and the release of much energy, anaerobic metabolism results in only partial breakdown of energy fuel and the production of considerably less energy for muscular contraction. Also, during anaerobic work, lactic acid, a by-product of muscle metabolism, collects in the muscles and interferes with muscle function. When oxygen supply is sufficient, lactic acid is oxidized and removed from the exercising muscles via the blood. Part of it is used to remake glycogen. Most of the remaking or resynthesis process takes place in the liver, and the glycogen formed is returned to the muscles. The lactic acid cycle continues only as long as the oxygen supply is adequate. When the oxygen supply falls behind oxygen demand, and work becomes anaerobic, lactic acid collects in the muscle and hampers its ability to perform work. Lactic acid buildup leads to fatigue and eventually cessation of the exercise.

When the body operates anaerobically, it is said to create an *oxygen debt*. Anaerobic activity can be viewed as a "function now, pay later" arrangement with respect to oxygen. The amount of debt depends upon the intensity and duration of the exercise engaged in. At the termination of exercise, any debt incurred must be paid. Payment of the debt is evidenced by continued accelerated respiratory and circulatory activity for a period after cessation of exercise. Those adjustments and other not so obvious adjustments continue for varying lengths of time depending on the amount of debt accumulated. Following periods of severe exertion, it may take the adjustment mechanisms over an hour to return the body to its pre-exercise level. According to A. V. Hill and associates, during severe muscular exertion such as sprinting, a person cannot possibly provide more than a fraction of the oxygen required for the task. As an example of the occurrence of oxygen debt, if an individual sprints 100 yards in 10 seconds, his oxygen requirement for the task is about 6 quarts. Since the maximum consumption possible is 4 quarts per minute, it follows that in the ten-second period

that person can, at most, provide less than one quart, which leaves him with an oxygen debt in excess of 5 quarts which must be made up following the exercise. If the body could not function without oxygen, it would be an extremely limited organism as far as its ability to perform work is concerned. It has been estimated that for you to incur maximal oxygen debt, you would have to engage in work or exercise equivalent to running at top speed for 40 seconds.

Efficiency

The efficiency with which you perform physical work is dependent upon your physical condition, the skill with which you perform the activities engaged in, and a knowledge of the pace, or rate, at which you must efficiently perform. Your physical condition is dependent upon the circulatory and respiratory systems and how well they perform the function of supply and removal, as well as many other factors about which volumes have been, and will be, written. The difference between performance of a task by the skilled and unskilled person centers on the muscles used by each in the performance of the same task. For every physical act, there are proper muscles for performing the act. The use of any other additional muscles will usually hamper performance. In endurance activities, the use of extra muscles is extremely costly since every muscle used must be supplied by oxygen. The additional muscles will merely use oxygen that would otherwise be available to the proper muscles. In some activities, the unskilled person may use additional muscles that actually work against, or resist, the desired outcome. A knowledge of pace comes from experience in the performance of physical work. Good physical condition, along with exercise experience, results in a knowledge of pace that allows you to perform within your physical capabilities for extended periods of time. The unfit person usually does not have a knowledge of pace because he lacks a backlog of physical work experiences to draw on and, therefore, often begins a task at a rate too rapid to assure its completion. Fatigue and an unfinished task are the usual results.

PERSONALITY

Recently, physical educators have been interested in the interrelationship between personality and physical activity. Primarily, they have been attempting to determine whether personality differences exist among athletes competing in different sports, between champions and nonchampions, between those competing in individual sports and those competing in team sports, and between athletes and nonathletes. That is, do certain personality traits influence a person in selecting one activity and rejecting another and do those same personality traits influence the success an individual will have in his chosen activity? In addition, the studies also sought to determine whether participation in sports caused changes in personality.

Personality and the Athlete

In 1952, Heusner, as cited by Dr. R. Cattell, administered the Sixteen Personality Factor Questionnaire to 41 British and American Olympic champions. He found that the personality profile of the athlete was different from the average adult. The athletes had greater freedom from general neurotic tendencies, they were more dominant or assertive, they were less easily inhibited and they were less likely to worry. As a result of this investigation, he suggested that a high level of physical fitness reduces anxiety and neuroticism and favors aggressive and extrovert adjustment. He proposed that, since the mind affects the body, an absence of neuroticism and anxiety leads to improved physical perform-

ance. Finally, he hypothesized that among persons with a high level of physical fitness, only those who were stable and low in anxiety would do well in intense training and competitive situations.

The relationship between physical fitness and personality traits of high school boys was investigated by Dr. K. Tillman. Those boys who demonstrated a high level of fitness were found to be less submissive, more dominant, more enthusiastic, more dependent socially, more interested in outdoor activities, and less tense than the boys with a low level of physical fitness. After a 9-month physical fitness program, the experimental group were found to have an improved level of physical fitness, but there was no significant improvement in their personality traits. However, it should be noted that their level of fitness was still 48 percentile points below that of the high fitness group.

Personality and the Cardiac Patient

In recent years, a number of studies have been concerned with the personality of post-cardiac patients. A study by O. Forssman and B. Lindegard used the interview technique to assess the personality of cardiac patients. The results indicated that there was evidence of a predisposition to periodic depression and aloofness. They also found that cardiac patients were predominantly engaged in occupations calling for a high degree of leadership. A need for dominance appeared to be a characteristic trait. The investigators found that patients of long survival differed from those whose heart attack had occurred within 18 months or less. The patients of long survival had a higher incidence of periodic depression, and a lower degree of dominance.

Recent studies have been concerned with the personality of potential coronary subjects. Drs. J. Brozek, A. Keys and H. Blackburn investigated the personality differences between potential coronary and noncoronary subjects. Of the 258 men studied over a fourteen-year period, thirty-one developed coronary heart disease. Those men who later developed coronary disease had at the outset significantly higher scores on the "Hypochondriasis" scale of the Minnesota Multiphasic Personality Inventory and were more "masculine" in their interests. In the Thurstone Temperament Schedule, the eventual coronaries had significantly higher scores on the "activity drive" scale.

In a recent study, B. McPherson found significant personality differences between sedentary groups of normal and cardiac adult men. Compared to noncardiac adult men of approximately the same age, the post-coronary patients were more tense, aloof, taciturn, fickle, emotional, hurried and aggressive. The normal and post-cardiac men were also compared with another group of adult men who had been on a fitness program for five years and, therefore, had achieved a high level of physical fitness. The group of highly trained men were more favorably disposed toward exercise and physical activity and exhibited a greater degree of self-control than either the normal or cardiac nonexercisers. As yet, it is not known whether it is the unique personality characteristics which caused the repeat exercisers to adopt exercise as a regular part of their life, or whether the personality differences existed because of their regular participation in exercise over an extended period. Discussions with those men revealed that they initially began an exercise program for recreation and weight control. However, they found that, in addition to the improvements in physical fitness, the exercise sessions resulted in decreased tension and increased alertness, patience, and self-confidence. Many of the subjects reported that the improved sense of well-being dissi-

pated during the summer months when the exercise course was not offered. It appears that, as a result of the noticeable changes in moods and feelings, a "need" for exercise was awakened in the men. The program satisfied the need and led them to continue to reenroll in the exercise course.

The study also indicated that personality changes occur after an exercise program. After a twenty-four week program of graduated exercises, the cardiac and noncardiac exercising groups and the cardiac group who engaged in a recreational swim showed a reduced level of anxiety. In contrast, a group of normal adult men who did not exercise increased their anxiety over the twenty-four weeks. In addition, both the cardiac exercisers and the cardiac swimmers showed comparable positive changes in mood states which occurred despite the higher level of activity and greater improvement in physical fitness by the cardiac patients who exercised. In comparison with the cardiac patients, the normal subjects who exercised experienced slight negative psychological changes. Thus, beneficial psychological effects appear to be related to the cardiac condition and to participation in a program appropriate to that condition.—*Barry D. McPherson*

PHYSICAL FITNESS

There is a great deal of confusion concerning the term "physical fitness." Some people think that physical fitness is the ability to do 50 push-ups, while others feel that physical fitness indicates the status of every aspect of the human organism. In reality, however, physical fitness is just one phase of the total fitness of the person which includes *intellectual fitness* (problem solving, memorizing, etc.), *moral fitness* (values, ethics, etc.), *emotional fitness* (hate, love, fear, etc.) *social fitness* (manners, mores, relationship with others), and *physical fitness* (motor fitness, appearance, and organic health and vigor). Although each of these five total fitness parts is a supposedly separate factor, they are closely interrelated and dependent upon one another. They are what make up the total being. For example, a lack of social fitness may be a factor in disrupting your emotional fitness, or an improperly functioning digestive system (a part of physical fitness) may affect your emotional or social fitness. Psychosomatic diseases also demonstrate the interrelationship and the interdependence of the many, varied and extremely complex facets of total fitness.

The American Association of Health, Physical Education and Recreation has prepared a list indicating the attributes a totally fit person will demonstrate.

1. Optimum organic health consistent with heredity and the application of present health knowledge.

2. Sufficient coordination, strength, and vitality to meet emergencies, as well as the requirement of daily living.

3. Emotional stability to meet the stresses and strains of modern life.

4. Social consciousness and adaptability with respect to the requirements of all of life.

5. Sufficient knowledge and insight to make suitable decisions and arrive at feasible solutions to problems.

6. Attitudes, values, and skills which stimulate satisfactory participation in a full range of daily activities.

7. Spiritual and moral qualities which contribute to the fullest measure of living in a democratic society.

Physical fitness itself has several basic components that must be developed and maintained if you expect to be physically fit. Included are motor ability, physique or appearance, and organic efficiency.

Motor Ability

Motor ability is the ability to execute any motor skills—athletic or not.

See MOTOR ABILITY. Typewriting, washing dishes, driving a car, hitting a golf ball, and running are all examples of motor skills. People have varying levels of ability in performing those motor skills. Some are quite good in almost all, while others have difficulty in any physical or motor skill. Most of us, however, fall somewhere between these extremes. Current research indicates that your ability or abilities in activity depend upon your experiences and practice in the sport, not in some inborn traits. It is apparent, however, that your capacity for physical activity is determined by heredity.

There are many skills involved in motor ability. The major components are speed, power, agility, balance, muscle strength, muscle endurance, circulo-respiratory endurance, flexibility, kinesthesia, reaction and movement time, motor educability and body type. Other components are arm-eye coordination, foot-eye coordination, rhythm, vision, arm and hand steadiness. For a more complete discussion of those specific skills and components, see the individual entries and MOTOR ABILITY.

Physique

Physique (appearance) should be robust and healthy looking, which means there must be good muscular development, good posture, good carriage, good bone, muscle, and fat proportion, and adequate flexibility because of proper development. If you have poor color and posture and inadequate development, you cannot be considered physically fit.

Organic Health and Efficiency

Organic health refers to normal sense organs, healthy heart and circulatory system; fit nervous, digestive, endocrine, excretory systems; normal sexual vigor; abundant energy and resistance to fatigue; and an ability to rest.

Other Components

If you are truly physically fit, you should also demonstrate the ability to perform such basic skills as walking, running, jumping, climbing, throwing, crawling and kicking. You should also demonstrate some ability or skill in a few recreational games such as ping pong, tennis, swimming, golf, archery, skiing, shooting, bowling, cycling and skating.

Specific Health Habits Necessary to Attain Physical Fitness

Here are several recommended steps to achieve physical fitness.

1. Get adequate and proper exercise through an enjoyable activity or exercise routine, at least four times a week.

2. Be certain that your daily diet receives your full attention and that all the necessary vitamins, minerals and foodstuffs are included.

3. Get adequate rest and relaxation daily.

4. Avoid or keep at a minimum those things which are harmful to the human organism—smoking, alcoholic beverages, caffeine stimulants and other unnecessary drugs.

5. Get a physical examination from your family physician every year. Carry yourself tall. That is a small thing, but it can mean a great deal to you. Simply standing tall and carrying yourself proudly will do wonders for your appearance.

6. Be certain that you balance your calorie intake and outgo to avoid gaining weight.

Amount of Exercise

You should exercise enough to adequately develop all the components of physical fitness, but especially the big four—muscular strength, muscular endurance, flexibility and circulo-respiratory endurance.

Muscular Strength—A reasonable degree of muscular strength is vital for several reasons. Sufficient arm, shoulder and back strength holds the upper part of the body in proper position. Sufficient abdominal strength is needed to help avoid a bay window and, therefore, possible low back pain. Sufficient muscle strength of the body is necessary for such tasks as carrying out the garbage, pushing the car when it is stuck in the mud or snow or meeting any other emergency. See STRENGTH.

Muscular Endurance—Although strength is mandatory to assume a correct posture, as mentioned above, muscle endurance is essential to maintain the posture throughout the day. You will find that many jobs require muscle endurance. A typist needs sufficient forearm, shoulder and back muscle endurance to type all day. A bricklayer needs a high degree of muscle endurance to perform continuously, and many of you need sufficient muscle endurance to stand or sit at your jobs all day long without becoming fatigued too rapidly. Without muscle endurance, you tire rapidly, and your efficiency level drops rapidly, thereby cutting down on your production level. See MUSCLE ENDURANCE.

Flexibility—An adequate amount of flexibility is necessary in all the major joints of the body to help avoid unwanted muscle pulls and strains. Lack of flexibility has been associated with low back pain and many other muscle and joint injuries that may occur simply by your attempting to reach for an object underneath the desk or on top of a shelf. See FLEXIBILITY.

Circulo-respiratory Endurance—You need a good degree of circulo-respiratory endurance to give you extra stamina for many daily tasks, thereby providing more efficient activity and enabling you to meet unexpected emergencies, i.e., shoveling snow or climbing several flights of stairs without placing a dangerous stress on the body. There is a considerable amount of evidence that circulo-respiratory endurance is related to the retardation of certain cardiovascular diseases. See CIRCULO-RESPIRATORY ENDURANCE.

Those four components are vital in society even if you never participate in any athletic activity. And if you want to participate in one or varied activities, you should develop some of the other motor ability or fitness qualities like balance, agility, speed and reaction time.

A physical fitness program should have two goals:

1. The improvement and maintenance of muscular strength, muscular endurance, flexibility and circulo-respiratory endurance.

2. The development of desirable health habits including checkups with your family physician.

The health habits and proper exercise program will aid in reducing disease, improve the physiological function of the various systems of the body and provide for a more efficient human organism.

PHYSICAL FITNESS INDEX

The Physical Fitness Index is a score derived from a series of PFI Tests, developed by Frederick Rand Rodgers. The tests are Lung capacity, Grip strength, Back lift, Leg lift, Pull-ups, Push-ups, or Dipping. The tests are proposed as a Strength Index, which is then compared to your weight, age and sex. Persons with exceptionally high PFI scores are considered "activity drunkards." See ACTIVITY DRUNKARDS and TESTS.

POSTURE

Traditionally, good posture was considered to be a static upright position almost akin to the exaggerated West Point position of attention. Recent opinions in the area of body mechanics has brought about the realization that posture is dynamic as well as static and is not rigid. There is not posture, but postures. Posture encompasses all

positions the body assumes in space as well as its movements through space. Good posture is the degree of efficiency with which you move. It is an

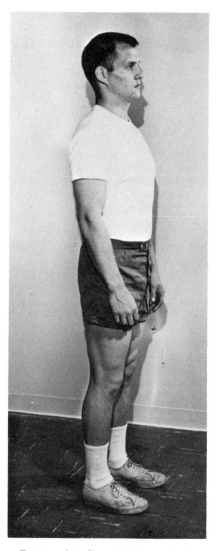

Proper Standing Posture. 1. Feet parallel, about 6″ apart. 2. Head high, as if balancing a book. 3. Chest out. 4. Stomach and hips firm. 5. Abdomen and back as flat as possible. 6. Knees very lightly flexed—not stiffly locked. 7. Weight evenly distributed on both feet— most of it on balls of feet.

individual matter, and all people do not fit a single mold. For every person there is a most efficient way to sit, stand, walk, run and otherwise move. That is posture. Obviously, some people are more efficient than others. That is, they have better posture.

The two basic elements of posture are *alignment* and *balance*. Alignment refers to the relationship between body parts. Balance is how the weight of the body is distributed over the supporting structures.

Many definitions have been proposed for posture. The following are a few of the more popular definitive ideas: Good posture is that body alignment which requires least muscular and skeletal effort and most favors function; good posture is that position or positions you assume to efficiently offset the force of gravity; and good posture is that state of balance which enables you to act efficiently with regard to work done, appearance, and, to a degree, health.

Overall body efficiency depends upon the coordination of the skeletal, muscular, nervous and visceral systems. The digestive system provides the energy material for the muscles which hold the bones in alignment. The nervous system sends messages on balance and position so the muscles can perform tasks efficiently. The skeletal framework affords the rigid support of the body and, with the muscular system, serves to support and protect the visceral organs. Good posture is the result of efficient interaction of those systems.

Line of Gravity

In an upright position, a vertical line, the *line of gravity*, is used as a frame of reference to determine postural deviations. Ideally, in a side view, a superimposed line connects the lobe of the ear, the middle of the shoulder, and the middle of the hip, passes just behind the knee cap (patella) and just in front of the lateral malleolus, the projection on the outside of the lower leg. In the back view, the line of gravity should bisect the head, neck and trunk. The spine should fall in line with the line of gravity. Below the waist the line should pass between the buttocks, the knees and the heels. The feet should point straight ahead. In that position, the postural muscles are under the least tension and are less likely to fatigue. Any deviations from the line of gravity can be possible sources of postural complications which may affect the efficiency of movement. At the same time, not all deviations necessarily result in the loss of efficiency or other related movement problems. Deviations can result from concentrated exercise on certain muscle

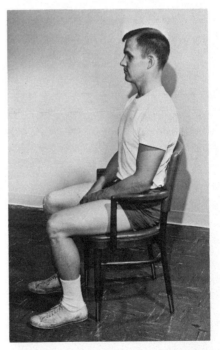

Proper Sitting Posture. 1. Sit tall and back, with hips touching the back of the chair, feet flat on floor. 2. Chest out, back of neck nearly in line with upper back. 3. When writing, lean forward from the hips so you keep head and shoulders in line.

groups. That type of deviation does not usually result in postural problems. As an example, in two activities, basketball and truck driving, quite often the muscles on the front of the chest are developed to such a degree that a muscle imbalance is created and a round-shouldered appearance may result. If the line of gravity were applied in those activities, the shoulders of some would fall slightly forward of the line, which technically, could be considered a postural deviation. But when related to function, no complications exist. That example shows why posture must be considered an individual matter. Two important considerations when dealing with posture are the causes of any deviations and their effect upon movement.

Postural Deviations

The human spine, or vertebral column, is the source of several postural problems. Aside from its own alignment, the spine may affect the align-

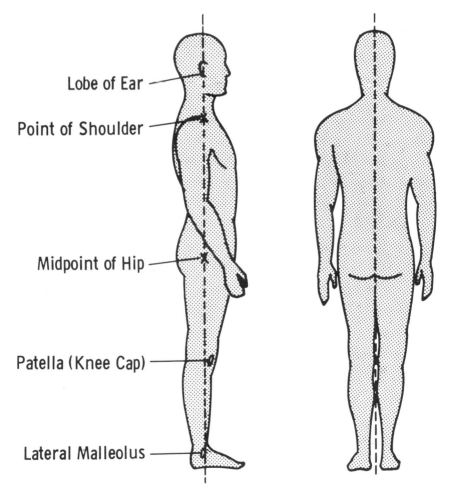

Lobe of Ear

Point of Shoulder

Midpoint of Hip

Patella (Knee Cap)

Lateral Malleolus

The line of gravity is used as a frame of reference to determine postural deviations.

ment of other body areas. It is possible for leg and foot deviations to be initiated by spinal complications. The spine is the base of posture and consists of four curves: cervical (neck region), thoracic (chest region), lumbar (low back region) and sacral. Spinal deviations are recognized as exaggerations or flattenings of those curves. There are five general types of spinal deviations:

1. *Cervical lordosis,* or *forward head,* is a condition in which the curve of the cervical area of the spine causes the lobe of the ear to fall forward of its normal position in relation to the lateral projection of the line of gravity.

2. *Kyphosis* is an exaggeration of the thoracic curve. The complication is often accompanied by a flat or hollow-chested appearance.

3. *Lordosis* is an exaggeration of the lumbar curve. That deviation, sometimes called swayback, is frequently caused by a weakness of the abdominal muscles.

4. *Flatback* is evidenced by a diminishment of the lumbar curve.

5. *Scoliosis,* which is recognized from a rear vantage point, is a lateral curve of the spine to one side or the other. It is possible to have a compound scoliosis in which the thoracic region may possess a lateral curve to one side while the lumbar area exhibits a curve in the opposite direction. See LOW BACK PAIN.

6. *Rounded Shoulders* frequently accompany kyphosis and are usually the result of muscle weakness or imbalance. If the muscles of the upper back responsible for stabilizing the scapulae are weakened, the shoulder blades (scapulae) and the shoulders will be pulled forward resulting in a round-shouldered appearance.

Leg Deviations

Aside from the line of gravity, the *anterior leg line* is used to help determine leg deviations. It is a vertical line that, in a normal situation, bisects the front of the thigh and the patella, and falls between the first and second metatarsals, the long bones of the foot just behind the toes.

1. *Bowed legs* is a condition in which the legs appear to "bow" to the outside. In a bowed-leg situation, the patella would fall to the outside of the anterior leg line.

2. *Knock-kneed legs* is the opposite of bowed legs. It is a deviation where the patella falls inside the anterior leg line. Bowed legs and knock-kneed legs are usually the result of faulty skeletal development.

3. *Hyperextension* of the knee joint is evidenced by straightening of the joint to more than 180 degrees. The patella would appear behind the lateral projection of the line of gravity.

Foot Deviations

1. *Eversions,* more commonly referred to as duck feet, is a turning outward of the foot from the normal straight ahead position.

2. *Inversion,* or pigeon feet, is a condition in which the feet are turned inward in relation to the normal position.

3. *Flat feet* result from the weakening, and subsequent dropping, of the long arch (longitudinal) of the foot.

Causes of Postural Deviations

Muscle Imbalance

The muscles of the body are arranged in pairs which are complementary to each other in function. That is, where there are muscles which flex a joint there is also a muscle or group which extends the joint. Muscles that perform opposing functions (flexion and extension, abduction and adduction) are called *antagonists.* For one reason or another, one set of the antagonists may become stronger in relation to the other set, creating a muscle imbalance in the postural (antigravity) muscles. Deviations in posture may result, which may or may not affect efficient movement depending upon activities engaged in as well as a combination of other factors. Muscle imbalance can be either the cause or the result of poor posture.

Poor Muscle Tone

There is an optimum muscle tone, or tonus, for keeping the skeletal components in correct alignment and balance. Poor muscle tone puts added strain on various joints throughout the body. Joints aside from their ligamentous support, depend on a certain amount of support from neighboring muscles. Without that muscular assistance, the ligaments are placed under severe and sometimes dangerous stress. People with poor muscle tone are more susceptible to joint and ligament problems than those with good muscle tone. Muscle tone is important for balance between groups of antagonistic muscles. The primary causes of poor muscle tone are laziness, lack of exercise and poor body mechanics habits.

Skeletal Complications

It is reasonable to expect that after a time muscle imbalance, poor muscle tone and poor mechanical habits will adversely affect the skeletal framework of the body. That effect is particularly true during the adolescent and early adult years when the skeletal system is undergoing rapid growth changes. Poor postural habits during the formative years when the bones are hardening result in permanent misalignment between adjacent bones. Once hardening occurs, resultant misalignments cannot be corrected except by surgical means. Skeletal deviations invariably affect muscle efficiency.

To a certain extent, the skeletal system is determined by heredity. It is possible that some skeletal misalignments can be traced to hereditary factors. Diet, particularly during the years of rapid growth, plays an important role in bone formation.

Other Factors Affecting Posture

Muscle Hypertension is a condition in which the muscles are too tense, resulting in jerky movement, fatigue, and, frequently, muscle soreness.

Kinesthesis is an awareness of balance and position within your self. A poorly developed kinesthetic sense could lead to postural problems.

Psychological Considerations—Psychologists have attempted to trace poor posture to factors like feelings of inadequacy, lack of pride, and other expressions of self. A relation seems to exist between posture and mental health.

Exercise and Posture

The muscles responsible for the position of the body are stimulated by the nervous system to contract and are supported by the skeletal system. Since the skeletal muscles move the body and maintain the many body positions, improvement in posture is dependent upon the development of muscular endurance and strength. For specific information on how to improve muscular endurance and strength, see MUSCULAR ENDURANCE and STRENGTH.

There are, moreover, several very important general principles you must follow to help prevent improper postural development.

1. Be certain that the entire body is involved in a great many activities, sport or nonsport. Such movement will allow the muscles and joints to develop properly and maintain their efficiency and will aid in avoiding unnatural development. The earlier the practice of exposure to many activities is begun, the better.

2. Pick out activities that will help you develop specific body areas, particularly those areas most often neglected. For example, hanging activities help to develop the arms and shoulder muscles, and balancing on a balance beam will help improve your balance.

3. Be sure that your activities em-

phasize extending the spine. Dancing, swimming and diving are all examples of extension activities.

4. Do not overemphasize developing one set of muscles of the body. For example, do not concentrate on developing the biceps muscles to such a degree that you neglect the triceps, thereby causing the arm to remain in a semi-flexed position. Also, do not spend all the time developing your abdominal muscles and neglect the back muscles.

5. Be sure that some time is spent relaxing. Besides assisting the mental state of the person, which may conceivably aid in improving posture, relaxing will aid in furthering the normal function of the muscles.

One of the most basic causes for poor posture is lack of abdominal muscle strength and resulting low back pain. See LOW BACK PAIN for a discussion of that relationship. Other related topics on posture are BODY MECHANICS and MUSCLE BOUNDNESS.

Importance of Good Posture

Good posture helps keep the various body segments in proper position over one another so that there is no undue fatigue on the many body parts. For example, leaning forward slightly at the waist may cause a feeling of low back pain because the muscles of the low back are forced to do extra work, and stress may be placed on the intervertebral discs of the spinal column.

Good posture allows for proper space of the internal organs. A crouched-over position can only result in a squeezing together of the abdominal organs, thereby inhibiting proper function.

Good posture allows for proper development of the musculature and bone structure, especially during the growing years.

Good posture is aesthetic. If you hold yourself properly, you present a desirable picture and actually look better.

POWER

Power, the ability to release maximum muscular force in the shortest period of time possible, is a term that is often confused with strength. Power, however, is composed of both strength and speed. For example, two men may have equal strength and be able to lift 200 pounds 3 feet off the floor, but one man does it twice as fast as the other. Both men have equal strength, but the man who can lift the weight twice as fast is twice as powerful.

Power is an extremely important component for success in most athletic activities. It is measured or most graphically demonstrated by explosive activities or movements. The vertical jump, the shot put, the softball throw, and the standing broad jump are all examples of explosive activities.

Your power can be improved by increasing your strength and/or speed for a particular movement. For example, if a shot putter wants to improve his power, he should concentrate on developing the strength of his extensor muscles or on increasing the speed of movement of his arm. To increase the speed of movement, the shot putter should concentrate on using a light weight or shot and trying to move his arm as rapidly as possible. The power is specific to the muscles involved so that an emphasis is placed on using the specific movement, in that case, the shot-putting action. An emphasis need not be placed merely on the arm movement but also on the entire body as it moves across the ring and the release is made.

That principle may be applied to virtually all activities where power is desired.

PREGNANCY

There are a great many misconceptions about pregnancy and exercise. Many people feel that exercise and sports, in particular, endanger a woman's chances for pregnancy or make childbirth more difficult. Such opinions do not have any justification, yet are currently held by many lay-people, educators, and even physicians.

Exercises and Chances for Pregnancy

A report made by the American Amateur Athletic Union revealed that fertility, pregnancy and pelvic measurements were all found to be within normal limits for women who engaged in vigorous athletics.

Exercise and Childbirth

Research has demonstrated that athletic women have quicker and easier deliveries than the normal population. A study conducted by W. A. Pfeifer revealed that the average duration of labor from rupture of membrane to delivery was 102 minutes in athletic women and 207 in nonathletes.

Pfeifer also noted that active women had a shorter labor period because of an ability to relax, better breathing control, strong abdominal musculature and an ability to reduce useless contraction of the arms and legs. Another study made by G. J. Erdelyi on Hungarian women athletes found a smaller incidence of complications during pregnancy and 50 per cent fewer Caesarian sections. He also found that the duration of labor of women athletes was shorter in 87 per cent of the women.

It is apparent, therefore, that exercise is desirable for preventing fewer complications during pregnancy and delivery.

Exercise During Pregnancy

Although some women have competed in their sixth to ninth month of pregnancy and followed with normal deliveries, any athletic competition, training, or vigorous sports participation should be forbidden during pregnancy. Bumps and falls are dangerous for fear of miscarriage. During preg-

nancy, the heart is taxed more than normal, and during exercise the additional work may be harmful to a heart that has an undetected defect. Likewise, during pregnancy the kidneys and the liver function with very little reserve capacity.

Those statements are not meant to discourage all exercise but only vigorous training and exercise that can cause hazards, bumps, strains, or falls. It is advisable that a pregnant woman walk every day, for at least 30 minutes or more. Generally, physicians recommend their patients do that along with additional light exercises.

Exercise After Childbirth

If the pelvic examination reveals normal involution, most obstetricians recommend resumption of regular exercise from 6 weeks to 3 months after childbirth.

Here are some exercises to follow to help regain your figure.

1. Lying on your back, take 5 deep breaths. Breathe from the abdomen.

2. Lying on your back with your arms out to the side at right angles to your body, lift your arms, keeping them straight, touch palms of hands, and return. Do 5 times.

3. Lying on your back, raise your head off the floor so that your chin touches your chest. Do 10.

4. Lying on your back, raise your left leg off the ground as high as possible. Keep the leg straight. Then lower the leg making full use of the abdominal muscles. Repeat with right leg. Do 10.

5. Raise your right knee, draw your thigh down on the abdomen and chest, and your lower leg against your thigh and buttock. Straighten your leg and lower it to the floor. Alternate with both right and left legs. Do 5 with each.

6. Starting gradually, walk 10-15 minutes per day until you reach at least 30 minutes. The exercises listed under EXERCISES, ISOMETRICS and

WEIGHT TRAINING may also be used to supplement the above. Concentrate on the muscles of the chest, abdomen, thighs and legs. Follow the basic principle of training. See TRAINING.

Childbirth and Subsequent Athletic Performance

Childbirth does not have an adverse effect on sport performance. Studies have indicated that women do not experience a decrease in physical performance as a result of pregnancy and childbirth.

For related discussions on pregnancy, see MENSTRUATION, VARICOSE VEINS and WOMEN.

PRE-TRAINING

There are two prerequisites before embarking on any exercise program. First, establish the purpose of your program. Second, have a physician evaluate your age and health status.

The purpose of the exercise program should be clear whether it is designed for improvement or maintenance of fitness, and what areas or components of fitness are going to be developed—strength, muscle endurance, circulo-respiratory endurance, flexibility, a combination of the four, or another specific area. See PHYSICAL FITNESS for specific components of physical fitness. Remember, tailor the program to meet your needs.

Evaluate your age and health status before engaging in an exercise program. The only way to effectively measure your current status is to have your physician give you a medical evaluation. Explain to him your intentions and goals. He may be able to make some valuable suggestions on the nature and intensity of the program. From the medical evaluation, you should be able to establish a realistic view of your present status and your potential development. See EXCESSIVE EXERCISE and INTENSITY OF EXERCISE.

It is also important to remember that you are an individual and that what may be good for you may be harmful for another, or vice versa. Progress at your own rate. Don't try to rush things. See TRAINING for specific program guidelines.

PROGRAMS

Many of our popular fitness programs are outshoots of programs developed by the Armed Services. That includes the 5BX, XBX and Aerobics programs as well as some other, less popular exercise schedules. Although most programs are similar in that they provide specific steps as you progress up the fitness ladder, other programs, less formally organized also exist. Those include such acceptable training procedures as Continuous Rhythmical Exercise, Isometrics, Weight Training, Circuit Training, Jogging and the LaSierra Program. The reader is referred to the individual entries under those headings.

Each program has its own technique for evaluating physical fitness. Many of them stress the role of diet and the inclusion of a specific exercise regimen as part of the daily living schedule.

Like most attempts to narrow the focus on a specific subject, these exercise programs are not complete, for they emphasize only a few of the many areas of physical fitness. Refer to PHYSICAL FITNESS and INTENSITY OF EXERCISE for a discussion of a complete exercise program.

Aerobics

Aerobics is a program developed by Dr. Kenneth Cooper of the United States Air Force Medical Corps. Dr. Cooper feels that the best forms of exercise are those activities that stress your cardiovascular system, causing your body to demand oxygen and forcing your body to process and deliver it. Running, swimming, cycling, walking, stationary running, handball, basketball and squash are aerobic activities and result in such bodily changes. Dr. Cooper calls it the training effect. For example the lungs are conditioned to process more air with less effort, the heart grows stronger and pumps more blood with each stroke, the number and size of the blood vessels carrying blood to the body tissues are increased and the tone of muscles and blood vessels is improved.

Through 4 years of studies on 5,000 officers and airmen Dr. Cooper has been able to scientifically measure the amount of energy all popular exercises cost the body. Translating those amounts into points, he has established that a basic minimum of 30 points each week is necessary to produce and maintain cardiovascular health. The exercise sessions must take place at least four times a week, or every other day. Moreover, you cannot earn the 30 points in one day and then forget about physical activity for the next six.

In Aerobics, Dr. Cooper lists complete conditioning programs for each aerobic exercise, including the number of points you can earn. But before you can start gaining points by following one of the conditioning programs, it would be a good idea to take the Air Force 12 Minute Fitness Test to determine your present condition. Your score on the test will establish how much or how long you have to exercise to gain your 30 points.

The 12 Minute Test

Get your doctor's permission to take the test, especially if you're over 30.

The test itself is simple and only requires that you run as far as possible within 12 minutes. Of course if your breath gets short, walk for awhile until it comes back and then continue running.

Now measure off a certain running area of up to 2 miles. You may want to get permission to use the track at your local high school or YMCA to take your test there. But wherever you begin, try to run the whole time at a pace you can maintain without excessive strain. After you have run for 12 minutes, check your distance on the preceding chart.

Now you're ready to accumulate your 30 points to keep in active and productive health. Six different progressive conditioning courses are listed in *Aerobics*. (See chart for details on the running program.) Take the 12 minute test, select the activity you prefer, and start exercising.

Aerobics is perhaps one of the best current programs on the market, because of its emphasis on getting a satisfactory pulse rate, 150 beats per minute, and on burning up sufficient calories in the workout. The program is also commendable, for Dr. Cooper directs his efforts toward activities rather than exercises on calisthenics which a great many people dislike. The program is progressive and has a test to gauge your improvement. The only drawback is that there is little emphasis on developing muscular strength and flexibility, which are essential for attaining physical fitness. You can rectify that situation very easily by including a few strength and flexibility exercises in the activity

Distance Covered	Fitness Category
Less than 1 mile	I. Very Poor
1 to 1¼ miles	II. Poor
1¼ to 1½ miles	III. Fair
1½ to 1¾ miles	IV. Good*
1¾ miles or more	V. Excellent

* For men over 35, 1.4 miles is Good; for women, 1.3.

RUNNING EXERCISE PROGRAM
Category 1

Week	Distance (miles)	Walk/run	Time Goal (minutes)	Freq/Wk	Points/Wk
1	1.0	WALK	13:30	5	10
2	1.0	WALK	13:00	5	10
3	1.0	WALK	12:45	5	10
4	1.0	W/R	11:45	5	15
5	1.0	W/R	11:00	5	15
6	1.0	W/R	10:30	5	15
7	1.0	RUN	9:45	5	20
8	1.0	RUN	9:30	5	20
9	1.0	RUN	9:15	5	20
10	1.0	RUN	9:00	3	
	and				21
	1.5	RUN	16:00	2	
11	1.0	RUN	8:45	3	
	and				21
	1.5	RUN	15:00	2	
12	1.0	RUN	8:30	3	
	and				24
	1.5	RUN	14:00	2	
13	1.0	RUN	8:15	3	
	and				24
	1.5	RUN	13:30	2	
14	1.0	RUN	7:55	3	
	and				27
	1.5	RUN	13:00	2	
15	1.0	RUN	7:45	2	
	and				
	1.5	RUN	12:30	2	30
	and				
	2.0	RUN	18:00	1	
16	1.5	RUN	11:55	2	
	and				31
	2.0	RUN	17:00	2	

Charts reprinted from *Aerobics* (M. Evans & Co., Inc.)

program, possibly as a warm-up and a variation as you are exercising.

5BX

This program was originally intended to provide a basis for the physical fitness of the men of the Royal Canadian Air Force, Royal Canadian Air Cadets and dependent children.

It involves no equipment and only a minimum of time—11 minutes. Therefore, it's well suited for the working man with limited time.

Although the publication which contains the program is concerned primarily with the five basic exercises (5BX), there is a discussion of weight control, diet, muscle power, physical capacity, the importance of physical fitness and physical fitness through daily activities and sports.

What Is It?

The 5BX Plan is composed of 6 charts arranged in progression. Each chart is composed of 5 exercises which are always performed in the same order and in the same maximum time limit. But as you progress from chart to chart, there are slight changes in each basic exercise with a gradual demand for more effort.

Here are some points of information:

Level—These are the Physical Capacity levels, each indicated by a letter of the alphabet.

Exercises—Exercises 1, 2, 3, and 4 apply to the first four exercises described and illustrated on the following pages. The column headed 1 represents exercise 1 (toe touch), etc. The figures in each column indicate the number of times that each exercise is to be repeated in the time allotted for that exercise. Exercise 5 is running on the spot. Two activities may be substituted for it, however, and if you prefer, you may run or walk the recommended distance in the required time in place of the stationary run of exercise 5.

Minutes for Each Exercise—The allotted time for each exercise is noted here. The times remain the same throughout all the charts. Total time for exercises 1 through 5 is 11 minutes.

Note—It is important that the exercises at any level be completed in 11 minutes. However, it is likely that in the early stages, you will complete certain exercises in less than the allotted time while others may require longer. In such circumstances, the times allotted for individual exercises may be varied within the total 11-minute period.

How Far Should You Progress?

The level of Physical Capacity to which you should progress is determined by your "Age Group." Levels for "Flying Crew" are listed separately.

Note: This chart is for illustration only.

How to Begin

Check your daily schedule and determine the time most convenient for you to do the exercises. It should be the same time each day.

Here are some suggested times: before breakfast; late morning or afternoon, at your place of employment; after your regular recreational period; in the evening just before you retire.

Regardless of the time you choose, START TODAY.

Maximum Rate of Progression Through Chart 1 According to Age

20 years or under, at least 1 day at each level

20-29 years, at least 2 days at each level

30-39 years, at least 4 days at each level

40-49 years, at least 7 days at each level

50-59 years, at least 8 days at each level

60 years and over, at least 10 days at each level

(If you feel stiff or sore, or if you are unduly breathless at any time, ease up and slow down your rate of progression. That is particularly applicable to the older age groups.)

A Note of Caution

Even if you are capable of starting at a high level and progressing at a faster rate than indicated—DON'T DO IT. Start at the bottom of chart 1 and work up from level to level as recommended.

For best results from 5BX, the exercises must be done regularly. Remember, it may take you 6, 8, 10 months or more of daily exercises to attain the level recommended for you. But once you have attained it, only 3 periods of exercise per week will maintain that level of physical capacity.

If for any reason (illness, etc.) you stop doing 5BX regularly and you wish to begin again, do not recommence at the level you had attained previously.

Drop back several levels—until you find one you can do without undue strain. After a period of inactivity of

PHYSICAL CAPACITY RATING SCALE

Level	Exercise					1 mile Run	2 mile Run
	1	2	3	4	5	In minutes	
A+	30	32	47	24	550	8	25
A	30	31	45	22	540	8	25
A−	30	30	43	21	525	8	25
B+	28	28	41	20	510	8¼	26
B	28	27	39	19	500	8¼	26
B−	28	26	37	18	490	8¼	26
C+	26	25	35	17	480	8½	27
C	26	24	34	17	465	8½	27
C−	26	23	33	16	450	8½	27
D+	24	22	31	15	430	8¾	28
D	24	21	30	15	415	8¾	28
D−	24	20	29	15	400	8¾	29
Minutes for each exercise	2	1	1	1	6		

AGE GROUPS
  12 YRS. MAINTAINS D+
  13 YRS. MAINTAINS C+
  14 YRS. MAINTAINS B+
  35-39 YRS. MAINTAINS B
  40-44 YRS. MAINTAINS C

FLYING CREW
  AGE 40-44 MAINTAINS A+
  AGE 45-49 MAINTAINS B

CHART 3

1 Feet astride, arms upward.
Touch floor 6" outside left foot, again between feet and press 6" outside right foot, bend backward as far as possible, repeat, reverse direction after half the number of counts.

2 Back lying, feet 6" apart, arms clasped behind head.
Sit up to vertical position, keep feet on floor, hook feet under chair, etc., only if necessary.

3 Front lying, hands interlocked behind the back.

Lift head, shoulders, chest and both legs as high as possible. Keep legs straight, and raise chest and both thighs completely off floor.

4 Front lying, hands under the shoulders, palms flat on floor.

Touch chin to floor in front of hands— touch forehead to floor behind hands before returning to up position. There are three definite movements, chin, forehead, arms straightened. DO NOT do in one continuous movement.

5 Stationary Run—(Count a step each time left foot touches floor.) Lift feet approximately 4 inches off floor. After every 75 steps do 10 "half knee bends." Repeat the sequence until required number of steps is completed.

Half Knee Bends—Feet together, hands on hips, knees bent to form an angle of about 110 degrees. Do not bend knees past a right angle. Straighten to upright position, raising heel off floor, return to starting position each time.

Keep feet in contact with floor—the back upright and straight at all times.

longer than two months, or one month if caused by illness, it is recommended that you start again at Chart 1.

How to Progress

Chart 1—Progress through all steps of the chart before moving up to Chart 2

Chart 2—Progress through all steps of the chart before moving up to Chart 3

Chart 3—Progress as in Charts 1 & 2

Start at the lowest Physical Capacity Level of Chart 1 (D−). Repeat each exercise in the allotted time, or do the 5 exercises in 11 minutes. Move upward on the same chart to the next level (D) only after you can complete all the required movements at your present level within 11 minutes. Continue to progress upward in that manner until you can complete all the required movements at level (A+) within 11 minutes. Now start at the bottom of Chart 2 (D−), and continue in that fashion upward through the levels and from chart to chart until you reach the level for your age group, i.e., age 35-39 (B Chart 3).

XBX

The XBX program was designed to help women develop and maintain physical fitness. The plan, which takes only 12 minutes to complete, is progressive and gives you an opportunity to progress at your own rate and achieve your own level of fitness.

The XBX (ten basic exercises) program is a physical-fitness plan that is composed of four charts of ten exercises. The charts are arranged in progression, with each chart becoming increasingly more difficult. The ten exercises are always performed in the same order in the same time interval. Each chart is divided into 12 levels, making 48 in all. The levels are numbered consecutively, 1 through 48.

Any exercise program should start at an easy level and progress to a more difficult level gradually. The XBX plan incorporates that concept into its structure by keeping the time limit the same for the exercise, even though there is an increase in the number of times the exercise is to be performed. It also makes the exercises more difficult from one chart to the next.

Purpose

The XBX will improve your general physical condition by increasing muscle tone, muscular strength, muscular endurance, flexibility and the efficiency of your heart.

The first Four Exercises are primarily to improve and maintain flexibility and mobility in those areas of the body which are usually neglected. They also serve as a warm-up for the more strenuous exercises which follow.

Exercise 5 is for strengthening the abdominal region and the muscles of the fronts of the thighs.

Exercise 6 exercises the long muscles of the back, the buttocks, and the backs of the thighs.

Exercise 7 concentrates on the muscles on the sides of the thighs. Those muscles get very little work in routine daily activities or in most sports.

Exercise 8 is primarily for the arms, shoulders and chest but, at the same time, exercises the back and abdomen.

Exercise 9 is partly for flexibility in the waist area and for strengthening the muscles of the hips and sides.

Exercise 10—the run-in-place with jumping—while exercising the legs, is primarily for the conditioning of the heart and lungs.

The two supplementary exercises are included for those who wish to do a little more. One exercise is for strengthening the muscles of the feet and the ankle joint. The other is for those muscles of the back and abdomen which assist in the maintenance of posture.

What the Charts Mean

Below is an explanation of what the chart pages mean. Check the para-

CHART II

	EXERCISE											
Minutes for each Exercise	1	2	3	4	5	6	7	8	9	10	8A	8B
24	15	16	12	30	35	38	50	28	20	210	40	36
23	15	16	12	30	33	36	48	26	18	200	38	34
22	15	16	12	30	31	34	46	24	18	200	36	32
21	13	14	11	26	29	32	44	23	16	190	33	29
20	13	14	11	26	27	31	42	21	16	175	31	27
19	13	14	11	26	24	29	40	20	14	160	28	24
18	12	12	9	20	22	27	38	18	14	150	25	22
17	12	12	9	20	19	24	36	16	12	150	22	20
16	12	12	9	20	16	21	34	14	10	140	19	19
15	10	10	7	18	14	18	32	12	10	130	17	15
14	10	10	7	18	11	15	30	10	8	120	14	13
13	10	10	7	18	9	12	28	8	8	120	12	12
Recommended number of days at each level	2				2	1	1	2	1	3	1	1

graph headings below with the sample chart.

Exercise

The numbers across the tops of the charts are the exercise numbers from 1 to 10. The column headed 1 refers to Exercise 1, and so on. The exercises are described and illustrated in the five pages following each chart. Exercises 8A and 8B are the supplementary exercises. If you choose those optional exercises, do them between Exercises 8 and 9.

Level

The numbers along the left side of the chart are the levels of the program, and each refers to the line of numbers beside it under the exercise headings. For example at Level 14, you do Exercise 3 seven times, Exercise 6 fifteen times and so on.

Minutes for Each Exercise

The exercises numbered 1 to 4 are the warm-up, and all four are to be completed within 2 minutes, or about a half minute each. Other examples: Exercise 5 takes 2 minutes, and Exercise 6 takes 1 minute. The total time for each level of ten exercises is 12 minutes. It is important that all the exercises be done within the total time limit. Do not move up to the next level until you can do your present level, without excessive strain or fatigue, in the 12 minutes.

Each group is given a physical fitness goal to attain, that is, a level which it should try to reach.

The goals indicated in the plan are based on the average achievement of girls and women who have participated in it.

Your goal, then, is the level of fitness that the average girl or woman of your age reached without undue stress, strain, or fatigue.

With every average, there are individuals who surpass it, and those who fall below it. In terms of the XBX plan and the goals, there will be some women who are capable of progressing beyond the goal indicated. On the other hand, there will be persons who will never attain that average level.

If you feel able to move further through the charts than your goal, by all means do so. If, on the contrary, you experience great difficulty in approaching that level, you should stop at a level which you feel to be within your capability. It is impossible to predict accurately a level for each individual who uses the program. Use the goals as guides, and apply them with common sense.

From time to time as you progress through the levels, you may have difficulty with a particular level or exercise. If so, proceed slowly but keep working at it. (The "plateaus" may occur anywhere in the progression.) Generally you will be able to move ahead after a few days at that level. If you cannot, then you have probably arrived at your potential physical fitness level in so far as the particular program is concerned.

Caution

If for any reason you stop doing XBX for more than two weeks because of illness, vacation, or any other cause—DO NOT restart at the level you had attained before stopping. DO drop back several levels or to the next lower chart until you find a level which you can do fairly easily. Physical fitness is lost during long periods of inactivity. That is particularly true if the inactivity was caused by illness.

Instructions for Using the XBX Plan

First select YOUR GOAL for YOUR AGE from the table below. Locate the level in the charts which follow.

Record the recommended minimum number of days at each level. For example, if you are 28 years of age, your goal is Level 30 on Chart III,

MY PROGRESS

LEVEL	STARTED	FINISHED	COMMENTS
24			
23			
22			
21			
20			
19			
18			
17			
16			
15			
14			
13			

MY AIM	DATE	HEIGHT	WEIGHT	WAIST	HIPS	BUST
Start						
Finish						

If Your Age Is	Your Goal Is Level	Recommended Minimum Number of Days at Each Level on			
		Chart I	Chart II	Chart III	Chart IV
7- 8 years	30	1	1	2	x
9-10 years	34	1	1	2	x
11-12 years	38	1	1	2	3
13-14 years	41	1	1	2	3
15-17 years	44	1	1	2	3
18-19 years	40	1	2	3	4
20-25 years	35	1	2	3	x
26-30 years	30	2	3	5	x
31-35 years	26	2	4	6	x
36-40 years	22	4	6	x	x
41-45 years	19	5	7	x	x
46-50 years	16	7	8	x	x
51-55 years	11	8	x	x	x

and you spend AT LEAST 2 days doing each level on Chart I, 3 days at each level on Chart II, and 5 days at each level on Chart III. Do not move faster than the recommended rate.

To Start and Progress

Start at Level 1, which is at the bottom of Chart 1. When you can do that level without strain and in 12 minutes, move up to Level 2. Continue through the levels and charts in this way until you reach the goal level recommended for your age group, OR until you feel you are exercising at your maximum capacity.

When You Reach Your Goal

Once you have reached your goal, you should require only three exercise periods a week to maintain it.

The 5BX and XBX programs are good programs because they are progressive and allow for a gradual improvement. The basic problem is that the program lasts only 11 to 12 minutes, that it does not burn up 300 to 500 calories (only around 170 and 200), and that several of the exercises used are undesirable. The authors do recommend, however, that additional exercises, such as walking, should be included.

RSP—A Minimal Program

A minimal development program that is unsurpassed for producing all-round results is the RSP—Running, Sit-ups, and Push-ups. There are five valid reasons for the selection of those three activities: (1) they provide a minimum program for *total* body development; (2) they require no fancy equipment; (3) progression of intensity is invidual, so that you—regardless of your physical condition—may gradually develop a high level of general fitness; (4) they have a built-in evaluation scheme so that progress may be measured from day to day; (5) a minimum amount of time—only 10 minutes a day at least 3 times a week—is required for significant results.

Running

The development of cardiovascular endurance is dependent upon your working at peak capacity for short periods of time in such activities as running and swimming, where the total body is involved. Here, *spot running*, or running in place, is used. In that exercise, you run for 10 seconds, rest for 10 seconds, and then repeat the run for 10 seconds. Ten reruns, each with a 10-second rest, are performed, requiring a total of 3 minutes and 10 seconds. If you have had little previous activity, you should take it easy at first. Over a period of 2 weeks, you should be able to exert more nearly maximum capacity for each 10-second run. Gradually, that "maximum" will produce greater efforts. Progress is accomplished by increasing the number of steps and by raising the knees higher during the run.

Sit-Ups

Abdominal muscles are usually very weak in people who lead sedentary lives. That weakness is a predisposing factor to low-back pain as well as the single most important factor contributing to the "watermelon" effect up front. Sit-ups are an effective way of strengthening abdominal muscles.

Perform sit-ups over a 2-minute period. Lie on the floor and place the hands behind the head. Flex the knees. Perform 1 cycle in about 2 seconds: up on count 1 and down on count 2. Rest when tired, and stop when 2 minutes are up. Try to improve by at least 1 sit-up each week. Forty sit-ups in 2 minutes is a reasonable goal. Intensity may be increased by increasing speed or by holding a heavy object behind the head while exercising. Always do sit-ups with the knees flexed, as straight-leg sit-ups may place an undue strain on the lower back.

Push-Ups

This exercise develops strength particularly in the arms and shoulders. Twenty push-ups from the floor are a desirable objective to work toward. Intensity may be increased by exercising faster and for a longer period of time. Perform 1 cycle in 2 seconds: down on count 1 and up on count 2.

If you are unable to perform that exercise, you may try a modification executing the movement from a chair or from the knees.

Adult Physical Fitness

The pamphlet "Adult Physical Fitness" was developed by the President's Council on Physical Fitness and Sports in an effort to direct the American population on how to get back into shape at home. It contains a series of specific facts about physical fitness, a program for women, a program for men, and a discussion of how to widen and broaden your program.

Women's Program

The women's program consists of an orientation program, a step test, and the exercise program.

Follow the orientation program to prepare yourself for the exercise program. It will help you in reducing the incidence of aches and pains. At least 1 week and possibly 2 or 3 weeks should be devoted to those mild exercises.

After following the mild exercise program for the stipulated time, begin to take the step test. The test involves stepping up and down on a 15-to-17 inch bench for 2 minutes, at 30 steps a minute. Immediately after the test, sit down for 2 minutes. After the rest, take your pulse for 30 seconds. Record the pulse, for that will be used as you progress in the program. Every 2 weeks, you will retake the test. As your physical condition improves as a result of the program, your pulse rate will decrease.

Now you are ready to start the actual program. The program consists of exercises that are of 3 general types —warm-up exercises, conditioning exercises, and circulatory exercises. The warm-up exercises are to limber up the body and prepare the circulatory system for the increased activity. They are the first 6 exercises of the orientation program. Next, come the conditioning exercises. They are designed to tone up the major muscles of the abdomen, back, and legs. Finally, you'll do the circulatory exercises to

ORIENTATION PROGRAM   GOAL

Conditioning Exercises	Repetitions
*1. Bend and stretch	10
*2. Knee lift	10 left, 10 right
*3. Wing stretcher	20
*4. Half knee bend	10
*5. Arm circles	15 each way
*6. Body bender	10 left, 10 right
7. Prone arch	10
8. Knee pushup	6
9. Head and shoulder curl	5
10. Ankle stretch	15

Circulatory activity (choose one each workout)	
Walking	½ mile
Rope (skip 15 sec.; rest 60 sec.)	3 series

* The first six exercises of the orientation program will be used as warmup exercises throughout the graded levels. *Step Test Record*—After completing the orientation program, take the 2-minute step test. Record your pulse rate here:_____. This will be the base rate with which you can make comparisons in the future.

stimulate the circulatory and respiratory systems.

The exercises should be done at least 5 days a week. There are 5 levels or charts, the first being the easiest and the fifth becoming the most difficult. Spend at least 3 weeks on each chart. Do not progress at a faster rate. You may actually find it necessary to go at a slower rate as you progress.

The President's Council also recommends that you direct your efforts to broadening your workouts. That includes the use of isometrics for building strength, water activities for improving heart and lung function, weight training for developing strength and sports for building circulatory endurance and proper posture.

The Adult Physical Fitness program lasts only about 15 minutes instead of a more preferred time of about 30 minutes. In addition, the program does not require you to burn up 300-500 calories, the normally recognized

SAMPLE   GOAL

Warmup Exercises	*Exercises 1-6 of Orientation Program*

Conditioning Exercises	Uninterrupted repetitions
1. Bend and stretch	10
2. Sprinter	6
3. Sitting stretch	15
4. Knee pushup	12
5. Situp (fingers laced)	10
6. Leg raiser	10 each leg
7. Flutter kick	30

Circulatory activity (choose one each workout)	
Jog-walk (jog 50, walk 50)	½ mile
Rope (skip 30 secs.; rest 60 secs.)	3 series
Run in place (run 100, hop 25—2 cycles)	3 minutes

Your progress record	1	2	3	4	5	6	7	8	9	10	11	12	13	14	15
Step test (pulse)													Prove-out workouts		

Men's Programs

ORIENTATION PROGRAM   GOAL

Conditioning Exercises	Repetitions
*1. Bend and stretch	10
*2. Knee lift	10 left, 10 right
*3. Wing stretcher	20
*4. Half knee bend	10
*5. Arm circles	15 each way
*6. Body bender	10 left, 10 right
7. Prone arch	10
8. Knee pushup	6
9. Head and shoulder curl	5
10. Ankle stretch	15

Circulatory activity (choose one each workout)	
Walking	½ mile
Rope (skip 15 secs.; rest 60 secs.)	3 series

* The first six exercises of the Orientation program will be used as warmup exercises throughout the graded levels. *Step Test Record*—After completing the orientation program, take the 2-minute step test. Record your pulse rate here:_____. This will be the base rate with which you can make comparisons in the future.

minimum for adequate improvement in physical fitness. For those reasons, the program represents only a very basic minimum, and must definitely by supplemented in order to derive maximum benefit.

PROGRESSION

The term *progression* is one of the physiological principles of training and is closely allied to the principle of adaptation. Since the body soon adjusts to the stress put upon it over a period of time (adaptation), it is necessary that the work be continually increased if improvement is desired (progression). For example, if you run a mile in eight minutes each day and find that the workout is no longer stressful to your body (overload), you should *progressively* increase the

SAMPLE   GOAL

Warmup Exercises	*Exercises 1-6 of Orientation Program*
Conditioning Exercises	Uninterrupted repetitions
1. Toe touch	20
2. Sprinter	16
3. Sitting stretch	18
4. Pushup	10
5. Situp (fingers laced)	15
6. Leg raiser	16 each leg
7. Flutter kick	40

Circulatory activity (choose one each workout)	
Jog-walk (jog 100, walk 100)	1 mile
Rope (skip 60 secs.; rest 60 secs.)	3 series
Run in place (run 95, hop 15—2 cycles)	3 minutes

Your progress record	1	2	3	4	5	6	7	8	9	10	11	12	13	14	15
													Prove-out workouts		
Step test (pulse)															

stress by running the mile in a little less than eight minutes, or running a greater distance than a mile in eight minutes. Progressively increasing the stress will present a new challenge to the body, thereby forcing it to adjust (adaptation) to the increased load.

Progression enables you to increase your work load gradually, which means muscles will not become sore. It also reduces the likelihood of over-taxing the body, guarding against permanent injury during the training period.

PSYCHOLOGICAL VALUES

In each individual, there is an innate drive toward activity. In a child, it is undirected, as exhibited by ever-changing play situations. As he matures, the drive becomes purposeful and directed; and he begins to participate in organized games and activities which have meaning and which give him pleasure. For adults, the meaning and purpose must be present before they will undertake a physical activity program. Thus, although the adult has an innate drive, he will not exercise unless the activity has meaning and value for him.

Recently, physical educators have been informing the public about the value and contribution that regular exercise can make to the development and maintenance of physical fitness, BUT the importance of the psychological component of fitness has not been promoted. For some, that may be the most important outcome of physical activity. The relationship between physical health and mental and social adjustment is reflected in the belief that there is an inherent unity and integration of the mind and body—known as the "whole man" concept. Therefore, an exercise program which influences the development of organic health may also improve mental and emotional well-being in many ways.

First, exercise or play serves as a diversion and an emotional release from everyday work. Studies have shown that the mentally healthy person participates in some form of activity to supplement his required daily work. In fact, psychiatrists have stated that, besides being fun, physical activity satisfies certain unconscious demands. It is likely that the euphoria or sense of well-being following physical activity is either caused by, or accompanied by, emotional changes. The changes, or mood states, may appear regularly or periodically and may be caused by external stimuli, such as other people. They modify considerable areas of personality and fluctuate in intensity and duration, lasting from less than an hour to more than a season. The intensity and duration of mood change depends on personality and the type and intensity of activity. In any activity, mood changes should be positive and healthy and should never result in the emotional destruction of either the individual or of others in the exercise or play setting.

The sense of well-being experienced during or after activity may also be important in man's adjustment to stress. Recent evidence indicates that regular exercise: (1) conditions the stress adaptation mechanism, requiring less adjustment of the nervous system in stressful situations; (2) increases an individual's sense of well-being; and (3) increases his capacity for enduring disappointments and frustrations.

Studies have also shown that a lack of activity often reduces the ability to withstand stress and results in a loss of integration between mind and body. That is, the individual becomes anxious and physically and mentally inert.

In recent years, psychiatrists have investigated the value of exercise for certain atypical adult groups. Psychiatrists have employed physical activity in the rehabilitation of mental patients. They have used activities like walking and swimming because of their potentialities for encouraging self-expression, promoting communication, developing socialized attitudes and habits, increasing the range of interests, improving self-confidence, gratifying narcissistic needs and facilitating relaxation. It is likely that physical activity causes similar psychological changes in normal adults.

Physicians, working with post-coronary men, recognize the psychological value of exercise for that group. Personality studies have shown that enforced inactivity after a heart attack is harmful to the patient since it is the antithesis of his aggressive and dynamic nature which was present before the attack. This enforced restriction deprives the patient of the medium whereby he can alleviate emotional tension and may also increase his anxiety. In a study completed by this writer, it was found that, at the conclusion of an exercise course, post-cardiac men had an improved self-confidence in their ability to live a normal life, a reduction in general anxiety, an improved attitude toward exercise and physical activity, and an improved sense of well-being. The sense of well-being was attributed to mood changes wherein they felt happier, more alert, relaxed, stable and carefree.

Physical activity benefits both the mind and body. The two are interrelated and neither should be neglected when you consider the meaning and purpose of physical activity. Thus, through participation in some form of physical activity, "psychological fitness" can and should be developed and maintained.—*Barry D. McPherson*

PUBLICATIONS

Most of the numerous magazines and journals that present information on physical fitness and related areas are concerned with describing the coaching aspects in athletics or discussing a particular activity, such as swimming. If you are interested in such publications, write to the various organizations mentioned under OR-GANIZATIONS or refer to the particular sport entries.

The magazines and journals discussed here include a good deal of information about physical fitness and its closely allied aspects. Many of the publications include: "hints" on how to stay in shape, to achieve fitness, or to organize a fitness program; research being conducted on fitness; and suppliers of fitness equipment.

General

Fitness For Living

Fitness For Living is a unique magazine that is directed specifically to the public. It includes articles about the effects and benefits of staying physically fit, the types of exercise, the relationship of diet to exercise, and the effects of proper exercise in the prevention of various modern day degenerative diseases. One feature is the summary of current research being conducted in the field of physical fitness. It includes advertisements of various fitness devices.

About two-thirds of the writers are free-lance writers, and the remaining are professionals actively engaged in research and teaching.

Publisher:
Rodale Press, Inc.
33 East Minor Street
Emmaus, Pa. 18049
Cost: $4.50 per year

Physical Fitness Newsletter

The *Physical Fitness Newsletter* is a 6 to 12 page mimeographed letter published monthly during the school year. The purpose of the newsletter is to provide a medium of exchange of ideas and experiences among physical educators actively involved in developing fitness programs. Summaries of research studies are presented. There are no advertisements.

Publisher:
Dr. H. Harrison Clarke
University of Oregon
Eugene, Oregon
Price: $1.50 per year

President's Council on Physical Fitness and Sports Newsletter

The Newsletter summarizes many of the activities of the President's Council. It also includes news briefs about fitness happenings throughout the country and the world. The Newsletter is very readable and compact, usually about 4 pages.

Publisher:
President's Council on Physical Fitness and Sports
330 C Street, SW
Washington, D. C. 20201

Sport International

This magazine presents material covering international aspects of sports including parachuting, military pentathlon, modern pentathlon, shooting, track and field, swimming, cross country, boxing, fencing, wrestling, judo, soccer, basketball, volleyball and hockey. Occasional articles also deal with other sports. It is directed toward readers interested in international sporting events and training methods. The articles are usually not of a very scientific nature.

Publisher:
CISM
Banque do Commerce
Place Royale, 6,
Brussels, Belgium
Cost: $2.00 per year (Quarterly)

Research

Index and Abstracts of Foreign Physical Education Literature

The *Index and Abstracts*, sponsored and published by Phi Epsilon Kappa

Fraternity as a service to the physical education profession, includes abstracts of research conducted about sports medicine, health education, recreation, rehabilitation, athletics, physiology of exercise and physical fitness. Publications from over 34 countries, other than the United States, are reviewed, abstracted and/or indexed.

Publisher:
Phi Epsilon Kappa Fraternity
3747 North Linwood Avenue
Indianapolis 18, Indiana
Dr. R. R. Schreiber, Executive Secretary
Cost: $2.00 per copy (published yearly)

The Journal of Sports Medicine and Physical Fitness

The *Journal* is devoted to the medical aspects of sports and physical training for the purpose of improving and maintaining health. Original papers covering the psychological, physiological and pathological effects of muscular activity on the human body are considered for publication. It is intended for use by professional people in the areas of physical education, physiology, medicine and psychology. This quarterly publication is the official journal of the International Federation of Sports Medicine.

Publisher:
Minerva Medica
Torino, Italy
Cost: $10.00 per year

Research Quarterly

The Quarterly publication originates research studies in the fields of health, physical education and recreation. It literally serves as a clearing house of research being conducted in those disciplines throughout the United States and Canada. The articles are technical and designed for the professional interested in such allied areas.

Publisher:
American Association for Health, Physical Education and Recreation
1201 North 16th St., NW
Washington, D. C. 20036
Cost: Available to individuals through professional membership in AAHPER

Journal of Applied Physiology

This journal emphasizes the "application" of scientific research to man in his normal environment. Intended for professional use, it includes 8 major areas of reported research: Circulation, Respiration, Renal and Electrolyte Physiology, Comparative and General Physiology and Neurophysiology.

Publisher:
The American Physiological Society
Journal of Applied Physiology
9650 Wisconsin Ave.
Washington, D. C. 20014
Cost: $20.00 per year (bimonthly)

Professional

Journal of Physical Education

Although primarily a publication for those engaged in the YMCA physical education program, this publication also includes articles, related to the fields of health and physical education. Laymen will find an article or two in each edition interesting. For there are many "experience papers" that concern successful programs for families and business. It is published by the Physical Education Society of the YMCA's of North America.

Publisher:
Robert C. Rule, Editor
Downtown YM-YWCA
600 Broad Street
Newark, N. J. 07102
Address for subscription:
Lloyd C. Arnold
P. O. Box 508
Princeton, N.J. 08540
Cost: $4.00 per year (6 per year)

Journal of the Canadian Association for Health, Physical Education & Recreation

This journal is dedicated to raise Canadian health, physical education and recreation standards. There are feature articles, newslines, book reviews, equipment, research reports, advertising, announcements and reports of conventions. Recently about one-third of the feature articles have been related to promoting physical fitness.

Publisher:
CAHPER
703 Spadiva Avenue
Toronto 4, Ontario
Cost: $5.00 (bimonthly)

Journal of Health, Physical Education and Recreation

A professional journal that strives to promote and improve the disciples of health, physical education, and recreation, the journal is aimed at the professional teacher. The lay person may also find some illuminating articles concerning fitness and closely allied areas.

Publisher:
AAHPER
1201 Sixteenth St., NW
Washington, D. C. 20036
Cost: Subscription with membership to AAHPER

Other

Many state organizations of Health, Physical Education and Recreation have publications that are similar to the Journal of Health, Physical Education and Recreation, except that they are devoted primarily to state news. Other publications such as the *Journal of the American Medical Association* and the *Journal of the American Geriatrics Society* occasionally publish articles on exercise and physical fitness and related areas.

PULSE RATE

The normal pulse rate, according to the American Heart Association, is extremely variable, ranging from 50 to 100 beats per minute. That range is arbitrary, and a pulse rate of even 38 or 108 can be considered normal for certain individuals. But any pulse rates outside of the range established by the American Heart Association should be investigated by your medical doctor to see if they are normal or abnormal.

The pulse rate of a healthy person can be affected by sex, age, food intake, time of day, emotions, body position, physical activity and physical condition.

Sex

The average pulse rate for men is 72 to 78 beats per minute, while for women the average is 78 to 84. Generally, the average pulse rates for women, in a true resting state, are 7 to 10 beats higher than for men.

Age

The pulse rate at birth may range from 130 to 140 beats per minute and drops progressively to adolescence, when the rate stabilizes. Generally, the pulse rate remains at that adolescent level until old age, when it rises slightly.

Food Intake

The intake or digestion of food causes the pulse rate to increase for two hours or more, an important point to remember if you are attempting to determine your pulse rate.

Time of Day

Pulse rates during sleep drop progressively during the first seven hours, after which there is a slight increase before waking. Upon waking, the pulse rate is the lowest of the waking day. During the day, the pulse increases gradually until late afternoon,

when the pulse rate may be six beats or more higher than the rate on awakening. The pulse then seems to start a downward trend in the evening. The reason for the increase and subsequent decline in late evening can be attributed to food intake and increased activity during the day. Toward evening, however, your activity usually decreases, thereby resulting in a lowered pulse.

Emotions accelerate the pulse rate considerably. If you can recall watching an exciting movie, witnessing an astronaut launching or being involved in a near accident, you will probably remember that your pulse rate jumped markedly. The space race has also served notice as to how emotions affect pulse rate. At the time of launch, the astronauts pulse rates are elevated considerably, sometimes 50 beats or higher than their normal level.

Body position plays a critical role in pulse rate. The lowest pulse rates are obtained when you are in a lying position. The pulse rate is elevated slightly in the sitting position and highest in the standing position. The amount of increase varies with each person. In a few rare instances, pulse rate may remain the same or decrease from the lying to sitting or standing positions. The pulse rate of the physically fit and nonfit increases from a reclining to a standing position about the same number of beats, usually 15 to 20 beats. The increase is desirable, for it compensates for the change in gravity from the change in position.

An excessive increase in pulse rate, on the other hand, may indicate an abnormal condition of being unable to adjust to a change in gravity. That often occurs if you have been subjected to prolonged bed rest and then attempt to stand.

The pulse rate increases rapidly at the onset of exercise. In fact, the increase may occur even before the exercising begins as you prepare for the exercise. That is particularly true for athletic events, where the pulse rate may almost double the resting rate prior to the event. The increase is normal and may be attributed to emotions and the cerebral center of the brain that controls the heart rate.

The acceleration at the onset of exercise increases rapidly during the first minute of exercise. After the rapid rise, the pulse rate usually reaches a plateau, although a continued increase may be observed in some forms of exercise.

The intensity of the exercise determines the response of the heart rate. In light exercise, the heart rate accelerates quickly, only to drop slightly and then level off until cessation of exercise. After exercise ceases, the pulse rate quickly returns to normal. In moderate exercise, the pulse rate again climbs quickly, only to a higher rate than during light exercise. The pulse rate then levels off and maintains a plateau until cessation of exercise. After you stop exercising, the pulse rate returns to normal, but the return is slower than in light exercise (see chart). In heavy exercise, the pulse rate rises quickly and continues to rise until you reach a point of exhaustion and are unable to continue. When you stop exercising because of exhaustion, the pulse rate drops quickly at first and then declines somewhat slower until the normal resting pulse rate is reached.

Some forms of exercise, however, vary in intensity during performance. For example, a soccer player may sprint after a ball for a few seconds only to slow down as the action drifts away from him. The pulse rate responds accordingly to the variance. If the work load or intensity increases, the pulse rate goes up. As the intensity decreases, the pulse rate drops.

The type of exercise plays a critical role in the rate and degree of pulse rate. The greatest acceleration occurs in exercises that involve speed, such as sprinting. Strength exercises, such as weight training and isometrics, involve the least amount of acceleration, while exercises of endurance like distance running involve a moderate acceleration of pulse rate. The reason is that, although the performance in sprinting is of shorter duration than in distance running, the work done is more intense and more oxygen is required so that the heart beats faster to meet the demand. In the short sprints, a great deal of oxygen is utilized, creating an *oxygen debt.* See OXYGEN DEBT. In the endurance activities, the respiratory and circulatory systems are able to keep up with the oxygen requirement. Therefore, the rise is not so dramatic.

Pulse rates taken immediately after exercise may serve as a guide indicating the intensity of the workout. The accompanying chart presents a resume of what various pulse readings might mean for a young adult.

PULSE RATE AND INTENSITY
OF WORKOUT

Pulse Rate	Intensity of Workout
120	Mild
140	Moderate
160	Good
180	Hard
200	Exhausting

As age increases, however, the elevated pulse rates of 180 or 200 are seldom seen. The January-February, 1965, issue of *The Heart Bulletin* showed how the average maximum attainable heart rates decline with age. The accompanying chart indicates R. A. Bruce, L. B. Rowell, J. R. Blackman and A. Doan's analysis of the decline with age.

Dr. M. F. Graham indicates that pulse rate should determine your work intensity. The rate should reach a peak of at least 60 per cent of its capability for several minutes. He cites the example of having a resting rate of 60

MAXIMUM PULSE RATE AND
AGE (MALE)

Average Age	Average Pulse Rate	Range of Pulse Rates From Sample
19	190	210-178
27	180	197-178
36	175	190-168
44	170	180-160
54	168	180-152
64	148	168-128

and an average maximum rate of 180. Your average maximum rate for your age can be determined from the chart above. Your capable range, therefore, in the example is from 60 to 180, or 120 beats. Sixty per cent of 120 is 72. Based on those calculations, you should strive for an increase in rate of at least 72 beats a minute above your resting rate, in this case 132. (60 + 72 =132). The rate must be maintained for several minutes.

Dr. Alan J. Barry, Lankanau Hospital, Philadelphia, Pennsylvania revealed that research has indicated a pulse rate of 130 to 140 beats per minute for several minutes is necessary for an improvement of cardiovascular function. Others have noted that 150 beats per minute is desirable.

However, pulse rate is not the only factor in determining the intensity of exercise. The calories consumed in a certain amount of time are critical. You should burn 300 to 500 calories in a half-hour period. Consumption of that amount of calories in a half hour produces an entirely different peak pulse rate than 300 to 500 calories in one or two hours.

Obviously, when you are in a low state of fitness and begin an exercise program, you will be unable to exhaust 300 to 500 calories by keeping your pulse rate at about 60 per cent of its range. The 60 per cent pulse increase and burning off of 300 to 500 calories will be a goal to achieve when better fitness is attained.

After cessation of exercise, the pulse rate usually begins to drop and returns to normal. The rate of return depends upon three factors—the work load (intensity), its duration and your physical condition. After a light workout, the pulse rate soon returns to the resting level. If the light workout is performed over an extended period (several hours), the pulse rate may be somewhat delayed in its return.

Moderate work affects the pulse rate in a similar manner as light work, except that the pulse rate returns to normal somewhat more slowly. In heavy work, however, the longer duration of exhausting work, the longer the return of the pulse rate to the resting level. The rate of return depends upon your physical condition, the amount of stress, and the oxygen debt incurred.

In exercise that is not continuous, but rather sporadic, the recovery rates are determined by the intensity of the work that preceded it. If the work is light or moderate, the recovery occurs in a relatively short time. In harder work, however, the pulse rate returns to normal at a much slower rate, and in particularly exhausting exercise, whether continuous or sporadic, the return to normal may take up to two hours or more.

For the most part, the descent to the normal "resting" rate is definite, although the declining rate may fluctuate considerably. There is usually a very rapid decline during the first few minutes and a more gradual drop thereafter. In older people, the pulse rate may rise immediately after exercise before the decline begins.

A drop in pulse rate, below the "resting" rate, may be expected in some people during recovery, and usually occurs if they did not have a true resting rate prior to the exercise. The elevated pulse rate may be a result of several factors, namely emotions, previous activity and lack of sleep.

Training or long-term exercise plays a critical role in pulse rate, for the resting rate of a person in good physical condition is invariably lower than that of a person in poor physical condition.

The type of training (endurance of strength), however, is also important in determining the resting rate. People who perform endurance exercises have lower resting pulse rates than those who perform strength-type exercises.

During exercise, or immediately after exercise, pulse rates are affected considerably by physical condition; for a person in good physical condition does not achieve as high a pulse rate as a person in poor physical condition, providing they have done the same amount of work. The difference is attributed, however, to the lower resting pulse rate of the well-conditioned person, for both types of pulse rates increase about the same number of beats. Also the recovery rate of people in good physical condition is faster than the recovery rate of those in poor physical condition provided they both perform the same amount of work.

A person in good physical condition can also accomplish more work over a longer period of time than a person in poor physical condition although their recovery pulse rates will be about the same.

Heart-Rate Monitoring

What is sufficient training stress for you may be too easy or too severe for another. How then can you determine appropriate training stress?

One solution is to monitor your own heart rate. The monitoring technique serves as an indicator of stress and has been featured in successful cardiovascular training projects at San Diego State College and at Simon Fraser University in Burnaby, British Columbia. It is simple, has demonstrated effectiveness, and can be adapted to running, swimming, or cycling.

How to Monitor Your Heart

Frequently in your running or other conditioning activity, pause and take your heart count for a ten-second period. The preferred position is with the left hand to the left chest wall. Wrist or neck pulse may also be used. However, in taking neck pulse, your fingers should not press so hard as to impede blood flow. Experiment with the different positions to find the one which is most convenient for you.

During the first few weeks of your exercise program, you may take as many as two dozen heart counts during each session. Later on in training, when you have learned to appreciate stress in terms of heart response, four or five counts during a session are sufficient to serve as an intensity guide.

The technique is simple. Begin counting five seconds after cessation of an exercise task, and start your count zero, one, two, three, etc., with zero marking the beginning of the time interval. If you are exercising with a group of friends, appoint an exercise leader who can use a watch with a sweep second hand to time a ten-second interval. Five seconds after stopping, the exercise leader gives a "ready—*count*" with the word "*count*" marking the beginning of the interval. The group count would then start with one, two, three, etc., and end on the command "ready—stop."

How Severely Should You Exercise?

Under laboratory conditions, it is possible to obtain a maximal heart rate. That value can be used as a guide to set training intensity levels. It may be convenient to classify your workouts as "easy" and "brisk." Early in training programs, "easy" represents an exercise intensity sufficient to evoke 65 per cent of the maximal heart rate, and "brisk" 80 per cent of that value. Later on, if the training response is good, the levels are raised to 70 per cent and 85 per cent.

When laboratory data is not available, you can use the values shown in the following table. Estimated maximal heart rates for various ages are shown with "easy" and "brisk" level for the first two-month and second four-month periods of training.

Figure it this way. If you are 40 years old, an "easy" exercise pace should evoke a heart rate of 20, and a "brisk" pace, a rate of 24. For the first two months, you should keep the running, cycling or swimming intensity within the 20-24 range. Initially, most of the time you should be following an "easy" pace and interspersing walk-recovery sequences where the heart rate may drop to 60 per cent of the maximal value, 18 in our example. As you start to improve, you can reduce the number of walk-recovery sequences and include more activity at the "easy" and "brisk" levels. Toward the end of the first two months of training and at least three times per week, you may be able to sustain a "brisk" pace throughout most of your workout. In the next four-month period, you can raise the "easy"-"brisk" range to 21-26 as indicated on the chart.

Using the chart, "easy" and "brisk" training pace intensities can be determined for any age level. However, remember age is only a general referent and that if you are grossly out of shape, you are physiologically older than your chronological age. For example, you might start training at an age-intensity level for men five years older than you are. You can always readjust to your proper age level when your training response warrants the change.

Heart-Rate Monitoring Puts You in Focus

As you become accustomed to the heart-rate monitoring technique, you soon learn to pace yourself with surprising accuracy. Even in group running or cycling, you can keep the exercise appropriate. By slightly lengthening a course or cutting corners, you can adjust the intensity of your activity to the group pace and enjoy your training with others.

The whole point in using heart-rate monitoring is to keep you in focus, to keep your exercise appropriate. That rules out incentive training such as mile-time trials, 100-mile total distance in training contests, or other such gimmicks which are detrimental to good exercise management.

Cardiovascular gains, of course, can be made by punishing training regimens if your musculo-skeletal tissues can withstand the stress and you are endowed with a temperament for enduring pain. However, such heroics are successful with only a small segment of the adult male population, and potentially hazardous to the vast

SUGGESTED "EASY" AND "BRISK" HEART RATES FOR
INITIAL 0-2 MONTHS AND 3-6 MONTHS TRAINING
(BEATS PER 10 SECOND INTERVAL)

Age	Heart Rate Max.	0-2 Month Training		3-6 Months Training	
		Easy	Brisk	Easy	Brisk
15	35	23	28	25	30
25	34	22	27	24	29
35	32	21	26	22	27
40	30	20	24	21	26
45	28	19	23	20	24
50	27	18	22	19	23
55	26	17	21	18	22

majority. Dr. Fred Kasch's counsel to his participants in the San Diego State College Program is more suitable— "Time is in your favor—allow at least one month of training for every year of sedentary living—aim for long-term gains from regular, enjoyable training —increase training intensity gradually."

A heart-rate monitoring training plan is consistent with those views. All habitually sedentary middle-aged males should give their tissues time to adapt to a gradually increased training stress. And the heart rate monitoring technique serves as a valuable individual guide.—*William D. Ross, W. Raymond Duncan*

RACES

Performance in American Negroes and American Whites

Anthropologists view "race" as a population differing in the frequency of certain genes in other populations. Central to that approach is the concept of human variability. Man is polytypic. Individuals and populations do in fact differ in a variety of biological features. Such differences enable an adequate understanding of the distribution and significance of human variability.

Researchers have discovered that external differences in body structure, particularly in the proportions of limbs and trunk, exist between Negroes and whites. Negro children and adults have shorter trunks, more slender pelvises, longer upper extremities (especially a relatively longer forearm), greater arm span and longer lower extremities (especially a longer lower leg). Such proportional differences appear early in prenatal life and persist postnatally into adulthood.

When compared with adult whites, adult American Negroes have greater skeletal weights, bone densities, and per cent of compact bone.

Subcutaneous fat as measured via skinfold thicknesses is less in Negro boys and young adult males. Newman reported a "remarkably narrower" distribution of skinfold thickness in young adult Negro males, suggesting, perhaps, racial differences in fat patterning.

Using radiographic techniques, J. M. Tanner noted composition differences in the extremities of Negro and white athletes. Negro-white differences in the composition of the upper arm and thigh were smaller than those noted in the lower leg. In the former, Negroes had slightly more muscle and bone, and less fat, while in the calf, Negroes had wider bones, narrower muscles, and less fat. Thus, Negroes have substantially smaller calf muscles relative to muscular development in the arm and thigh.

Motor Development

Evidence indicates a tendency toward motor advancement in Negro children during the first three years of life, the differences between Negro and white children in early motor development being more pronounced at the younger ages. J. E. Sessoms suggests a persistence of the Negro-white difference in manual skills through four years of age, while A. Rhodes suggests little, if any, difference between Negro and white children (2½- 5½ years) in speed of walking a path and three fine motor skill tasks.

In children of elementary school age, several studies indicate higher levels of performance among Negro as compared to white children. A. Espenschade, for example, noted a greater percentage of Negro males passing all items of the Kraus-Weber test than white males at the fourth-grade level. Differences between Negro and white girls of the same grade level, however, were not evident. Using the 35-yard dash, P. W. Hutinger found fourth, fifth, and sixth grade Negro boys and girls faster than their white grade and sex peers. N. A. Ponthieux and D. G. Barker reported fifth and sixth grade Negro males superior to white males of the same grade levels in five of seven items of the AAHPER fitness test, while Negro females exceeded the white females in four of the seven items.

At the older age levels, the available studies are limited to rather specific test batteries. J. E. Codwell attempted to analyze the effects of American Negro hybridity on performance, using skin color as a classification device. Generally greater levels of motor ability (McCloy's battery) were noted in high school boys classified as "dominantly negroid" as compared to those classified as "intermediate" and "strong evidence of white," with the "intermediate" boys resembling the "dominantly negroid" in performance more closely than they did the "strong evidence of white" group. L. M. Fraley reported higher levels of performance in the total battery of the Cozens' general athletic ability test for Negro Civilian Conservation Corps enrollees compared to white enrollees of the same age. A. Espenschade found no differences between the total Brace motor ability test scores of Negro and white tenth grade girls, but noted within specific items of the battery, greater levels of balance in white girls and greater arm strength in Negro girls.

Regarding more specific skill items, Negro males exceed white males in vertical jumping ability at the high school and college levels, but are equal in measurements of their flexibility.

Comparative studies of strength performance in American Negroes and whites are few. A. Hrdlicka reported a tendency towards greater grip and traction strength in Negro compared to white children of both sexes from 6 to 16 years of age. Relative to body weight, the Negro children showed greater proportionate strength. R. R. Montpetit *et al.* found significantly greater grip strength in Negro compared to white girls from 9 through 17 years of age. Among boys, however, greater grip strength was evident among Negroes from 9 through 11 years, with the white boys significantly stronger in grip thereafter through age 14 years. Among adults, A. Hrdlicka found Negro males slightly stronger in grip and traction strength relative to stature, while M. A. Ohlson *et al.* reported greater grip strength in Negro females from 50 through 89 years of age.

Implications and Speculations

Researchers have studied rather thoroughly the differences between Negroes and whites. They suggest that Negroes excel in running and jumping events. That is likewise reflected in the large percentage of Negro athletes who excel in the sprints and jumping events, especially the high jump and broad jump, in competitive track and field athletics. Hence, it is logical to inquire whether structural or compositional differences between Negroes and whites may contribute to the apparently greater levels of performance in the Negro.

J. M. Tanner says that the American Negro, whether athletic or nonathletic, is generally linear in build with relatively longer arms and legs, a narrower pelvis, and more slender calves. Hence, mechanically speaking, a Negro performer with legs identical to a white performer would have a lighter, shorter, and slimmer mass to propel, implying a greater power-to-total weight ratio at any given size. The power-weight ratio would thus be advantageous in events in which the body is propelled; for example, the sprints and jumps, events which require relatively short bursts of muscular power rather than prolonged effort. However, the skeletal weight and density of the Negro appear to offset that general advantage.

Tanner's data indicates greater musculature in the arm and thigh, and less in the calf for the Negro. Muscle size, however, is only moderately related to muscular strength. Further, because strength of a muscle is physiologically related to its cross-sectional area, it is difficult to assume that the Negro calf musculature produces more power enabling him to excel in the sprints and jumps. Perhaps there are qualitative differences in the muscle tissue between Negroes and whites. There is, however, no evidence for that indicating the need for biochemical research to supplement the evidence of external structure and body composition in searching for the factors underlying superior function of the human machine. Nevertheless, there is more to performance than sheer muscle and bone. It is the individual who eventually must perform, and the words of M. Smith summarize the situation very appropriately:

Every athletic performance depends on what the individual brings to the contest. The sprinter, tensed in the starting blocks, must rely upon a whole complex of human factors to take him across the finish line—muscle and sinew, and mind and heart, too.—*Robert M. Malina*

REACTION TIME

Reaction time is technically defined as the period from the stimulus to the beginning of the overt response. It's the time required for you to begin to react, not the time occupied by the execution of the response. The stimulus could be anything that stimulates you to react, such as the starter's gun for the sprinter, the realization by the western gun fighter that the bad guy is starting to draw or an opening in an opponent's defense as seen by the boxer. Following that stimulus, there is a latent period while the impulse or message is transmitted from the receiving sense organ to the central nervous system and then back to the muscles. Those actions are not instantaneous. There is a measurable period

of time while the impulse travels from the eye to the brain and then to the muscles. Probably most of the time is taken in the motor areas of the brain. That delay is particularly true if any decision making is required, i.e., if you have to decide what type of response to make.

Movement Time

In order to understand your total response in a rapid-action situation, the term movement time has been developed. *Movement time* refers to the period from the beginning of the overt response to the completion of a specified movement. Movement time, therefore, begins where reaction time ends, at the beginning of the response. That movement, of course, is the action that you observe when evaluating the speed of an individual's response.

It has been assumed that there is a high relationship between reaction time and movement time. That is, the individual with a fast reaction time was believed to be able to move more quickly or to run faster than a person with a slower reaction time. That particular question has been investigated quite thoroughly during the past few years. The majority of research indicates that there is little, if any, relationship between those two components. Contrary to general opinion, therefore, the individual who is able to initiate movement rapidly will not necessarily be able to move faster once he gets started.

Improving Reaction Time

Is it possible to *improve reaction time* and movement speed? An analysis of the two aspects of that question reveals differing results. The reaction time phase, or speed of starting movements, cannot be appreciably shortened. That component, which is dependent upon efficiency in the nervous system, is an inherited trait. The movement phase of reaction speed, however, is based on muscular force and is, therefore, modifiable through practice and conditioning. Consequently, although reaction time in the technical sense cannot be improved through practice, effective speed of movement associated with specific sports skills can be heightened. Thus, by practicing such activities as starting from the blocks in sprinting, face-offs in ice hockey, bulleys in field hockey, racing dives in swimming or rapid movements in wrestling or fencing, you can improve your effective speed in those activities. However, it has not been established that practicing one type of movement will improve the speed of a different movement, or with a different body part. Improvement in speed is not accomplished on a general basis but is restricted to the particular type of movement being practiced. Therefore, the best way to improve the speed or efficiency of a movement with the right hand is to practice that particular response with the right hand, not a different movement, nor the same response with the left hand or with the feet.

Individual Differences

Reaction and movement time varies with different individuals. The potential for speed is obviously not the same for all persons. Within individuals, however, there are several factors which contribute to differences in speed of reaction. Those factors may be external, dealing with the stimulus; or they may be internal, dealing with the state of the individual. Among the external variables are the identity of sense organs stimulated and the intensity of the stimulus. Several authors have reported that the particular *sense organ* stimulated makes a difference in speed of reaction. Hearing elicits a slightly faster response than does vision. It has generally been established that those senses are followed in order by pain, taste, smell and touch. Responses seem to be speeded when several of the senses are stimulated simultaneously. Aside from the sense organ, the *intensity of the stimulus* is a factor in reaction time. A very loud noise, for example, will result in a faster reaction than a milder sound. The sharp sound of a starter's gun in track should, therefore, produce a quicker response than would the oral command, "Go." Similarly, a vivid or brilliant color will result in a faster reaction than softer shades. The same principle regarding intensity applies likewise to the other senses. However, it appears that above a certain maximum, additional increases in intensity do not prove beneficial.

The *height of readiness* for reaction is an internal variable which has been of interest to investigators. Your peak of attention does not last indefinitely. If the foreperiod (the time between the "ready" and the "go" signals) is too short, you will not have time to get sufficiently ready. If it is too long, the readiness will gradually wane. Most researchers have reported that the point of maximum readiness lies between one and three seconds. Coaches or other individuals who are interested in quick starts should take advantage of that period of peak readiness. From a strategy standpoint, the short or the long count in football, or similar timing by the pitcher in the stretch position in baseball, may be designed to avoid the opponent's period of maximum readiness.

During the developmental years, *age* appears to play a part in the determination of reaction time. Peak speed in both reaction and movement time is attained during the late teens and early twenties. Following that period, there is a leveling off with practically no drop-off in reaction time up to the age of sixty. However, the slowing of reaction time occurs rapidly when you approach feebleness. Movement speed deteriorates earlier and is, contrary to reaction time, closely related to your physical fitness.

Reaction and movement speed

varies somewhat according to *sex*. Most studies in which comparisons have been made report that males are faster in both of those components than are females.

Alcohol and *drugs* have a variable effect on your reaction speed. Above a certain minimum, the greater the amount of alcohol in the blood system, the more the reaction time will be slowed. Many such studies have been conducted in relation to traffic safety. Most drugs, when taken in normal doses, do not have an appreciable influence on reaction time. When large doses are absorbed, however, the same drugs slow your reaction and speed of movement. Certain drugs have recently been found to speed reaction time slightly. Nevertheless, the use of those drugs for the purpose of improving speed in sports activities has been strongly discouraged by authorities. Since the possibility of harmful or habit-forming effects has not been determined, such drugs have no place in fitness programs at this time.— *Joseph B. Oxendine*

RECONDITIONING

Reconditioning programs are corrective and adapted programs for people who have problems or special needs. Literally, the word reconditioning means to condition again. To be effective, reconditioning programs must meet the following objectives.

1. To help participants develop their physical capabilities to the fullest.

2. To protect the participants' condition from further aggravation.

3. To speed the rehabilitative process and prevent reinjury.

4. To provide satisfying and rewarding physical experiences for the participants.

5. To help participants understand and accept their physical or mental limitations.

6. To develop enjoyable recrea-

tional skills commensurate with the individuals' limitations.

7. To make the participants aware of good body mechanics and efficient movement.

Categories of Participants

People who benefit from reconditioning programs are classified into the following categories:

Permanent Disabilities—Amputees, paraplegics, post-polio cases, individuals with certain neuro-muscular afflictions and those with permanent heart and lung conditions.

Temporary Physical Disabilities—People with healing injuries and those recovering from extended illnesses or surgery.

Mental Disturbances—Normally people with low I.Q.'s or some form of diagnosed mental illness.

Special Needs—People who are not handicapped by injury or mental problems but lack muscular strength and endurance or certain physical skills to meet the demands of their environment. Normally, they cannot meet the minimum standards of regular physical education.

Programs for individuals with permanent physical or mental disabilities are designed from a knowledge of their limitations, capabilities and needs. Only from that base can effective programs be developed. There can be no set formula for designing reconditioning programs, but if you are interested in working with such individuals, you will find the following activities quite beneficial.

SPECIFIC PHYSICAL DEVELOPMENT PROGRAMS

A. *Frequency*—Perform weight training, calisthenics, isometrics, and running every other day. Perform isometric exercises on each non-lifting day.

B. *Warm-up*—Prior to beginning any of the workouts listed below, you should warm up with light calisthenics commensurate with your disability.

1. Trunk Twisting—Perform 10 trunk rotating movements attempting to stretch the back, abdominal, and hamstring muscles.
2. Arm Circles—Perform 20-30 seconds of arm circles. Alternate rapid small circles with slow larger ones.
3. Wrestler's Bridge—Assume a bridge position on the back and roll the neck for approximately 20 seconds.
4. Sit-ups—Perform 10-15 bent-legged sit-ups without any additional weights.
5. Run In Place (or jog)—Run in place or jog for 30-45 seconds.

C. *Pull-Up Conditioning Program*—Develops biceps and shoulder muscles.

1. Pull-Ups—Every workout, 3 sets of as many pull-ups as you can perform. Get help when you can no longer perform 3 good pull-ups.
2. Lat Machine—Approximately ⅓ body weight, 3 sets of 30-35 repetitions (reps).
3. Curls—⅓ body weight plus as much weight as you can handle, 3 sets of 8-10 reps.
4. Rowing—⅓ body weight plus as much weight as you can handle, 3 sets of 8-10 reps.
5. Military Press—⅓ body weight plus as much weight as you can handle, 3 sets of 8-10 reps.
6. Push-Ups—Every workout, 2 sets of as many push-ups as you can perform.
7. Run—Six (6) laps of a 150-yard track at 26-28 seconds with five (5) push-ups and a brisk walk between each lap.

D. *Standing Broad Jump Conditioning Program.* Develops explosive power of the legs.

1. Toe Extension—Body weight plus 20 lbs. or more, 3 sets of 20-25 reps.
2. ¾ Squats—½ body weight plus 20 lbs. 3 sets of 8-10 reps.
3. Standing Broad Jump—Every workout perform 3 sets of 10 practice jumps and record distance. (Work up to that amount of jumps.)
4. Leg Press—Body weight plus as much weight as you can handle, 3 sets of 8-10 reps.
5. Sit-Ups—One set of straight legged sit-ups should be performed with a 10 lb. weight held behind the head. Perform *as many as possible,* minimum of 15.
6. Run—Six (6) laps of a 150-yard track at 26-28 seconds with 5 push-ups and a brisk walk between each lap.
7. Isometrics—Perform isometric exercises after the workout and on all nonweight lifting days.

E. *Push-Up Conditioning Program*—Develops triceps and back muscles.

1. Push-Ups—Every workout, 3 sets of as many push-ups as you can do.
2. Dips—Dip five times on parallel bars and walk the length on your hands, then do 4 more dips. Try to increase the numbers.
3. Military Press—½ body weight plus 10 lbs., 3 sets of 15-20 reps.
4. Bench Press—½ body weight plus as much weight as you can handle, 3 sets of 15.
5. Run—Six (6) laps of a 150-yard track at 26-28 seconds with 5 push-ups and a brisk walk between each lap.
6. Isometrics—Performed after each workout and on all non-workout days.

F. *Sit-Up Conditioning Program*—Develops the abdominal muscles.

1. Sit-Ups—Three (3) sets of

bent-legged sit-ups should be performed with a 10 lb. weight held behind the head. Perform as many as possible.

2. Supine Leg Raiser—Lie on your back with legs fully extended. Lift your heels 12 inches off the floor and hold for 10 seconds. Continue to raise legs to the vertical, then lower to the floor (3 sets of 5).

3. Trunk Twister—Two (2) sets of 10.

4. Run—Six (6) laps of a 150-yard track at 26-28 seconds with 10 sit-ups and a brisk walk of one lap between each lap.

5. Isometrics—To be performed after each workout and on all nonworkout days.

G. *600-Yard-Run Conditioning Program*—Develops leg muscles and circulo-respiratory functions.

1. Time one 600-yard run at the beginning of the workout and record.

2. Toe Extension—Body weight plus 20 lbs. or more—3 sets of 10 reps.

3. Squats—¼ body weight plus 20 lbs.—3 sets of 8-10 reps.

4. Sit-Ups—Three (3) sets of 20 using a 10 lb. weight.

5. Interval Running—Run ten laps of a 150-yard track in 26-28 seconds. Between each lap, walk briskly the same distance run. (Work up to that number of reps. and pace.)

6. Isometrics—After each workout and on nonworkout days.

GENERAL PHYSICAL DEVELOPMENT PROGRAM

A. Suggested for individuals with no physical impairment for the purpose of general strength development.

B. *Frequency*. Perform weight training, calisthenics, isometrics and running every other day. Perform isometric exercises on each non-lifting day.

1. Trunk twisting—10 reps. (warm-up).

2. Sit-ups—20 reps. (warm-up).

3. Push-ups—15 reps. (warm-up).

4. ¾ squats with body weight—20 reps. (warm-up).

5. Isometrics exercises.
   a. Hold each contraction for at least 6 seconds.
   b. Perform exercises on non-workout days.

6. Two-man neck isometrics or wrestler's bridge.

7. Two-hand curl with barbells—8-10 reps. with as much weight as you can handle.

8. Bench press with barbells—8-10 reps. with as much weight as you can handle.

9. Leg press—8-10 reps. with as much weight as you can handle.

10. Rowing—8-10 reps. with as much weight as you can handle.

11. Sit-ups with 10 lb. weight held behind the head, knees bent—20 reps.

12. Running in place—75 steps (count on right foot only).

13. Repeat prescribed exercises 5 through 12.

14. Run six (6) laps of a 150-yard track at 26-28 seconds—walk briskly one lap between each run.

15. Swim ten (10) 25-yard laps at approximately 30 seconds each—rest 30 seconds between laps.

CONDITIONING PROGRAM FOR PEOPLE WITH UPPER BODY INJURIES

A. Suggested for individuals with arm or shoulder impairments.

B. *Frequency*. Perform weight training, calisthenics, isometrics and running every other day. Perform isometric exercises on each non-lifting day.

1. Trunk twisting—10 reps. (warm-up).
2. Sit-ups—15 reps. (warm-up).
3. ¾ squats with body weight—20 reps. (warm-up).
4. Isometric exercises.
   a. Hold each contraction for about 6 seconds.
   b. Perform exercises on non-workout days.
5. Two-man neck isometrics.
6. Leg press, 8-10 reps. with as much weight as you can handle.
7. Curls with good arm, 8-10 reps. with as much weight as you can handle. Use dumbbell.
8. Bench press with good arm, 8-10 reps. with as much weight as you can handle. Use dumbbell.
9. Hamstring exercise, 8-10 reps. with as much weight as you can handle.
10. Repeat exercises 4 through 9.
11. Run 6 laps of a 150-yard track at 26-28 seconds—walk briskly one lap between each run.

or

12. Swim ten (10) 25-yard laps at approximately 30 seconds—rest 30 seconds between laps.

CONDITIONING PROGRAM FOR PEOPLE WITH LEG INJURIES

Frequency. Perform weight training, calisthenics, isometrics and running every other day. Perform isometrics exercises on each nonlifting day.

1. Trunk twisting—10 reps. (warm-up).
2. Sit-ups—15 reps. (warm-up).
3. Push-ups—10 reps. (warm-up).
4. Isometric exercises.
   a. Hold each contraction for at least 6 seconds.

   b. Perform exercises on non-workout days.
5. Two-man neck isometrics or wrestler's bridge, 1 minute of work.
6. Rowing, 8-10 reps. with as much weight as you can handle.
7. Bench press—8-10 reps. with as much weight as you can handle. Adjust weight so that 8-10 reps. are difficult.
8. Two hand curls—8-10 reps. with as much weight as you can handle.
9. Sit-ups with 10 lb. weight—maximum reps. (sit-ups should be done with knees bent if possible). Wrap weight in towel to prevent discomfort.
10. Straight arm pullovers—8-10 reps. with as much weight as you can handle.
11. Pull-ups—as many as possible.
12. Lateral arm raising—8-10 reps. with 12½ lb. dumbbells or 10 lb. weight in each hand.
13. Repeat exercises 4 through 12.
   —*Patrick H. McHargue*

RECREATION

Recreation is any activity apart from your occupation done for pleasure. Recreational activities aid in relaxation, alleviate worries and problems, and stimulate the human organism physically and mentally. For an activity to be truly recreational, it must lead to complete personal involvement. But what is one man's work may be another man's pleasure. There is no one activity that is a pleasure for all. Activities that are too competitive, aggressive, or uninteresting may cause you to withhold tensions and, in fact, accumulate additional stress.

People in different jobs and with different personality make-ups will need varying amounts of recreation. For example, the person who is in a low-pressure job with a great deal of variety and who has a basically calm personality will need much less recreation than another who is high strung and deadline conscious and holds a high-pressure job.

Because of the reduced work week, extended vacations, and earlier retirements, it is necessary that a great majority of the population develop desirable recreational habits—habits that will recreate. A further problem is that automation has taken the creativity out of many of the jobs, resulting in boredom and a lack of motivation. Recreation can play an important role in such cases with activities that are enjoyable and creative. See CARRY-OVER SPORTS, COMMUNITY, LIFETIME SPORTS, RELAXATION and SCHOOLS.

REHABILITATION

According to Dr. E. Delagi and others, rehabilitation can be defined as a process (1) to prevent or reverse the harmful effects of inactivity, (2) to minimize disability and (3) to train the person who has residual permanent disability in the techniques of overcoming his handicap. In order to accomplish that rehabilitative process, a multidisciplinary team from the medical doctor and the physical therapist to the vocational counselor is involved.

In recent years, there has been a consistent increase in the number of physical medicine and rehabilitation departments in the hospitals. New approaches have been developed which include early ambulation and exercise programs for the post-surgery and post-coronary patients. The growth has been a result of medicine's changing concepts from a passive to a dynamic approach in the management of patients. Prolonged bed rest, inactivity and immobilization were the customary procedures for patients at one time. However, it was found that the limitation of activity during prolonged bed rest had debilitating effects causing significant deterioration of multiple organ systems including the cardiovascular, neuromuscular, respiratory, skeletal and urogenital systems. F. J. Kottke has reported that neuromuscular and emotional control and intellectual performance are all impaired by prolonged bed rest. The neglect of a disability in its early stages, according to Rusk, is far more costly than an early aggressive program of rehabilitation. E. Jokl has stated that the diagnostic and therapeutic clinical effects must be supplemented by physiological methods to restore the patient's fitness. It appears that medicine has acquired an increased understanding of the role of exercise as well as other types of physical activity in the treatment of aftercare patients.

Exercise and Rehabilitation

Exercise, with its attendant fitness benefits, is applicable to the clinical situation in neurological, orthopedic and general medical and surgical conditions. Drs. J. Wessel and W. Van Huss report that the therapeutic objectives for which exercise is prescribed in the clinic fields generally include maintaining and/or augmenting strength, power, tone, range of motion, and coordination; and maintaining and/or improving general body and muscular endurance. F. H. Krusen states that passive, active-passive, active, resistive, reeducation, coordination, and relaxation are all types of therapeutic exercises that may be utilized. However, there is a specificity of effect based upon the particular form of exercise used. Therefore, in order to obtain the desired therapeutic results, Dr. Janet Wessel and Dr. Wayne Van Huss advocate careful exercise prescription and administration of the prescribed exercises. For example, training and assistance with walking is often an important part of a patient's rehabilitation. Preliminary strengthening (resistive) exercises may be needed by

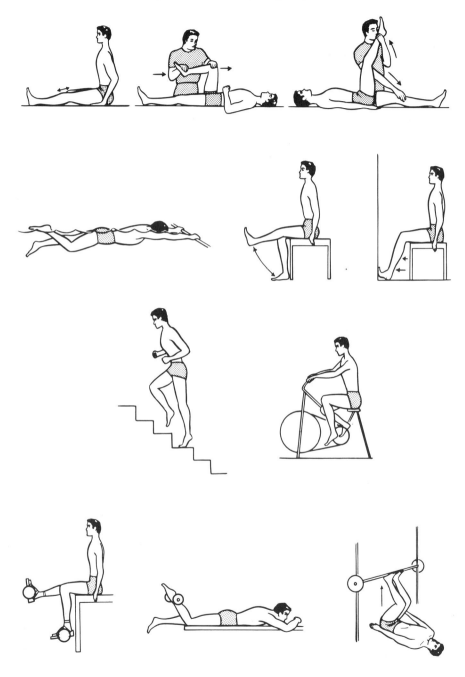

These illustrations show a typical sequence of exercises for rehabilitating the knee. Initially, the exercises are easy, but as the condition of the knee improves, more strenuous exercises are selected.

the patient in preparation for a cane, crutches or braces. Military hospitals have employed strengthening exercise programs at bedside even before the patient was able to be moved from his bed.

Many of the principles applied in therapeutic exercises have direct application to other forms of exercise. According to Wessel and Van Huss, swimming, dancing and other sports have certain clinical applications. The greatest impetus for use of therapeutic exercises and other types of physical activity occurred during World War II in the convalescent and rehabilitation programs in the military hospitals. The successful use of sport activities as a phase of the patient's rehabilitational experience was considered unique. Frequently the rules were changed and the game simplified so that the individual would meet with success. Those basic concepts involving sport activities are still being employed today in many of the adapted physical education programs in colleges.

Exercise as Prevention

In addition to acting as a therapeutic agency, exercise has potential as a preventive medicine. Authorities on aging believe that individuals who maintain a relatively high degree of fitness seem to suffer less from degenerative disease and may even live longer than one who follows a sedentary life. An important cause of athletic injuries in sports is the lack of an adequate physical fitness level which is necessary for the particular sport activity. Following an athletic injury, the training and conditioning program carried on during the period of rehabilitation assumes an equally important role in the prevention of reinjury. According to M. B. Howorth, backache is primarily a product of soft muscles, abuse and a soft life. Aside from obesity, the most common major factors in backache are weak muscles, poor patterns of physical performance

and irregular activity for which the person is not trained or conditioned. The trauma is rarely seen in people who are well-conditioned in the occupation or sport they are practicing and who use the back every day. It is Howorth's professional opinion that a vast majority of backaches of mechanical origin can be relieved (1) by correcting obesity, (2) by appropriate trunk-muscle exercises and (3) by training in good posture.

E. Jokl has pointed out that a well-conditioned athlete will recover from disease normally at a faster rate in comparison to the poorly physically conditioned individual. In regard to surgery, he contends that the athlete is considered a good "risk" to the physiological stress placed upon him during the operation, and the athlete should be able to return to activity in a short period of time. Jeff Farrell, a 1960 Olympic swimmer in the 400 meter medley relay for the United States, exemplifies the rapid postoperative recovery of a well-conditioned athlete. Three and one-half weeks after an emergency appendectomy, he placed fourth in the Olympic Trials. Under certain conditions, exercises are recommended to patients prior to surgery in order to maintain or improve their fitness. The author has been associated with military hospitals in which a series of "bed exercises" were prescribed for the presurgical patients. Those exercises were generally of the resistive type and involved the unafflicted area(s) of the body.

H. H. Clarke has shown that individuals, especially children who are adequately nourished and free from any visible defects and handicaps may still exhibit physical deficiencies. The individuals with muscular weakness and the lack of circulatory-respiratory endurance for their age, sex, weight and somatotype are classified in a low physical fitness status. To overcome that condition, a rehabilitation program stressing general developmental and conditioning activities should be prescribed.

For man to cope with the interacting stresses of life, he should develop the physiological functioning capacity of his body. Proper exercise causes the necessary physiological adaptations which result in increasing the functional capacity. For the permanently disabled individual, it means making the most of his remaining capacities, through maximum physical restoration so that he can achieve the fullest possible life compatible with his abilities. The post-surgery, the post-coronary, the athlete and the low fitness person should all be able to reestablish their normal daily living activities and occupational skills. In fact, some individuals will find success and enjoyment in areas in which they previously had failure. Thus, exercise with its obvious physical fitness implications plays an important part in the total rehabilitative process. Finally, it is important to remember that exercise should be engaged in judiciously and that it is not a remedy for all illnesses and injuries.—*H. H. Merrifield*

RELAXATION

Physical fitness is but one aspect of your total fitness, and is entwined with your emotional, mental and social fitness. Each affects the other. In fact, thought, emotion and motor activity are functions of the central nervous system, which is but one of the systems of the body.

Emotions and Health

Most disfunctions of the body are reflected by some disturbances of emotional reaction and thought processes, and vice versa. Witness the emotional depression which accompanies some disorders of the liver or the abdominal cramps from the spastic colons of many nervous, tense people.

All thoughts are accompanied by some degree of emotion and also by minute tensions in those muscles which are used to execute that thought. Both reactions occur simultaneously, are part and parcel of the same thing and form a functional unity. You cannot control your emotions or thoughts directly but can learn to control your skeletal muscular activity, thereby bringing the other aspects of that functional unity under greater control.

The ability to habitually relax your musculature has far-reaching effects on the entire organism. It conserves energy, reduces the work of the heart, tends to reduce blood pressure, reduces spasms in various parts of the digestive tract and contributes to a general feeling of well being. Also it tends to quiet the entire nervous system so that your general readiness to respond is reduced. You are much slower to anger, do not become upset over inconsequential things, do not experience the constant sense of urgency and are better able to perform daily tasks without the unnecessary fatigue but with the necessary reserve to meet an emergency. Consequently, your emotions will influence your thinking to a much lesser degree so that you will see things more realistically than emotionally.

The ability to relax comes naturally to some people, but most can attain such ability to relax the musculature only through systematic training or relearning.

Learning to Relax

Research and development of the techniques of relaxation training were begun by Dr. Edmund Jacobson some 50 years ago and entitled "Progressive Relaxation." Dr. Jacobson has continued his research and refinements of his techniques to the present day.

The basic procedure in teaching muscular relaxation is as follows. You may be instructed to contract the extensor muscles of the hand in the forearm by bending the hand backwards. That contraction causes a shortening of thousands of tiny muscle fibers which represent work, effort and the expenditure of energy. The contraction is the result of your "doing" a conscious and voluntary action. When the muscle fibers are shortened, they send signals to the brain indicating that they are shortened and to what degree. You perceive those signals as a sensation from the area of the contracted muscle which is different from any other sensory experience. You are asked to maintain the contracted state until you perceive some sensation which is different from that in your other, inactive forearm. When you do feel such a sensation, referred to in the future as "tenseness," you are told to "go off with the power," by *allowing* the hand to drop at rest. That state of rest, or the absence of the sensation of tenseness, will hereafter be known as "relaxation." The term "relaxation" is used in its scientific sense, which means the absence of neuromuscular activity, and not in its everyday sense of diversion or recreation.

You repeat the contraction in the forearm several more times, separated by periods of relaxation. Each time that you bend your hand back, you bend it to a lesser degree than the previous time, hold it until you feel any degree of the sensation of tenseness, and then allow the hand to drop. You are asked to practice for an hour each day until the next training session. Through the repetition in practice, you become more and more aware of even very faint sensations of tenseness and your ability to relax them.

Here are two practice schedules from Dr. Jacobson's pamphlet on *Self-Operation Control*, designed for distribution to patients as a guide for home practice sessions. Notice how the schedules give you an idea of how to release tension and acquire a relaxed state.

In the same general way, every major muscle group of the body is covered including those muscles which control the eyes and speech.

Effects of Relaxation

Throughout the years, Dr. Jacobson found that individuals trained in relaxation develop a general feeling of calmness and well being and lost much of their general nervousness, irritability, tendency to worry, insomnia and other such disturbing symptoms. Also, he found that, when the general tension level of the musculature was reduced, many physical symptoms improved or disappeared, such as those associated with spastic colon, mucous colitis, esophageal spasm, peptic ulcer,

ARM PRACTICE

In each hour-practice period, perform the tension indicated 3 times at intervals of several minutes. These are NOT exercises. Interest yourself in becoming familiar with the control sensation in each part so that you can learn really to run yourself properly relaxed under all conditions.

PERIODS	LEFT ARM	PERIODS	RIGHT ARM
1.	Bend hand back.	8.	Bend hand back.
2.	Bend hand forward.	9.	Bend hand forward.
3.	Relax only.	10.	Relax only.
4.	Bend at elbow.	11.	Bend at elbow.
5.	Press-wrist down on books.	12.	Press wrist down on books.
6.	Relax only.	13.	Relax only.
7.	Progressive tension and relaxation of whole.	14.	Progressive tension and relaxation of whole arm.

PERIOD No. 1

Select a quiet room, free from intruders and phone calls.

1. Lying on your back with arms at sides, leave eyes open 3 to 4 minutes.
2. Gradually close eyes and keep them closed entire hour.
3. After 3 to 4 minutes with eyes closed, bend left hand back, observing the control sensation 1 to 2 minutes and how it differs from the strains in the wrist and in the lower portion of the forearm.
4. Go negative for 3 to 4 minutes.
5. Again bend left hand back and observe as previously.
6. Once more go negative 3 to 4 minutes.
7. Bend left hand back a third and last time, observing the control sensation 1 to 2 minutes.
8. Finally go negative for remainder of hour.

PERIOD No. 3

Lie quietly on back as previously, arms at sides. In this *and in all subsequent periods lying down,* leave eyes open several minutes, then gradually close them and *keep closed* for entire hour. Throughout this period go negative only: Do not bend, extend or stiffen the arm; but if you should do so, awaredly or unawaredly, note the slight control sensation which will thereupon appear in the left arm and go negative there at once.

Do not tense to relax.

In General

Period No. 3 is called a zero period.

Hereafter, every third period is to be a zero period. In other practice periods, specialize on one tension only, performing the three times.

and high blood pressure, (only) to mention a few.

You may ask how learning to relax the skeletal musculature could so affect the nervous system as to cause those changes. There are three fundamental physiologic facts which go a long way towards explaining the phenomena. The first is that the skeletal muscular system is the only system in the entire body over which you have conscious voluntary control. (Note that tenseness means that the musculature is tense.) But, since those muscles are under conscious control, they can be trained not to be tense, i.e., to be relaxed. The second is that muscular tension is an integral part of any emotion. Therefore, it is impossible for you to be angry, worried, anxious or emotionally upset in any way and be completely relaxed because those two states are physiological opposites and cannot exist in the same person at the same time. Furthermore, the

type of thinking you engage in at any particular time is dictated largely by the existing emotional state. If you are anxious, your thoughts are frightening. If depressed, you are unable to have pleasant or happy thoughts. Therefore, training in muscle tension control can indirectly affect your thinking.

Thinking occurs as mental images and verbal symbols. Whenever you are thinking in mental images, the eyes are active as though to look at the images and thus directly involve the muscles that control the eyes. Whenever you imagine or enact some activity in fantasy, minor tensions occur in those areas of the body which would be used to actually carry out the activity. For example, it is impossible to imagine doing something with an arm and, at the same time, to allow that arm to remain completely relaxed. Whenever you think in verbal symbols, which is much of the time, tensions are present in the chest, throat, vocal cords, tongue, lips, jaws, cheeks and eyes as though to actually say the words. Such thinking is usually referred to as "sub-vocal" or "inner speech."

Faulty Tension-Producing Habits

It is not difficult to see what effect a great conservation of energy would have on the entire organism. Most people, however, have formed many faulty habits of tension which they practice throughout the day, without even realizing that they are wasting a tremendous amount of energy.

A simple example of faulty tension habits is the businessman who sits down at his desk to write a letter or a memorandum. He is likely to raise his shoulders, grip his pencil firmly, hold the paper too tightly, grimace and look at what he is doing too intently. His abdomen is likely to be tightened, his back not resting against the back of his chair, and very likely his legs are pulled back under his chair with his feet entwined. The man is expending several times the amount of energy necessary to do the job at hand. Some tensions are necessary for every activity of the day, but there is an optimum level of tension for efficiency. When the tension level rises above the optimum, efficiency itself suffers.

Our hypothetical businessman's general excessive tension would undoubtedly show itself in additional ways. He would probably light a cigarette with one already burning in the ash tray, show other signs of poor concentration and distractability, and possibly be irritable and short with those employees under him. By noon he requires the aid of two martinis to "relax" sufficiently to eat his lunch and even then probably continues to talk business. How much healthier, happier and more efficient that man would be if he could learn to stop expending the tremendous amount of energy in

useless and destructive secondary tensions. Those tensions can be unlearned through relaxation training.—*Bruce Kendall*

REPETITION TRAINING

Repetition training is an attempt to stimulate the stress involved in an actual race. The training technique involves completing a given distance at a fast speed, and then resting until you are completely recovered. The normal criteria for the resting interval is that the pulse rate should return to normal, or very close to it. When that happens, you repeat the training distance again at the same fast speed. As training progresses, the distance covered is gradually increased until it reaches the actual racing distance. Normally, repetition training covers longer distances than interval training, which does not allow as long a rest interval between efforts. See INTERVAL TRAINING and FARTLEK.

RESPIRATION

Exercises cause two increases in the respiratory system—the rate at which oxygen is used by the cells of the body during oxidation, and the rate at which carbon dioxide is formed. Changes must take place in the respiratory system to meet the demands caused by the increase in oxidation rate. The demands are more oxygen for the cells and faster removal of carbon dioxide.

The efficiency of gaseous exchange and transfer depends on a number of factors; rate and depth of breathing, efficiency of lung ventilation and the condition of the blood and the circulatory system.

The most obvious change brought on by increased oxidation is an increase in the rate and depth of breathing. The increase results in greater minute respiratory volume, or the amount of air breathed into and out of the lungs per minute. More air is made available from which the blood can receive oxygen.

The nature of the stimuli which cause changes in breathing patterns during exercise has been the subject of much experimentation and speculation. It is felt that much new information will come from future studies.

When the breathing center of the brain receives stimuli informing it of greater oxygen need, it in turns sends nerve impulses to the chest muscles whose function is to cause alternate inspiration and expiration. The result is an increase in the rate and/or depth of breathing and, therefore, an increase in the minute respiratory volume.

An increase in minute respiratory volume is meaningless if there is not a corresponding increase in lung ventilation. Lung, or pulmonary, ventilation refers to the gaseous exchange between the alveoli and the blood stream. During exercise, alveolar activity increases to aid ventilation. The well-conditioned person does not rely so much on greater minute respiratory volume or greater lung volume, but on greater efficiency of ventilation. The more inspired air that can be made to take part in gaseous transfer, the more efficient is ventilation.

During increased oxidation, the respiratory and circulatory systems must work together to make the necessary adjustments.

How much oxygen can be taken into the blood stream and how efficiently this oxygen can be delivered to the cells depends on the condition of the blood and the circulatory system. While respiratory activity is increased, the rate of the heart beat and the stroke volume of the heart are increased. (Stroke volume is the volume of blood the heart pumps at each stroke.) These changes result in an increase in the speed of the blood flow between the lungs, the heart and the body cells, making more blood available for transportation of oxygen, carbon dioxide and other substances.

The minute volume of breathing during exercise is influenced by the physical condition of the subject and by training. According to Morehouse and Miller, a person in good condition will have: (1) a decrease in the minute respiratory volume required for the performance of a given work load, which indicates an improvement in the efficiency of lung ventilation, and (2) an increase in the maximal, or greatest minute respiratory volume which can be achieved during very strenuous exertion.

As the depth of breathing approaches the limit imposed by lung capacity, subjective feelings of discomfort develop. That stage is reached sooner by the untrained man than by the trained man, and the subject is said to be "out of breath" or "winded." Most researchers believe that there is a difference between the breathing patterns of trained and untrained men. The untrained man tends to breathe more frequently in order to attain a given minute respiratory volume. That is probably due to his inability to achieve both rapid and maximal expansion of the chest cavity because of the lesser strength of his respiratory muscles.

Aftereffects of Exercise

The time required for breathing to return to normal, or pre-exercise level depends upon the severity and duration of the exercise and your physical condition. Work of moderate intensity may be performed over a period of time in a condition of steady state, which is that situation when the oxygen supply and oxygen usage are equal. During a period of steady state, increased rate and depth of breathing and subsequent lung ventilation are sufficient to supply the oxygen necessary for the task. Following work performed at steady state, the minute volume of breathing falls off rapidly.

That is, breathing rate and depth return to pre-exercise level quickly.

When you can't maintain the steady state because of an increase in the intensity or duration of work, you will incur an oxygen debt. Oxygen debt is the difference between the oxygen requirement and the oxygen intake during the performance of a task when the requirement is greater than the intake. Oxygen supply does not parallel oxygen demand. Following very severe exercise, the return of breathing to the pre-exercise level may be greatly delayed in proportion to the magnitude of the oxygen debt which must be repaid. The greater the oxygen debt incurred, the longer it will take the increased respiratory activity to return to the pre-exercise level. The depth of breathing usually returns to normal before the rate of breathing.

For a given work load, the less fit individual will incur a larger oxygen debt than the fit individual. That debt results in a greater delay in the postexercise return of breathing to normal in the unfit person. The more fit person is capable of maintaining a steady state at a higher level and for a greater duration than the unfit person during the performance of similar tasks.

Some researchers feel that exercise can reach a point of intensity where pulmonary ventilation becomes excessive. Ventilation then exceeds oxygen consumption in the cells. Since the delivery of oxygen to the tissues is limited by the maximal output of blood by the heart, the excessive ventilation serves no useful purpose. Other possible limitations of oxygen supply to tissues lie in the inability of the blood to carry enough oxygen to the tissues or the inability of the tissues themselves to accept and use the oxygen at the rate it is being supplied. For additional information see AEROBIC EXERCISE, ANAEROBIC EXERCISE, CIRCULO-RESPIRATORY ENDURANCE, CIRCULO-RESPIRATORY SYSTEM, ENERGY COST OF ACTIVITIES, ENVIRONMENT, METABOLISM, OXYGEN SUPPLEMENT, OXYGEN DEBT, OXYGEN INTAKE, OXYGEN REQUIREMENT, SECOND WIND and SMOKING.

RETROGRESSION

The term retrogression refers to one of the physiological principles of training. When you engage in a program of training that is rather rigorous, you may find that your performance levels off or decreases. The retrogression usually lasts from a few days to a week. A typical example of retrogression occurs when you have run a mile in 6 minutes and are beginning to aim for a 5:45 mile. For no apparent reason, your time falls off. You cannot even get below 6:30. Try as you might, you seem to have lost your ability and have actually become worse. In a few days, however, you are back to your regular 6-minute level and are making progress toward your next goal.

The reason for the decline is usually a result of a delay in the body's ability to mobilize its resources for meeting the overload imposed upon it. When the body adjusts, you then begin to reach your typical level of performance. Occasionally, retrogression is the result of poor diet, inadequate sleep or rest, lack of motivation and/or improper conditioning or training.

Regardless of the cause, it is important that you take inventory of your current condition. Be certain that your nutritional status is adequate, that your rest and sleep are sufficient, and that your training techniques are proper. If the retrogression is significant, it is a good idea to reduce the degree of overload for a few days or switch to another activity. After the reappraisal and tapering-off, improvement will follow when you attempt to return to old performances. Retrogression, however, is not to be confused with staleness or overtraining. See OVERTRAINING, STALENESS IN TRAINING AND RACING and TRAINING.

ROLLER SKATING

Indoors or outdoors, people of all ages may enjoy roller skating. Skates that are worn outdoors for the most part have steel wheels and are clamped to your shoes. Indoor skates have wheels made of wood, fiber or plastic and are either clamped to your foot or are attached to a shoe (boot-type).

Roller skating has been organized into various sports which include artistic roller skating, speed skating, roller derby and roller-skating hockey.

Recreational roller skating is considered to be a high-energy activity and is recommended, therefore, to improve circulo-respiratory endurance, provided that it lasts 30 minutes. Leg muscle endurance and balance are also improved as a result of roller skating.

Roller skating can be enjoyed by all people despite their level of fitness. To attain benefits, they merely gear their rate of skating with their fitness level.

Associations:

Roller Skating Foundation of America, 515 Madison Avenue, New York, New York 10022.

United States Federation of Amateur Roller Skaters (USFARS), 20600 Woodward Avenue, Detroit, Michigan 48203.

United States Amateur Roller Skating Association (USARSA), 120 West 42nd Street, New York, New York 10036.

Below is a roller skating program that takes into account the important principles of training.

If you desire to improve your strength and power, see WEIGHT TRAINING and ISOMETRICS. The weight training and isometrics exercises may also be used to prepare your body for athletic competition.

°ROLLER SKATING PROGRAM (Vigorous)°°

Chart 1		Chart 2	
1.	5 minutes	1.	21 minutes
2.	8 minutes	2.	23 minutes
3.	10 minutes	3.	25 minutes
4.	12 minutes	4.	26 minutes
5.	15 minutes	5.	28 minutes
6.	16 minutes	6.	30 minutes
7.	17 minutes	7.	32 minutes
8.	18 minutes	8.	35 minutes
9.	20 minutes	9.	36 minutes

°See ENDURANCE and ENERGY COST OF ACTIVITIES for an explanation of these charts.

°°Doesn't include rest periods, times out, etc.

Fitness 1

If you achieved a score of poor or low average on the *Harvard Step Test* or a score of very poor or poor on the *12 Minute Run*, start on Chart 1-Level 1 and spend 1 week at each level until Chart 2-Level 9 is reached. It is recommended that you participate 4 to 5 days a week. When Chart 2-Level 9 is reached, 4 days a week is sufficient.

Fitness 2

If you achieved a score of high average on the *Harvard Step Test* or fair on the *12 Minute Run*, start on on Chart 1-Level 1. Spend 1 week on Chart 1-Levels 1, 3, 5, 7 and 9, and Chart 2-Levels 1, 3, 6, 8 and 9. It is recommended that you participate 4 to 5 days a week. When Chart 2-Level 9 is reached, 4 days a week is sufficient.

Fitness 3

If you achieved a score of good or excellent on either the *Harvard Step Test* or *12 Minute Run*, continue your current program or select Chart 2-Level 9 as your level of participation. Four days a week is sufficient.

ROPE SKIPPING

Rope skipping is one of the simplest activities for acquiring a high level of fitness with a minimum of equipment and space. To begin rope skipping, find a piece of rope about 10 feet long and set aside about 15 minutes a day. That's all you need to start. In some cases, however, you may have to acquaint yourself with the proper techniques of rope skipping before beginning a program. Children seem to have a natural knack for skipping, but adults may find it difficult at first.

On your first few attempts, you may find that you are all arms and legs and that you just cannot seem to coordinate the proper action. You may only be able to place the rope behind your body and to swing it over your head. Repeatedly practicing that movement and then finally attempting to jump over the rope as it passes under your feet will eventually bring victory. If that doesn't work, merely go through the motions without the rope until you have mastered the proper timing, coordination and rhythm.

Research demonstrates that brief periods of rope skipping will improve your physical condition. A study reported in the May, 1962 *Research Quarterly* illustrates the improvement. The authors of the study engaged 7 untrained women, ages 19 to 42 years, employed in sedentary occupations in a rope-skipping program. The 7 women participated Monday through Friday in a 5-minute rope-skipping program for a period of 4 weeks. They skipped one minute and rested for two, until they had a skipped total of 5 minutes. They jumped rope at a rate of 76 skips per minute. After the 4-week training program, the researchers found that the exercise pulse rates of the women declined, that their maximal oxygen intake (breathing intake) had increased, and that their physical work capacity had increased 25 per cent. All those findings indicate an improve-

ment in physical condition. A control group of women who did not engage in the exercise program but had similar occupations did not show the changes.

A second research study on rope skipping, reported in the booklet *Physiological Aspects of Sports and Physical Fitness*, examined the effect of rope skipping on the physical work capacity of sedentary college women. The investigators, Spencer, Youmans, Shumen and Rodhal, compared 68 college women. One group engaged in a rope-skipping program like the one described in the *Research Quarterly*. A second group participated in physical education classes that were held twice a week for 50 minutes and involved swimming, soccer and tennis. A third group acted as controls and did not participate in physical education classes or in the rope-skipping program. The study revealed that the women in the physical education classes and the rope-skipping program improved their physical work capacity significantly while the control group did not. The study also indicated that the women involved in the rope-skipping program improved their physical work capacity to a greater extent than the women who participated in the physical education classes.

More recently, John A. Baker compared rope skipping and jogging as methods of improving cardiovascular efficiency in college men (*Research Quarterly*, May, 1968). The results showed that ten minutes of rope skipping and 30 minutes of jogging will result in significant improvements in cardiovascular efficiency, and that the 10 minutes of rope skipping is equivalent to 30 minutes of jogging. It must be noted, however, that the intensity of rope skipping is greater than the intensity of jogging.

Techniques

The establishment of a rope-skipping program will vary considerably

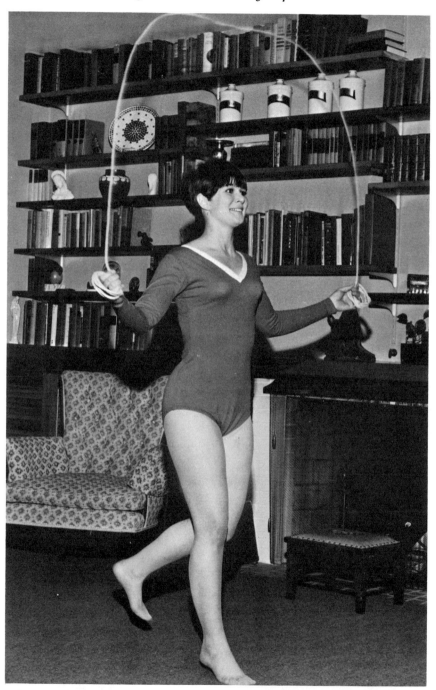

For coordination and cardiovascular fitness, rope skipping is an extremely valuable activity. Because it requires little space, it can be done indoors as well as out.

depending upon your physical condition and ability. Some techniques that have been used successfully are to skip 3 minutes and rest one minute, skip three minutes, rest one, until a 9, 12, or 15 minute exercise period is completed. Naturally, you may not be able to start out at such a level so that you may begin by skipping one minute and resting one, constantly increasing the exercise time in each subsequent session until you reach the 3-minute time period.

A second program used successfully is to try skipping rope for one minute at 100 turns per minute. If you are able to do that, the next day set your goal for 200 skips in two minutes. Continue increasing each day, if possible, until you are able to skip 1,000 times in 10 minutes. Ideally it will take you ten days. But since most of us are not in the best physical condition, it may take several weeks or even months to reach that goal.

If your physical condition does not warrant your improving at the above rate, you may find it necessary to adjust the schedule so that you increase at a rate of 75 skips per minute. Eventually you should be able to skip 750 times in 10 minutes. To reach 750 or 1,000 skips in 10 minutes, you should jump rope 6 days a week. Once your goal is achieved, you may reduce the number to 4 or 5 days a week.

Skipping 1,000 times in ten minutes is by no means the end of the line. Some proficient people have continued to improve beyond the 1,000 level. A group of graduate students at the University of Illinois followed a rope-skipping program similar to the 100 skips per minute program described above. As a result of their program, they set up an achievement scale for rope skippers. Below is their scale:

1,000 skips in 10 minutes—Poor
1,200 skips in 10 minutes—Fair
1,400 skips in 10 minutes—Good
1,600 skips in 10 minutes—Excellent

Those standards may not be applicable to all people, but it certainly gives you an idea of how far a rope skipper can go.

How many skips you can do in a minute and the number of minutes you will be able to skip depends upon your motivation, interest, physical condition, age, body type and present health.

Avoiding Boredom

To help avoid boredom and fatigue, there are several techniques that will aid you in your skipping program. The basic motion of rope skipping is to keep your legs together as you skip. If you find that way fatiguing or boring, a change in position will help. Change to skipping on only your right leg and then on only your left, or alternating with each foot. Or try running in place as you are skipping. Another technique is to cross the arms over your body as you skip. To make the exercise more demanding, try making two foot contacts with each skip. Finally, as you are skipping, you may find that your legs became fatigued or tighten up as a result of the great demand placed upon them. To help alleviate that problem, swing the legs back and forth as you skip. The leg which is not on the floor should be swung either backward or forward. While in that position, it may be shaken vigorously to help relax the muscles while you are skipping.

Some people jump rope following music, watching television or listening to the radio. They claim that it keeps them from getting bored and helps them keep their rhythm.

If you select a rope that does not have any wooden handles, you will find it to your benefit to wear gloves while skipping. The constant rubbing of the bare rope against the forefinger may cause blisters or abrasions of the skin.

Benefits Derived from Rope Skipping

A rope-skipping program can be quite a challenge and a pleasure. The varieties of rope jumping are as many as the programs. The appeal of rope skipping is that it is an individual exercise program that may be done in the privacy of the home, in any type of weather. Participating in the exercise program on a regular basis and in the manner described previously will result in an improvement of circulo-respiratory endurance, leg muscle endurance and, in some instances, arm and shoulder endurance because of the repetitive movements required to swing the rope.

ROWING (SCULLING)

Row, row, row your boat
Gently down the stream
Merrily, merrily, merrily, merrily
Life is but a dream!

That familiar stanza describes the common attitude toward the old, enjoyable pastime of rowing. During the warm months of the year, thousands of families descend upon streams, rivers and lakes to go boating. Their rowing consists of leisurely gliding around the water or moving to a good fishing or napping spot. The physical benefits from that type of rowing are relatively nil, other than offering an excellent means of relaxation.

The actual sport of rowing or sculling, however, contributes greatly to your physical fitness for it is vigorous and exhausting competition that places great stress on many of your body's muscles. Sculling differs from rowing in that the oarsman has an oar in each hand, whereas rowers use only one oar.

The origin of rowing goes back thousands of years when the chief means of international transportation and war was propelling vessels throughout the waterways.

Down through the centuries the Thames River in England became the center of rowing as a competitive sport and a universal pastime. Dating as far back as the 15th century, rowers competed against each other on the waters of the Thames. The first English regatta took place there in 1775. Later, in 1817, the Leander Club for rowing was founded which stressed the highest standards of rowing and sportsmanship.

Naturally, rowing as a sport had spread to other countries. During the 19th Century, Canada, Australia and the United States had organized rowing contests between the larger cities and developed a rather elaborate system of rules for amateurs and professionals.

In the United States, the National Association of Amateur Oarsmen is the governing body. The world governing body with headquarters in Switzerland is the Fédération International des Sociétés d'Aviron (F.I.S.A.). Present-day rowing, therefore, is an international sport which provides for competition by crews in seven categories, using specially designed racing craft or shells.

A crew consists of the oarsmen and, in some events, a coxswain who is responsible for steering and giving commands. The man nearest the stern is called the stroke and is responsible for setting the pace or stroking rate. The boats are variable in size and design; but they must be rigged to suit the crew. That means gearing the stroke correctly so that the crew rows at the right rate with the right length, eliminating unnecessary exhaustion. Rigging involves adjusting the distance between the rowing pin and the center of the boat, the movement and height of the sliding seat, the position of feet, the height of oar supports and similar requirements.

Contribution to Physical Fitness

Rowing makes very high demands on cardio-respiratory efficiency and on strength and endurance of most large muscle groups of the body—thigh extensors, back extensors, shoulder adductors, arm flexors, wrist flexors and extensors and trunk flexors.

The qualities of strength, endurance, and heart-lung efficiency are developed in the course of training for rowing, particularly for competition, which may average as much as two hours daily. Competitive rowing is heavy exercise and calls for superlative efforts of stamina.

Conditioning Programs

Much of the conditioning occurs through practice in the boat, singly (if for sculling), or with other members of the competitive crew. The principles of interval training have been adapted to rowing by most successful crews, but training will also include long rows and variations of stroke rating (strokes per minute).

Supplementary training includes weights (squats, reverse curls, sit-ups, shoulder shrugs, high lift, chinning), but heavy weights should be avoided. Light weights with many repetitions are more profitable. Running, skipping and jumping exercises producing near maximum heart beat are useful for developing heart-lung efficiency.

Physical Qualities Needed Before Competition

Rowers are big men, averaging between 180 and 200 lbs. in weight and not less than 6 feet tall. They have long trunks rather than long legs which give them maximum range of movement for rowing. Arm span is longer than height by several inches. They have well-developed biceps and big hands.—*A. S. Lewis*

Associations:

Amateur Athletic Union (AAU). See ORGANIZATIONS.

American Rowing Association, 4 Boat House Row, Fairmount Park, Philadelphia, Pennsylvania 19130.

Intercollegiate Rowing Association (IRA), Hotel Manhattan, New York, New York 10036.

School-Boy Rowing Association of

* ROWING PROGRAM
Vigorous, but not racing
(20 Strokes/Minute)

Chart 1		Chart 2	
1.	5 minutes	1.	22 minutes
2.	7 minutes	2.	25 minutes
3.	9 minutes	3.	27 minutes
4.	10 minutes	4.	30 minutes
5.	12 minutes	5.	32 minutes
6.	14 minutes	6.	34 minutes
7.	16 minutes	7.	36 minutes
8.	18 minutes	8.	38 minutes
9.	20 minutes	9.	40 minutes

* See ENDURANCE and ENERGY COST OF ACTIVITIES for an explanation of these charts.

Fitness 1

If you achieved a score of poor or low average on the *Harvard Step Test* or a score of very poor or poor on the *12 Minute Run*, start on Chart 1-Level 1 and spend 1 week at each level until Chart 2-Level 9 is reached. It is recommended that you participate 4 to 5 days a week. When Chart 2-Level 9 is reached, 4 days a week is sufficient.

Fitness 2

If you achieved a score of high average on the *Harvard Step Test* or fair on the *12 Minute Run*, start on Chart 1-Level 1. Spend one week on Chart 1-Levels 1, 2, 4, 6, 8, and 9 and Chart 2-Levels, 2, 4, 6, 8, and 9. It is recommended that you participate 4 to 5 days a week. When Chart 2-Level 9 is reached, 4 days a week is sufficient.

Fitness 3

If you achieved a score of good or excellent on either the *Harvard Step Test* or *12 Minute Run*, continue your current program or select Chart 2-

Level 9 as your level of participation. Four days a week is sufficient.

*SCULLING PROGRAM (RACING)

Chart 1		Chart 2	
1.	5 minutes	1.	15 minutes
2.	6 minutes	2.	16 minutes
3.	7 minutes	3.	17 minutes
4.	8 minutes	4.	18 minutes
5.	9 minutes	5.	20 minutes
6.	10 minutes	6.	21 minutes
7.	12 minutes	7.	23 minutes
8.	14 minutes	8.	24 minutes
9.	15 minutes	9.	25 minutes

*See ENDURANCE and ENERGY COST OF ACTIVITIES for an explanation of these charts.

Fitness 1

Same as Rowing Program.

Fitness 2

If you achieved a score of high average on the *Harvard Step Test* or fair on the *12 Minute Run,* start on Chart 1-Level 1. Spend 1 week on Chart 1-Levels 1, 3, 7, and 9 and Chart 2-Levels 1, 4, 5, 7, and 9. It is recommended that you participate 4 to 5 days a week. When Chart 2-Level 9 is reached, 4 days a week is sufficient.

Fitness 3

Same as Rowing Program.

America (SRAA), 4 Boat House Row, Philadelphia, Pennsylvania 19130.

United States Rowing Society (USRS), 4 East River Drive, Philadelphia, Pennsylvania 19128.

Since rowing and sculling are high or very high-energy-cost activities, they may be used to help improve your fitness level, especially your circulo-respiratory and muscle endurance. Below are two training programs that take into account the important principles of training.

If you desire to improve your strength and power for those activities,

see WEIGHT TRAINING and ISOMETRICS. The weight training and isometrics exercises may also be used to prepare your body for athletic competition.

RUNNING

Each day, before or after work, thousands of people put on a sweat suit and a pair of sneakers or running shoes and take to the roads or country for an exhilarating jaunt. Although many of those runners are in training for weekend long-distance races, the majority forget about the word training and are out for the fun of it. It's amazing how the miles click by, especially if you're running with a partner. Many adhere to the 30-60 minute session and find that, in addition to the fun aspect, the workouts lead to a slimmer figure, toned-up muscles, lower blood pressure, better sleep, greater work production and more relaxation.

Starting a personal program of endurance running means following one general rule, "train, don't strain." For example, don't make the mistake of running up grades in the early sessions. Such overenthusiasm may result in a pull of the calf muscle and a long disability.

The neophyte should start slowly by alternately walking and jogging a quarter mile for a period of about two weeks. At that point, start jogging a mile at a speed which would permit you to talk easily with a running companion. That pace may turn out to be quite slow for the first 6-9 minutes or until a "second wind" develops. Signalled by the onset of sweating and a slowing of the respiratory rate, the new burst of energy, or second wind, will mean that you can try longer distances, perhaps even three to five miles.

Running until the second wind develops is a sort of warm-up exercise which signifies an ability of endurance. Elite athletes reach that stage in three minutes, then shift into high gear, and you will start thinking of running 20 miles. However, that feeling of elation gradually fades as you put on running mileage. And then when you think you just can't run another inch—after about 35 to 40 minutes—you get another lift which keeps you going for another 10-20 minutes.

Adolph Gruber, the Australian long-distance champion, once said that even a girl could run a marathon by observing this rule: "Hold back for the first seven miles, use it as a warm-up, and then gradually increase your rate but never strain." For the person just starting out, however, seven miles is in itself a marathon. Few of the experienced runners even try the marathon, and most are content to get the physical, mental and spiritual benefit from an ordinary 30-60 minutes in motion.

Another method to keep interest high in the early stages of a running program is to select different running routes. Bill Bowerman, who has been so successful in coaching track at Oregon State, has 5 to 6 different cross country courses for his runners. Running the same route or track constantly can be boring, so change your route and scenery often.

One precaution—don't run on a full stomach. Wait at least two or three hours after a meal. And if possible, visit the bathroom before starting the training session. If not, abdominal pain may develop, especially if you are determined to run quite a distance.

Time of training is a matter of personal preference. Of course, in the hot weather and in periods of high humidity, morning or evening workouts would be better. If you're not used to the heat, running in hot weather can lead to heat exhaustion or heat stroke. Once acclimated, you will find that the sweat has a very low salt content and

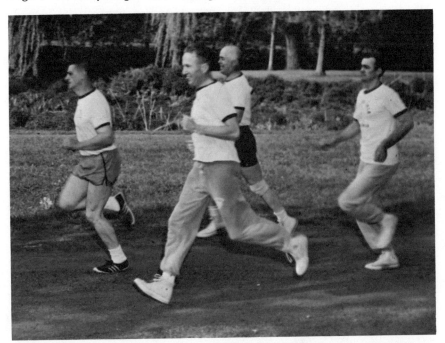

When you run with others, the miles click by and the fitness benefits build up. Many people have found running to be a satisfying and rewarding physical activity.

that you can go long distances without using much water. In fact, you can actually douse your body liberally before starting to run.

Cold weather requires special clothing. Thermal underwear is excellent. Wear warm gloves and cover your ears. Occasionally in very cold weather, you may need a ski mask. For very cold or rainy weather, a light nylon parka is rain proof and retains body heat. Some people also use liniment on their legs in cold weather.

Injuries

No matter how careful you are, you are bound to run into some problems. However, a runner who trains and doesn't strain automatically cuts down on the occurrence of injury. Tom Ossler, a leading Eastern distance man, says that all injuries are unnecessary and result from carelessness or fatigue. It is the tired runner who makes a misstep and turns an ankle or gets a bone bruise. Using slow warm-ups and avoiding speed in workouts usually cancels out muscle pulls especially of the large thigh muscles, the quadriceps, the hamstrings and even the calf muscles.

Perhaps the most common injury is the heel cord (Achilles' tendon) pull. Luckily, however, such an injury usually gives warning for days or weeks before it actually becomes disabling. A heel lift inside the shoe or a heel on the running shoe is a simple way to avoid the problem. Another aid is a warm-up exercise designed to stretch the hamstring and "quadriceps" muscles before a workout. Incidentally, investment in a good road running shoe, preferably with a heel, and arch supports, is worthwhile. Since running is the least expensive sport in terms of needed equipment, investment in good shoes should be a must.

A final note on that old bugbear, blisters. As soon as a blister is suspected, stop running. Painting with tincture of benzoin and taping with light Zona tape will clear up the blister if the original shearing action within the shoe is prevented. Wearing two pairs of socks is a good preventive, plus taping of the susceptible areas before long runs. A felt pad which provides a vacuum where the blister is will also do the trick. But the pad may have to be put in place by a podiatrist or trainer. Avoid the use of sponge rubber.

Another hazard awaits the individual who is serious about his running. Many a runner has had to overcome the psychological roadblock resulting from the reaction of friends, neighbors and even family. However, as soon as they see that your running is not a passing fancy, jokes and jibes stop, and you can go on your way in peace.
—*George Sheehan*

Further Comments

Running is the best activity to be used to get back into shape and to maintain good physical condition. It is natural and yet strenuous enough to cause the pulse rate to increase appreciably and to burn up 400-500 calories in a half hour.

Sample Running Program

As with any exercise program, it is essential that you begin at a low level and gradually work up to the desired level of activity. Here's a sample program for running.

1. Start gradually by walking one mile.

2. After you feel comfortable covering that distance, increase your walking to two miles in thirty minutes.

3. Next progress to walking 1½ miles and running ½ mile.

4. Continue by walking 1½ miles and running 1 mile.

5. When adjusted to that pace, work into walking 1 mile and running 1½ miles.

6. Then, progress to walking ½ mile and running 2 miles.

7. Next, advance to walking ½ mile and running 2½ miles.

*RUNNING PROGRAM

Chart 1	Chart 2
1. Walk-Run ¾ mile in 10 minutes	1. Run 2 miles in 22 minutes
2. Walk-Run ¾ mile in 9 minutes	2. Run 2 miles in 21 minutes
3. Walk-Run 1 mile in 12 minutes	3. Run 2¼ miles in 24 minutes
4. Run 1 mile in 11 minutes	4. Run 2¼ miles in 23 minutes
5. Run 1¼ miles in 14 minutes	5. Run 2½ miles in 26 minutes
6. Run 1¼ miles in 13 minutes	6. Run 2½ miles in 25 minutes
7. Run 1½ miles in 16 minutes	7. Run 2¾ miles in 28 minutes
8. Run 1½ miles in 15 minutes	8. Run 2¾ miles in 27 minutes
9. Run 1¾ miles in 18 minutes	9. Run 3 miles in 30 minutes

*See ENDURANCE and ENERGY COST OF ACTIVITIES for an explanation of these charts.

Fitness 1

If you achieved a score of poor or low average on the *Harvard Step Test* or a score of very poor or poor on the *12 Minute Run*, start on Chart 1-Level 1 and spend 1 week at each level until Chart 2-Level 9 is reached. It is recommended that you participate 4 to 5 days a week. When Chart 2-Level 9 is reached, 4 days a week is sufficient.

Fitness 2

If you achieved a score of high average on the *Harvard Step Test* or fair on the *12 Minute Run,* start on Chart 1-Level 2. Spend 1 week on Chart 1-Levels 2, 4, 6, 7, 8, and 9, and Chart 2-Levels 1, 3, 5, 7, 8, and 9. It is recommended that you participate 4 to 5 days a week. When Chart 2-Level 9 is reached, 4 days a week is sufficient.

Fitness 3

If you achieved a score of good or excellent on either the *Harvard Step Test* or *12 Minute Run,* continue your current program or select Chart 2-Level 9 as your level of participation. Four days a week is sufficient.

8. Finally, progress to running 3 miles.

All of the above should be performed in 30 minutes if possible.

An alternate technique is to start off by walking briskly as far and as long as you can, assuming that you can do that for 5 minutes. Remain at that level for one week. The next week walk the 5 minutes but add 5 minutes of easy running. If that is impossible perhaps 3 minutes of walking and 2 minutes of easy running is the answer. Gradually increase in that manner until you are able to run 3 miles in 30 minutes. If you are unable to reach that goal, be satisfied with doing less. But if you can do more—do it! Run the 3 miles in 25 minutes or even 20 minutes.

Running 3 miles in 30 minutes is the desired objective for most of the population, because that's the intensity of running that burns up sufficient calories and elevates the pulse sufficiently, (140 beats and above), to produce beneficial changes to the circulo-respiratory system.

The major benefits derived from running are improved circulo-respiratory endurance and muscle endurance of the legs, arms and shoulders.

Since running is a high- or very high-energy-cost activity, it may be used to help improve your fitness level, especially your circulo-respiratory and muscle endurance. Below is a running program that takes into account the important principles of training. Also see JOGGING.

RUNNING IN PLACE

For those who prefer to exercise in the privacy of their homes or want an exercise routine to follow that is beneficial when the weather is inclement, running in place may be the answer. Running in place is the basic ingredient in the XBX, 5BX, and the President's Council's Programs. (See PROGRAMS.) To run in place, raise each foot at least 4 inches off the floor and jog in place. Count 1 each time the left foot touches the floor. As you do this stationary run, be certain that you move your arms vigorously.

The number of times that you run in place is up to you, naturally. But to gain optimum benefits, a program similar to the one developed by the Air Force School of Aerospace Medicine will be helpful. Here it is:

Run in place lifting the feet well off the floor, counting one step each time the left foot hits the floor.

Individuals with a high level of physical fitness exceeding the optimal values for testing should continue an active daily exercise program. Ideally daily exercise should exceed 1,500 steps twice daily and should include 30 minutes to one hour of vigorous exercise. This level of physical fitness should be achieved by a gradual daily effort. It is dangerous to proceed too rapidly in developing physical fitness.

The rate of progress should under no circumstances be more rapid than recommended above.

Some people may find running in place without a change quite boring. After every 100 steps, therefore, do 10 or 20 jumping jacks, in place of the running in place. Another idea is to run listening to the stereo or watching television.

One of the most famous and ardent men who incorporate running in place as the basic part of their exercise routine is Dr. Wilhelm Raab. Dr. Raab, a noted cardiologist, is on the faculty of the University of Vermont. Now 74 years of age, he runs in place 1,500 times every day. He also does a good bit of walking. A very sedentary person until his mid-fifties, Dr. Raab now claims that he never felt better in his life.

SAILING

Sailing has three basic positions in relation to wind direction: beating, reaching, and running free. Beating is a means of sailing upwind by alternating courses in a zig-zag manner at angles approximately 45° off the relative wind direction. Reaching, which is usually the fastest position in plain-

RUNNING IN PLACE PROGRAM

100 steps	2 Xs (A.M. & P.M.)	4 days	1 min.
150 steps	2 Xs (A.M. & P.M.)	4 days	1½ min.
200 steps	2 Xs (A.M. & P.M.)	4 days	2 min.
250 steps	2 Xs (A.M. & P.M.)	4 days	2½ min.
300 steps	2 Xs (A.M. & P.M.)	4 days	3 min.
400 steps	2 Xs (A.M. & P.M.)	4 days	4 min.
500 steps	2 Xs (A.M. & P.M.)	4 days	5 min.
600 steps	2 Xs (A.M. & P.M.)	4 days	6 min.
700 steps	2 Xs (A.M. & P.M.)	4 days	7 min.
800 steps	2 Xs (A.M. & P.M.)	4 days	8 min.
900 steps	2 Xs (A.M. & P.M.)	4 days	9 min.
1,000 steps	2 Xs (A.M. & P.M.)	4 days	10 min.
1,100 steps	2 Xs (A.M. & P.M.)	4 days	11 min.
1,200 steps	2 Xs (A.M. & P.M.)	4 days	12 min.
1,300 steps	2 Xs (A.M. & P.M.)	4 days	13 min.
1,400 steps	2 Xs (A.M. & P.M.)	4 days	14 min.
1,500 steps	2 Xs (A.M. & P.M.)	4 days	15 min.

ing hulls, consists of courses sailed perpendicular to wind direction. The third position, running free, is sailed at courses in common with the wind direction. Running free is referred to as sailing with the wind, while beating is sailing against it, and reaching is sailing across it. By using the three positions, it is possible to sail to any destination as long as there is wind and water.

The forces which drive a sailboat through the water are primarily generated from wind pressure on the sails and spars and water pressure on the hull, keel or centerboard, and rudder. The role of the skipper and crew of the sailboat is to use those forces with the greatest degree of efficiency possible.

The effect of sailing on cardio-respiratory endurance, for the most part, is low. In small boat handling, the sailor spends most of his time sitting down. The major contribution of sailing to physical fitness is muscular endurance. Hiking, steering, and trimming can place parts of the body un-

der stress for the full length of the sail or race.

Hiking is a means of stabilizing the sideward push, or capsizing effect, of the wind on the sails by applying as much of your weight as practical (and crew's weight if there is any) on the windward side of the boat. In some cases, it is accomplished by sitting on the windward deck. However, in some boats, a more efficient method of stabilization is required. In that type of hiking, the feet are usually placed under a hiking strap inside the boat; and the back of the legs rest on the edge of the deck, while the upper body is suspended over the water. The knees, hips, trunk and ankles are bent. The primary muscle groups involved are the flexors of the trunk, hips and ankles, and the extensors of the knees. In sailboats a skipper may hike almost an entire race, which may last two or more hours. During that time, he projects the upper body over the water at an angle approximately 45°. The body weight from the head to the thighs is supported by the mus-

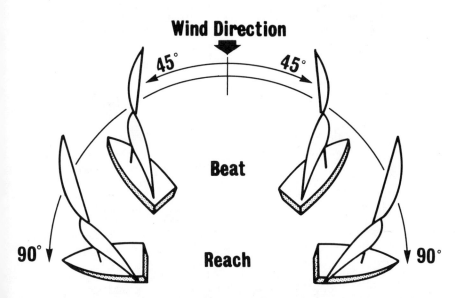

By using appropriate nautical skills even weekend sailors can sail upwind.

cles between the thighs and the ankles. The abdominal muscles and hip flexors are also involved by controlling the angle between the trunk and the legs. The greater the angle, the greater the mechanical advantage of hiking and the greater the stress on the supporting muscle groups.

Trimming involves primarily the flexors of the forearm, hand and fingers, along with most shoulder muscles. Trimming refers to the adjustment of the ropes responsible for sail setting or positioning. The adjustment becomes progressively more stressful as wind velocity and wind fluctuation increases. The highly skilled sailor may reset his lines every time he sails up or down the crest of a wave, or every time there is the slightest variation in relative wind direction or wind velocity. While trimming, the fingers are closed firmly around a rope. The primary joint actions are wrist and elbow flexion and extension, with shoulder movement in all directions. The actions usually originate in the shoulder area and proceed outward to the hand whether the sailor is pulling ropes inboard or letting them out. The tension on the lines is always outboard and depends on the wind velocity and the efficiency of each boat's rigging. Therefore, the stress on the muscle groups involved in trimming is directly proportional to wind velocity and indirectly proportional to the mechanical advantage of the rigging.

Steering involves the same muscle groups as trimming with the addition of the elbow and wrist extensors. Unlike trimming, steering doesn't demand a constant outward tension on the ropes. Therefore, you will need a forceful, rather than a controlled, extension of the wrist and elbow. In steering the fingers grip a tiller, or tiller extension, which is connected to the rudder. By controlling the movement of the tiller, using the arms, forearms, hands and fingers, the skipper can control the direction of the boat. That activity almost necessitates constant attention and, therefore, places constant stress on the involved muscle groups. As in trimming, the degree of muscular endurance achieved depends upon wind velocity and fluctuation, the efficiency of the rigging, and the individual preferences of each skipper. All three activities, hiking, trimming, and steering, can be performed simultaneously. While the skipper is hiking, he is usually steering with one arm and trimming with the other. The advantage is obvious for better quality in sailing as well as for better muscular endurance.

Each activity can require, or produce, a large amount of muscular strength. By increasing the angle between the upper body and the legs while hiking or by adding wet sweat shirts, the pounds supported by the legs and abdominal muscles can approach total body weight. Trimming and steering can also increase muscular strength as the speed of the activities is increased. Valuable seconds are gained while racing as a result of fast trimming and steering. Some beats demand abrupt, jerky arm actions for maximum efficiency. In many instances, the sailor who works the hardest wins the most.

As a result of the range of shoulder motion required for proper steering and trimming, there is a substantial amount of shoulder flexibility developed. However, the shoulder area is usually the only area where a good deal of flexibility is obtained as a result of sailing. The leg action in hiking and the actions of steering and trimming (other than shoulder movements) are primarily functions of flexion. The emphasis on flexion isolates the range of motion in body joints and. does not enhance the development of flexibility.

To aid the muscle groups responsible for trimming and steering, appropriate isometric exercises are bent arm hangs from a bar and bent arm pushes against a wall or doorway. To condition the muscle groups used in hiking, half leg lifts and half sit-ups held for varying lengths of time are very valuable.

Almost any weight training is advantageous for sailing as are general exercises such as sit-ups, push-ups, leg lifts and pull-ups.

Before attempting to sail, you should have a fair amount of muscular strength and endurance. That doesn't mean that you have to be extremely muscular to sail, but you can't be a weakling either. A substantial level of muscular strength and endurance should also be accompanied with good coordination. Sailboats are often unstable; and therefore, quick and accurate work is sometimes needed to keep them afloat. The most important and essential physical ability required by the sailor is swimming. A person has no right being in a sailboat unless he is a competent swimmer.—*Carl Patterson, Thomas Patterson*

Associations:

Alcort Sailfish-Sunfish Class, P. O. Box 1345, Waterbury, Connecticut, 06720.

Aqua-Cat Catamaran Sailing Association (ACSA), P. O. Box 297, South Norwalk, Connecticut 06852.

El Toro International Yacht Racing Association (ETIYRA), 2820 Telegraph Avenue, Berkeley, California 94705.

SALT TABLETS

The well-known belief that summertime discomfort is caused by humidity rather than high temperature has a strong basis in scientific fact. A few years ago, a high school football player died of heat stroke on a day when the air temperature did not exceed 68.0° but the relative humidity was 100%. Only five deaths occurred among competitors during the modern series of Olympic Games; but two of those were due to heat stroke occurring on days when both air temperature and humidity were high.

The body demands a certain amount of salt to function properly. Exercise that occurs in a humid environment causes the body to sweat profusely. As a result of the sweating, there is a great deal of salt lost. It is impossible to replenish the salt naturally so it is necessary to take on additional salt to avoid adverse effects to the body.

Three types of problems may result from exposure to conditions of high air temperature and relative humidity when a person is exercising vigorously —heat cramps, heat exhaustion and heat stroke. Each presents a different group of symptoms and findings, and each is entirely preventable. Since young and old may equally be involved, everyone should know how to prevent and treat all three. The main factors involved in those conditions are excessive losses of body salt and water.

Heat cramps are due chiefly to loss of body salt. The person who is not in good physical condition or who has not become accustomed to vigorous exercise in a hot humid climate may lose as much as 5.0 gm. of salt in the first quart of sweat from the body. After prolonged training or repeated exposure to hot, humid conditions, the loss of salt may be as little as 0.05 gm. in the same volume of sweat. Until the body learns to conserve its salt supply in that way, it is necessary to make up the deficit by taking sodium chloride, ordinary table salt. To begin, you should take 5.0 gm. daily (10 salt tablets if each is 0.5 gm.) spread out over the three meals of the day. Too much salt taken at once may upset the stomach. As conditioning progresses, the amount is gradually reduced. When cramps occur, they affect the legs first, then abdominal muscles and finally the arms. They may be almost immediately relieved by drinking a solution which contains 1.0 gm. of salt in a quart of water or taking salt tablets. Massaging legs for heat cramps only makes them worse.

Heat exhaustion results chiefly from loss of body water. The body cools itself when it is working hard or exercising chiefly by sweating. Sweat is principally water but contains salt, some lipids and protein. Although the rate of water loss ordinarily remains constant during exercise, the loss of salt decreases. When body water is depleted, the volume of blood in the circulation is reduced and blood pressure falls. Weakness, fainting, and shock may occur. Heat exhaustion is completely preventable by taking water and other liquids freely before, during and after exercise. Alcoholic liquids should be an exception, since they tend to increase dehydration. When heat exhaustion occurs, the remedy is water, supplemented with some salt.

Heat stroke hits when the control of body temperature by sweating fails. That happens when the skin is soaked with sweat and the atmosphere is so humid or clothing so restrictive that perspiration cannot be completely absorbed. The openings of the sweat glands become swollen and close off. Sweating stops, and body temperature rises sharply if exercise continues. The skin becomes warm and dry; mental confusion occurs and coma quickly follows. Treatment must begin instantly by immersing the victim in a tub of ice water or placing him under a cold shower. If treatment is not started within a few minutes from the onset of symptoms, death may result. Heat stroke is prevented by careful conditioning, taking salt regularly before exercises, drinking adequate amounts of water and other liquids during exercise, changing sweat-soaked clothing as required, and stopping exercise at the first sign of cessation of sweating or mental confusion.

General precautions to be taken in hot weather include the following:

1. Wear light-colored, loose-fitting clothing.

2. When working hard or exercising vigorously, take rest breaks in the shade.

3. Drink water and other liquids (except alcoholic ones) freely before and during exercise.

4. Take extra salt until fully acclimated.—*Allan J. Ryan*

SAUNA

Sometime ago Drs. Antonio Fornoza and Carlos Gutierre Salgado evaluated the effect of the Sauna or Finnish Bath on the leukocytes (white blood cells) of the blood. The sauna in their study consisted of a room with ceiling, walls and floor made of Finnish Red Pine. The heating unit was an electric heater.

The doctors concluded from their research and previous studies that the sauna was stressful because it caused an increased secretion of hormones. They also noted that there is an individual difference among people in regard to their tolerance to heat. When the heat is related to the person's ability of adaptation, the sauna is apparently beneficial and improves general physical condition. But if the temperature and the humidity are not related to the residence time and if the bath is repeated without the necessary rest, the effect can be detrimental to the body. For those reasons, rigid medical control is essential when using a sauna.

Another study conducted by M. Huikko, P. Jouppila, and N. T. Karki reported that almost every Finn takes a sauna once a week. The majority of them find it an emotionally pleasant, relaxing experience. They also note that the sauna produces *major* changes in the circulatory system. The average time spent in a sauna is from 30 to 60 minutes. In that time, body temperature may increase 3° F. The blood vessels dilate and the peripheral resistance falls significantly. The cardiac output increases 73 per cent and the pulse rate 61 per cent. Systolic and diastolic blood pressure remain practically unchanged.

One danger of remaining in a sauna for long periods of time is that your body begins to absorb and store the heat. If unchecked a heat stroke may result.

A second danger is dehydration. The sweat loss can adversely offset the body causing heat exhaustion. Plenty of liquids should be taken before entering and after leaving the sauna.

If the temperature is elevated long enough it is possible that chronic irritation of the mucous membrane may occur.

Here are some of the erroneous claims made by promoters of the sauna: (1) Saunas help you lose weight sensibly. No! What you lose when you are in the sauna is water weight. The weight is put back immediately when you take on additional liquids. To lose body weight you must balance your calorie intake and outgo, see CALORIES. (2) Saunas develop fitness. No! To develop fitness you must do the work. Proper exercise is necessary to place demands on the body to achieve fitness, see MECHANICAL DEVICES.

SCHOOLS

Physical fitness occupies a strange place in our modern culture. Nearly everyone preaches its virtues. At the same time, almost no one is willing to maintain it within themselves or lend meaningful support to programs that will allow our children in school to experience this highly beneficial phenomenon. That attitude toward physical fitness is as prevalent among educational administrators and physical educators as it is among the general public.

The dual attitude among those responsible for what goes on in our schools underlies the problems faced by people who sincerely wish to establish meaningful physical fitness programs. Those problems usually manifest themselves as insufficient allotment of time, lack of provision of sufficient facilities or parental pressure against strenuous work by the students. Substantiation for the latter position usually comes from some pseudo-scientific information on the dangers of physical exertion to the heart of the growing child or that such activity is not in keeping with desired feminine qualities.

The reluctance of educational administrators to commit themselves to the sufficient emphasis for a meaningful physical fitness program is not surprising. They are merely reflecting a cultural hierarchy of values in which predominantly physical occupations are placed at the lower end of the scale and predominantly mental occupations receive the majority of accolades. The negative influence on school policy and on the individual child created by skeptical parents is a measure of the profound lack of understanding on the part of parents involving the benefits of physical fitness. In many cases, that ignorance can be laid at the feet of the physical educator, whose job it is to educate his local public toward the urgent need for attaining those benefits. Even among athletes, the attitude is prevalent that getting in shape for their particular sport represents an unpleasant task, and many of them make little or no effort to maintain their conditioning once the season is over.

While many physical educators are also unwilling to either campaign for more emphasis on physical fitness within the schools or to place that emphasis in their own programs, the reasons behind their practices are somewhat different. While it must be realized that physical education must contain more than just physical fitness in order to fulfill its potential as an integral part of total education, many physical educators utilize that factor as a basis for either drumming physical fitness out of the physical education program or relegating it to a very minor role. Those individuals will point to carry-over activities, socializing values, aesthetic enrichment or some other alleged value as the primary aim of physical education.

All of those positions in opposition to physical fitness within the school are extremely vulnerable to attack. If you really believe that children learn through experience, how can you expect them to learn about physical fitness without experiencing it? Increased fitness will naturally encourage people to be more physically active, and therefore, they will be more likely to participate in activity throughout life, which is the carry-over people strive for anyhow. The socializing and aesthetic values of activity increase as the vigor of the activity and the keenness of competition increase. Both of the elements require physical fitness. And finally, how can we expect the concepts which undergird fitness to be meaningful to students who have never experienced physical fitness? That approach is similar to teaching an appreciation of music without allowing the students to play or hear music.

Such a bleak picture of the battle that physical fitness must fight in today's schools is not a hopeless one. There are many encouraging signs for the future. In some situations, like the La Sierra program in California, a school and community philosophy has evolved that has placed a high value on physical fitness, and an effective program to attain it has evolved within the school. The President's Council on Physical Fitness through both its fitness tests and its awards program has helped to provide guidance to physi-

cal educators in planning their physical fitness programs and has also promoted public support for such programs. The advances currently being made in programmed instruction provide means for overcoming the deficiencies in both facilities and time that face many devoted physical educators.

The bright hope for a more physically fit nation lies in the future. If today's students are to exert a meaningful influence in behalf of adequate fitness programs, they must believe in the value and benefits of physical fitness. Therefore, they must understand and experience the satisfying benefits through attaining and maintaining fitness themselves.—*Jay Arnold, Laurence McDermott*

SCUBA DIVING

Man has always yearned to explore the unknown. Through the fascination and challenge of scuba diving he has an efficient and thrilling means of discovering the wonders of the deep. In addition to sport and exploration, scuba diving opens the underwater worlds to photography, treasure hunting, salvage and extended research.

In effect, scuba diving means using Self-Contained Underwater Breathing Apparatus (SCUBA). It enables the diver to stay underwater longer and explore the strange environment more leisurely and carefully. Compressed air is delivered from the scuba cylinder by an air hose, and a regulator enables the diver to obtain air at various pressures. Other standard scuba gear includes a diving mask, fins, snorkel, rubberized suit, weight belt and an inflatable life vest.

Obviously, you are in a new environment when you dive—like a fish out of water. You will experience great freedom of movement (weightlessness), encounter strange fish and vegetation and be subjected to the squeezing effects of increased pressure. You must give careful consideration to your diving activities due to a limited air supply. How well you succeed depends on how well you can adjust. Naturally, the factors of health, physical condition, mental stability and a usable knowledge of oceanology and limnology become the determinants for your safety and pleasure. *Ignorance is the diver's worst enemy.*

Contribution to Physical Fitness

Even though scuba diving requires a high level of physical fitness, it does not necessarily contribute to the continued maintenance of fitness. The movements of the diver are slow and easy, since overexertion could deplete his air supply and physical reserve. As a consequence, fitness benefits are minimal.

In general, the better your circulo-respiratory fitness, the longer you will be able to remain under water and enjoy your activity. At first, you will acquire the ability to extend your underwater time considerably. Thereafter, you must use supplemental conditioning programs (swimming, running, stair climbing) to increase cardio-respiratory fitness.

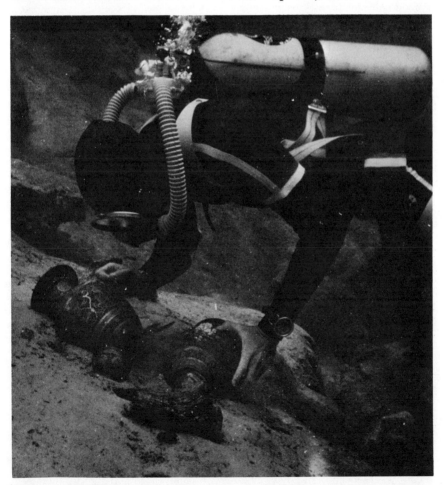

Through the use of special breathing apparatus, scuba divers can conduct extensive underwater explorations. Scuba diving requires a high level of cardiovascular fitness.

A certain amount of muscular strength is necessary to carry equipment to and from the diving areas, to complete the dive and also to maintain a reserve in case of a diving emergency. Muscle strength and endurance are generally not increased through diving.

Conditioning

Swimming for short periods daily, or at least two or three times a week, is better than one long workout a week. Practicing different swimming and survival skills is beneficial for all-around development. Some concentrated work should be devoted to leg strokes and to the skin and scuba diving skills.

When swimming facilities are not available, such activities as running, cycling, climbing, rope jumping, and walking are helpful; but, obviously, those activities have limitations. Practicing controlled breathing throughout the day is also beneficial.

If you are unable to participate in various recreational activities, you will need to follow a general physical conditioning program. Such a program should include the development of muscular strength and endurance and flexibility of the total body.

It is strongly recommended that you join a credited diving club. A scuba club practices safe diving procedures, has a regular schedule of swimming and diving sessions and provides motivation and guidance.

Physical and Mental Qualities Needed

Prior to starting, be sure you receive a thorough physical examination. Circulo-respiratory, ear, nose, throat, vision, or sinus problems may eliminate scuba diving as an activity.

Mental well-being and emotional stability are essential. A person that takes chances, ignores safety rules, panics when encountering new or different situations or tends to be a show-off not only jeopardizes himself but places tremendous responsibility on his partner. In this strange, new environment, traumatic experiences often occur during initial dives.

To understand all the implications of diving safety requires serious examination of scuba diving and how it affects the diver. It is absolutely essential to take a scuba course or study it thoroughly with an experienced diving instructor.—*Larry Good*

Associations:

Underwater Society of America (USA), Bourse Building, Room 492, Philadelphia, Pennsylvania 19106.

SECOND WIND

In his book, *Physiology of Muscular Activity,* Dr. Peter V. Karpovich notes that, "During violent exercise, such as running or rowing, a feeling of distress frequently develops which is associated with considerable breathlessness. If, however, the exercise is continued, that distress disappears and may be replaced by a sense of great relief. When the change occurs, we say we have our 'second wind.'

"The symptoms that precede 'second wind' are varied. There may be a look of distress on the face, often thought of as an anxious expression. Breathing is rapid and comparatively shallow; the pulse is rapid and fluttering or irregular. You may feel a sense of constriction around the chest; your head may throb and 'swim'; but outstanding among the symptoms is a feeling of breathlessness. Muscle pains sometimes occur. The minute-volume of breathing and the percentage of carbon dioxide in the alveolar air are higher before than after 'second wind' has occurred. With the onset of 'second wind,' breathlessness and discomfort sometimes disappear suddenly. The look of distress vanishes; the head becomes clear; and the muscles seem to act with renewed vigor. Breathing becomes easier; the minute-volume is usually reduced, the frequency decreased and depth increased. Even the heart observers find that sweating also accompanies 'second wind.' The man can now continue his exertion with comparative comfort. There are individual differences in the way adjustments are made: in some persons the sensation of relief coming with 'second wind' is definite, while in others it may be so indefinite as to pass unrecognized."

The second wind usually occurs within the first five or six minutes of exercising.

To some people, the passage of the initial stages of exercising to the second wind may occur with a very minor adjustment; while others feel extreme stress; and still others do not appear to get their second wind at all. The trained individual seems to achieve his second wind more easily than the untrained.

There are several factors that influence the second wind. They are: the rate of exercise, type of exercise, temperature and physical condition.

There are, furthermore, several factors that help you get "second wind." Those are: getting a good warm-up or keeping the body warm until the starting time and starting the activity rather gradually instead of rapidly.

Dr. Laurence Morehouse and Dr. Augustus Miller (*Physiology of Exercise*), present the objective and subjective changes that occur with second wind.

1. Respiration:
   (a) Relief of a feeling of breathlessness.
   (b) Reduction in rate and minute volume of breathing.
   (c) Reduction in alveolar pressures of carbon dioxide and oxygen.
   (d) Decrease in oxygen consumption and achievement of steady state (oxygen intake is equal to oxygen requirements).
2. Heart:
   (a) Decrease in heart rate and more regular rhythm.
3. Muscles:
   (a) Relief of swelling that often occurs, which may be delayed.
   (b) Relief of muscle pain.
4. Temperature regulation:
   (a) Rise in temperature of active muscles.
   (b) Appearance of sweating.
5. Brain:
   (a) Disappearance of sensation of dizziness.

Analyzing those changes may provide some indication regarding the physiological basis of second wind.

The disappearance of the feeling of breathlessness may be a result of stimulus traveling from the exercised muscles to the respiratory center in the brain. When vigorous exercise begins, there is an increase in the release of the lactic acid in the exercising muscle, thus signaling a demand for more oxygen. When a steady state (oxygen intake equals oxygen demands) is achieved and the metabolic conditions of the exercising muscles begin to stabilize, the stimulus is sent to the respiratory center in the brain. The rate and minute volume of breathing, therefore, decrease. The additional lactic acid released at the onset of exercise, moreover, causes a temporary increase in the output of carbon dioxide; and when the steady state occurs, there is a decrease in the carbon dioxide production. The reason for the decrease in oxygen consumption is not clear, except that the muscles may be exercising more efficiently, thereby reducing their oxygen demands. The decreased heart rate and the establishment of a more steady rhythm may be concerned with increased stroke volume (blood pumped with each beat). Research, however, has not demonstrated a valid reason.

The changes occurring in the muscles may be a result of the increased body temperature. Again, research is lacking in that particular area.

The disappearance of dizziness may be a result of the return of blood to the brain. At the onset of vigorous exercise, a great deal is required by the exercising muscles; therefore, the brain may not receive a sufficient amount. When the oxygen demands steady themselves, the blood is sent to the brain and the feeling of dizziness disappears.

Second Wind When Exercising

There are two techniques to enable you to get your second wind when exercising or participating in a sport. Momentarily slowing down or calling a time out at the first sign of severe pain or distress—with a few seconds of relaxation—may aid in your second wind. If the contest or situation does not warrant a time out or slowing down, then a vigorous warm-up prior to the competition may enable you to achieve second wind before the actual event.

SEX

In his book *Sexercises,* Edward O'Relly points out the obvious fact that sexual performance is a physical act. No amount of rationalizing or moralizing can change that fact. Although there may be mental and emotional involvements, the sexual union itself, he points out, is physical, involving physical people who use physical muscles.

We need not be astonished or ashamed by that truth. We need only to recognize it and recognize too, that the muscles involved in sexual union are also involved in other daily activities—or not involved as our level of inactivity dictates. That means that the muscles used in the sexual act are subject to the same deterioration and disuse that is prevalent in all the other

muscles of the normally senile modern man. They will normally lose their strength, stamina, vigor and endurance unless they are not allowed to deteriorate by the use of a comprehensive, scientific exercise program.

Of course there's another, more obvious affirmation for exercise—it's a necessity for the aesthetic, attractive body. Every man and woman strives to be sexually attractive to members of the opposite sex. But a flabby disproportionate figure can be a drawback to a successful marital union. Too many people eat, drink and smoke too much and exercise too little, particularly after marriage. A well-proportioned, sexually attractive body can be obtained through systematic exercise.

Some physical educators have recommended that specific exercises can be used to enhance the sex act. Bonnie Prudden was one of the first to discuss those various exercises (*How to Keep Slender and Fit After Thirty*). Her basic exercises emphasized the "belly dancer" movements and exercises to develop and strengthen the muscles of the low back, gluteal muscles and abdomen. Here are a few of those exercises:

Pelvic Tilt—Lie on your back and bend your knees. Place your feet 18 inches apart. Keeping your seat and shoulders tight on the floor, arch your back slightly. Do 10 times.

Hip Swing—Stand with your feet apart and knees stiff. Shift your hips as far to the right as possible. Then swing to the left.

Pelvic Tilt on Knees—Start by kneeling on the floor. Rest your seat on your heels. To do that, you will have to push your seat way out. Then without raising your head more than a few inches, bring your seat under the pelvis and forward. Return to the starting position and relax.

Those exercises are directed toward increasing the efficiency of those muscles that are specifically involved in the sex act. More important, however, is the necessity for developing complete physical vitality. To do that requires endurance activities such as walking, running, jogging, swimming and cycling. They are the activities that will condition your heart, arteries and lungs. Your circulo-respiratory systems will improve in endurance. That's critical in preventing possible damage to the heart as a result of inactivity because sex can place a serious load on the sedentary heart. The large muscle activities will also aid in reducing your weight, a very important consideration in obtaining a more attractive figure.

SHIN SPLINTS

A shin splint is recognized as a pain on either side of the lower third of the shin bone. In some instances a roughened area can be felt along the bone.

The cause of a shin splint may vary. Here are some of the most common. (1) The arch may drop somewhat, thereby setting up a reaction in the five tendons of the lower leg. (2) The membrane (interosseous) between the tibia and fibula may be irritated. (3) Inflammation of the tibial periosteum. (4) Tearing of the muscles of the lower leg from the bone. (5) A muscle spasm caused by the swelling of the anterior tibial muscle. (6) A hair-line fracture of one of the bones of the lower leg. (7) A muscle imbalance caused by the "toeing out" of the feet. The above are by no means complete, for other causes have been recognized and discussed by sports medicine personnel.

Care and Prevention—The best care is complete rest and heat (almost constantly). You cannot "run out" shin splints. Taping will provide some relief.

The prevention of shin splints involves:

1. A gradual conditioning program to get "into shape."

2. In the beginning, wearing tennis shoes.

3. Running on the grass, not hard surfaces.

4. Reversing your direction when running, especially track men.

5. Avoiding running on your toes—run lower.

6. Using a sponge heel pad.

SHOOTING

The relation of fitness to shooting is in some ways indirect. The act of firing a rifle, pistol or shotgun for short periods of time does not require more than average strength or endurance. Women, children and old people compete successfully in shooting matches. Also, many thousands of sedentary people count shooting and hunting as an occasional hobby, and they manage to be quite successful at those avocations.

An interest in shooting, particularly hunting, can promote fitness, however. In most country areas, fall is generally considered to be the season for walking expeditions into the field, and the pursuit of game with a gun creates the excuse for such outings. Millions of people who ordinarily never walk more than they have to, cover miles of ground on foot while hunting. The contribution of that activity to the general level of fitness in a community is probably significant.

It is also true that the once-a-year hunting trip—if too vigorous—can overtax an untrained heart and result in death or injury. A number of deaths from heart attacks while hunting are reported each year, and the American Heart Association and other groups have publicized the need for both caution and physical training prior to exertion. Walking up and down hills in warm clothes and heavy boots creates a dangerous strain on the bodies of people accustomed only to light activity. A man or woman of normal weight who has followed a moderate fitness program will usually be strong enough to go on extensive hunting trips without undue risk.

The role of physical conditioning in the preparation of a competition shooter has been best described by the Russian author A. A. Yur'yev in the book *Competitive Marksmanship With Rifle and Carbine*, State Publishing House for Physical Culture and Sport, Moscow, 1957. That book was translated into English by the Department of the Army for the use of the U.S. Army Advanced Marksmanship Unit. The principles of physical training described by Yur'yev have been used since then by U.S. shooters to produce continued success in international and Olympic competition.

The Physical Preparation of a Competition Rifleman

"Not so long ago, the opinion was prevalent among certain riflemen and coaches that physical training and allied sports were not at all necessary, that the model for a rifleman ought to be a person who is a little plump, that a well-developed musculature is sometimes even harmful for a rifleman because powerful muscles—since they are in a contracted state—flutter more and prevent the body from remaining immovable in the ready position.

"Experience has demonstrated the utter absurdity of such views. But the consequences of the scornful attitude of some coaches and their underestimation of the value of physical training as a part of the total training of a competition rifleman are, to a certain extent, still with us. The clinical observations on a rifle team in training for one of the most important tournaments by Dr. A. A. Sokolov merit attention in this connection. (*Clinical Observations on Sportsmen in Training*, Physical Education and Sports Publishing House, 1954, p. 157.) He notes: 'The significance of physical training is fully appreciated by coaches and riflemen. However, coaches do not

personally supervise such exercises because they do not know how to conduct them. Some riflemen have done physical exercising on their own with great harm to themselves. But nevertheless, riflemen who systematically do physical exercise get better scores in tournaments than those riflemen who ignore them.'

"In spite of the fact that shooting is considered basically as an exercise in endurance, there is much about it that requires brute strength. The standard international free rifle match, which lasts five or six hours and during which a rifle weighing seven or eight kilograms is lifted many times, makes great demands on a rifleman's energy. During such an exercise, a rifleman may lift the equivalent of more than three tons, to say nothing of the work performed by the muscles in holding the rifle for so long a time. According to the observations of Dr. A. A. Sokolov, which agree with the data of Ye. V. Kukolevskaya, a rifleman may lose as much as three or four kilograms in the course of that match, in spite of the fact that there is not much moving around in a shooting exercise. In addition, the execution of rifle exercises requires holding the breath. Thus, for example, a rifleman who aims an average of two or three times for each shot in a free rifle match holds his breath for a total of 50 to 75 minutes in the course of five or six hours' shooting. That causes a definite oxygen starvation of his body, bringing with it premature fatigue.

"It should be obvious from all that has been said that physical training as an integral part of a rifleman's technical development is extremely important.

"A competition rifleman must possess the following basic physical and psycho-physiological characteristics:

an adequately developed muscular system (this is especially true for the muscles of the abdomen, arms and legs) and the endurance to fire many shots without perceptible worsening of results;

the ability to relax completely and to keep from exercising all those muscles which are not required to hold the body in the ready position or while squeezing the trigger;

strong breathing muscles so that breathing is easy in the prone position when the chest is compressed somewhat;

strong lungs with a high oxygen assimilation factor so that long pauses between inhalations will not cause oxygen starvation;

precision and coordination;

quick reflexes;

a well-developed sense of equilibrium, and so forth.

"The physical training of a rifleman must be directed to the development of these qualities. If one is mindful of the fact that the successful execution of a rifle exercise requires an all-round physical development, such training will have a complex nature.

"The most common, the best developed, and most readily accessible kind of physical exercises for a rifleman are:

morning gymnastics (drills);

fast-moving games (especially basketball and volleyball);

skating and skiing;

rowing and swimming;

track and field athletics (especially running for medium and short distances);

bicycle riding and others.

"It is most important that physical training not have a haphazard character nor should it be timed to coincide with some particular period when a rifleman is in training for a tournament. A rifleman should perform physical exercises regularly both during the preparatory period between shooting seasons and during the principal training period when he is training directly for tournament participation. Morning exercise drills are very important in this connection, and they should become a part of a rifleman's daily routine. Morning athletics and a cold rubdown or shower should be a part of his daily regimen.

"Morning athletics must consist of enough exercises of a general nature directed toward strengthening the muscles, toward proper breathing, and toward developing body flexibility and precision of movement. The specific requirements of marksmanship are such that drills must consist of exercises which develop the muscles—the flexors of the arms and fingers, the muscles of the shoulders, and the muscles of the waist. Along with dynamic exercises, a certain amount of static exercise is valuable if it is not overdone. For example, the muscles be made to do some work which does not require movement (supporting oneself in a hanging position for short periods of time) because this facilitates the best muscle development and accustoms the muscle system to the sort of work which it must do in holding the ready position.

"It is especially desirable during the preparatory period (between shooting seasons) that a rifleman spend some time at other sports in addition to his periodic rifle training.

"Fast-moving games merit attention in this connection. Of these, the most valuable is volleyball, a game that is not physically too taxing. The movements involved in volleyball are sufficiently varied and are very useful from a rifleman's point of view. The short runs, jumps, bends, turns, and the movements of the arms are examples. This game requires mobility and develops precision from whence it derives its value for a rifleman.

"In the wintertime, a rifleman will find it very useful to go skiing because this sport helps to teach proper breathing, to increase the capacity of the lungs, and to acquire physical endurance. Ice skating and figure skating are also very important because these sports are proven methods for train-

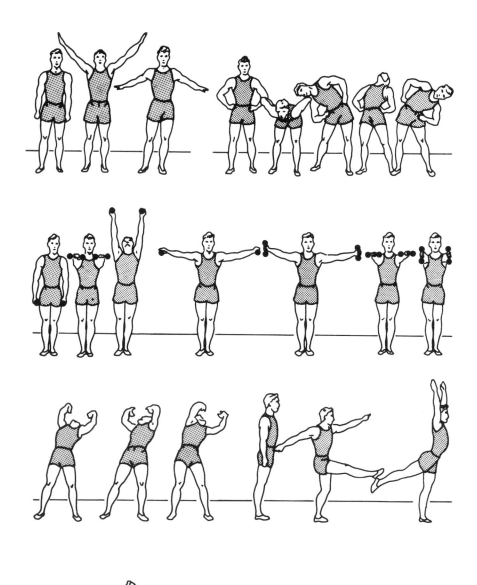

A series of morning exercises (drills) for a rifleman.

ing the aural vestibule and thus for developing and sharpening the sense of equilibrium which is so necessary for successful shooting from a standing position.

"In the summertime, field and track sports, especially running with rhythmical breathing, and swimming and rowing are good sports for a rifleman because they develop his lungs, help him to acquire endurance, and strengthen his whole muscular system. Many riflemen have observed useful results from bicycle riding, which, in addition to the physical development which it encourages, helps to train the aural vestibule. According to the observations of some riflemen, after a moderate ride on a bicycle and a rest period of approximately an hour or two, shooting from the standing position goes much better. Bicycle riding is a good means of limbering up, helping to bring about the most advantageous condition in which an equal, almost unnoticeable, tiring of the leg, abdominal and arms muscles assures the steadiest ready position. A rifleman ought to avoid certain sports which are, so to speak, antagonistic to shooting. Examples of these are heavy athletics and climbing exercises."—*Robert Rodale*

Associations:

National Skeet Shooting Association, 2608 Inwood Road, Dallas, Texas 75235.

Amateur Trapshooting Association, Vandalia, Ohio.

National Rifle Association, 1600 Rhode Island Ave., Washington, D. C. 20036.

SHOULDER

Here are some of the muscles of the shoulder area together with some exercises that you can use to develop them. The short, thick muscle located at the shoulder girdle is the *deltoid*. It looks almost like a cap for that area.

The muscle helps to raise the arm from the side of the body and acts with other muscles to move the arm forward and backward. You can develop the deltoid isometrically by standing in a doorway with your palms out and pressing against the doorjamb. Exert a maximum force for 10 seconds. Pull-ups are also good as a deltoid developer.

The *supraspinatus* is only one of several muscles located on the back part of the shoulder. It can be found at the back of the collar-bone and the upper portion of the scapula. Other muscles include the *infraspinatus*, which lies immediately below the spine of the scapula, and the *teres major* and *minor*, which lie farther down the back. Those muscles act to hold the arm in the shoulder socket. The *teres major* also draws the arm backward and toward the body.

To develop those muscles, lie flat on your stomach with books or dumbbells in each hand. Place your arms at right angles to your body, then raise your chest from the floor and lift your arms, holding them at right angles to the floor.

SKIING

Skiing is a vigorous sport but also lots of fun. More and more people are learning how to ski. New ski areas are constantly being developed to meet the demand for better facilities. Because skiing is a challenging sport, it requires a well-developed form and technique.

There are basic steps to learn as you progress in your skiing ability. Skiing becomes a dangerous sport when you ski out of control and cannot stop or turn at will. A skier is considered an expert when he can ski under all terrain and snow conditions. There is an excitement and thrill which captivates you as you glide down a mountain side. The air seems to sparkle and the white surroundings of the

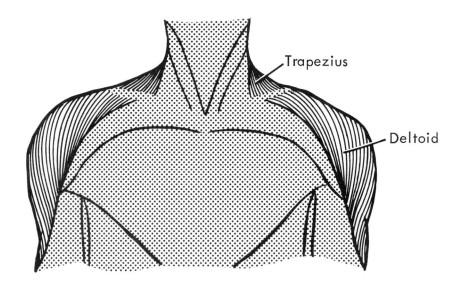

Muscles of the Shoulder
Front View

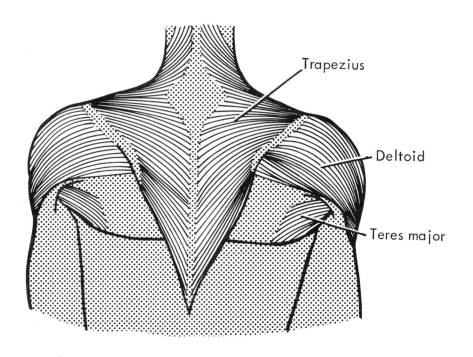

Back View

mountains make cares and frustrations of normal living vanish. An exhilarant sensation takes over.

The stamina needed and the physical fitness required depends on how you want to ski. A very high degree of cardio-respiratory endurance is needed for a competitive skier, an advanced skier and a person who skis for hours at a time. Fatigue of the legs will occur in an hour or two if you are not in good physical condition. Most people set their own pace, ski in their own manner and style and at their own speed without overtaxing their bodies. Like any sport, skiing becomes dangerous if you push yourself when tired or if you ski under icy conditions or on slopes or trails which are too difficult.

Skiers need especially strong thigh and calf muscles, for when those muscles tire, it is difficult to control the skis. Condition those muscles *before* the skiing season to improve the muscle tone and endurance. Skiers need a great deal of relaxation and flexibility in the shoulders, abdomen and hips. There is much twisting and rotating of the upper trunk area. The arms are used a great deal in poling, thus there should be some degree of strength in the upper torso.

Conditioning Program for the Skier

Endurance-stamina exercises:
1. rapidly repeated jumps on both feet with knees bent
2. rapidly repeated sit-ups to bent knee position
3. running in place
4. squat position with one leg extended and then other leg in rapid succession
5. burpees done rapidly
6. jumping rope
7. running laps and sprinting
8. jumping jacks
9. double treadmill

See ISOMETRICS and WEIGHT TRAINING for additional exercises.

Before you start to ski, get yourself in good general physical condition. When you tire easily and your muscles don't respond, you're ripe for an accident. Develop good muscle tone by starting an exercise program early and continuing it. Exercise should be done before and throughout the season.

Try to develop a high degree of cardio-respiratory endurance which will enable you to ski better and for longer periods of time. You are less likely to become injured if you condition the whole body. Anyone who experiences a great deal of knee trouble may find difficulty in skiing because bending and twisting of the knees are quite necessary.

Learning basic fundamentals from the very beginning is of the utmost importance. Know how to stop, how to execute a turn and even how to fall properly. Take a few lessons to learn the fundamentals in the event you do not have a friend to teach you properly. It is not impossible to learn on your own, but it will take much longer to progress and may produce bad habits. At first, you may feel a lack of balance, but with confidence, you will learn how to control balance and motion.

The most common injuries are leg, ankle and wrist sprains, pulled muscles and torn ligaments. A National Ski Patrol System is usually found in the area where you are skiing, and a member can be summoned if you are injured. They are trained in first aid techniques and in transporting injured skiers. Since more serious injuries do occur than those listed above, caution is needed in skiing. Note the safety advice and adhere to the rules of safety.—*Jean A. Hecht*

Associations:

United States Alpine Cub (USAC), The Broadmoor, Colorado Springs, Colorado 80906.

United States Ski Association

(USSA), The Broadmoor, Colorado Springs, Colorado 80906.

*DOWNHILL SKIING PROGRAM**

Chart 1		Chart 2	
1.	10 minutes	1.	38 minutes
2.	15 minutes	2.	40 minutes
3.	18 minutes	3.	43 minutes
4.	20 minutes	4.	45 minutes
5.	23 minutes	5.	50 minutes
6.	25 minutes	6.	53 minutes
7.	30 minutes	7.	55 minutes
8.	33 minutes	8.	58 minutes
9.	35 minutes	9.	60 minutes

*See ENDURANCE and ENERGY COST OF ACTIVITIES for an explanation of the charts.

**Doesn't include rest periods, time outs, riding back to top, etc.

Fitness 1

If you achieved a score of poor or low average on the *Harvard Step Test* or a score of very poor or poor on the *12 Minute Run*, start on Chart 1-Level 1 and spend 1 week at each level until Chart 2-Level 9 is reached. It is recommended that you participate 4 to 5 days a week. When Chart 2-Level 9 is reached, 4 days a week is sufficient.

Fitness 2

If you achieved a score of high average on the *Harvard Step Test* or fair on the *12 Minute Run*, start on Chart 1-Level 2. Spend one week on Chart 1-Levels 2, 4, 6, 7, and 9; and Chart 2-Levels 2, 4, 5, 7, and 9. It is recommended that you participate 4 to 5 days a week. When Chart 2-Level 9 is reached, 4 days a week is sufficient.

Fitness 3

If you achieved a score of good or excellent on either the *Harvard Step Test* or *12 Minute Run*, continue your current program or select Chart 2-Level 9 as your level of participation. Four days a week is sufficient.

Since skiing is a high-energy-cost activity, it may be used to help improve your fitness level, especially your circulo-respiratory and muscle endurance. Below is a skiing training program that takes into account the important principles of training.

Ski Touring (Cross Country)

If you want to get the "whole body" out-of-doors exercises of skiing but cannot afford the time, expense or risks of downhill skiing, try "instant skiing."

Interest in instant skiing—or ski touring—is rising because of its varied attractions: It is inexpensive—a complete outfit costs $50 to $75. You can ski tour almost anywhere—no hills or tows are required. You can start without elaborate lessons or training—it is nearly as easy as walking. It is safe. And you can participate as a family with all ages joining in.

Ski touring, or Nordic skiing, will never replace the thrill of pointing a pair of skis downhill and racing to the bottom at speeds of 40 miles an hour or more. That kind of skiing (called Alpine skiing) is exciting, demanding and challenging to the skill and daring of even well-conditioned athletes. However, ski touring has a growing appeal for every one—especially those who are taking up skiing for the first time.

Anyone in reasonably good condition is ready to start. It is about as simple as hiking. The skier sets his own pace by the distance he goes, by the difficulty of the terrain he covers and by the speed at which he travels.

For skiers interested in competition, cross-country skiing represents a field in which U.S. skiers have not been as strong as people from other nations; and therefore, a special opportunity to excel exists. Even devoted Alpine skiers find that Nordic skiing is an ideal conditioner and expands their interest and understanding of their sport.

You Can Tour Almost Any Place, Anytime

Ski touring is as near as the nearest park, trail, country club, or woods path. Unplowed roads or bridle paths make an especially fine trail. There is no need for a long drive to the mountain or tows. Suitable terrain can even be found as near as your own backyard; just step out, strap on the skis and go off across lots. Many commercial ski areas, state and national parks have opened and maintain special ski touring trails, usually well mapped and marked.

Snow conditions do not make any difference as long as there is some. When the downhill areas are closed for lack of adequate snow cover, the chances are the ski tourer will still have sufficient snow for a very pleasant outing.

Equipment Is Inexpensive

Ski touring equipment does not cost much because it is simple, not susceptible to the vagaries of style, and lightweight (weighing only about one-third as much as a standard downhill skiing outfit).

Touring skis are slightly narrower than the downhill type and do not have the familiar metal edges. They are a laminate of selected woods—soft on the bottom to hold wax, hard on the edges for wear, and strong in the center for long service. Pick a pair that reaches the heel of your hand held over your head. Heavier or more experienced skiers can use a slightly longer pair. Beginners should select shorter skis.

Cable binding is best for touring. It lets the heel lift normally as in walking but can be adjusted to hold the whole boot flat to the ski for extended downhill runs. Another type of binding used by cross-country skiers, especially those interested in racing, is the Rotefella or "rat trap." Using four prongs matching holes drilled in the boot, it clamps the toe of the boot with a trap-like action but leaves a great deal of freedom to the rest of the foot. It is firmer, faster to put on, lighter, but cannot clamp the heel for the control sometimes desired on a downhill run.

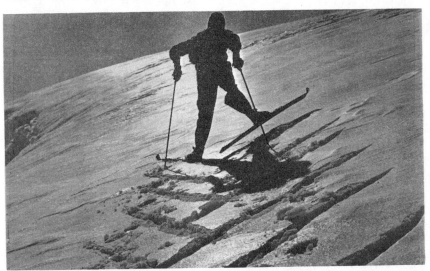

Cross-country skiing is more vigorous than downhill skiing. It's also less popular. Cross-country skiers don't rely on lifts or tows to get up steep hills.

Special ski touring boots are recommended but not an absolute necessity. Any good stout boot with a heel and sole that will take the strain of a cable binding will serve. However, ski touring boots with heels grooved for the cables and toes reinforced for clamps are better. Even ankle-high touring boots are as light as a pair of men's street shoes and very flexible. Regular stiff, heavy, downhill boots will definitely not do.

Poles used in touring are of light bamboo and have a curved tip to be more useful in the push and glide of cross-country skiing. They are usually slightly longer than poles for downhill skiing, the recommended length being from armpit to floor plus three inches.

Clothing Is Strictly Practical

No special clothing is required. Wear about what you would wear if you went for a winter walk in the woods or fields. You will be plenty warm while running (that's a tourer's word for any progress over the snow). Even at a walking rate, you fly along at running speed. Have clothes loose and in layers that you can take off and tie around your waist or slip into a pack. Remember that you will cool quickly when you stop; and it is well, too, to have enough to cover up when taking a break or pausing to enjoy the scenery.

Make sure that you provide for ventilation—"fishnet" underwear, for example, is ideal—and that you guard against accumulation of perspiration. Wear a soft wool or synthetic cap that ventilates, gloves or mittens and a shell parka. If you get warm, try taking off your hat and gloves, like opening a window. If you are still warm, try taking off your parka and put on the hat and gloves. Make adjustments to suit your comfort.

Knickers make the best touring pants, but any loose fitting pants— preferably wool—are satisfactory. Don't get tight stretch pants.

Depending upon the length of time you will be out and where you are going, a light pack and additional equipment can be a wise precaution. You might carry a lunch, dark glasses, tan lotion, matches, compass, waxes, a map of the area and a piece of nylon line.

Technique Is Simple

Start on the flat and ski ahead by sliding one foot in front of the other. Your toe will stay on the ski. The motion is almost like shuffling along in a pair of loose bedroom slippers. The pole in the hand opposite to the foot being advanced is used for push and balance. Use a simple walking rhythm, and as you progress in confidence, the stride is increased and the movements become a series of long smooth glides.

Going uphill is not quite so easy and takes more practice; but climbing is fun because it usually earns you a view and a ride down. Try these four basic ways of climbing. First, you can traverse or criss-cross your way uphill. Using push and glide as on the flat, you climb in a series of slants across the face of a hill. At a flattened, angle, it is easier and you do not slide back. Second is sidestep. Turn your skis perpendicular to the slope and go directly up the steepest angle of the slope in a series of parallel sidesteps. Dig in with the ski edges so as not to slip down sideways.

The third method is the herringbone. Again you go straight up the steepest part of the slope, walking with your skis out at 45° to the incline making a pattern of tracks like a herringbone. It requires a strong push with poles and edging of the skis. It is fast and a little tricky at first, but with practice it gets rhythmic. It is the best way to get up fairly steep short slopes.

Finally, if the slope is short or not too steep, you can get up a little extra speed and run directly upward using the momentum of your speed to keep

°CROSS COUNTRY SKIING PROGRAM

Chart 1	Chart 2
1. ½ mile in 6 minutes	1. 1½ miles in 17½ minutes
2. .6 mile in 7 minutes	2. 1.6 miles in 19 minutes
3. ¾ mile in 8 minutes	3. 1.7 miles in 20 minutes
4. .8 mile in 10 minutes	4. 1¾ miles in 21 minutes
5. .9 mile in 11 minutes	5. 1.9 miles in 22½ minutes
6. 1 mile in 12½ minutes	6. 2 miles in 24 minutes
7. 1.1 miles in 14 minutes	7. 2.1 miles in 25 minutes
8. 1¼ miles in 15 minutes	8. 2.2 miles in 26 minutes
9. 1.4 miles in 16 minutes	9. 2.3 miles in 30 minutes

yourself from sliding back. That is, of course, the fastest and most energetic of all, but also the technique most commonly used by the Scandinavians and all racers.

Waxing

Downhill skiers who want to slide all of the time use a permanent polyethylene plastic base, but ski tourers need a running surface that will hold them or let them slide. The right waxes come separately or in complete kits with base waxes, tools for application and a complete selection of running/climbing waxes suitable for different snow conditions. With kits, you get a chart showing the best wax for each type of snow condition. When touring, it is a good idea to take your wax along with you if you plan to be out very long.

Additional Information

One of the fine things about ski touring is the enthusiasm of the participants. They are anxious to introduce others to touring which makes it easy for a beginner to get the guidance and help he wants. There are many places you can turn to for further information on equipment, places to tour, techniques and organized tours.

John S. Day is National Director of the United States Ski Association touring program. Write to him at USSA, Broadmoor, Colorado Springs, Colorado, for information on local ski touring organizations and trails.

°See ENDURANCE and ENERGY COST OF ACTIVITIES for an explanation of the charts.

Fitness 1

If you achieved a score of poor or low average on the *Harvard Step Test* or a score of very poor or poor on the *12 Minute Run,* start on Chart 1-Level 1 and spend 1 week at each level until Chart 2-Level 9 is reached. It is recommended that you participate 4 to 5 days a week. When Chart 2-Level 9 is reached, 4 days a week is sufficient.

Fitness 2

If you achieved a score of high average on the *Harvard Step Test* or fair on the *12 Minute Run,* start on Chart 1-Level 4. Spend 1 week on Chart 1-Levels 1, 3, 5, 7, & 9, and Chart 2-Levels 1, 3, 5, 7, 9. It is recommended that you participate 4 to 5 days a week. When Chart 2-Level 9 is reached, 4 days a week is sufficient.

Fitness 3

If you achieved a score of good or excellent on either the *Harvard Step Test* or *12 Minute Run,* continue your current program or select Chart 2-Level 9 as your level of participation. Four days a week is sufficient.

There are at least three books with more information on ski touring. The best and most useful for the beginner is "The Cross-Country Ski Book" by

John Caldwell. Other books are the "Manual of Ski Mountaineering," edited by David Brower, and "Nordic Training and Cross-Country Skiing," by Michael Brady.

Touring is a pleasant and healthful activity in which you can vary the amount of exercise to suit your own needs and ambitions. Because you glide over the snow, five miles is a relatively easy tour.

But those of us bound to a desk, whose principal exertion is pushing paper and lifting the telephone, touring is exercise, solitude and poetry. Getting exercise is important but so is it vital to get out-of-doors next to nature and to be alone.—*Weston B. Haskell, Jr.*

Since cross-country skiing is a high-energy-cost activity it may be used to help improve your fitness level, especially your circulo-respiratory and muscle endurance. Below is a skiing training program that takes into account the important principles of training.

SKILL

The term skill is related to the physiological principles of training. Much of the improvement that takes place during training is a skill improvement. In the beginning, for example, you may find that noticeable changes appear to be taking place in your physical condition. A great deal of the improvement is a result of learning how to do the exercises or activity more efficiently. Becoming more efficient means you are making noticeable physical performance increases as a result of improved coordination. See TRAINING and MOTOR LEARNING.

Skill and Condition

A skilled person is one whose performance approximates closely his intention—the greater the skill the closer the performance resembles the intention. Skill differs from habit in that it is characterized by the absence of stereotyping. The skilled performer is adaptable and able to make adequate adjustments to the varying conditions of the environment in which he performs. A games player does not merely learn a series of skills but rather how to make the appropriate reaction, according to the position of all players and the flight of the ball, assessing its speed, height and direction.

Skill and condition are closely interwoven in athletic performance. In the past twenty-five years, attempts have been made to determine which factors are required for successful participation in particular sports. Three qualities have emerged as fundamental in most sporting activities: skill, strength and endurance. Quite naturally, considerable attention has been given to each of those areas separately in order to investigate the optimum methods for their individual development. Most training programs attempt to improve the factors to varying degrees. All too often, there has been an unfortunate tendency to separate the skill training (or practice of skills) from the program designed to develop the requisite strength and endurance. Only in recent years have attempts been made to integrate the skill and conditioning programs which should be closely related.

At certain stages in the training of athletes, skill and conditioning will be developed separately; but during the competitive season, the two facets should be progressively integrated, with the emphasis changing according to the actual performance of the people in competition.

The following points are emphasized in drawing up a suggested framework of a training session in which skill training and conditioning are integrated:

1. Progressive fatigue affects the performance and particularly the learning of skills. The player should be given an opportunity to maintain

as much as possible his level of skill as he becomes progressively fatigued. His skill will be practiced within the framework of stress that occurs within the actual game situation.

2. Maintain the intensity of effort at a higher level during the training than is required during the match play.

3. Players should be given tests measuring their level of skill (kicking, marking, etc.) when they are fatigued. They should indicate which skills "break down" more quickly than others in the later stages of match play. The training may then develop proficiency in those areas, and individual players may be advised to avoid attempting those particular skills in the later stages of the game.

Changes Associated with the Acquisition of Skill

Steinhaus has pointed out in "The Chronic Effects of Exercise" (*Physiological Reviews,* 1933) that skill is characterized by precision and economy.

"Perfection of movement is the most prominent result of training. It is also the most specific. . . . A most important by-product of the development of skill is the economy of effort which the more purposeful use of the muscle entails, thus reducing the total load and at once postponing fatigue."

The smooth, coordinated action of the skilled performer impresses with its grace and fluency. It is a commonplace observation to hear spectators comment upon the apparent ease of the successful performer: for example, the successful sprinter often looks as though he could have run faster if only he had tried.

Training reduces the amount of oxygen required to perform a specific task. With an increase in skill, subjects are able to perform the same amount of work with greater efficiency, using less oxygen which results in a lower rate of breathing and a lower heart rate.

Fewer muscle fibers are called upon to contract at one time. Lundervold reported the results of electromyographic studies (in which the electrical activity of muscles is picked up and recorded) in a paper entitled "The Measurement of Human Reaction During Training." He found that untrained subjects who lacked skill in the performance of even a simple skill, such as tapping with one finger, contracted more muscles, more forcibly and for a longer time than skilled persons. Furthermore, the untrained subjects fatigued more rapidly than trained subjects, demonstrating the interdependence of skill and condition. In the case of a more complex skill, such as running, Lundervold pointed out that muscles can be trained in such a way that the highest speed can be produced with less muscle activity.

Steinhaus has indicated in "Metabolism of Exercise—A Measure of Skill" that oxygen consumption is an objective measure of skill on the basis of information presented by physiologists. The skilled runner uses less energy, per kilogram of body weight, than the less skilled, clumsier runner, for the same amount of work. Improvements in economy are associated with increases in skill and not condition as might be expected. Successive tests of the energy cost, in terms of oxygen consumption, for a standard amount of work, showed improvements in economy before but not after a month of very strenuous training.

A complex mixture of skill and condition will enable a person to perform more efficiently and more effectively for a longer period which surely must be the major objective of training. See MOTOR LEARNING, SKILL and TRAINING. —*E. R. Sandstrom*

SKIN DIVING

The popularity of diving underwater with face mask, snorkel and fins (skin diving) has been growing tremendously in the last decade. Public awareness of the potential of skin diving has been influenced greatly by entertainment mediums as well as the documentation of oceanography and limnology research and the prolific accounts accruing from the growing school of sport divers.

Unlike the sportsman at the surface, the skin diver takes his body, consisting of solids, gases and liquids, into an environment that is nearly incompressible and is heavier and more viscous than air. That creates unusual demands on the underwater diver.

The safety and pleasure of the skin diver will be directly affected by his health, physical fitness, emotional stability, level of competency in swimming and skin diving skills, and knowledge of the marine environment. Skin diving should always be practiced with a partner, and a diver jeopardizes both his partner and himself when he is deficient in any of those areas. The higher the competency, the more assurance (insurance) of enjoying the dive with a greater measure of safety.

Fitness Benefits

Swimming underwater for extended periods of time and making repetitive dives, typical of skin diving, requires unusual physical prowess. The diver must acquire a high level of cardiorespiratory endurance through supplemental conditioning programs to enable him to safely enjoy skin diving. Without it, he cannot dive as long, exhausts quickly, must rest more often, and will not have the reserve to han-

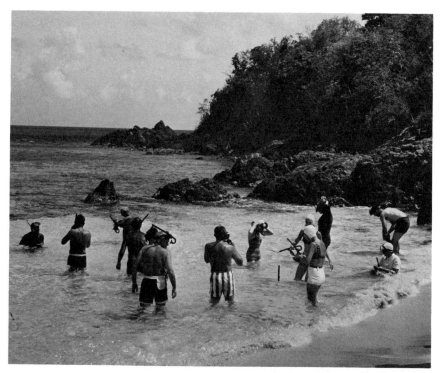

Skin diving promotes swimming skills and physical fitness. Here an instructor helps a class don snorkels and masks prior to exploring the underwater sea world.

dle himself or his buddy in an emergency.

The diver uses slow and relaxed movements when skin diving. If he is tense, swims fast, becomes chilled or stays underwater too long on his initial dives, he seriously limits his diving activity. Once submerged, the only air supply that the muscles of the body can utilize is the amount the diver carries with him in his lungs.

Free of the gravitational pull experienced on land, the underwater movements of the diver promote increased neck, upper-back and shoulder flexibility.

Muscular leg endurance is enhanced to some degree by skin diving. The legs are the most important motor unit in skin diving, but overall physical fitness is necessary for the many and varied tasks required of the diver. Equipment has to be carried to and from the diving area, a one-quarter to one mile swim may be necessary to get to a desirable diving area; and, of course, the divers must be able to get back to shore safely.—*Larry Good*

Now don't think that you have to be an expert swimmer or live near a sea coast or in some sub-tropical region in order to skin dive. If you are a fair swimmer and not afraid of the water, you're ready for your first lesson in skin diving. And you can do your diving in lakes, streams, ponds, rivers, oceans, quarries and springs. Professional divers go down for lobsters, fish, gold, ship wrecks, shells, treasure, photographs, you name it. I dive and explore to take my mind off the effort of swimming.

Technically, a skin diver is anyone who swims underwater with or without breathing equipment. But let's differentiate between "skin" and SCUBA divers. SCUBA (Self Contained Underwater Breathing Apparatus) divers use an aqualung, breathe compressed air and remain underwater from 10 minutes to an hour, depending upon water depth. See SCUBA DIVING.

The skin diver simply floats or swims on the surface of the water, sometimes taking a deep breath and diving for as long as he can hold it. With a little practice, almost anyone can reach a depth of 25 to 30 feet and remain on the bottom for about 30 seconds.

Naturally, you must be in good health to skin dive. A physical examination is recommended for everyone. Stay away from the sport if you have a cardiac condition or a history of lung or sinus disorders.

Skin Diving Uses Muscles

Skin diving like swimming utilizes almost all of the muscles of the body. The large and small muscles of the legs are especially exerted during the actual dives. They also get a good workout while you are snorkeling on the surface. Most skin divers use the head-first descent, executed by jack-knifing the body at the surface. That places the head and shoulders under the water. Then you straighten your legs sharply, raising them so they are at right angles to the surface. Keep knees stiff and toes pointed. The weight of the legs pushes the body below the surface. When you are completely submerged, use your usual swimming strokes.

The jack-knifing of the body benefits the hips, stomach and back muscles. The swimming strokes—usually the breast stroke or Australian crawl, work on the muscles of the arms and chest, especially the pectorals. It's easy to see that almost all of the body's muscles are activated in skin diving.

The body is also physically affected in other ways. Circulatory and respiratory systems are conditioned by the stress of the swimming, diving and breath holding combinations. The heart beat quickens, the lungs expand and as adrenalin increases, reflexes quicken. Although the heart seems to take on the major strain, it does not overwork itself if you try hard to maintain a relaxed easy diving procedure. Something like this: a nice easy breath, a simple jack-knife, a few gentle kicks, a look-see at the bottom, a few more kicks—back to the surface, an expelling of stale air, then floating on until ready for the next dive. Most divers, like runners, come upon a "second wind" which enables them to stay down longer and swim farther.

Best of all, skin diving drains little from the family budget. All you need is a mask, a snorkel and a pair of swim fins. All can be purchased for less than $20. But choose your mask carefully. A good one is made of fairly soft rubber, has a sturdy headstrap, metal binding rim and a feather-edge seal. Testing a mask for proper sealing is simple. Place it on your face without using the headstrap. The bottom of the mask should fit against your nose. Inhale gently through the nose. That should cause a partial vacuum inside your mask. If it stays on without your holding it, you have a proper fit—no air or water will be able to enter.

Why Fins?

It is difficult to explain to someone who has not tried them, but fins do boost swimming ability. A fair swimmer usually becomes a much better swimmer onces he gets used to using fins. They increase forward motion and maneuverability, and enable good swimmers and divers to tread water almost indefinitely. Take the same care in your choice of fins that you would in buying a pair of dress shoes —tight fins will cause muscle cramps and restrict blood circulation. Loose fins will raise painful blisters. You can choose either buoyant or nonbuoyant fins. The floating fins are easily retrieved at the surface should you decide to remove them. Nonbuoyant fins are stiff, but with just a few hard kicks, you can glide an amazing distance.

However, they do require very strong, hard leg muscles.

The snorkel is a simple tube which allows you to breathe under water. It should be about 16 inches long with a comfortable mouthpiece that won't irritate the gums. Hold the mouthpiece of the snorkel by biting firmly on its two rubber prongs, forming a water-tight seal around the flange with the lips. Fancy snorkels with corks or ping-pong balls are neither practical nor safe. A simple, "J" snorkel is the best.

If you're going to dive in water over your head, make sure you have a flotation device. Ideal ones are made of neoprene, rubber or rubber-impregnated fabric with both a carbon dioxide cartridge and a mouth inflation tube. Use the cartridge only once— then it must be replaced. A float makes it easier to return to shore when you are tired, and it also acts as a safety device in case of cramps or undue fatigue.

One more precaution—don't dive with earplugs. They can be pushed into the eardrum by the greater outside water pressure. If a pocket of air is formed between the plug and the eardrum, and the plug doesn't move inward, the eardrum may rupture outward.

Just like in any other sport, skin diving is best learned from a qualified instructor. Your YMCA usually offers basic instruction. Many skin diving ships also sponsor large group or individual classes. Begin in a pool—it's safe and it's fun. It's also a good place to learn to use the snorkel. Then, when you're ready, try first descent in a nearby pond or river. There's a feeling of great accomplishment after a 10-foot dive and most people can do that the first time out! In the beginning you'll be able to stay underwater for only 10 to 15 seconds. Then, you'll increase it to half a minute, then perhaps to a full minute. That's when the fun begins.—*Ellsworth Boyd*

Association:

Underwater Society of America (USA), Bourse Building, Room 492, Philadelphia, Pennsylvania 19106.

SLEDDING

Long before the invention of the wheel, early man used flat wooden "sleds" to move heavy objects across snow, sand and almost any other surfaces. Once the wheel was invented, the sled became impractical except on ice and snow. Today sleds are used primarily for sport and recreation, although in the Far North they are still used for transportation. Such sleds as the *Nome Sledge* pulled by a team of dogs, the *Nansen Sled* lighter but wider than the Nome, and the Russian *Troikas* pulled by horses or reindeer are examples.

The two most popular forms of sledding are toboggans and double runner sleds. Traditionally, children used the large majority of sleds; but more recently, people of all ages have been actively engaged.

Various forms of sledding have become very popular in the Olympic Games. Presently, there are two types of competition—bobsledding and luge. Luge is often called tobogganing; but it is not the tobogganing that is familiar in the United States. The Olympic luge has runners on its sleds and is shorter in length.

Sledding is an activity that may be enjoyed by almost any age group. It is not very demanding, although walking back up the hill numerous times after descending will require that you have a healthy circulo-respiratory system. The majority of the benefits derived from normal recreational sledding are primarily psychological rather than physiological. In Olympic competition, naturally, the benefits derived and the physical condition are increased appreciably because of the speeds reached and body movements required.

If you wish to make sledding a fitness activity, you can do so by walking vigorously up the hill after descending. Walking on hard or soft snow greatly increases the energy-cost of sledding. It can range from moderate to high-energy-cost depending upon the speed of walking, whether the sled is carried or pulled, hardness of snow and grade of hill.

SLEEP

Sleep is extremely important for the human organism. The human body can be compared to a machine or engine. It can generate power, and its source of power is food. Like any other engine, the body is continually wearing out. The wearing out process is very gradual and, to most of you, unnoticeable until you get into the advanced years. Even then, there is considerable variation from person to person.

Each day the body wears out a little bit, but it has one saving device that keeps it from wearing out too soon. That device is sleep. Sleep is extremely important for the human organism. It replaces the worn parts, and as a result, the body can work a lifetime without incurring serious damage, provided some other condition is not cause for disease. The body works at a certain rate during the day without noticing that it is slowing down; but after a certain point is reached, you have a safety device, fatigue or tiredness, that warns you and finally forces you to stop. See FATIGUE.

Generally, every muscle of the body is an engine that receives fuel from glycogen and oxygen. If the work is slow and steady, the pace can be maintained for a long period of time because the body can supply the muscle with the necessary sugar and oxygen. However, if the work is too intense or continues for a long period of time, the muscles cannot be supplied with those necessary nutrients.

Also there is a buildup of waste products in the muscles which reduce their efficiency and finally cause the muscles to stop working entirely. Rest allows the muscles to rid themselves of the lactic acid and to be resupplied with oxygen and sugar.

Fatigue may not just be a result of work or muscle contraction. It may occur from emotional problems, body ailments or a rather intangible form — boredom. Of those four forms of fatigue, that which occurs from physical exertion is the healthiest and the most desirable.

What Happens When We Sleep?

When the body becomes tired, there is a tendency for the whole organism to let go. You lose consciousness and several other changes take place. The heart slows from 75 to 60 beats per minute, the breathing rate slows from 16 to 12, blood pressure falls, basal metabolism is reduced, the body temperature falls slightly and the liver stores glycogen during sleep. For some unknown reason, however, the sweat glands increase their activity. During sleep, the kidneys continue their unending job of filtering metabolic poisons out of the blood.

Relaxation the Necessary Ingredient

Relaxation is the key to sleep. Tense muscles present a very serious obstacle to sleep. Many times, those muscles are tense because they have not been exercised enough during the day or because the brain is so active as a result of emotional problems or other stimulations. To relax, you must reduce tension; the most effective technique to relax was developed by Dr. Edmund Jacobsen. Called progressive relaxation, it is the ability to learn to completely control the muscles. See RELAXATION.

How Much Sleep?

How much sleep you need cannot be generalized, for there are many variations from one person to another. Traditionally, 8 hours for young adults has been the standard, yet there are many well-known people (Thomas Edison, for example) who are accustomed to only 3 or 4 hours a night.

The world is geared to an eight hour night. Most people turn in between 10 and 12 and rise between 6 and 8. It may be desirable for you to cat-nap during the day, rather than taking all the sleep at one stretch. Those naps aid the body in reducing fatigue or tiredness. Two well-known cat-nappers of the twentieth century are Dr. Michael DeBakey, world famous vascular specialist and the late President Kennedy. Dr. DeBakey is able to sleep at the drop of a hat. When traveling, he is able to buckle himself in a seat of an airplane and be asleep before the plane leaves the runway. President Kennedy was able to "micro-sleep" very easily. During a busy day, he was able to sit down in a chair, close his eyes, and fall asleep almost immediately. In five minutes, he would wake up fully refreshed and ready to delve into the tasks ahead. The important point is that the sleep should be sufficient to allow you to wake up spontaneously and refreshed.

How to Sleep

Insomnia has become almost a way of life in the United States. Practically every family has one or more members who suffer from an inability to get to sleep. Many times, that lack of sleep is due to overstimulation.

A recipe for sleep is as follows:

Good sleep habits must be formed and learned. Do not eat a heavy meal before retiring, do not take stimulating drinks, do not listen to the radio or watch TV just before retiring and do not read exciting books. Some positive steps to be taken are to retire at the same time every evening, drink warm milk or take a warm bath just before retiring, count sheep or progressively try to relax the muscles. In the evening occupy yourself with some quiet, creative hobby.

Another important consideration is not to let yourself get too tired during the day. If you feel fatigue coming on, try to "micro-sleep" by closing your eyes for a short time or just momentarily forgetting your troubles, work and assignments for the day by literally blanking out for a few seconds.

Exercise and Sleep

The relationship between exercise and sleep is two-fold. (1) exercise helps in bringing on sleep; and (2) sleep is necessary for adequate exercise and development of physical fitness.

Moreover, the typical American is overstimulated, underexercised, and tension ridden, see HYPOKINETIC DIS-EASE. Exercise helps to reduce that overstimulation and tension which causes a great many physiological and emotional problems in our society. It helps to tire the muscles adequately and reduce the level of tension. By increasing the physical fatigue and reducing the tension levels, sleep is achieved much easier. The exercise need not be done just before retiring; it can be done anytime during the day.

Sleep is also very important for proper exercise and physical fitness. If you are run-down physically and mentally from improper sleep, you will not be able to exercise at the desirable level. In fact, the exercises may be harmful. Physical fitness cannot be achieved without adequate sleep because of the detrimental effects it has on the human organism.

SMOKING

Statistics continue to show that smoking is on the upswing. More people are smoking more tobacco products, particularly cigarettes. Youth is losing to the smoking habit and in-dications are that, unless something is done, the trend will continue. In 1961, statistics showed that 61 million people consume 488 billion cigarettes (an average of over 20 cigarettes per person daily). Over 7 billion dollars literally went up in smoke on tobacco products.

Almost all research done on the effects of smoking on the human body indicates that smoking, particularly cigarettes, is hazardous to health. Smoking has been linked to lung cancer, poor nutrition, ulcers, increased resting heart rate, high blood pressure and other health problems. In addition, smoking may contribute to heart disease, since the existing information shows that the disease is more common among smokers than nonsmokers.

Man's breathing apparatus is a fascinating structure. Breathing is a continuous process that goes on as long as you are alive. Barring interference, it may go on for as long as 70, 80, or even 90 years without your being aware of it. See RESPIRATION. The respiratory apparatus (the lungs and the passages leading to them) is responsible for providing oxygen for the cells and tissues of the body so that they can carry out their specific functions.

The lungs are adapted to receive atmospheric air, a mixture of three gases: nitrogen, oxygen and carbon dioxide. During the inhalation phase of external respiration, atmospheric air is drawn into the lungs. Any other substances present in the air will also be inhaled, some are harmful and can cause damage to the respiratory system, particularly the lungs. In addition to being a threat to the lungs, some of those foreign substances that manage to enter the blood stream may prove to have a damaging effect on other cells, tissues and organisms.

Among the dangerous substances are certain gases, dust, smoke and other chemicals. Cigarette tobacco smoke falls into the category of substances that can have harmful effects on the respiratory system as well as other parts of the body.

Normally you breathe through your nose. The nasal passages act as filters and air conditioners; they screen out impurities from the inhaled air and adjust the temperature of the air so that it will not "shock" the other respiratory passages and the lungs. When smoking, you inhale the tobacco smoke through the mouth, bypassing the protective features of the nasal passages. Breathing through the mouth is a poor practice with fresh air, let alone doing it with smoke-filled air. Just the temperature of cigarette smoke is enough to cause irritation to the mouth, throat and other respiratory components. The heat of the smoke, furthermore, is sufficient to cause itchiness in the throat and coughing.

The cough is a physiological protective mechanism which is the body's attempt to reject some undesirable element and keep it from entering the lungs. If the smoker was aware of that, he would realize that the "smoker's cough" is a sufficient indictment against smoking; the respiratory system does not want smoke.

Aside from the heat of the smoke, there are substances present in the tobacco which pose a threat to health. Two in particular, nicotine and benzopyrene, are highly suspect as troublemakers. Nicotine in its pure state is a colorless poison, which if injected directly into the blood stream in a small amount could cause instant death. In laboratories, small animals have gone into instant shock as a result of merely coming into contact with a single drop of nicotine. In industries where pure nicotine is used, care must be taken by the workers to avoid contact with the substance. In smoking, the strength of the nicotine inhaled is considerably less than in the pure state since much of it is burned off.

The body exhibits an ability to adjust to small amounts of some poisons. Nicotine is one of them. Despite that ability, the amount that does reach the lungs can cause problems. Moreover, nicotine affects the coordination of the heart by activating the sympathetic nervous system. Ironically, people who smoke to relax actually cause the opposite result since nicotine acts as a stimulant. Benzopyrene is a chemical component of tobacco that irritates the respiratory passages.

The effects of smoking seem to be cumulative. That is, the more you smoke and the longer you smoke, the more severe are the complications and risks. Studies conducted by K. Cooper and others showed that smoking led to chronic problems with respect to endurance performance, but it also affected the smoker's ability to improve his performance through training. Those who smoked more performed more poorly than those who smoked less or not at all. Those who had a longer history of smoking did more poorly than those who had smoked for less than six months. Smoking cigarettes without inhaling was found to have no appreciable deleterious effect on endurance performance.

Other findings by Cooper and associates revealed that the smokers had increased pulse rate at rest, increased blood pressure, constriction of certain blood vessels, increased oxygen consumption at rest, decreased diffusing capacity (ability of the lungs to exchange gases with the blood stream), decreased lung capacity and a larger oxygen debt incurred during exercise. Other investigators have found that cigarette smoke causes a slight bronchoconstriction (constriction of the tubes leading into the lungs) upon inhalation.

All of those findings indicate that smoking leads to decreased overall body efficiency. Not only does the body of the smoker work harder at rest, but its capacity to do work is not as great as that of the nonsmoker.

Smoking has also been connected to poor nutrition, temporary night blindness, ulcers and bronchitis. It has long been common knowledge that smoking affects the appetite. Some smokers feel that smoking is a good way to lose weight. Even though weight loss often does accompany smoking, it is not a good way to lose weight because it interferes with good nutrition. Cigarettes do still the pangs of hunger temporarily. Hunger is signaled by, among other things, rhythmic contractions of the muscles of the stomach wall; and smoking quells those contractions.

Smoking seems to have another unpleasant effect on the digestive system. It can cause gastritis and possibly the formation of ulcers. Smoking can initiate the secretion of excess stomach acids, and ulcers develop and thrive in that type of environment. When you smoke, the digestive acids are secreted, and at the same time, hunger is suppressed. Then the acid, with no food to digest, begins to digest the stomach wall. Result? An ulcer. Normal eating habits would result in utilization of the digestive acids. Doctors strongly recommend that their ulcer patients who smoke either stop smoking or, at least, cut down on their smoking. In numerous cases, the cessation of smoking has resulted in the elimination of ulcer symptoms.

Dr. Charles Sheard of the Mayo Clinic has stated that nicotine in cigarette smoke can cause a 15-30 minute delay in the time required for the eyes to adjust to darkness. For that reason, Army Air Forces training manuals advise against smoking before night flights. Tests have also shown that smoking affects steadiness and coordination.

Smoking and Health, an exhaustive report, mentioned that sixteen substances capable of initiating cancer in animals have been identified in cigarette smoke. Furthermore, the report said:

"Cigarette smoking is a cause of lung cancer and bronchitis, and probably contributes to the development of coronary heart disease and various less common diseases.

"Cigarette smokers have the greatest risk of dying from these diseases, and the risk is greater for the heavier smokers.

"The many deaths from these diseases present a challenge to medicine; insofar as they are due to smoking they should be preventable."

Most smokers, when first introduced to smoking, find it offensive, and only after a concentrated effort do they acquire a taste for it. Quite often this "taste" becomes a reliance, an unhealthy reliance.

If through education people could be made more aware of the dangers involved in smoking, many more might not smoke. In the Royal College report, some specific recommendations were made with regard to preventive measures for individuals as well as national governments:

1. More public education, particularly of school children concerning the hazards of smoking.

2. More effective restrictions on the sale of tobacco to children, and wider restrictions on smoking in public places.

3. Raising the tax on cigarettes, and possibly lowering taxes on pipe tobacco and cigars since pipe and cigar smokers incur a much smaller risk than do cigarette smokers.

4. Testing the various filters on cigarettes and including the results on the package label.

Recommendations have been voiced for those who cannot break the smoking habit:

1. Try to smoke less or change to pipe or cigar smoking.

2. Smoke more slowly; in that way, less nicotine is inhaled and the smoke is not as hot.

3. Do not smoke to a short butt; that part of the cigarette has filtered the already smoked part and is laden with undesirable substances.

4. Do not inhale; in that way none, or nearly none, of the harmful ingredients of the tobacco smoke reach the lungs.

Exercise can prove valuable to the smoker. Through a planned program of physical exercise, particularly running, the smoker, like anyone else, can increase his capacity to do work. But the smoker cannot increase that capacity to the degree that the nonsmoker can. He will still be frustrated by this ugly habit.

Through exercise, it may be possible to stop smoking. See JOGGING.

SOCIAL CONTEXT

Modern man functions in a given geographic environment or context. He also functions within a given social context; that is, he is surrounded by other persons including family, friends, fellow students or co-workers and those persons in his neighborhood, town or city, state and nation. His attitudes and behavior regarding all of his life's activities including his fitness are influenced in varying degrees by (1) his perceptions of his role and status in the society, (2) those members of the society with whom he interacts, and (3) his role and status as perceived by the society.

Age

Early childhood (birth to five)

For the young child, the family exerts the strongest influence on his development. The family's ethnic background, religious views and geographic location inevitably affect the child's attitudes toward and practices in physical fitness. Some stress spiritual values, while others place more emphasis on physical health and vigor. From a geographic standpoint, families may be differentially affected by location in areas that are: (1) urban, suburban, or rural, (2) warm, cold, rainy or dry, (3) proximity to bodies of water and indoor and/or outdoor recreational facilities, and (4) mountainous or flat.

As the child grows older, he begins to move out from the home base and encounter persons outside the family. To some extent, his fitness orientation will be influenced by his playmates, his playmates families and other persons outside the home.

Later childhood (five to puberty)

During this period, the child enters school and is exposed to a whole new and complex set of values and experiences. The school is the agency of the community charged with preparing the individual to become a happy and productive member of the society. In its attempts to accomplish that task, it includes a formalized study of physical fitness. Information on nutrition and health practices is part of the curriculum. In addition, the school provides opportunities for children to practice fitness in its sport and physical activity programs. The exposure to the many and varied students will also influence his fitness orientation. He will come into contact with widely varying attitudes toward and practices in fitness and will have to discard or incorporate them into his own system of values and behavior.

Adolescence (puberty to physical maturity)

As the individual moves into puberty, the physical and psychological changes taking place affect him in ways that are often confusing to his perceptions of his role and status in the society. As he acquires greater independence from the family, he has more opportunity to ignore those tenets of fitness learned in earlier years and elect to behave in a manner detrimental to his health.

On the other hand, the interaction he is now having with the opposite sex may motivate him to use the principles of fitness to improve his appearance and physical abilities. Of all the avenues open to adolescents to achieve status in their peer group, sport offers the most rewarding alternative. The negative side is that as the school encourages students into the formalized patterns of interscholastic sport, many candidates for teams are excluded from participation. That pattern of participant and spectator may make it difficult to identify with participation and fitness in later life.

By the end of adolescence, the individual's perceptions of himself, the people with whom he has interacted and the society's perceptions of him combine to establish the role, status and fitness orientation he will carry into the larger adult society.

Adulthood

The majority of adults who take their place in the society are concerned with earning a living and/or maintaining a home and family. His society may vary considerably in its emphasis on fitness. National characteristics combine with a given status vis-a-vis war or the threat of war to establish a set of values regarding the relevance of fitness to the maintenance of the society.

It is during this stage of life that man begins to notice the physical changes that take place as he grows older. How he reacts to the changes depends partially on his fitness orientation. Many reach a stage of poor fitness, recognize it, and take steps to remedy it. Still others move on through life making little or no effort to maintain and/or improve their physical condition. Most excuse their lack of fitness through rationalization, revolving around the demands of a job, lack of time or lack of access to facilities.

At times, physical fitness may be attained in ways that are unintended. For many, it is only developed when demanded by circumstances such as occupations requiring varying levels of fitness, given conditions of health, or membership in the armed forces. For others, fitness may accrue as an unintended side effect of a commitment to a given leisure time pursuit such as an outdoor activity, a recreational sport or an avocational activity that requires fitness.

As man moves through middle age, his commitment to fitness, depending on the norms of his society, may decrease with age. Many societies accept the often heard contention that as you grow older, you should "slow down." Acceptance of that viewpoint, combined with advancing years, can result in an extremely low level of physical condition by the end of middle age.

Old Age

The point at which man moves into old age depends on his physiological condition, his state of mind and the norms of the society in which he lives. Portions of given societies hold that, as man reaches a specific age, he should cease all vigorous work or activity and retire to a purposeless existence in an institution for the aged. In essence, his society may have discarded him as no longer needed. In this case, it is difficult for the older person to find the motivation to maintain his fitness at a high level.

On the other hand, some societies hold that older persons should stay in the family, have an active part in the maintenance of that society and, consequently, stay fit. In that case, social norms support the older person's attempts to retain vigor and a youthful appearance. There are societies that are in the process of attempting to establish those circumstances that lead to older people being a relevant and active part of that society. To the extent these societies succeed, their aged will be motivated to retain the abilities and appearance needed to fulfill their social roles.

Sex

From the time he can perceive cues from others, the male child is exposed to stimuli that are constantly shaping his perception of himself as a male. The manner in which he is handled, how he is dressed and expectations for his behavior combine to create a role that he fills to given degrees of success. He is influenced by varying expectations for behavior from his parents and siblings, his playmates, the schools he attends, the male and female friends he acquires and eventually, the vocation he selects and the adult society in which he lives. As he grows, the male child is increasingly expected to develop physical abilities that are needed in those activities agreed upon as proper for boys. As he moves into puberty, more specified standards are applied to measure his maleness. Adolescence is the time of a male's life when speed, agility, strength and endurance are the most relevant to social success in his age group. To a varying degree, depending on the society and the man's position in it, that emphasis declines as adult status is reached. The demands of the role of breadwinner take precedence. As the male continues to move through his life, those expectations for fitness continue to decline until, at old age, the standards for the male are usually little different from those of the female.

In a manner identical to the male, the female is also shaped by her social environment. As she moves through adolescence into adulthood, social expectations change and, in comparison with those of the male, decline. To varying degrees from society to society, the sexually mature female is not expected to meet the same standards demanded of the male. Traditionally, the female qualities most likely to be valued are those of grace of movement, charm, beauty and the ability to establish and maintain a home and family. Again, in comparison with the male, the adult female social role usually does not stress the values of physical fitness.

As they have moved into a level of status more nearly equivalent to that of men, women have increasingly rejected their traditionally passive role and have elected to enjoy a life more in keeping with the standards of physical vigor and youth expected of men.

Socio-economic Status (SES)

Sociologists have determined SES by having informants that represent all sections of a society rank such things as occupation, neighborhood or home type, life style, education and family background. The different levels of those dimensions are given numerical values. Thus, a person with a given occupation, home location, life style, education and family background can be assigned a place on the SES hierarchy by totaling his scores for any or all of the SES dimensions.

In a more informal way, SES is assigned to each member of a society by all other members of that society by an almost unconscious process of evaluating any or all of the SES dimensions that can be perceived during interaction with that person. Thus, a person driving a given car, dressed in a particular way, and working in a specific job is assigned a given status by those with whom he interacts.

The different categories—lower, lower-middle, upper-middle and upper status—are discussed from the perspective of two dimensions. The first, "life chances," refers to the degree of access a given class has to the wealth, facilities and positive attitudes needed to actually get involved in the process of attaining and maintaining fitness. The second, "life style," refers to the manner in which a given class lives—how it dresses, how it allots its

income and, in general, how it be-
haves.

Lower class

The life chances of the lower class
have a great deal to do with its fitness orientation. Traditionally, because
of a combination of lack of access to
facilities, low income, and culturally
motivated negative or neutral attitudes, the lower class has little incentive to practice physical fitness. Other
problems are lack of proper nutrition,
health habits and medical care. Even
those lower class members who are
usually unemployed, and as such have
the time, rarely look upon fitness as
an end in itself. Generally, their main
concern is recreational rather than the
improvement and maintenance of fitness. Conversely, when working, members of the lower class regard fitness
as more or less of a pragmatic concern that relates to the specific needs
of the job.

The life style generally revolves
around the maintenance of appearance
or the minimal patterns of survival.
Consequently, most of its income is
used for purposes other than those
related to physical fitness.

Lower-middle class

In comparison with the lower class,
the improvement in the life chances
of the lower-middle class give it a
better opportunity to practice good
fitness. The life style of this group
tends to be more conservative. Consequently, more of their income may
be allotted to the purchase of goods
and services related to fitness. To a
certain extent, however, as with the
lower class, much of the fitness orientation of the lower-middle class again
revolves around the demands of a job,
rather than from a commitment to
the values of fitness as an end in itself.

Upper-middle class

The upper-middle class, roughly
consisting of members of the professions, high level business and owners
of businesses, apparently has a high
level of commitment to physical fitness as relevant to the maintenance
of health, vigor and a youthful appearance. The life chances enable it
to be the major consumer of physical
fitness literature and equipment. The
life style includes a trim and fit appearance to go with its wealth of material possessions.

Upper class

In a way similar to those in the
upper-middle class, members of the
upper class appear to have inculcated
the values of fitness. Their life chances
give them unlimited access to leisure,
facilities and positive attitudes. A life
style that has traditionally included
participation in all kinds of physical
activities gives more support for the
contention that while their activities
are not as visible as those of the upper-
middle class, members of the upper
class are committed to and practice
physical fitness.

Historically, attitudes toward and
practices in physical fitness have been
related to the social context in which
they have occurred. The fitness orientation of modern man is influenced by
(1) his perceptions of his role and
status in the society, (2) the members
of the society with whom he interacts,
and (3) his role and status as perceived by the society. When those
three factors are looked at through
the perspectives of age, sex and socio-
economic status, it is apparent that a
knowledge of the social context in
which man lives can help in understanding his physical fitness attitudes
and practices.—*John Newell Sage*

SOMATOTYPE

See BODY TYPE.

SPECIFICITY

The term specificity, one of the
physiological principles of training, is

the concept that improvements made in training are specific to the type of training followed. For example, a strength training program does not necessarily result in an increase in endurance; nor does a flexibility training program improve strength and endurance. Furthermore, a flexibility exercise program for the shoulder will not improve the flexibility of the ankle joint. Likewise, training for one sport does not result in an improvement for another sport.

Many athletes have experienced this phenomenon when they have concentrated on one sport, swimming, for example, and considered themselves to be in reasonable condition. Then they walked onto a basketball court and attempted to play a rigorous game of basketball. Rapid fatigue was often the result. The reason for that apparent lack of condition for basketball is due to the physiological principle of specificity.

As a result, the principle of specificity is one of the best arguments for practicing the skills exactly as they will be used in the sport. See TRAINING.

SPEED

Speed is total body movement from one place to another and is an extremely important factor in athletics. Like many other facets of physical fitness, speed is very specific. It is difficult, therefore, to make a generalization and label a person as fast or slow. Although he may be a fast runner, he may not be able to throw a fast ball in baseball. Ability to cover a prescribed distance in a certain amount of time is a result of two factors. The first is how fast you can accelerate from a standstill, the acceleration involves the first 5 or 10 yards of action and is basically reaction time. The second is the maximal movement rate or the ability to sustain movement once top speed is reached.

According to Dr. Herbert deVries, those two factors of speed are not related. You may be a good 100-yard

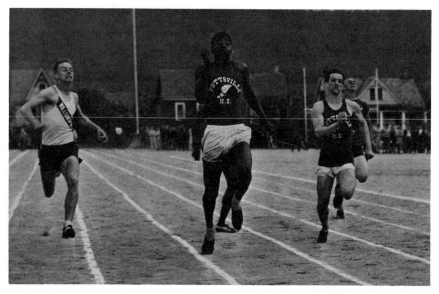

Speed is only one of several specific facets of physical fitness. People with a high degree of speed usually combine proper body mechanics, flexibility and strength.

dash man with a poor start because you have good maximal movement rate, or you may be a good 100-yard dash man with a good start and only an average maximal movement rate. Consequently, some people are proficient in football, tennis and badminton (quick starts) and yet poor in the 100-yard dash. That point was illustrated in the May 22, 1967, issue of *Sports Illustrated*: Frank Deford discussing Tommie Smith, the phenomenal 220- and 440-yard sprinter, noted that Smith is "the fastest *moving* human the world has ever known . . . (He), in a word, does not burst. He can only uncoil after he comes out of the starting blocks. His every race is a finishing kick, all the way, great liquid strides, faster and faster, in a relentless drive. For unlike other runners, Smith reaches no peak; he is accelerating to the end." Here, then, is the phenomenon of an individual who with a poor start is a record

holder in the 220 (19.5 in the straightaway) and a contender for the records in 440- and 100-yard dash.

Factors That Influence Speed

Body Mechanics. Proper body mechanics are important in speed. The proper arm action, leg action, angles of body and many other factors play a critical role in the correct kinesiological pattern so that the movement is efficient. Wasted motion is reduced or virtually eliminated. Speed is generally improved with an improvement in body mechanics.

Flexibility. Logically, flexibility may play a role in improving speed, because better flexibility appears to permit more efficient movement, which indicates more speed. That generalization, however, has not been demonstrated by research.

Strength. There is a strong relationship between a gain in strength and a gain in speed. In *Physiology of Ex-*

COMPARISON OF WORLD RECORDS FOR MEN AND WOMEN
(July 10, 1963)

Event	Women	Men	Per Cent
Swimming (Meters)			
100 free style	59.5	53.6	90
200 free style	2:11.6	1:58.4	90
400 free style	4:44.5	4:13.4	89
800 free style	9:51.6	8:51.5	90
1,500 free style	18:44.0	17:05.5	91
100 breaststroke	1:18.2	1:07.5	86
200 breaststroke	2:48.0	2:29.6	89
100 butterfly stroke	1:06.1	57.0	86
200 butterfly stroke	2:29.1	2:08.2	86
100 backstroke	1:08.9	1:00.9	88
200 backstroke	2:28.2	2:10.9	88
Running (Meters)			
100	11.2	10.0	89
200	22.9	20.5	90
400	53.1	44.9	85
800	2:01.2	1:44.3	86
Field Events (Meters)			
High jump	1.91	2.28	84
Long jump	6.62	8.31	80

(*Physiology of Exercise for Physical Education and Athletics,* Dubuque, Iowa: Wm. C. Brown Co., Publishers, 1966, p. 407.)

ercise for Physical Education and Athletics, Dr. Herbert A. deVries reports that "gains in strength, whether brought about by isometric or isotonic training, are associated with significant gains in speed movement."

Sex. The difference between speed in men and women is appreciable. As any comparison of performance will reveal, however, the differences are primarily a result of strength differences.

SPORTS

It is traditionally assumed that if you engage in a sport you will improve your level of physical fitness and consequently, your general health. However, there is a wide difference

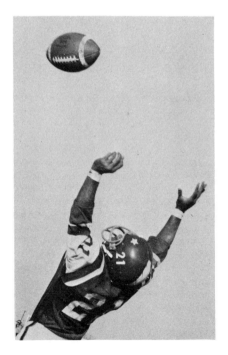

Although spectator sports like football are often more popular, many fitness seekers have turned to other, less violent, sports as their personal route to fitness.

among various sports in their contribution to physical fitness. Some sports such as swimming place a great stress on the circulatory and respiratory systems of the body and, for that reason, help you develop a high degree of that vital component. Other activities, such as weight lifting, increase strength, while still others stress flexibility, such as floor exercise in gymnastics.

Moreover, it is true that many sports do not have a training effect on the body. That is, they do not allow the body to be overloaded sufficiently to improve fitness. Or they may take you only so far on the fitness scale and then stop.

Some investigators have found that athletic teams are in the same physical condition at the end of the season as they were at the beginning. Some even found that the fitness of athletic teams deteriorates with time during the season. That indicates the body may have adapted to the overload or the exercise, resulting in no more improvement and instead in a slow decline; or it may indicate that the training phases of the program—wind sprints, grass drills, and general exercises—contributed more to fitness rather than to the activity itself.

If you desire maximum fitness benefits through sports, find an activity that burns up a high number of calories and increases the pulse rate and oxygen consumption enough to have a training effect on the body. See ENERGY COST OF ACTIVITIES.

Furthermore, you should take into account the several training principles set forth under TRAINING. In this book a training program for many sports is included in the listing. Remember, those activities develop circulo-respiratory endurance, and usually muscle endurance, especially of the legs, hip flexors and diaphragm.

If you want to develop the other vital components of fitness—strength and flexibility, you may find it necessary to use weight training exercises or isometrics for strength development and stretching exercises for flexibility. They will then supplement your program of fitness through sports.

Another problem encountered in using sports as a vehicle for fitness is the changing weather. It seems that just when you have gotten into the swing of the activity, your intentions are interrupted by Mother Nature. The result is that you have to give up your activity and fall back into a loss of fitness and creeping obesity.

Properly planning your program of fitness through sports, however, can eliminate that problem. Planning for the changing seasons includes organizing your outdoor activities so that you are working with, not against, nature. Below are a series of selected sports that may be used in the various seasons for helping you to develop and maintain physical fitness.

Winter

Skiing	Ski Touring
Ice Skating	Winter Canoeing
Sledding	Basketball
Handball	Roller Skating
Volleyball	Ice Hockey

Spring

Cycling	Orienteering
Tennis	Golf
Badminton	Volleyball
Rowing	Canoeing

Summer

Rowing	Canoeing
Swimming	Tennis
Volleyball	Cycling
Badminton	Basketball
Handball	

Fall

Cross Country	Badminton
Cycling	Basketball
Handball	Squash
Tennis	Soccer
Playground Football	

One of the biggest drawbacks of fitness through sports is that it is dif-

ficult to measure improvement in fitness. In running or cycling, for example, you see the improvement because you can cover a greater distance in a shorter time. The charts devised for the various sports may help you in that regard. Another method is to periodically check your fitness level with a fitness test. See TESTS.

Another limitation is that a specific sport may not develop all the vital components of fitness. As a result, the sports fitness program requires a supplement. Although sports may be used to develop a high degree of circulo-respiratory endurance and muscle endurance, it is advantageous for you to consider adding further training to your program. Coaches have been doing this for years with their athletes. They do not simply insist on game play but include conditioning drills such as wind sprints, calisthenics, grass drills and guerrilla drills. They also recommend weight training in the off-season to develop strength and/or power; those fitness components may not be developed through the sport but are vital for participation.

SPORTS MEDICINE

Sports medicine is a wide and varying science that encompasses the realm of sports and fitness. Here are a few of the areas that are included under a general listing:

Physiology—(especially the physiology of exercise) included are the implications of exercise, immediate and long range effects, causes of muscle soreness, etc.

Applied anatomy and physiology—This category includes the effect of using muscular leverage on the efficiency of performance, together with the muscular and mechanical analysis of activity.

Anthropology—This elusive heading includes the classification of body build and its inherent limitations, the

FITNESS BENEFITS OF SELECTED SPORTS

H–High, M–Medium, L–Low, M-H–Depends whether recreation (M) or Vigorous (H)

Sport	C-R Endurance	Muscle Strength				Muscle Endurance				Flexibility			
		Arms	Legs	Abdomen	Back	Arms	Legs	Abdomen	Back	Shoulder	Hip	Elbow	Knee
Australian Football	H	L	H	M	M	M	H	M	M	L	M	L	H
Baseball	L	M	M	L	L-M	L	M	M	M	H	M	H	H
Basketball	H	L	H	L	L	M	H	M	M	M	M	M	H
Bobsledding	L	L	M	L	L	L	L	L	L-M	L	L	L	L
Boxing	H	H	H	H	H	H	H	H	H	L-M	M	H	H
Cross Country Running	H	M	H	M	M	L	H	H	H	L	M	L	H
Cricket	L	L	M	M	M	L	M	M	M	H	M	H	H
Diving	L	L	L	H	M	L	L	L	L	H	H	L	L
Fencing	M-H	M	M-H	M	M	M	M	M	M	M	H	H	H
Field Hockey	H	M	H	M	M	M	H	M	M-H	M	H	H	H
Football													
a. Tackle	H	M-H	H	H	H	M	H	M	H	L	H	L	M
b. Playground	H	M	H	M	M	M	H	M	M-H	L	H	L	H
Gaelic Football	H	M	H	M	M	M	H	M	M	L	M	L	H
Gymnastics													
a. Balance Beam	L	L	H	M-H	M-H	L	L	M	M	L	H	L	H
b. Floor Exercise	M	H	H	H	H	H	M	M	M	H	H	H	H
c. Horse	L	H	L	M-H	M-H	M-H	L	M	M	M	H	H	L
d. Horizontal Bar	L	H	L	H	H	M-H	L	M	M	H	L	H	L
e. Long Horse	L	M	M	L	M	M-H	L	M	M	L	L	L	L
f. Parallel Bars	L	H	M	H	H	L	L	L	M	H	H	H	H

Activity															
g. Rings	L	H	M	H	H	M-H	L	M	M	L	H	H	H	H	L
h. Trampoline	M-H	L	M	M	M	L	L	L	L	H	M	H	M	L	H
Hauling	H	M	H	M	M	M	H	M	M	H	M	M	M	H	H
Ice Boating	L	M-H	L-M	L	L	M	L	M	M	L	L	L	L	M	L
Ice Hockey	H	H	M-H	M-H	M-H	H	H	M	M	H	M	H	M-H	M	M
Jai Alai	M	H	M	M	M	H	H	M	M	M	M-H	L	M	L	H
Judo	H	H	H	H	H	H	H	H	H	H	H	H	H	H	H
Karate	H	H	H	H	H	H	H	H	H	H	H	M	H	H	H
Lacrosse	H	H	M	M	M	H	H	M	M	H	M-H	M	M-H	H	H
Lumberjack Activities	H	H	H	H	H	M-H	M	M	M	M	M	L-H	M	H	M
Motor Sports															
a. Boat	L	L	L	L	L	M	L	L	L	L	L	L	L	L	L
b. Car	L	L	L	L	L	M	L	L	L	L	L	L	L	L	L
c. Cycle	L	L	L	L	L	M	L	L	L	L	L	L	L	L	L
d. Plane	L	L	L	L	L	M	L	L	L	L	L	L	L	L	L
Parachute Jumping	L	L	L	L	L	L	L	L	L	L	L	L	L	L	L
Polo	M	M	L	M	M	M	M	M	M	M	M-H	M	M	H	L
Rodeo	M	H	H	H	H	M	M	M	M	M	M-H	H	H	H	H
Rugby	H	M-H	M	H	H	H	H	M	M	H	M	M	M	L	H
Scuba Diving	M	M	M	L	L	M	M	M	M	M	M	H	M	M	M
Soccer	H	L	M	M	M	M	H	M	M	H	H	M	M	L	H
Softball	L	M	M	L	L	L	M	L	L	L	L	H	M	L	H
Speedball	H	L	M	M	M	M	H	M	M	H	M	M	M	L	H
Surfing	L	L	L	L	L	L	L	L-M	L-M	L	L	L	L-M	L	M
Tennis	H-M	M	H	M	M	M	H	M	M	H	H	H	M	H	H

FITNESS BENEFITS OF SELECTED SPORTS

H–High, M–Medium, L–Low, M-H–Depends whether recreation (M) or Vigorous (H)

Sport	C-R Endurance	Muscle Strength				Muscle Endurance				Flexibility			
		Arms	Legs	Abdomen	Back	Arms	Legs	Abdomen	Back	Shoulder	Hip	Elbow	Knee
Track & Field													
a. Sprints	M	M	H	M	M	M	M	M	M	L	H	L	H
b. Middle Distance	H	M	H	M	M	M	H	M	M	L	H	L	H
c. Long Distance	H	M	H	M	M	M	H	H	H	L	H	L	H
d. Marathon	H	M	H	M	M	H	H	H	H	L	H	L	H
e. Walking	H	M	H	M	M	M	H	H	H	L	H	L	H
f. 35 lb. weight throw	L	H	H	M	H	L	L	L	L	M-H	H	H	H
g. Shot Put	L	H	H	M	H	L	L	L	L	M-H	H	H	H
h. Pole Vault	L	H	H	H	H	M	M	M	M	H	H	H	H
i. Triple Jump	L	M	H	H	H	L	L	L	L	M	H	L	H
j. Hurdling	M	M	H	H	H	L	L	L	L	M	H	L	H
k. Discus Throw	L	H	H	M	H	L	L	L	L	M	H	H	H
l. Hammerthrow	L	H	H	M	H	L	L	L	L	H	H	H	H
m. High jump	L	M	H	M	H	L	L	L	L	M	H	L	M
n. Javelin	L	H	H	M	H	L	L	L	L	M-H	H	H	H
o. Long Jump	L	M	H	H	H	L	L	L	L	M	H	L	H
Volleyball	M-H	M-H	M-H	L-M	M	M-H	M-H	M	M	H	M	H	M
Water Polo	M-H	H	M	L-M	L-M	H	H	M-H	M-H	M-H	M	M	M
Water Skiing	M-H	H	M-H	L-M	M	H	H	M-H	M-H	L	M	L	M
Weight Lifting	L	H	H	H	H	L-H	L-H	L-H	L-H	M	M	M	M
Wrestling	H	H	H	H	H	H	H	H	H	M-H	H	H	H

effect of age on performance and the influence of race and physique of sports participation.

Hygiene—Health, diet, vitamin requirements, sleep, fatigue, and drugs and their effect on physical performance are included here.

Pathologies as related to sport

Clinical sports medicine—Included here are the relationships of heart function, exercise therapy, obesity, dermatological problems and other medical knowledge to exercise and sports.

Application of physical medicine to sports—Physical medicine includes exercise therapy as well as heat, light and massage to improve performance.

Surgery and orthopedics—Included is the study of posture, bone structure and all types of sports injuries.

Exercise therapy—This classification takes in the wide scope of exercise as a therapeutic aid in homes, schools and hospitals.

Psychology of sports—Includes the use of psychological devices to improve sports as well as the effect of sports on the personality of the participant.

Girls and women in sports—This includes the effects of body culture and the hygienic and aesthetic effects of sports on the female.

Techniques of training—This category incorporates the physiological principles underlying training and the effects it produces.

Pedagogy of sports—The best methods and techniques of teaching sports to all ages and classes.

The trainer—The responsibilities and limitations of the trainer and the procedures and techniques he can use.

Tests and measurements in sports and sports medicine—The measurement of speed, strength, endurance and other athletic capacities.

Research in sports medicine—Although there are research problems inherent in every general area of sports

medicine, this catch-all category includes the basic research that is being conducted by the world's scientists and medical personnel.

General and miscellaneous—Various publications, including periodicals, textbooks and records are included here.

SPOT EXERCISES

Spot exercising is the process of attempting to overcome a physical problem of one area of the body. Many people ask medical doctors, physical therapists, and physical educators: "How can I firm up my flabby thighs?" "What can I do for my weak back?" "How can I build up or maintain my physique or figure?" Those are questions that plague many of us. There are numerous misconceptions about the benefits of spot exercising; many have persisted for years and are difficult to eliminate.

Spot exercises are performed for one of three reasons: to reduce body measurements, to increase body measurements, or to strengthen a weak area.

Spot Exercises to Reduce Body Measurements

The underlying concept in reducing body measurements is that the caloric outgo (energy consumption) must exceed the caloric intake (food consumption). For example, assuming that you are presently maintaining your weight, you have balanced your caloric outgo and caloric intake. To make the caloric outgo exceed the caloric intake, you can do one of three things: (1) you may increase your activity level (caloric outgo) without increasing your caloric intake; (2) you may decrease your caloric intake without increasing your activity level; or (3) you may increase your activity level and decrease your caloric intake. If you eliminated 100 calories a day by any of those methods, the result would be a 10-pound loss a year.

When the caloric outgo exceeds the caloric intake, the result is a loss of body fat; for in weight loss, the fat is the first to go. Interestingly, fat comes off the areas of greatest concentration such as the hips, thighs and abdomen.

Effective spot reducing then, requires that the exercises be of sufficient intensity and duration to cause a metabolism of the fat. For example, if you weighed 150 pounds and were going to do a series of sit-ups to reduce the girth of your abdomen, it would be necessary for you to do 20 sit-ups a minute for 25 minutes to burn up 100 calories. Yet if you walked for 20 minutes or ran for about 8 minutes, you would achieve the same effect!

Since exercises or activities such as cycling, walking, running, jogging and swimming are more efficient and perhaps more enjoyable for reducing girth measurements, what good are spot exercises? Spot exercises are effective in firming up the musculature underneath the fat so that when the fat disappears there is nice definition of the muscle that contributes greatly to an attractive appearance. And spot exercising may be effective in reducing girth measurements if it's poor muscle tone causing the protruding stomach. The improvement in the musculature of the abdomen will undoubtedly help to hold or push the abdominal viscera and organs in their proper place, thereby reducing the girth measurement. Likewise, the protrusion may cause a sway back condition that will give the appearance of a pot belly.

Spot Exercises for the Abdomen

1. Abdominal Compression—Stand and retract your abdomen as much as possible. Attempt to suck your stomach to your backbone. A variation is to lie on the floor and perform the same exercise.

2. Abdominal Curl—Lie flat on your back and, keeping your lower back in contact with the floor, curl your head and upper part of your body forward and upward. Return slowly to the starting position by lowering your upper trunk and body to the floor.

3. Rowing Curl—Assume a supine position with the arms extended overhead. Then sit up, curl your head, arms and upper back toward the legs. At the same time, raise your legs to the upper body, so that you are sitting up with your knees next to your shoulder and your arms partly extended at the sides of the knees. Then return to a supine position.

4. V-Seat—Start by sitting on the floor with your hands interlocked behind the head and your legs fully extended. Lean back until your legs are slightly off the floor and you are balanced on your buttocks. Hold that position for several seconds. Then return.

5. Sit-up—Interlace your fingers behind your head while lying on your back. Put your heels close to your buttocks with your knees together. Get a partner to hold your feet or lock your feet underneath some sturdy object. In that position, attempt to sit up so that your chest or shoulder touches your knees.

6. Side Lying Sit-ups—Assume a side-lying position on the floor. Have a partner hold your feet down. Place your arms above your head, or place your bottom arm under your head and the top arm across your chest. Attempt to sit up sideways. At first, you may find the exercise very difficult. Be content with coming up just a few inches. As the muscles are strengthened, you will be able to raise up higher. Repeat on the other side.

7. Side Leg Raiser—Lying full length on your left side with your head resting in your left hand, rapidly whip your right leg up and down as high as possible. If that is too strenuous, do not whip the leg but perform

gradually. As your condition improves, you can progress to supporting your body with only your left foot and left hand. Repeat to the other side.

8. Knees-up—Lie on floor on your back, with your knees bent and feet flat on the floor. Raise your knees to your chest, while lifting your hips off the floor. Return to the starting position.

Spot Exercises for Increasing Size

Research has indicated that if a muscle is adequately overloaded, it will increase in size (hypertrophy) and in strength. The maximum increase in strength and size, however, is limited by heredity. The process is reversible; for when there is no longer an overload, the muscle will lose its strength and size. If you are interested in building up muscles, weight training is an excellent technique. See WEIGHT TRAINING.

Spot exercises can also be used to develop the strength of a muscle that may have decreased as a result of being in a cast or immobilized for a long period of time. For related discussions, see EXERCISES, MUSCLE, SKELETAL, OVERLOAD, STRENGTH and TRAINING.

Spot Exercises for Strengthening a Weak Area

Spot exercises are particularly effective in helping a person improve weak musculatures. A person who has weak arm and shoulder muscles will find it helpful to select specific exercises to improve the weak musculature. See also RECONDITIONING.

SQUASH

Squash is a fast, demanding sport, offering a complete workout in a matter of minutes. Because of the need for a four-walled court, however, it tends to be confined to private clubs, colleges and universities which can provide the adequate playing space.

Furthermore, squash has an elaborate system of rules, swinging procedures, and game strategy that are essential for play. Few high schools and athletic clubs provide such training in squash, which explains why the sport is not universally accepted.

Each player uses a long handled racquet to hit a soft rubber ball against a four-walled court. Only two or four players can play at one time.

After tossing for service, the server stands with one or both feet inside either service box. The ball must hit the front wall above the cut line without bouncing first; it may fall into the opposite half of the court or hit either of the other three walls on the way.

If the serve is a fault, the receiver may either play the ball if he feels he may gain an advantage or order another serve. If the second serve is a fault, the service passes to his opponent. The receiver may hit the ball any time after it has struck the front wall, but the ball may not bounce on the floor more than once. It must be returned to the front wall between the play line and the out of court line either directly or via any other walls and must not touch the floor. Play continues until one player fails to return the ball. If the server wins the rally, he gains one point, changes sides and serves again. If the receiver wins the rally, he becomes the server but does not score a point. The first player to reach 15 points is the winner, except when the score is 13 or 14 all; then the receiver may decide to play to either 15, 17 or 18. A match is usually the best of 5 games.

The game is excellent for the development of cardio-respiratory endurance, especially between two players of equal skill. It requires great agility because the ball travels extremely fast from side to side as well as from the back and front court. Arm, shoulder and wrist strength are required together with shoulder flexibility.

* SQUASH PROGRAM **

Chart 1	Chart 2
1. 5 minutes	1. 33 minutes
2. 10 minutes	2. 35 minutes
3. 13 minutes	3. 38 minutes
4. 15 minutes	4. 40 minutes
5. 20 minutes	5. 43 minutes
6. 23 minutes	6. 45 minutes
7. 25 minutes	7. 48 minutes
8. 28 minutes	8. 50 minutes
9. 30 minutes	9. 55 minutes

* See ENDURANCE and ENERGY COST OF ACTIVITIES for an explanation of the charts.

**Doesn't include rest periods, time outs, etc.

Fitness 1

If you achieved a score of poor or low average on the *Harvard Step Test* or a score of very poor or poor on the *12 Minute Run*, start on Chart 1-Level 1 and spend 1 week at each level until Chart 2-Level 9 is reached. It is recommmended that you participate 4 to 5 days a week. When Chart 2-Level 9 is reached, 4 days a week is sufficient.

Fitness 2

If you achieved a score of high average on the *Harvard Step Test* or fair on the *12 Minute Run*, start on Chart 1-Level 4. Spend 1 week on Chart 1-Levels 4, 5, 7, and 9, and Chart 2-Levels 2, 4, 6, 8, and 9. It is recommended that you participate 4 to 5 days a week. When Chart 2-Level 9 is reached, 4 days a week is sufficient.

Fitness 3

If you achieved a score of good or excellent on either the *Harvard Step Test* or *12 Minute Run*, continue your current program or select Chart 2-Level 9 as your level of participation. Four days a week is sufficient.

There are two opposing schools of thought on the best training techniques. One emphasizes skills practice, the other cardio-respiratory fitness. The former suggests that as you practice the skills during a game, sufficient endurance is gradually built up. The other favors a program of endurance training similar to long distance runners. Possibly a blend of the two extremes would prove the better method for the above-average player.

General flexibility exercises (particularly for the back and shoulders) are also recommended. You may also benefit from racquet swinging, together with exercises designed to strengthen the wrist and fingers.— *Colin P. Davey*

Associations:

U. S. Squash Racquets Assn., 200 E. 66th St., New York, N. Y. 10021.

National Intercollegiate Squash Racquets Association (NSRA), c/o C. C. Chaffee, Williamstown, Massachusetts 01267.

National Squash Tennis Association (NSTA), 200 Park Avenue, New York, New York 10017.

United States Women's Squash Racquets Association (USWSRA), 42 Dudley Lane, Milton, Massachusetts 02186.

Since squash is a high-energy-cost activity, it may be used to help improve your fitness level, especially your circulo-respiratory and muscle endurance. Below is a squash training program that takes into account the important principles of training.

If you desire to improve your strength and power for the activity, see WEIGHT TRAINING and ISOMETRICS. The weight training and isometrics exercises may also be used to prepare your body for athletic competition.

STALENESS IN TRAINING AND RACING

The human organism, as expressed in human individuality, varies to a remarkable degree. There are some athletes, of whom Dan Waern of

Sweden and Wes Santee of the U.S.A. are typical, who can deliver a high performance, week after week, and month after month, sometimes competing on world class levels, setting world records, and occasionally racing as often as three times in a week. Other athletes, Roger Bannister being a typical and self-expressed example, have said it is only possible to obtain world-class performances three or four times a year.

That statement suggests that some athletes have a capacity for efforts sustained at a high level of performance that some other athletes do not have. As an example, Herb Elliott, the great Australian miler, even if he raced weekly, could arouse himself so that, he was never beaten in the 1500 meter race. Furthermore, he never avoided a race in order to keep his record intact. In his short career, Elliott accepted the challenge of all-comers, and *always won!* Staleness never interfered with his endeavors. Elliott instinctively understood the necessity for change and variety. While being a dedicated athlete in his attitude to training, and above all, to racing, he would instinctively understand the necessity to "give it all away," to forget athletics, and to remove himself for a day, or a week, from the daily grind of training and racing.

Here, then, is the key to staleness. Staleness is both physical and mental since, in the ultimate, the two are one.

An athlete will become "stale," or lose strength, power, speed, incentive and the capacity to dominate and to excel, when his bodily cells become jaded, tired and bored with the ceaseless effort thrust upon them.

The feelings of fatuity, of lack of drive, of lack of the desire to excel or win are both physical and mental. They are the result of the over-exercise of the will, of the driving of the physical, the heart, lungs and legs beyond capacity.

When the athlete runs within his ultimates and without the extreme pressures, when he is not subjected to the demands of ambitious coaches, officials or promoters, he will not become stale.

Staleness is the result of being pushed, either by personal or outside pressures, to a point beyond which the athlete can respond. It is a kind of physical and mental satiety mixed with boredom. Life and excelling has ceased to have meaning. It is Nature's way of telling you to let-up, to change, to add some variety or other experiences.

The symptoms are easily recognized: lassitude; lack of desire; an indifference to our fate, or future; a loss of weight; a loss of interest in food.

You may not know what is wrong. You may claim to feel O.K. but are irritable. No suggestions or urges please you. Life and athletics have come to a standstill. You are alive but feel half dead. What then is the cure for staleness? Certainly emphatically it is not by an overdose of training nor of will or dedication.

The cure is by a giving away to an abandonment, for the time, of all that you desired.

After all, acceptance is as important as determination.

So, we conclude, staleness is due to pushing the physical and mental processes of an athlete to a point greater than what the athlete can sustain. It occurs when the whole organism, physical and mental, has been submitted to stresses that cannot be indefinitely sustained. The cure is a partial, or temporarily complete, cessation of all the activities that induced the condition, whether those be conditioning, training or racing.—*Percy Wells Cerutty*. See OVERTRAINING.

STRENGTH

A muscle has the possibility of working in two different ways. The contraction of the muscle can be an isometric contraction, that is, the muscle develops only tension without changing the length of the muscle; or an isotonic contraction, the muscle changes its length, indicating work in the physical sense (work = strength × way). Each movement is a mixture of isometric and isotonic contraction. In practice, there is never a real isotonic contraction. On the other hand, sometimes you can find a typical isometric contraction. That is a compression of the blood vessels during contraction of muscle fibers; causing the blood flow to stop. Oxygen cannot go into the muscle. Lactic acid in the muscle arises, and the result is a very fast fatigue of the muscle. In isotonic contraction, contraction time and rest periods change; the optimal is a relation from 1:1. In the rest period, new oxygenized blood can go into the muscle. The muscle can work much longer than in isometric contractions.

In the histological sense, the different muscles in the body do not have the same structure in their cells. Red and white fibers are mixed in a muscle and different in relation. A muscle may be dynamic (isotonic), like the muscles of the arms and legs; or static (isometric), like the muscles of the trunk. It seems that the mixture of red and white cells does not have to be the same in different peoples.

Strength is directly correlated to the cross section of a muscle. Here are some physiological facts of strength.

(1) The strength of the muscle shows a relationship to the muscle length. In most muscles, it is in a relation 1:3, up to 1:4.

(2) The muscle strength in the same man is different from muscle group to muscle group.

(3) The muscle strength is related to the cross section of the muscle. For the voluntary isometric muscle contraction, 1 cm² = 4 kp. 4 kp is the psychological value for maximal muscle strength.

(4) The absolute muscle strength (physiological) is about 6 kp per 1 cm². The difference in strength between the relative and absolute strength, divided by the "mobilization-border," is available only in stress-situations.

(5) The "mobilization-border" can be moved, for example, in the training of the athletes. It seems to be a psychological influence.

(6) The fatigue in muscle is primarily connected in the central nervous system and not in the muscle itself.

(7) The muscle strength in women, in average, is about ⅔ of the men.

(8) The difference in muscle strength between male and female is related to the trainings conditions of the muscles and the use of the muscle in the daily life in relation to their muscle capacity. The difference in masticate muscles is relatively small (about 20%) and relatively high in the lower arm flexors and extensors (about 45%).

(9) There is also a direct relationship between muscle strength and age. The highest strength in man equals 100% at age 20-30. In youngsters, there is no difference between girls and boys. Then the strength in boys increases very fast, until about 20 years of age, there is a steady period between 20-30 years of age; and then the strength starts to drop. At 60 years, the strength in the male is about the same as at 14 years. In youth, the strength increases, without special training, about 5% from year to year. The strength in girls also increases but slower than in boys.

Those facts are true to the "normal" strength, or the strength build up in relation to the "normal" daily life. According to the studies by Morpurgo in 1897, strength training resulted in muscle hypertrophy, which means the cross section of the muscle fibers of the muscle increased. A short time ago, van Linge and Reitsma demonstrated that in muscle training both hypertrophy and hyperplasia—the increase in the number of muscle fibers —take place. Reitsma found hyperplasia effects when the diameter of muscle fibers is higher than 20-50. Furthermore, they found that, in training, the number of blood capillaries also increased.

As reported by Peder, Petow and Siebert and the review by DeLorme and Watkins in 1945, there are three important points regarding strength training:

1. Increase in muscle strength can be accomplished by a few repetitions against strong resistance.

2. Increase in performance of the circulatory system can be accomplished by many repetitions against slight resistance.

3. The two methods are not interchangeable; one cannot replace the other.

The biological law of training for all systems in the body is the same; the training stimulus has to be greater than their usual daily use.

In 1953, the first paper in the field of muscle training, by Hettinger and Muller, tried to answer three primary questions in relation to the adequate training stimulus.

A muscle tension or strength of about 40-50% of the maximum obtainable was enough to produce the maximum training effect. Using a training strength between 30-40% of the maximum strength in a voluntary isometric muscle contraction resulted in a lower training effect, and using only 20-30% of the maximum showed no change at all in muscle strength. The indication is that the 20-30% of muscle strength is about equal to the muscle tension used in daily activity. If the training strength is lower than 20% of the maximum strength, a decrease in muscle strength was found.

Those studies demonstrated that, in the physiological sense, a muscle tension of 40-50% of the maximum gives the maximal training effect obtainable.

Nevertheless, in electromyograph studies made by Stoboy et al., it was indicated by training experiments that the economy to training by maximum strength will be higher than training by lower muscle tension. Therefore, muscle training with maximal contractions seems to be more successful.

It is unnecessary to train to the point of complete muscular fatigue in order to achieve increased muscle strength. That statement has been supported by findings in experiments with athletes, who rarely push themselves to the point of complete fatigue in training. A muscle contraction of about 20-30% of the possible maximum duration will achieve the maximal training effect obtainable. On the other hand, very short contractions such as in ordinary reflexes do not show any effect in increasing muscle strength. A contraction held for a certain length of time seems to be necessary to start the chemical condition for increasing muscle strength.

What is the number of training stimuli necessary for the maximal training effect? Studies have shown that one training period in 14 days does not appear to increase muscle strength. One training stimulus per week, provides about 35-40% of the maximum training effect. A training stimulus, given once a day, shows about 85% of the maximal training effect obtainable; and about 5 training stimuli per day gives 100%, the maximal training effect obtainable. Josenhans has given up to 600 training stimuli daily, but the effect is according to 1 training stimulus per day. It looks as if the muscle, after one training stimulus, is unresponsive to the next stimulus for about the next 24 hours. On the other hand, if the time between 2 training stimuli is more than one day, the training effects diminish.

Therefore, for an isometric exercise to be effective in increasing muscle strength the exercise must:

1. exert about 40-50% of maximum isometric tension
2. be held for about 20-30% of the time required to produce complete muscle fatigue, and
3. be repeated five times each day to give the optimal training effect.

A maximal, voluntary isometric muscle contraction can be held about 10-15 sec., which means that for a muscle strength training, the muscle contraction should be held at maximum strength for not more than about three seconds.

In atrophied muscles, the training effect is about four to five times greater than in normal muscles; while in athletes with extremely hypertrophied muscles, the effect is much lower than in normal muscles. Furthermore, there is a large variation in training effect on the different muscle groups in the same individual. The lowest effect is in finger flexors, in lower leg extensors and so on; on the other hand, trunk flexors and extensors and foot extensors show a very high training effect.

The trainability can change from man to man according to their daily activity in their job. In athletes, however, most muscle groups resulted in a high strength standard. That means the training effect must be lower than in "usual" people.

In studying the reasons for the relationship of trainability in limb muscles to age and sex, researchers have found a parallelism in the production of male sex hormones and trainability. In experiments with animals—as in human experiments, the positive effect of male sex hormones, in the form of testosterone, was proved. In animal experiments, it was possible to demonstrate clearly that in training, following the application of sex hormones, the mass of muscle protein increased at the same rate as the increase in the cross section of the muscle. The percentage of muscle fat was lowered. The weight of muscle increased, also the cross section of muscle fibers and the number of nuclei.

In human experiments in older men from 65-75 years of age, the training effect was two-three times higher after giving testosterone during a training session than in "normal" conditions. Here the question arises, is it possible to increase the trainability of muscles in athletes with male sex hormones? The demonstrated effect in trainability by giving testosterone is called an anabole effect of the sex hormones. It is evident in older men, in whom production by their own glands is reduced. In younger men, giving testosterone by injection, the anabole effect can change in a katabole (negative) effect. Giving a patient male sex-hormones has to be ordered by a physician in a pathological case.

In many athletes, strength training by isometric muscle contractions takes place as an important part of the whole training program. The reason for promoting isometric muscle training is that it gives more efficient training. Without strength, a high performance in most sports is not possible. Even though strength is only one part, it is as important as the training of the circulatory system or the nervous system. The short time of training that is needed in isometric muscle training makes more time available for training the other systems of the body. Isometric muscle training can be done without special equipment and does not require any space. That means it can be performed by athletes in their home, next to the normal training program. It can be done by our youngsters at school, if it is rainy weather and they cannot go on the playground. It can be done while traveling in a train or plane, or when sitting in meetings, without being noticeable to other people.

With tensing the muscles, primarily the extensor muscles, a stimulus is given—via nervous system—to the cerebrum next to the hypothalamus, in the area of the center of regulation sleep and awake. That stimulus is an awake stimulus, making one more alert. This is demonstrated in dogs and cats which, on arousing from sleep, stretch their legs for a few seconds and then are fully awake. Isometric muscle training should be done with maximal voluntary isometric muscle contraction against a resistance, given by other muscle groups or equipment. Maintain the contraction for about 3 seconds, for each of the muscle groups. No abrupt contractions should be done. Furthermore, there is no need for stopping ventilation; breathe in usual way. Isometric muscle training is the optimal method to make muscle strength, but it will be impossible to make an athlete by only training the muscles isometrically. Only the best condition of all the body systems, in relation to another, will give the best result in sports and in "usual" life. The atrophy of one of your body systems has a negative effect on your physical fitness. All of your body systems are important in the same way.—*T. Hettinger*

STRESS

Life is stressful yet stress is part of enjoyable living. Physical fitness contributes to enjoyable living; however, stress results from physical exertion and is generally considered antagonistic to living enjoyably. The physical, social and psychological facets of living each contribute to a stressful life. Without those multinumerous stressors, life would be nothing more than a negative, dull existence. By his own initiative, man has self-imposed a very pressurized, tension-filled life. His struggle to achieve a mechanized, technically easier existence while attempting to hustle through more than twenty-four hours of living in a single day signifies continual confrontation with stress.

Physical fitness, though a stressor itself, actually can combat the effects of many tension sources by serving as a diversion and by strengthening the body through adaptation at a higher fitness level.

A simple, meaningful definition of stress explains stress as the process of exposure to physical, psychic, and social pressures of life with resulting physiological and psychological alterations known as aging. Regardless of the exact meaning assigned to stress, it is ever present; and everyone must cope with it to varying degrees.

Sources

Sources of tension and stress pressure arise from many phases of life which range from chronic and gradual to acute and violent. Social interactions such as crowded city living or rejection from a peer group; emotional involvement in various situations by fearing, hating or loving; environmental alterations in temperature, altitude or humidity; and physical activity during work or play represent only a cross section of possible stressors. Those or similar stresses can individually or collectively be acting upon a person at any one time.

The rookie, major league pitcher striving to hurl his first win on a hot, July afternoon before a crowded stadium is a complex, stress-packed panorama. At various times, everyone is confronted with a similar quantity of stress as the major league rookie, even though the quality may be somewhat lacking. The weekend athlete or the physical fitness advocate is often subjecting himself to a combination of stressors.

Symptoms

The feelings of extreme alertness, a tight, unreceptive stomach, and uneasiness are usual preactivity symptoms which indicate the presence of stress. Often the early indications of stress are indistinct and difficult to distinguish.

Physical adjustments in preparation for "fight or flight" closely precede stress; namely, an elevated heart rate and respiration rate, a concomitant increase in blood flow and blood sugar, and a shift in blood flow from the viscera and skin to the skeletal muscles. Those changes are associated with the increased activity of the adrenal glands as they release adrenalin into the blood stream. A complete blood count examination would reveal an increase in red blood cells, platelets, and an increase in all white blood cells except the eosinophiles which mysteriously disappear during stress exposure. Recently, researchers have noted the reduction and sometimes complete absence of eosinophiles in the blood of fatigued athletes, especially those who have been under considerable stress. They have concluded that the eosinophile count serves as a fairly reliable indicator of the exposure to stress although the exact mechanism causing their disappearance remains uncertain. Generally speaking, metabolism is temporarily elevated during stress exposure.

Following exposure to tension and emotional pressures, a person is sometimes left with a headache and a feeling of tiredness and loss of weight. The proportion of those feelings are in direct relationship with the length and degree of stress exposure.

As a result of long term stress from a single cause or a combination of sources, subtle but far reaching effects are experienced. The adrenal cortex, or outside portion of the kidneys, hypertrophies due to its overactivity in manufacturing adrenalin. Lymphatic tissue tends to shrink during stress exposure. Thirdly, ulcerations of the intestinal walls appear as a result of increased acidity. Selye has identified the dramatic changes as the triad response.

Stress and Physical Fitness

The achievement of physical fitness necessitates physical and psychological stress. As the fitness participant physically indulges, dramatic physiological and psychic changes, discussed elsewhere in this book, occur which will enable him to withstand normal, daily stresses. Even though he has given up some "wear and tear" as a result of exercise stress, he can now participate in a day's activities with less total wear and tear due to improved physiological efficiency.

Strength and endurance training programs advocate gradual, progressive exposures which will lead to adaptation by the body to a greater strength or endurance level. Selye feels that you inherit a given quantity of "adaptation energy," and when that is depleted, you have aged to the point where death results. Physical fitness permits you to use less adaptation energy per given task, thereby providing for a more efficient usage of the "fuel for living." In other words, stress adaptation results.

A person can change from one stressful environment to another and, as a result, benefit from the switch. The wife-angered husband can gain release and a satisfying diversion by striking a golf ball as he engages in a game of golf. The businessman, involved with pressurized decisions, can find diversion through the stress of a handball game during his lunch hour. Following the change of stress, i.e., diversionary activity, the participant usually finds himself relieved and facing his problems with new vigor, sometimes with a heretofore hidden solution now quite obvious.

Stresses sometimes accumulate to the point where they collectively lead to exhaustion. That occurs when the body fails to adapt. Instead of satisfactorily finding a release through activity, the person retains his tensions from living within himself, and they continue to mount to the point of mental or physical failing adaptation.

Stress Combatants

Many times, rest in the form of sleeping or simply relaxing serves as a means of combating stress, but occasionally more extravagant methods are necessary. As mentioned previously, tension can be alleviated by activity of another type. Usually that works best when some type of mental activity is engaged in to combat physical stress products or by using physical activity to eliminate mental or emotional fatigue. Vacationing or some other way of gaining a restful change of scenery can serve as an effective procedure to combat mental stress. Finally, talking about your problems and bringing them to the surface can alleviate stress symptoms caused by mental strains and tensions. Generally there seems to be two means of combating stress, depending upon its nature. Physical activity works best to attack mental and emotional tension, and rest and relaxation are most effective in fighting physical stress.

A general plan of attacking stress is to strike a balance between work and play, slow down your speed of living and occasionally loaf a little. The plan can achieve remarkable success by cultivating the habit of participating in restful and diversionary activities. Likely opportunities occur in the evenings and weekends when you can pursue a hobby or give attention to your own children.

Note how children are very capable of obtaining release from stress with their knack of alternating rest with play activities. Unfortunately society forces a life of continual stress with "hurry-up" being the password. In retaliation, it would be wise to rebel and periodically revert to acceptable child-type rest and play activities as a means of achieving a fuller and richer life.—*Alan J. Stockholm*

SURFING

Not many years ago, the super sport of surfing was restricted to the Hawaiian Islands and a few miles of sloping coastline in southern California. But now, with the acceptability of East Coast surfing and the radical "scoop nosed" boards for small surf, at least a million people are enjoying this healthy form of recreation. And although you must be in excellent physical shape to surf, the sport itself supplemented with a bedroom exercise course will bring the very fitness you need.

Just as water skiing is not limited to those who can safely navigate the tough racing slopes, surfing offers benefits to the beginner, the intermediate and the expert. Actually, the beginner has more available surf and surfing areas than the intermediate or top surfer because any breaking wave, no matter how small or shapeless, will present a challenge for the first months.

There is no question that the teenage male dominates the surfing scene, but the popular surfing magazines are continually sketching profiles of many successful business and professional men who surf. *Newsweek* magazine reported recently that over one million Americans were riding the breakers. The progressive popularity and the surfers' desire to share enthusiasm, plus thousands of miles of available coastline linked by high speed freeways to the cities, promise to rank surfing along with other sports that do not require an opponent. Years ago skiing may have held that distinction, but since the introduction of the T-bar tow and lifts, its benefits do not compare to the exercise the surfer gets paddling out through the swells.

Fitness Features

First and most important is the general overall tone-up that occurs during the surfing hours. The emphasis is directed toward the entire respiratory system. The effort required to lay flat or kneel on the board and paddle through the incoming set of waves can be compared to sprinting. While surfing in a moderate to large surf, it is important to move the board quickly in the relative calm between large sets. Too slow and the surfer, already nearly exhausted, is caught in the "soup," or white water of a large breaking wave, and is wiped off his board. To avoid that occurrence, surfers stretch their lungs and shoulders in a last possible effort to dash up and over the face of the last wave before it breaks. Reaching the safety outside the "line," they can sit and catch their breath before

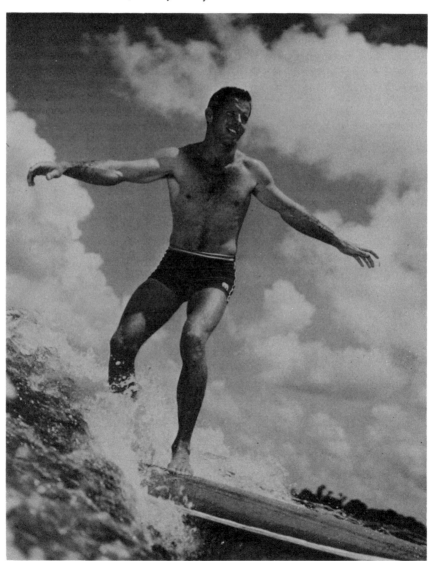

To the beginning surfer, any breaking wave presents a challenge.

selecting the right wave for the speedy ride back.

During the paddle out, all of the back, chest, shoulder and arm muscles are stretched in the lying position as the back is arched for greater paddling leverage. One of the generally accepted tests for overall fitness is to lie on your stomach, feet pinned to the floor and fingers laced behind your neck. The test requires that you raise your chin until it is 18 inches from the floor. Surfers will have no difficulty passing that one. A stretching of the lower back muscles is also an excellent relief from tensions—another reason why business and professional men can benefit from the sport.

Take a brief look at the major muscles that are helped by surfing.

1. Arm—The triceps in the upper arm get some benefit paddling, but the real test comes during the fast push-up to jump to your feet.

2. Forearm—The flexors and extensors work hard to grip the rail, especially during the wrist action which occurs while paddling.

3. Chest—The pectorals really get a buildup from paddling both in the kneeling and lying position. Most surfers become quite muscular through the whole chest region.

4. Shoulders—The deltoids and the trapezius along with the triceps of the upper arm become very well developed, strong, lithe and sinewy. This whole upper back, neck and shoulder area takes the bulk of paddling work and derives the most benefit.

5. Lower Back—This region needs exercise to prevent back trouble that comes with aging. The muscle set is called *erector spinae,* and surfing keeps them strong and supple.

6. Respiratory System—To a surfer, paddling is much like a runner's sprinting, and the demands on lungs are strong. Circulatory and respiratory systems are taxed forcibly.

7. Legs and Thighs—They are probably not helped too much by surfing,

although there is some benefit from the balancing exercises which occur during the ride.

The surfing enthusiast who is interested in an all-round conditioning program must supplement his surfing activities with a few leg exercises. The leg muscles receive a brief isometric-type workout during the ride as the surfer seeks continuous control of the board, but it is not sufficient to keep the legs in good shape.

Balance, another standard measurement of overall fitness is, of course, a constant part of surfing. The lightning-fast adjustments that the body must accomplish to maintain it contributes to overall body tone.

It's Easy to Learn

It is difficult for the beginner to find a teacher, at least on the Northeast Coast, but there really is very little a teacher could help you with anyway. The best way to start is to watch other surfers and try to judge their wave timing. The next step is to take your board into shallow water and stand right in the area where the white water, or "soup," still has some forward momentum after the waves have broken. Lie flat on the board in front of a small breaking wave and paddle as hard as you can toward the beach. You must develop a bit of your own momentum before the wave hits you. Now, if you are adjusted on the board properly, not too far forward or back, you will have your first surfing thrill—riding into the beach. Even as tame as that is, you'll be amazed at the feeling of speed.

A word about "trimming." If you are too far forward on the board, the nose will go under and you will "pearl," too far back and your board will just wallow. The wave won't push you anywhere at all. The correct trim varies from board to board and with the weight and height of the surfer. A good starting place to experiment is with the nose of your board only about one inch out of the water. After you've "bellied in" a few times, try to jump to your feet. Some surfers try kneeling as an interim step. However, that practice may develop the bad habit of dragging a knee when a fast "kip up" is necessary to control the board on the crest of larger waves. You keep moving further and further out into the breaking surf until you are beyond the "line," or where the surf is starting to crest. Then try to get "locked" onto the smooth face of a wave just before it breaks; and by control of speed and direction, stay just ahead of the "soup." Again just like our beginner, the speed of the board increases as the surfer moves toward the nose; and the board slows as the surfer moves back toward the tail.

One of the most talked about small surf maneuvers is to "hang ten," that is to put all ten toes over the nose of the board while "locked" in the curl of the wave, or "tube," without "pearling." It requires a good amount of speed and control. Conversely, the surfer can stop, or "kick out" of a wave, by stepping back into the tail-block of the board. There are a lot of other small surf maneuvers. The performance of the whole group is referred to as "hot-dogging."

Just as in any active sport, people get hurt surfing. The most prevalent injuries occur when surfers get hit with their own board or fall on it. A loose board in the water also represents a potential danger and, even in the small surf, can leave nasty bruises. Never stand between a breaking wave and a surfboard and never let go of your board in the water if you can help it. However, when you do fall, try to stay clear of your board.

The other dangers are really more likely to occur with improper conditioning before surfing. Anyone contemplating surfing should run through this 10-minute exercise program every day for at least a month before starting.

1. Sit-ups—30. (Make sure that the back curls on the way up.)
2. Chin Lifts—10. (Lie on stomach—fingers laced behind head—lift chin from floor.)
3. Push-ups—15.
4. Jump-ups—30. (Lie on stomach—jump to feet as quickly as possible by any means without touching knee to floor.)
5. Jog ½ mile with a heavy sprint at the end, or run in place 400 steps, counting each time the left foot hits as one complete step, lifting feet at least 4 inches high.
6. Deep breathing and breath holding. Try to develop the ability to hold your breath for ever-lengthening periods of time. That, of course, can be practiced any time during the day.

Surfing demands health. Yet the hours spent surfing and preparing to surf can bring you into the peak of condition in an enjoyable and thrilling way.—*Robert Horstman*

Association:

United States Surfing Association, P. O. Box 59, Redondo, California 90277.

SWIMMING

Don't miss the fun and fitness of swimming. Even if you've never learned water skills, it's not too late to get in the swim of things.

Here is a fitness through swimming program based on 3 principles which are being used to develop swimming champions. Of course, gold medals aren't promised, but you'll probably feel better than you have in years.

Principle No. 1. An adequate warm-up prior to vigorous physical activity improves performance and reduces the possibility of injury.

While you're not trying to break any records, you will find swimming more enjoyable if you warm up properly. Swimming is not a high-injury activity, but pulled muscles can result from unaccustomed exercise. A warm-up for any vigorous exercise should elevate body temperature and stretch muscles. Stretching is especially important when the activity involves quick movement. But since you will be starting out slowly—no racing yet!—concentrate only on raising body temperature. That is done either by standing in a warm shower for several minutes prior to swimming, or simply getting into the pool and swimming slowly.

Principle No. 2. Cardiovascular and respiratory efficiency can be regained through a graduated exercise program.

Put another way, a fitness through swimming program can help regain some of that zip and go you've lost if you have been living a sedentary life. Tests on middle-aged men by Dr. Thomas K. Cureton, professor of physical education at the University of Illinois, showed that vigorous swimming drills can help lower pulse rates, improve breath-holding ability, improve leg and strength endurance and reduce body fat. The men swam 50 minutes per day, 6 days a week for 8 weeks. If you spend less time than that, you will reduce your benefits. That is only natural. But, remember that any time spent will produce gains that are worthwhile.

One final word before starting your own swimming program. If you are going to have to force yourself to do it just to become fit—forget it. Find yourself another sport or activity. Swimming, like any other exercise, should be pleasurable with the fitness benefits being a by-product.

Don't overdo it the first few times and especially the first day. If you haven't swum for years, do just one length of a standard pool slowly and use your best stroke. Most indoor pools are 25 yards long, but outdoor public or private pools may be much longer. Check with your lifeguard if you're not certain about the length. If you have a backyard pool, it's probably 10

yards long. So perhaps two lengths would be just right.

It will make a difference, of course, how often you swim. Daily activity is best but significant gains can be attained by swimming 2 or 3 times a week.

For the first 4 weeks add about 10 yards to your distance each day. That is about a half length of the standard pool and one length of your backyard pool. After the fourth week you can begin to add 25 yards each time you swim. Remember, at that point in your program, increased distance is your objective, not speed.

If certain muscles really get tired as you increase your distance, try changing strokes at the end of each lap or two. You'll bring different muscles into use and get some relief for those under stress.

Setting Up Goals

Your immediate goal should be to swim 450 yards, changing strokes when necessary. Eighteen lengths of a 25-yard pool equals 450 yards. Your second objective is to swim the same distance using just one stroke. That stroke should be the one which requires breathing between strokes such as the breast stroke or the overhand crawl stroke. The overhand crawl is more demanding than the breast stroke. That switch to one stroke can be done gradually as in your original buildup to the quarter-mile-plus distance. The added stress imposed by breathing between strokes will help to improve your respiratory efficiency. Eventually, you'll reach a plateau and be able to swim the 450 yards with little difficulty.

Principle No. 3. Once the body has adjusted to a higher level of activity, no further gains in efficiency will occur until new demands are placed on it.

That is the overload principle. Your muscles and your cardio-respiratory systems only respond when they are pushed beyond the accustomed normal load.

To increase the demands upon the body, try swimming the same distance in less time. In swimming 450 yards, a reduction in your total time of one or two seconds per week is a substantial improvement. Do that by increasing your speed or pace slightly in the last 25 to 50 yards. A word of caution —don't try to be a Don Schollander as you start that first lap or two, or you will become too tired to complete the 450 yards.

Interval Training

If after a period of weeks you have improved your time for the 450 sufficiently to swim the distance in 12 minutes or less, you're ready for a different type of training.

It's called interval and repetition training—swimming a distance moderately fast, resting, and then repeating the sprint. Because the element of speed is being introduced, you'll want to add stretching exercises to your warm-up.

Here is an appropriate set of exercises. First, stand erect with your hands on your thighs. Swing your arms overhead in a circular motion. Do that slowly at first and then increase your speed slightly. Ten circles are sufficient. Second, place your hands on your hips, bend forward at the waist and rotate your trunk, to the right, back, left and forward again. Repeat the rotations 10 times, starting slowly

and increasing your speed moderately. For the final flexibility exercise, bend forward with knees straight and reach toward your toes. Do that 5 times, reaching just far enough to feel some tightness in the back portion of your lower leg. Don't force it.

You're now ready for the interval and repetition training. First loosen up by swimming 200 yards very leisurely. Next try just one length of the 25-yard pool or two lengths of your backyard pool. The pace should be moderately fast, faster than you've been swimming your 450 laps, but not all out.

Repeat that procedure for a week or two. Then, swim 25 yards, take a 3 minute rest and repeat a second 25 yards. Gradually, over a period of 8 to 10 weeks, add repetitions until you are doing 10 repeats. If on any day you feel uncomfortably tired during your workout, stop. Or if you don't feel up to the interval and repetition training on a given day, swim the 450 at normal pace instead. See INTERVAL TRAINING.

The times listed under No's. 2 and 3 are suggested times for men in the 40-plus age group. You may find you're able to swim faster than that without strain or that it is too fast a pace. It is important to establish your own starting point and then gradually increase the stress on your body. Your body will respond, but not like that of an 18-year-old.

By this time you may feel like chal-

Your workout schedule looks like this:

Time	In a 25-Yard Pool	In a Backyard Pool (10-13 yards)
5 min.	1. Warm-up or flexibility exercises	1. Same
6-8 min.	2. Loosening swim (200 yards)	2. Same
25-35 secs.	3. Sprint 1 length	3. Sprint 2 lengths
3 min.	4. Rest	4. Same
25-35 secs.	5. Sprint 1 length	5. Sprint 2 lengths
3 min.	6. Rest	6. Same
	Continue to 10 repetitions	Same

lenging your teenage son to a race. Don't do it! Just enjoy your new-found vigor and keep swimming.—*Richard T. Mackey*

Swimming Competition

In competition, there are four popular strokes. They are the free style, backstroke, breast stroke and butterfly. In meets, the free style events range from 40 yards to 1500 meters. Here a swimmer is allowed to use any technique, but normally the "crawl" is used. The backstroke, breast stroke, and butterfly competition is usually confined to 100 meters or yards and 200 meters or yards.

Competition is held in either 20- or 25-yard indoor pools or Olympic size, 50-meter outdoor pools.

The swimming rules are simple. A starter shooting a pistol begins the race, at which point the swimmers commence. If a performer leaves before the gun is fired, he commits a false start. Three false starts result in disqualification. Other means of disqualification are not using proper stroke, touching a competitor during a race, and not touching the end of the pool on a turn.

There are numerous weight training and isometric exercises that may be used to develop strength and power. See WEIGHT TRAINING and ISOMETRICS.

Techniques that are used for conditioning are INTERVAL TRAINING, FARTLEK TRAINING and REPETITION TRAINING. Sometimes they are used separately or in combination.

Associations:

National Collegiate Athletic Association (NCAA).

Amateur Athletic Union (AAU).

National Federation of State High School Athletic Association (NFSHSAA). See ORGANIZATIONS for addresses of the above.

Since swimming is a moderate high-to very high-energy-cost activity, it may be used to help improve your fitness level, especially your circulorespiratory and muscle endurance. Below is a swimming training program that takes into account the important principles of training.

If you desire to improve your strength and power for the activity, see WEIGHT TRAINING and ISOMETRICS. The weight training and isometrics exercises may also be used to prepare your body for athletic competition.

Here are some of the more popular swimming strokes.

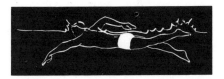

The crawl, above, and the back stroke, below, are good conditioners for the shoulders and the arms.

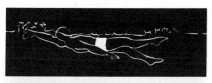

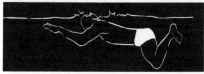

The breast stroke, above, works out the legs and chest, and the side stroke, below, aids the thighs.

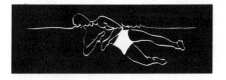

*SWIMMING PROGRAM
Back, Crawl, Breast stroke

Chart 1	Chart 2
1. 2½ minutes (100-150 yds.)	1. 19 minutes (701-750 yds.)
2. 5 minutes (200 yds.)	2. 20 minutes (751-800 yds.)
3. 7½ minutes (300 yds.)	3. 22 minutes (851-900 yds.)
4. 7 minutes (300 yds.)	4. 23 minutes (901-950 yds.)
5. 10 minutes (400 yds.)	5. 25 minutes (951-1000 yds.)
6. 9½ minutes (400 yds.)	6. 26 minutes (1001-1050 yds.)
7. 12½ minutes (500 yds.)	7. 27 minutes (1051-1100 yds.)
8. 15 minutes (600-650 yds.)	8. 29 minutes (1101-1150 yds.)
9. 18 minutes (651-700 yds.)	9. 30 minutes (1151-1200 yds.)

Fitness 1

If you achieved a score of poor or low average on the *Harvard Step Test* or a score of very poor or poor on the *12 Minute Run,* start on Chart 1-Level 1 and spend 1 week at each level until Chart 2-Level 9 is reached. It is recommended that you participate 4 to 5 days a week. When Chart 2-Level 9 is reached, 4 days a week is sufficient.

Fitness 2

If you achieved a score of high average on the *Harvard Step Test* or fair on the *12 Minute Run,* start on Chart 1-Level 2. Spend 1 week on Chart 1-Levels 2, 4, 6, 7, 8 and 9, and Chart 2-Levels 2, 4, 5, 7, and 9. It is recommended that you participate 4 to 5 days a week. When Chart 2-Level 9 is reached, 4 days a week is sufficient.

Fitness 3

If you achieved a score of good or excellent on either the *Harvard Step Test* or *12 Minute Run,* continue your current program or select Chart 2-Level 9 as your level of participation. 4 days a week is sufficient.

*SWIMMING PROGRAM
Side Stroke

Chart 1	Chart 2
1. 3 minutes (100 yds.)	1. 40 minutes (1301-1450 yds.)
2. 6 minutes (200 yds.)	2. 45 minutes (1451-1600 yds.)
3. 9 minutes (300 yds.)	3. 50 minutes (1601-1750 yds.)
4. 12 minutes (400 yds.)	4. 55 minutes (1751-1900 yds.)
5. 15 minutes (500 yds.)	5. 60 minutes (1901-2050 yds.)
6. 20 minutes (600 yds.)	6. 65 minutes (2051-2200 yds.)
7. 25 minutes (700-900 yds.)	7. 70 minutes (2201-2400 yds.)
8. 30 minutes (901-1100 yds.)	8. 75 minutes (2401-2600 yds.)
9. 35 minutes (1101-1300 yds.)	9. 80 minutes (2601-2800 yds.)

Fitness 1

See previous chart.

Fitness 2

If you achieved a score of high average on the *Harvard Step Test* or fair on the *12 Minute Run,* start on Chart 1-Level 2. Spend 1 week on Chart 1-Levels 2, 4, 6, 7, 8, and 9, and Chart 2-Levels 2, 4, 5, 7, and 9. It is recommended that you participate 4 to 5 days a week. When Chart 2-Level 9 is reached, 4 days a week is sufficient.

Fitness 3

See previous chart.

* See ENDURANCE and ENERGY COST OF ACTIVITIES for an explanation of the charts.

TARGET TRAINING

Origin and General Description

Target training is a modern system of fitness training which was first developed by A. S. Lewis at the University of Canterbury (New Zealand) to meet the needs of students. It is now widely used in schools and colleges throughout New Zealand and in some educational institutions in America, Australia and Great Britain. Apart from general fitness training, it is adaptable as a conditioning program for almost any sport.

Its appeal lies in its progressive nature, its economy of apparatus required, its ease of administration, and the sense of personal achievement gained from each performance. It is probably the only system of fitness training where it is possible to record and measure progress from day to day, simply and meaningfully.

The system derives its name from the fact that an attainable "target" in the form of a completion time is established for a standardized set of exercises or workload. The aim is to achieve a fitness level which will enable you to "beat the target." In working toward that level, you will establish further personal targets by recording the time you take to complete the set of exercises and by trying to better that time on the next attempt. Even when you have surpassed the "official" target, your objective will continue to be an improvement of the working time.

Target training is unique in the use of a time factor to achieve progressive overload. Whereas other systems employ greater resistance or increased repetitions, target training uses speed. Just as it is harder to run up stairs than to walk up, it is more difficult to perform any physical work quickly than slowly. Speed is a highly individual and subtly adjusting reflection of fitness. One person may run up a flight of stairs faster than another, but each,

through gains in fitness, can improve on his performance, or, conversely, through trying to improve can make gains in fitness.

The Exercise Program

The original and still most commonly used set of target training exercises contains 18 different exercises and a precise number of repetitions for each in 3 separate grades. A target for the total working time is given for each grade. The three grades and three targets provide for additional incentives, more progressions and a greater scope for individual abilities.

You should commence on the Beginner's level or Light Grade. That level provides a demanding work-load and satisfies the needs of a good level of general fitness. Many, especially those whose training time is limited, do not feel the necessity to progress to the higher and more demanding grades, but step up the intensity and toughness of their conditioning by striving for continued improvement of their working time for the Beginner's Grade.

The Standard or Middle Grade may be attempted after the Target Time for the Beginner's Grade has been bettered at least three times consecutively. Work in that grade is more demanding than for the Beginner's Grade and produces a level of fitness that should provide adequate training for most sports. Probably only the first-class sportsman who has a dedicated attitude toward training will make use of the Super or Heavy Grade.

Instructions for Use:

1. Read the description of each exercise carefully so that you understand it thoroughly.

2. On the first attempt, do not bother about timing, but treat it as a familiarization run-through with only half work loads attempted.

3. Check that all necessary apparatus is ready.

Target Training for Fitness (Indoors)

TARGET TRAINING EXERCISES	Number of Times		
	Beginner	*Standard*	*Super*
1. Running-lengths of gymnasium	30	40	40
2. Climb rope to touch beam	1	2	3
3. Squat with 50 lb. barbell	2 sets of 10	2 sets of 12	2 sets of 18
4. Alternate punch upwards with 7 lb. dumbbells	60	80	100
5. Double skips	15	20	30
6. Backward arch from lying face down	12	15	20
7. Press barbell 50 lbs.	2 sets of 7	2 sets of 10	2 sets of 12
8. Splits jump. Jump from squat, one foot forward	20	30	40
9. Heave to chin bar from arms stretch	8	10	12
10. Standing broad jump (height) plus standard	5xht + 15 in	6xht + 15 in	8xht + 18 in
11. Press-up to arms straight from lying	15	20	25
12. Sit-up from lying on back	20	24	30
13. Step up on double bench	25 each leg	40 each leg	50 each leg
14. Barbell curls 50 lbs.	8	10	15
15. Jump from side to side over medicine ball	20	30	40
16. Duck walking	length	length	length
17. Squat thrust (burpees)	15	20	25
18. Shoot baskets	10	15	20
TARGET TIMES	22 min.	24 min.	26 min.

Enter completion times on score sheet below.

Dates			
Beginner			
Standard			
Super			

4. When ready to commence, start stop watch or note time on wrist watch.

5. Begin with the first exercise—the run. That acts as a warm-up.

6. Perform the exercises in any order, but it is not advisable for similar ones to follow each other, e.g., rope climb and chinning.

7. Complete the full work load or number of repetitions for each exercise before progressing to another exercise even if it means several attempts, e.g., there must be a total of 8 chin-ups even if they cannot be achieved in one attempt.

8. When completely finished, note elapsed time to nearest quarter minute, and record it with date.

9. Try to beat the Target set but, whether attained or not, try to better the previous best time.

Equipment

For a group of 30, the following equipment is sufficient: 1 or 2 hanging ropes, 5 barbells at 50 lbs., 3 or 4 pairs of dumbbells (7-10 lbs.), 5 skipping ropes, 2 or 3 large medicine balls, 4 benches stacked two high (N.Z. school benches are 11 inches high and 10 feet long), 2 or 3 basketballs and 2 basketball backboards, 2 heaving bars for chin-ups, floor area marked in feet and inches for long jump, wall bars for anchoring feet for sit-ups and back arching (bars are desirable but not vital).

Stop watches are necessary. It is best to have several. The whole group can start together using only one watch, or small groups can be started as they arrive, each using a different watch. Individuals may use their wrist watches if they are suitable, i.e., have a sweep second hand.

Description of Exercises

1. Running. Lengths of gymnasium. Run from one end of the gymnasium to the other. The exercise acts as a warm-up and heart-lung conditioner.

2. Climb rope. Climb to touch rope attachment. If you do not have the strength to climb to the top (usually 15-20 feet) you must make one determined attempt and try to climb a little further each time until you succeed. The exercise is for gripping strength, arm and shoulder strength.

3. Squat with barbell. The bar is placed across the shoulders. The feet are slightly apart and kept flat on the floor. The exercise strengthens the quadriceps or thigh extensors.

4. Alternate punch upward. Stand with dumbbells at shoulder level. Stretch first the right and then the left arm upward in a continuous punching movement. The exercise develops strength and endurance of shoulder muscles and arm extensors (triceps).

5. Double skip. That is skipping, turning the rope twice each jump. The exercise develops agility and heart-lung efficiency.

6. Backward arch. Lie face down with hands clasped behind neck. Arch the back by lifting chest and legs off the floor. The exercise strengthens back muscles.

7. Barbell press. Lift the set barbell and stand with the bar under the chin. Raise the bar as high as possible and lower to start position for the required number of repetitions. The exercise develops upper body strength, especially shoulders and arm extensors.

8. Splits jump. Squat with buttocks over heels but with one foot six inches (half a shoe) in front of the other so that nearly all the body weight is over the one foot. Spring upward high enough to permit the body and the legs to stretch straight with the toes pointed downward. Land in deep crouch as for start but with the other foot slightly forward. Spring without pause for the required number of times. Strengthens ankles and knees, develops springing ability and endurance of thigh muscles.

9. Chin-ups. Hang with overgrasp on bar. Pull up until the chin is level with or touches the bar. Lower to full arm extension. This develops arm flexors (biceps) and pulling muscles of the shoulders and back.

10. Standing broad jump. To your height, add the standard (15 inches for beginners). That is the distance you must attempt to clear for the required number of times (5 for beginners). The exercise develops jumping ability and explosive action.

11. Press-ups. From front support (press-up) position, lower the body, held rigidly straight until the upper arm is horizontal. Push up until elbows lock. The exercise develops shoulder, chest, and arm (extensors) strength.

12. Sit-ups. Lie on back with feet anchored slightly apart under the wall bar. Clasp hands behind the neck and sit up to touch the opposite knee and elbow. Return to lying and repeat touching the other knee and elbow. This exercise is for abdominal strength and endurance.

13. Step-ups. Step on to double-stacked bench with the right leg leading. Step down with the right leg leading and continue in a brisk rhythm. Change to the left leg leading after the required number of steps. Strengthens knee joint and thigh mus-

cles. It also increases heart-lung efficiency.

14. Barbell curls. Use the under grasp and hold the bar with your arms extended downward. Bend the elbows to lift the bar under your chin and then try to lift elbows forward before lowering. The exercise strengthens wrists and arm flexors.

15. Jump from side to side. Stand with the medicine ball at the side of your foot. Jump sideways over the ball and back again without rebound or pause. The exercise is useful for strengthening ankles for most sports.

16. Duck walking. Squat on heels and walk the required distance. The exercise strengthens ankles and knee joints.

17. Burpee. Squat with your hands on floor, shoot the feet backwards, jump the feet back to squat, stand up straight. The exercise increases body agility.

18. Shoot baskets. Put the ball through the hoop from any position with any style. The exercise provides light relief. See EXERCISES for a further description of the exercises.

A Challenging Experience

In Target Training, there are easily recognized challenges. First, there is the challenge to complete a varied and demanding exercise program. Second, there is the challenge to better the target time that has been imposed to provide the incentive for improvement. Third, there is the challenge to make a steady improvement on personal best performance irrespective of the Target Time, and, fourth, to progress to a higher grade as a result of improved physical efficiency.

Each exercise provides an amount of work that is well within the capabilities of all. The penalty of loss of time acts as a spur to those who cannot perform all the required number of repetitions in a single attempt. For example, a person who can produce double skips only as single efforts can

before long repeat as many as 20 or 30 in one continuous attempt.

Numerous Target Training programs have been devised to suit various sports, but enough information has been given to enable those interested to devise their own programs using time as the basic principle for creating load and measuring progress. The original program has proved highly suitable for most general conditioning purposes and is particularly attractive to students in colleges and universities. Women as well as men find satisfaction and benefit from use of the Target Training system of improving fitness.—*A. S. Lewis*

TAPERING OFF

A cooling-off period should always follow a workout. The cooling off or tapering off is merely a gradual slowing down from maximum (high) muscle contractions to minimum (low) muscle contractions or from high activity to low activity.

When you are exercising, the heart is pumping blood at a faster rate in order to supply the active muscles with oxygen and life-sustaining nutrients. The blood is pumped into the muscles by the forceful contractions of the heart, but there is no similar force to remove the blood from the muscles to the heart via the veins. The blood, therefore, is pushed back to the heart by means of the "milking action" of the veins. The veins are not as heavily muscled as the arteries and, moreover, are easily compressible. When the veins are filled with blood, the exercising muscles literally massage the vessels and push the blood toward the heart. That is called the milking action. To aid in that process, the veins have valves to help trap the blood as it is pushed back to the heart.

When you immediately stop exercising, the heart continues to pump blood at a vigorous rate to the muscles. But since the muscles are no longer active, there is less action to send the blood back to the heart. The blood then has a tendency to pool in the muscles and veins. By tapering off gradually, you avoid the delay in return of the blood to the heart and aid in helping the body adjust to the new situation of less activity.

The tapering off also allows for proper heart dissipation, or sweating, and avoids cooling off too quickly so that chills do not develop.

Allowing your muscles to cool down gradually by reducing the activity gradually is an excellent means of tapering off. To supplement the lessened activity, you may find it beneficial to take a shower or bath to help taper off.

A hot shower or bath gradually reduced to a cold shower will aid in the cooling down process, the reason being that the more superficial blood vessels constrict because of the cold and force the blood back into the large vessels. That process makes more blood available to circulate throughout the body via those large vessels to the critical organs of the body, i.e., brain, stomach and kidneys.

TENNIS

Tennis can meet the needs and desires of just about anyone. It offers wholesome enjoyment for all ages; a degree of physical activity which can be regulated to the needs of the individual; inexpensive equipment and courts which are usually convenient; only two people needed for a match; universal rules and camaraderie among tennis players; extreme demands on the expert player involving skill, self-discipline, endurance and tactical analysis.

The effect which tennis has on cardiorespiratory endurance will depend on the manner in which you wish to compete. A high degree of cardiorespiratory endurance is demanded for a competitive player. A participant will need to condition his body with activities such as running or rope jumping so that he will be able to withstand the physical demands of a long and difficult match. On the other hand, it is very possible for people to continue playing tennis throughout life with a minimal amount of cardiorespiratory endurance. It is not unusual to see many people over 60 playing tennis with their own level of competition just because they enjoy it.

Tennis itself will not greatly increase your muscular strength, although there is a certain amount of strength necessary in the legs, racket arm and shoulder, and chest. Even though strength is not gained to any great degree through playing tennis, strength will certainly contribute to better tennis play. Most great Australian tennis players have long recognized that fact and included weight-training exercises in their training programs. In better tennis tournaments, the winner is likely to be the player with a com-

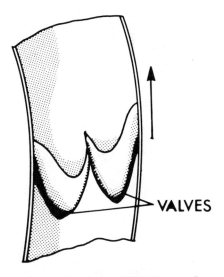

The veins of the body have valves which assist in pushing the blood back to the heart. Tapering off assists the veins and valves to do their job effectively.

bination of superior strength and skill.

Muscular endurance in certain body areas is enhanced through tennis participation. The endurance of the legs will gradually increase as you play more, and the main muscles used in the serve and ground strokes will certainly need muscular endurance in order for you to carry out the given movements as many times as necessary during competition or recreational play. The muscles involved are mainly the triceps, pectorals, deltoids and brachioradialis. The biceps are utilized as a supporting muscle in the forehand and backhand shots, but its flexion movement is not a primary part of tennis strokes. Furthermore, it is very helpful to supplement actual play with an appropriate exercise program for strength and endurance. Many a recreational tennis match has been spoiled by unnecessary fatigue or muscle soreness caused by inadequate physical preparation.

Conditioning Programs

General Exercises
a. Chin-Ups
b. Shoulder Dips (parallel bars)
c. Running (jogging and sprinting)
d. Rope-Jumping
e. Squat Thrusts
f. Squeezing tennis ball in racket hand
g. Side-Stepping (shuffling)
See WEIGHT TRAINING and ISOMETRICS for additional programs.

Physical Qualities Needed Before Participation

Before beginning participation in tennis, the most important physical at-

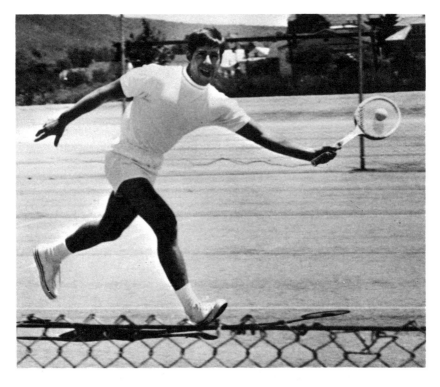

One requirement for tennis success is to develop adequate racket-eye coordination.

tribute to possess is a good degree of hand-eye coordination. Most people don't have much trouble hitting the ball with the strings of the racket, but there are some who seem to need extra work on that basic aspect before attempting to really play tennis. It can be quite frustrating to swing and miss the ball completely time after time. It is necessary to become accustomed to a longer arm, which is actually what a player has when you consider the added length of the racket to the existing length of the arm. Usually only a short amount of time is needed in order to master that basic aspect of tennis, but you can avoid many later problems by developing the basic physical skill in the first place.

Several drills may be used to develop hand-eye coordination. One is to "choke up" on the racket so that you can easily move it. Then, you should attempt to bounce or dribble the ball, on the floor, with the racket held about waist height. Or you may bounce the ball continuously in the air without permitting it to touch the ground. There are more advanced drills, such as dropping the ball and hitting it into a wall or fence.

Once basic racket-eye coordination is developed, it is necessary to possess at least minimal levels of muscular strength and endurance as well as cardiorespiratory endurance. With the basic levels of physical capacity, you will find that you will be able to enjoy tennis more and also continue to increase your physical capacities at the same time.

Most Common Injuries

Tennis is not a game in which there are very many injuries. The tennis elbow is associated with tennis quite commonly, even though it does not seem to occur very often. It is characterized by pain in the elbow and forearm and appears to result from repeated forceful twisting of the extended arm as required in tennis. There does not seem to be a general

*TENNIS PROGRAM (Competitive)**

Chart 1	Chart 2
1. 10 minutes	1. 38 minutes
2. 15 minutes	2. 40 minutes
3. 18 minutes	3. 43 minutes
4. 20 minutes	4. 45 minutes
5. 23 minutes	5. 50 minutes
6. 25 minutes	6. 53 minutes
7. 30 minutes	7. 55 minutes
8. 33 minutes	8. 58 minutes
9. 35 minutes	9. 60 minutes

* See ENDURANCE and ENERGY COST OF ACTIVITIES for an explanation of these charts.

**Doesn't include rest periods, times out, etc.

Fitness 1

If you achieved a score of poor or low average on the *Harvard Step Test* or a score of very poor or poor on the *12 Minute Run*, start on Chart 1-Level 1 and spend 1 week at each level until Chart 2-Level 9 is reached. It is recommended that you participate 4 to 5 days a week. When Chart 2-Level 9 is reached, 4 days a week is sufficient.

Fitness 2

If you achieved a score of high average on the *Harvard Step Test* or fair on the *12 Minute Run*, start on Chart 1-Level 2. Spend 1 week on Chart 1-Levels 2, 4, 6, 7, and 9, and Chart 2-Levels 2, 4, 5, 7, and 9. It is recommended that you participate 4 to 5 days a week. When Chart 2-Level 9 is reached, 4 days a week is sufficient.

Fitness 3

If you achieved a score of good or excellent on either the *Harvard Step Test* or *12 Minute Run*, continue your current program or select Chart 2-Level 9 as your level of participation. Four days a week is sufficient.

agreement as to the pathology involved.

Tennis thumb is the name given to an inflammation of a tendon of the thumb. It occurs frequently among tennis players and appears as a small lump under the thumb of the playing hand. At first the lump may go unnoticed, but in time it increases in size and becomes red and tender. The lump becomes so irritating that it is difficult to hold the racket. Movement of the joint is limited and painful.

Care involves rest and immobility. Massage and/or movement are quite harmful. The pain may be relieved somewhat by diathermy.

Associations:

United States Lawn Tennis Ass'n., 51 E. 42nd Street, New York, New York 10017.

Division of Girls' and Women's Sports (DGWS). See ORGANIZATIONS. —*Clint E. Bruess*

Since tennis is a high-energy-cost activity, it may be used to help improve your fitness level, especially your circulo-respiratory and muscle endurance. Below is a tennis program that takes into account the important principles of training.

TENSION

See STRESS.

TESTS

There are numerous tests that are used to measure man's physical performance. Some of those tests are attempts to evaluate all or several of the various components of physical fitness, some measure only those components the tester feels are the most important, and still others measure only one component of physical fitness.

Some tests are superior to others in ease of administration, validity (does the test measure what it is supposed to measure?), reliability and objectivity (will you get similar results if you or someone else gives the test again?), norms (can test scores be compared?), and economy of time and effort.

The following list of "physical fitness" tests is divided into various categories including several fitness components, test batteries and tests that are administered in the laboratory and are of a highly sophisticated nature. Some of these tests can be administered in your school. Others you can take right in your backyard.

Some of the test items may be undesirable as indicated under EXCESSIVE EXERCISE. The majority of the tests were designed several years ago before research revealed that some of the exercises are possibly detrimental.

Individual Fitness Components

Circulo-respiratory Tests

Circulo-respiratory tests measure the capacity and endurance of the circulo-respiratory system. A high score on the tests indicates a capacity or ability of the body to continue muscular exertions which place a stress on the circulatory and respiratory systems for a prolonged period of time. Some of the tests measure the ability of the body to adapt to the stress and then to recover from that work or stress.

There are circulo-respiratory tests that may be performed at home with a minimum of equipment. Further circulo-respiratory tests will be found under the LABORATORY TESTS in this chapter. Also, there will be a few circulo-respiratory tests listed under the TEST BATTERIES. That section includes the circulo-respiratory tests to measure your fitness. For example, in the AAHPER Test there are a series of tests to be administered. One of the tests is the 600 Yard/Run Walk, a test designed to measure circulo-respiratory endurance.

Harvard Step Test

This is one of the most well-known tests used to evaluate cardiovascular condition and is constructed for measuring the ability of the body to adapt itself to hard work and recover from that stress.

There are two forms of the test, the long and the short form.

Long Form

Step up and down thirty times a minute on a bench 20 inches high. The stepping is done in four counts. Try to exercise, at that rate, as long as possible up to five minutes. The stepping rate is very important because a decrease to 28 steps per minute changes the effort considerably.

Upon completing the exercise, sit down immediately. Then take your pulse at every minute interval from one to three minutes after cessation of exercises.

An index of physical efficiency is computed from the following formula:

Physical Efficiency Index (PEI) = Duration of Exercise in Seconds × 100

2 × Sum of Pulse Counts in Recovery

Here's an example. If you exercise for five minutes, or 300 seconds and your recovery pulse counts are 75 for one to one and one-half minutes, 60 for two to two and one-half minutes, and 50 for three to three and one-half minutes. Addition of the three figures totals 195.

Substituting in the formula:

$$PEI = \frac{300 \times 100}{2 \times 195}$$

$$= \frac{30,000}{390} = 77$$

The figure obtained (77) means little until applied to the norms established on 8,000 college students. Here they are:

Below 55: Poor physical condition
From 55-64: Low Average
From 65-79: High Average
From 80-89: Good
Above 90: Excellent

On the basis of those norms, your score of 77 would then fall into the category of high average, 65 to 79.

Short Form

In this form, the exercise routine remains the same with five minutes of

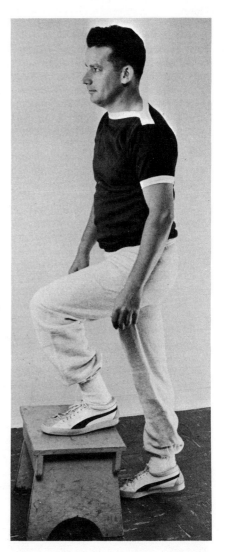

The Harvard Step Test is an effective measurement of cardiovascular condition that is easily self-administered. Use a sturdy bench about 30 inches high and make every effort to maintain a rate of 30 times per minute for several minutes.

bench stepping. The pulse count, however, is recorded from only one to one and one-half minutes after the exercise.

The formula in that instance is:

$$PEI = \frac{\text{Duration of Exercise in Seconds} \times 100}{5.5 \times \text{Pulse Count}}$$

If you had decided to use this form of the test, your results would be as follows:

You exercised for five minutes, or 300 seconds, and your pulse count in recovery was 75 for one to one and one-half minutes. Your score, therefore, was:

$$PEI = \frac{300 \times 100}{5.5 \times 75}$$
$$= \frac{30,000}{412}$$
$$= 73$$

The norms for the short form are as follows:

Below 50: Poor physical condition
50-80: Average
Above 80: Good

With a score of 73, you would fall into the average category.

Dr. Peter Karpovich has prepared the following scoring table chart to avoid computations on the short form.

There are many variations of the test to make it less demanding. For example, a bench of 16 to 17 inches may be used, the pace may be reduced to 24 steps a minute, and the test may be performed for only 3 minutes. The pulse is taken one minute after exercise for 30 seconds. Repeat the test every two or three weeks and each time record the pulse. A decrease in pulse rate after exercise is an indication that the circulo-respiratory endurance is improving.

Carlson Fatigue Test

H. C. Carlson in an article "Fatigue-Curve Test" (Research Quarterly, 16, October, 1945) discussed a test that is designed to place severe stress on the individual being tested. It is a test that makes use of the general fatigue curve, an accepted physiological principle.

Essentially, the test is as follows:

1. Run in place as fast as you can for ten seconds, rest ten seconds, run in place for ten seconds, rest again for ten seconds, and so on. That is done ten times.

2. When running in place, raise and lower your feet far enough to clear the floor as fast as possible.

3. Count the number of right foot-contacts only and record them.

Duration of Effort	\multicolumn{11}{c}{Heart Beats from 1 Minute to 1½ Minutes in Recovery}
	40-44	45-49	50-54	55-59	60-64	65-69	70-74	75-79	80-84	85-89	90-Over
0 - 29″	5	5	5	5	5	5	5	5	5	5	5
0′30″-0′59″	20	15	15	15	15	10	10	10	10	10	10
1′0″ -1′29″	30	30	25	25	20	20	20	20	15	15	15
1′30″-1′59″	45	40	40	35	30	30	25	25	25	20	20
2′0″ -2′29″	60	50	45	45	40	35	35	30	30	30	25
2′30″-2′59″	70	65	60	55	50	45	40	40	35	35	35
3′0″ -3′29″	85	75	70	60	55	55	50	45	45	40	40
3′30″-3′59″	100	85	80	70	65	60	55	55	50	45	45
4′0″ -4′29″	110	100	90	80	75	70	65	60	55	55	50
4′30″-4′59″	125	110	100	90	85	75	70	65	60	60	55
5′	130	115	105	95	90	80	75	70	65	65	60

4. Pulse rates are also taken to indicate the stress placed upon the body. The following five pulse rates are taken for ten seconds, multiplied by six, and recorded:

a. Before exercise, sitting on the floor

b. Ten seconds after the ten bouts of exercise

c. Two minutes after the ten bouts of exercise

d. Four minutes after the ten bouts of exercise

e. Six minutes after the ten bouts of exercise

5. The scoring for the test involves counting the right foot-contacts and the five pulse rates. The results are plotted on graphs.

6. The right-foot contacts indicates production. If you go "all-out," fatigue will cause a drop in the contacts with each subsequent inning. If fatigue does not occur, you probably are not really applying yourself or there is an error in your counting.

7. Merely using the foot-contacts means little unless the pulse rates are also plotted for the pulse rates indicate what stress is being placed on the body. Fewer heart beats required for more work (foot-contacts) indicates better conditioning.

8. When you are taking the test, you may find it rather cumbersome to do it by yourself. Therefore, a partner is recommended to help time the bouts and record your results. If a partner is not available, however, you can do the test by yourself with a little ingenuity. You may find a method to your liking, or the following procedure may be helpful.

a. Place a watch or clock with a sweep second hand directly in front of you.

b. Take a three by five card and number from one to ten on the card. On the other side, make provision for recording your pulse rates as shown on the illustration in the graph.

c. Hold a pencil in your hand and place the card beside the watch.

d. As soon as you finish each exercise bout, immediately record the number of foot contacts along the corresponding number designating the exercise bout.

e. Take your post-exercise pulse rate.

f. Plot your scores on the graph side of the card.

g. Evaluate your performance according to the previously described procedure.

Cooper's 12 Minute Test

Dr. Kenneth Cooper in his book *Aerobics* presents the 12 minute run/walk test. The test itself is simple and only requires that you run as far as possible within 12 minutes.

The 12 minute test is a maximum test. Therefore, you should run to a point of near exhaustion. Since the test is strenuous, your physician should give you a physical examination and permission to take a maximum physical test. Remember, if you become tired in the test, you are permitted to walk.

It is best to run on an indoor or outdoor track if possible. If one is not available, get in your car, find a level country road, and mark off a two-mile distance as measured by your car's odometer. Once your track is selected, you are ready to take the test. Get a stop watch or a wrist watch with a sweep second hand to record the twelve minute time. It might be helpful to have someone else, such as your spouse, record the time.

Start by running, but if your breath becomes short, walk for a while until it comes back and then run some more. Keep going for the entire 12 minutes. When the 12 minutes are up, check the distance you have run. Once you have established your distance, compare it with that of the chart to determine your physical fitness category.

Distance Covered	Fitness Category
Less than 1 mile	Very Poor
1 to 1¼ miles	Poor
1¼ to 1½ miles	Fair
1½ to 1¾ miles	Good*
1¾ miles or more	Excellent

* For men over 35, 1.4 miles is good; for women, 1.3 miles.

If you fall in one of the first three categories, you are not in very good physical condition—about 80 per cent of the American population falls in those three categories. Only categories 4 and 5 are considered to be passing. See CIRCULO-RESPIRATORY ENDURANCE.

Strength Tests

Muscular strength refers to the measurement of the maximum strength applied with a single muscular contraction. Time is not a factor. Muscular strength is not to be confused with power or muscle endurance. The measurement of strength is very difficult without instruments. Some instruments measure the tension of the muscle group, and other strength test instruments measure the force that the group can develop.

A rough estimate of strength is sometimes obtained by lifting your body a number of times. For example, if you can do only *one* push-up or *one* pull-up, then you have only enough arm and shoulder strength to do one of the exercises. If you can do more, then the variable of muscle endurance enters the picture, and strength alone is not measured.

The importance of endurance (local circulation) increases with the number of repetitions until it becomes the dominant factor. Some experts feel that endurance becomes more important than strength if you do 10 or more push-ups or pull-ups. Another method of measuring strength consists of mechanically isolating a muscle group and then lifting a weight or other resistance with a specific group of muscles. For example, to measure the strength of the left elbow flexors, you should increase the weight of a dumbbell until you can do just one repetition. That is called one repetition maximum (1 RM), which is a common term used in testing strength during rehabilitation from injury. Although absolute strength is not measured with that technique, you can determine when your strength has increased. Many weight lifters estimate their strength by checking one RM or 3 or 5 RM on specific types of lifts.

There are two types of strength—static and dynamic. Although they are related, they are tested and developed differently. Static strength is the greatest effort given by a muscle or muscle group in which there is no movement—an isometric effort. Dynamic strength is the force required to move the greatest resistance through the complete range of motion of the muscles. See STRENGTH.

Muscle Endurance

Muscle endurance is the ability of the muscle or muscle groups to persist in an activity or movement. Local muscle fatigue causes the stopping of the activity, not the entire body, as would be expected in circulo-respiratory endurance. There are two types of muscle endurance—dynamic and static. Dynamic endurance is conceived with the number of repetitions of a contraction given movement. Static endurance involves the amount of time a continuous contraction of a certain magnitude can be held. There are many tests that may be used in the home to measure the muscle endurance of specific muscle groups.

Tests of Dynamic Endurance

Arm and Shoulder Endurance

Pull-ups (Chin-ups)—All that is needed for this test is a horizontal metal or wooden bar, approximately 1 to 1½ inches in diameter. The bar must be placed high enough so that the feet will not touch the floor when hanging with the arms fully extended.

To perform the test, jump up and grasp the bar with thumb around the bar and palms facing away (pull-ups). From the hanging position, pull yourself up so that your chin can be placed over the bar. Then lower yourself until your arms are fully extended. Do not pause to stop at either the top or the bottom of the movement. Avoid swinging the body or kicking the legs. Perform as many repetitions as possible. If you perform a pull-up incorrectly, i.e., kicking or not going all the way up or down, give yourself credit for only ½ a pull-up (chin-up). Only 4½ pull-ups (chin-ups) are permitted in most of the official tests. A score of 8 pull-ups or 10 chin-ups is a satisfactory score for men.

Women should do a modified pull-up test. In that test, the bar is lowered so that it is at chest height. Slide your feet under the bar until the body and arms form approximately a right angle when the body is held straight. The weight should rest on the heels. The test is to pull up with the body held perfectly straight as many times as possible. If the body sags or there is movement of the body, ½ credit is given. Only 4 half pull-ups are permitted. A satisfactory score is 25.

Push-ups—Men should be expected to perform 25 to achieve a satisfactory score for arm and shoulder endurance. Women are to perform the *bent knee push-up*. Eighteen is a satisfactory score.

Abdominal Endurance

Bent Knee Sit-ups—To measure the endurance of the abdominal muscles, you can do the knee sit-up. In that exercise, lie with your back flat on the floor. Interlock the fingers behind your head. Bend your knees so that the back of the upper leg and the back of the lower leg form a 90° angle. Then without letting your feet leave the floor and keeping your hands

locked behind your head, sit up and touch your right elbow to your left knee, return, and then sit up and touch your left elbow to your right knee, and return. Each time you sit up counts 1. To achieve a satisfactory score, men should perform 40, women 20.

Tests of Static Endurance

Arm and Shoulder Endurance

Flexed Arm Hang—Use the bar that was used for the pull-ups. Grasp it so that the hands are shoulder width apart. Have someone boost you up until your eyes are level with the bar. Then have your partner let you go. Hang as long as possible. 50 seconds is satisfactory for men, for women 40 seconds.

Abdominal Endurance

V-Seat—Sit on the floor so that your upper body and legs form a right angle. Your arms are beside your body. Lean back with your upper body and keep the right-angle position. That will cause your legs to rise up off the floor. Hold the position with all your weight resting on your buttocks. Your hands are to be extended and pointing toward your toes. Hold the position for 60 seconds. See MUSCLE ENDURANCE.

Flexibility

Flexibility is the ability to move the body parts through their full range of motion at the joints. The range of motion is restricted by the muscles, tendons, ligaments and bones. Flexibility is very specific. That is, each joint has its own desirable and possible range of motion. You can be quite flexible at one joint and have poor flexibility at another joint. Each limb or joint should be tested. Just because you have an adequate range in one wrist does not indicate that you have the same range in the other. You can estimate whether you have adequate flexibility by observation, or you can use a piece of paper, pencil and pro-tractor to make your evaluation more scientific. For example, to measure ankle flexion and extension, tape a piece of paper and then sit down next to that paper with your knees extended and adjacent to the paper. Have someone mark the paper indicating the position of your foot when it is perpendicular to the floor. Then extend your foot downward as far as possible, have your partner mark the paper at the point of greatest extension, and then pull your toes toward your face and mark for flexion. To measure the flexibility at the joint, consider the total range of movement in degrees. Other flexibility tests are listed under Test Batteries and Laboratory Tests. See also FLEXIBILITY.

Agility

Agility, the ability to change directions quickly and correctly while moving at full speed, is a very important component in many sport activities.

It is a component that is very difficult to measure and is the subject of great controversy. Dodging run tests are usually considered agility tests. Other specific agility tests are listed under the Test Batteries. See also AGILITY.

Balance

Balance involves your reflexes, vision, cerebellum, skeletal-muscular system and inner ear (kinesthetic senses). There are many tests that have been used to measure balance. There are, however, several different forms of balance. See BALANCE. One of the most popular tests of gross body balance is to walk on a balance beam for a distance of 8 to 10 feet. The beam is about two inches wide. The height off the ground need only be a few inches, and it becomes harder rapidly as the height is increased. One of the best progressive balance tests is this one devised by Dr. T. K. Cureton at the University of Illinois.

Power

Power is the ability to release maximum muscular contractions in a short period of time. It is sometimes confused with strength. Power, however, involves both strength and speed. See POWER.

There are several tests that have been used to measure power. The

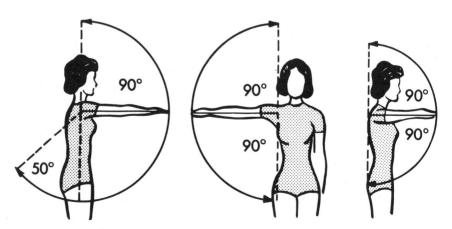

These tests of shoulder flexibility, show the limits of normal range. Left, flexion and extension; middle, abduction and adduction; right, internal and external rotation.

PROGRESSIVE BALANCE BEAM TEST

Preliminary: Execute three successive forward somersaults on the mats, then return the complete distance log-roll fashion, get up and do in succession the following balance stunts. If one stunt is missed, go right on to the next one, accumulating points for each test passed.

Scoring: Stunt passed on first attempt—Score = 3 × points.
Stunt passed on second attempt—Score = 2 × points.
Stunt passed on third attempt—Score = 1 × points.

Items	*Specifications*	*Points*	*Score*
1. Diver's Stance	Standing on toes, eyes open, hands horizontally forward, 10 secs.	1	
2. Walk One Length on Balance Beam	Straight walk in sneakers or shoes.	1	
3. Turn 180° at End of Beam	Quick right-about turn.	1	
4. Walk One Length and Turn 180°	Straight walk and turn.	1	
5. Walk One Length Touching One Knee Then the Other	Take long steps so there is room to touch the rear knee behind the forward foot.	1	
6. Cross Walk, One Length	Skip sideways on the beam.	2	
7. Half-Turn Jump	Jump 180° in a half-twist and hold balance 5 seconds on the beam after the jump.	3	

Total Score ....

Physical Fitness Research Laboratory
T. K. Cureton, Jr., Director
University of Illinois
Urbana

most common are those that are involved with leg power.

Standing Broad Jump—The standing broad jump is used to measure your leg power and can be done with equipment such as a take-off board and jumping pit, or a very minimum of equipment. Mark a spot on the floor as your take-off point. Be certain that both of your feet are behind that line. Your feet should be apart slightly. Then spring forward with both feet. The nearest point touched by any part of the body is recorded as the distance jumped. It is important, therefore, not to fall backward. It will be helpful to have someone mark your jumping distance for you. It is also advisable to jump on a mat or on a surface that will not allow slipping. A satisfactory distance for men is 7 feet 3 inches; for women, 5 feet.

Vertical Jump—The vertical jump is done by standing beside a wall, right or left shoulder toward the wall. Place your arm along the wall so that you are reaching upward as high as possible. Mark the wall at that point to indicate your maximum reach while jumping. Have someone record the height. Measure the distance between your first mark and your second mark, giving you an indication of the height you jumped off the floor. A man should jump 20 inches for a satisfactory score, and a woman 13 inches.

Speed

Speed, although not important in most aspects of daily living, is extremely important in many sports, particularly in football, sprinting and baseball. Speed is very specific to the various limbs of the body. For example, you may have fast arm movements but not have particularly fast leg movements. Speed may also depend upon the task being performed. A person may be a very poor runner, yet he may be very fast in placing a series of blocks into various compartments.

There are many tests of speed, most of them concerned with the running speed. Those types have been used because the speed in running is important in many sport activities.

50-Yard Dash—An excellent test for measuring running speed is to run the 50-yard dash. To perform the test simply requires that you mark off a 50-yard distance, have someone as an official timer, and get someone to start you. Any type of start can be used.

Other tests of speed are complicated and usually very specific, an example is the wrist-finger speed test of speed of movement.

Test Batteries

AAHPER Youth Fitness Test

The American Association for Health, Physical Education and Recreation started a Youth Fitness Project in 1957. To evaluate the youth a battery of tests were administered to a national sampling of boys and girls from grades 5 through 12. From that representative group, national norms were established. Below are the test items included in the original battery.

1. Pull-ups—The pull-up test for boys employs the palms-forward grip. One point is allowed for each pull-up completed. For girls, the flexed arm-hang test is used.

2. Sit-ups—The sit-up test is done by having the student clasp his hands behind his neck. His knees are kept flat on the floor during the exercise. Upon sitting up, he twists his trunk and touches the right elbow to the left knee. On the next sit-up, he alternates. One point is awarded for each sit-up. A maximum of 50 for girls and 100 for boys is the cut-off point. Provided more than one sit-up is performed, the test is a measure of abdominal muscle endurance (iliopsoas). In the revised version of the test, the subject performs with his knees bent for a time limit.

Shuttle Run—The shuttle run is conducted over a 10-yard course. Two parallel lines are drawn 10 yards apart. A pair of wooden blocks (2" x 2" x 4") are placed on one of the lines. The student starts to run from the opposite line, picks up one block and brings it back where he began, and then returns for the other block, running across the finish line as soon as possible. The test is recorded to the nearest tenth of a second, and the better of two trials is recorded. The test is a measure of agility.

50-Yard Dash—The 50-yard dash, scored in seconds to the nearest tenth of a second, is a test of speed.

600-Yard Run-Walk—The 600-yard run-walk is recorded in minutes and seconds. It measures circulo-respiratory endurance.

Standing Broad Jump—The standing broad jump is scored to the nearest inch. The best of 3 trials is recorded. It measures leg muscle power and overall coordination.

Softball Throw—The softball throw for distance is done in an overhand method. The best of 3 trials is recorded. The student must remain between two parallel lines that are 6 feet apart. The test measures arm and shoulder muscle power. (It is being transferred to the Softball sports skills battery and being dropped from the fitness battery.)

The battery of tests has been used on American children to measure their fitness level. The test battery was first administered in 1957-58 and was recently administered again. Below is a resume of that investigation.

During the 1957-58 school year, thousands of boys and girls, representing a cross section of American society, were tested to develop national norms for a seven-item physical achievement test. A similar group was given the same tests in 1964-65. Comparison of the scores recorded by the two groups provides dramatic proof of the improved physical fitness of America's youth.

In only one case (out of 104 direct comparisons) was the mean score for 1964-65 less than 1957-58 mean. In most cases, the difference between the two test groups was so pronounced that youngsters turning in average scores in 1964-65 would have ranked in the upper 25 or 30 per cent of the 1957-58 group.

Other test results support those statistics. In 1961-62, 200,000 youngsters were given a simple three-item screening test designed to detect the physically undeveloped. Only 6 of 10 passed. Today, approximately 8 of every 10 youngsters taking that test pass.

Comparison of the mean scores for the 1957-58 and 1964-65 study groups on the seven-item physical achievement test follow on pp. 504 and 505.

Cureton's 18-Item Motor Efficiency Test

Dr. Thomas K. Cureton at the University of Illinois designed a test to measure six major aspects of motor fitness—balance, flexibility, agility, strength, power and endurance. The tests are either pass or fail. On pp. 506–7 are the 18 test items that will help you determine your motor fitness. In determining your percentile ranking, total all of the test areas that you passed and then interpret your class result.

Kraus-Weber Tests for Minimum Muscular Fitness

The Kraus-Weber Strength Tests were conducted over a period of 18 years of clinical study. They are designed to measure the *minimum* fitness of a person and the level of strength and flexibility of certain key muscle groups. Without the proper functioning of those muscle areas, the whole body as a healthy organism is endangered. The tests represent the very least degree of strength and flexibility necessary for healthy living.

1. Take off your shoes and relax. Lie flat on your back and place your hands behind your neck. Have someone hold down your legs. Now roll up into a sitting position. You pass if you can do one sit-up. Test measures the strength of the hip flexors and stomach muscles.

2. Lie flat on your back, hands behind the neck and knees bent. Have your partner hold down your ankles. Now roll up into a sitting position again. Test measures strength of the stomach muscles.

3. Lie flat on your back with hands behind the neck and legs extended. Keeping your knees straight, lift your feet ten inches off the floor and hold that position for 10 seconds. Test measures strength of hip flexors.

4. Lying prone, with pillow under abdomen, raise your hands behind the neck. Your partner should hold down on the small of your back and on your ankles. Raise your trunk and hold that position for 10 seconds. Test measures the strength of your back muscles.

5. Lying prone over the pillow, have a partner hold your back and hips. Lift your legs up and hold for 10 seconds. Test measures the strength of your low back muscles.

6. Put your feet together, keep the knees straight and lean down slowly. Do not strain. See how close you can come to touching the floor with your fingertips. If you touch the floor, you

BOYS

Test	Year	10	11	12	13	14	15	16	17
Sit-ups	1958	32	34	38	40	44	45	50	48
	1965	48	51	57	65	70	73	73	69
		(82)	(83)	(84)	(88)	(85)	(85)	(80)	(83)
Pull-ups	1958	2	2	2	3	4	4	6	6
	1965	3	3	3	4	5	6	7	8
		(80)	(75)	(65)	(70)	(75)	(75)	(70)	(70)
Shuttle run	1958	12.2	12.0	11.6	11.3	10.8	10.8	10.5	10.5
	1965	11.3	11.2	11.1	10.7	10.1	10.1	10.0	9.9
		(78)	(75)	(60)	(65)	(65)	(70)	(65)	(68)
Standing broad jump	1958	4'6"	4'9"	5'1"	5'5"	5'10"	6'2"	6'7"	6'10"
	1965	5'0"	5'2"	5'5"	5'10"	6'4"	6'9"	7'0"	7'3"
		(80)	(70)	(65)	(70)	(72)	(75)	(65)	(63)
50-yard dash	1958	8.9	8.6	8.2	7.8	7.6	7.2	7.0	6.8
	1965	8.3	8.1	7.8	7.5	7.2	6.9	6.7	6.7
		(75)	(70)	(70)	(65)	(70)	(70)	(65)	(55)
Softball throw	1958	88	98	114	123	139	155	164	176
	1965	97	110	123	141	155	172	181	187
		(69)	(70)	(69)	(74)	(72)	(71)	(71)	(62)
600-yard run	1958	2.55	2.51	2.45	2.37	2.30	2.19	2.11	2.11
	1965	2.36	2.32	2.28	2.15	2.06	2.00	1.55	1.55
		(72)	(71)	(67)	(75)	(78)	(78)	(73)	(70)

AGE

GIRLS

Sit-ups	1958	22	23	24	21	20	18	20	19
	1965	33	32	33	32	30	28	28	28
		*(80)	(78)	(84)	(87)	(85)	(85)	(82)	(83)
Shuttle run	1958	12.9	12.7	12.5	12.3	12.2	12.2	11.9	11.9
	1965	11.8	11.8	11.7	11.6	11.5	11.5	11.5	11.4
		(80)	(77)	(70)	(70)	(70)	(65)	(60)	(63)
Standing broad jump	1958	4'3"	4'5"	4'7"	4'8"	4'10"	4'11"	5'0"	5'1"
	1965	4'8"	4'11"	5'0"	5'0"	5'2"	5'3"	5'4"	5'5"
		(75)	(75)	(75)	(65)	(70)	(70)	(68)	(65)
50-yard dash	1958	9.2	8.9	8.8	8.6	8.6	8.8	8.6	8.9
	1965	8.5	8.4	8.3	8.3	8.3	8.3	8.4	8.4
		(80)	(70)	(65)	(58)	(60)	(60)	(50)	(60)
Softball throw	1958	44	54	62	70	72	76	79	80
	1965	52	61	67	72	77	81	79	79
		(73)	(68)	(63)	(55)	(64)	(61)	(54)	(50)
600-yard run	1958	3.17	3.12	3.16	3.15	3.18	3.19	3.19	3.19
	1965	2.49	2.55	2.55	2.58	2.55	2.50	2.51	2.58
		(80)	(66)	(69)	(65)	(72)	(80)	(76)	(72)

* Figures in parentheses are the approximate percentile scores of the 1964-65 means, based on the 1957-58 tables.

18-ITEM MOTOR EFFICIENCY CLASSIFICATION TEST
WITHOUT APPARATUS
(Men and Women)

		Pass = ✔ Fail = X	Check Result Pass	Check Result Fail	Ring Result Passed	Ring Result Percentile	Class
BALANCE	1.	Divers Stance, on toes, eyes closed, 20 seconds			18	100	Superior
	2.	Squat Stand, 10 secs., balance.			17	94.4	
	3.	Dizziness Recovery, after 10 turns around finger on floor, walk 10' line, 5 secs.			16	88.9	
FLEXI-BILITY	4.	Floor Touch, knees straight, (women touch palms flat).			15	83.3	Good
	5.	Trunk Flexion Forward, sitting position, knees held down, forehead slowly to within 8" of floor, (2 fists, 1 on top of other).			14	77.8	
	6.	Trunk Extension, Backward, lying on front, buttocks held down with hands behind neck, raise chin 18" from floor.			13	72.2	
AGILITY	7.	Kneeling Jump, spring to feet, hold balance for 3 secs.			12	66.4	Above Average
	8.	Jack Spring, touching hands to toes at least waist high, 5 times in succession.			11	61.1	Passing
	9.	Agility 6-Count Exercise, squat, extend legs backward, extend legs forward, flip over, return to squat-rest position, return to standing position (times in 20 secs.).			10	55.5	Failing
STRENGTH	10.	Man Lift, pick up partner of own weight and place on shoulders for carry in 10 secs.			9	50.0	Below Average
	11.	Stick Body, hold 30 secs., head on partner's knee, hands on hips.			8	44.4	

18-ITEM MOTOR EFFICIENCY CLASSIFICATION TEST
WITHOUT APPARATUS—*Continued*
(Men and Women)

		Check Result		Ring Result		
	Pass = ✔ Fail = X	Pass	Fail	Passed	Percentile	Class
	12. Extended Press-Ups, from hands and toes without using elbows. (Women do forearm press-ups, 20 secs.)			7	38.8	
POWER	13. Standing Broad Jump, Height + 1 ft.			6	33.3	Poor
ENDUR-ANCE	14. Floor Push-Ups, 15 times (women do 30 from knees)			5	27.7	
	15. Straddle Chinning, 20 times (women do 10)			4	22.2	
	16. V-Sit, 60 seconds.			3	16.6	
	17. Breath Holding, 30 secs. after running in place 120 secs. at 180 steps per min.			2	11.0	Very Poor
	18. Endurance Hops, in succession, 200 up and down, 200 straddle jump, 200 alternate stride, 50 on left foot, 50 on right foot and as many full squat-jumps as possible.					

have sufficient flexibility in your back muscles and hamstrings.

There are no failures permitted on the Kraus-Weber Tests. You must be able to pass all the test items to be considered to have a minimum level of fitness for healthy living.

President's Council Fitness Tests

The President's Council's Physical Fitness Tests are very similar to the tests items for the AAHPER Youth Fitness Test, except there are fewer test items. The girls' test items include the Bent Arm Hang (Flexed Arm Hang), Sit-ups, Standing Broad Jump, 600-Yard Run-Walk and Endurance Swim. For boys, the test items include the Pull-up, Sit-ups, Standing Broad Jump, 600-Yard Run-Walk and Endurance Swim.

Laboratory Tests

Many laboratory tests used to measure physical performance require expensive equipment that is restricted to laboratory use. A few schools are fortunate to have some of this equipment, particularly the PFI testing equipment, at their disposal.

Circulo-Respiratory Tests

The typical measures of standardizing stress or exercise in the laboratory are the treadmill and the ergometer.

1. Treadmill

The motor driven treadmill is the best device for standardizing the work load during exercise. The speed of the treadmill can be regulated for walking, jogging, running or sprinting. The incline of the treadmill can also be increased so that you can be forced to walk or run up a certain "grade." While a person is exercising on the treadmill, all types of measurements can be taken before, during and after exercise depending upon the sophistication of equipment. That includes pulse rates, blood pressure, electrocardiograms and oxygen uptake (oxygen taken in).

2. Ergometer

An ergometer is similar to a stationary bicycle. You ride the ergometer and pedal at a certain rate against a designated resistance until you are not able to keep the proper pace. In some tests, the resistance is increased in steps as you pedal, until fatigue sets in and you are no longer able to continue at the proper pace.

Like the treadmill, the ergometer is used for standardizing the work load. While you are pedaling, heart rates, electrocardiograms, oxygen intake and blood pressure readings may be taken.

3. Pulse Rates

Pulse rates are taken at rest, before, during and after exercise. It is an excellent measure of determining the amount of stress that you are experiencing. A pulse rate of 200 is usually considered to be exhausting. The pulse rate, taken at intervals after exercise, is very important, for it indicates how well you recover from the stress imposed upon you. For more information, see PULSE RATE.

4. Blood Pressure

Blood pressure before, during and after exercise has also been used to measure cardiovascular fitness.

At rest, systolic blood pressure (the top number) may be used as a general indicator of cardiac stress to which the arteries are subjected. Unfitness is associated with resting systolic pressures below 90 and above 160 mmHg.

At rest, diastolic blood pressure (the bottom number) should be between 70 and 96 mmHg. A person who demonstrates a reading between those measures for both systolic and diastolic pressures can be considered normal. But a systolic or diastolic reading cannot distinguish whether you are fit or unfit.

THIGHS

See LEGS

TRAINING

Physical training and conditioning are interchangeable terms that apply to the procedures of systematically preparing people to perform strenuous work in the most efficient manner and to recuperate from that work as quickly as possible. The process of training or conditioning is a deliberate one and should follow specific principles for the most efficient results.

Principles of Training

Adaptation—The principle of adaptation refers to the body's attempt to adapt to stress placed upon it. Simply stated, it means that if you make your body work harder, it will soon adjust and be able to work harder. See ADAPTATION.

Overload—The overload principle implies that people being trained do more work than they normally would be called upon to perform. Consequently, there is an improvement in physical condition. Overload can be accomplished in three general ways:

1. Increase the work being done, i.e., lift or carry more weight.

2. Increase the work done in a certain length of time; i.e., walk one mile

in 14 minutes rather than three-quarters of a mile in 14 minutes.

3. Do the work in a shorter period of time; i.e., walk one mile in 12 minutes rather than one mile in 14 minutes.

The increased stress is called overload. As you can readily see, after a period of time, that increase is no longer an overload; for your body adapts to the work (adaptation). That's when the third principle of training comes into play. See OVER-LOAD PRINCIPLE.

Progression—The progression principle is a combination of adaptation and overload. Since the body adjusts to the stress placed on it, the amount of work must be increased, periodically, for improvement to occur. For example, if you start an exercise program that involves running one mile a day in eight minutes—to improve your cardiovascular function—in the beginning you would probably find the workout stressful (overload). You would, therefore, improve your cardiovascular function for the next several weeks. But if you continued to perform at that level, run the same distance in the same time, cardiovascular improvement would stop (adaptation). To continue improving you would increase your stress by (1) running the eight-minute mile with weights, such as heavier shoes; (2) running a mile-and-a-quarter in eight minutes; or (3) running a mile in seven minutes. That would place additional stress on your cardiovascular system, and, therefore, the overload principle would go into effect again. In a few weeks or months, additional stress would have to be added. See PROGRESSION.

Specificity—The specificity principle implies that the improvements made in training are specific to the type of training undertaken. For example, a strength program will develop strength, but not an appreciable amount of endurance. Perhaps the best illustration is the person who has trained for a

sport such as swimming and considered himself to be in good condition, but when he participates in basketball or some other sport, he becomes fatigued during the play and sore afterwards. Each activity requires specific demands. Performance in the sport, therefore, is the best way to train for the event. See SPECIFICITY.

Retrogression—When following a training program, you may find that at certain levels of the program you reach a plateau or slip somewhat. Try as you may, you are unable to regain or surpass your previous level. Then suddenly, for no apparent reason, you seem to surge ahead improving all previous performance levels. The reason for such retrogression is not clear except that the body may be making adjustments to meet the demands of the overload. When the adjustments are effected, then progress or improvement is made. See RETROGRESSION.

Use and Disuse—The sixth principle of training is that of use and disuse. Simply stated, it means that if you train, there will be improvement. If not, you will decline in physical performance. Use stimulates the function of the organism, and disuse results in a deterioration. See USE and DISUSE.

Skill—Much of the improvement that takes place during training is improvement in skill. In the beginning, for example, you may find that noticeable changes occur in your physical condition. A great deal of the improvement is a result of learning how to do the exercises or activity more efficiently. Such efficiency means you are making noticeable physical performance increases as a result of improved coordination. See SKILL.

Individual Rates of Response—Each person will have his own level of response to a training program. Many people who participate on athletic teams seem to arrive at a high level of condition long before others. The reason is probably dependent upon many factors, some of which are emotional and others that are hereditary. A few of the variables may be (1) present physical condition; (2) age; (3) body type; (4) weight; (5) rest, sleep and relaxation; (6) nutrition, (7) freedom from disease; (8) proneness to injury; (9) motivation; and (10) ability to learn new skills. See INDIVIDUAL RATES OF RESPONSE.

Types of Training

There are four distinct types of training. They are (1) strength, (2) endurance, (3) flexibility and (4) skill. In all of those forms, the eight basic principles of training apply, although some may be emphasized more than others.

Strength Training—Strength is the ability, or inability, to lift an object, such as a one hundred-pound weight. It is only *the force* exerted in a simple muscular contraction.

To increase the strength of a muscle or muscle group requires that the muscle(s) be progressively overloaded. That is, they must be exercised against an increasing amount of resistance. Each time the body adapts to a certain resistance, additional resistance must be placed on the muscle so that it is overloaded. The resistance may be isotonic (movement) or isometric (no movement).

Weight training is a form of isotonic exercise concerned with building muscle strength or endurance. There are several methods of weight training. See WEIGHT TRAINING. Essentially, the idea is to find a desirable weight for each exercise, so that 6 repetitions of a maximum weight can be lifted. You work at that level on an alternate-day basis until 10 repetitions maximum can be executed. Then more weight is added so that only 6 repetitions maximum can be executed, and the entire cycle is repeated. As the muscle is overloaded, it adapts, more weight is progressively added, and it is overloaded again. Research indicates that

low repetitions (6 to 10) and high resistance on alternate days produces the best strength improvements.

A second form of isotonic exercises to build strength increases the resistance against which the muscles work. Many popular exercise programs make use of that principle. For example, the starting level of the sit-up for abdominal strength involves just raising the head from the floor to look at the feet. The exercises progress, however, to the level where the knees are bent, the hands are behind the head, and the upper part of the body is lifted from the floor.

The second major type of strength training is done with isometric exercise. Here a muscle is exercised against an immovable object which may be a wall, a bar or another muscle. Since the resistance is so great, no movement occurs, but, because the muscle is overloaded, it grows in strength. See ISOMETRICS.

Once a sufficient amount of muscular strength has been developed to perform a particular movement, it may be advantageous to work on increasing the speed of the movement. The concentration on increasing movement speed is called *power training* and it emphasizes explosiveness. Generally, the technique employed is using weighted shoes in jumping, using a heavier shot in shot putting or swinging a heavier bat in baseball.

Endurance Training—Endurance is the capacity to perform work of moderate intensity for a prolonged period. There are two types of endurance—muscular and circulo-respiratory endurance. Muscular endurance is the ability to perform repeated submaximal muscular exertions. As with strength training, those muscular exertions can be isometric or isotonic. An example of isotonic muscular endurance of the arm and shoulder muscles is the ability to do as many push-ups as possible—provided you can do more than a few. You could build isometric muscular endurance by maintaining an "up" position of the push-up for as long as possible.

The maximum performance level in either the isotonic or isometric muscular endurance is usually indicated by pain (or fatigue) of the muscles involved and the eventual inability to continue. Therefore, muscular endurance is a phenomenon of the nervous and muscular systems. See MUSCLE ENDURANCE.

The second type, circulo-respiratory endurance, is the ability to persist in strenuous tasks for a relatively long period of time in which many muscles of the body are involved. Circulatory-respiratory endurance is concerned with the pumping capacity and efficiency of the heart, the blood flow to the muscle cells (skeletal and cardiac), the efficiency of transfer of gases in the lungs and the number of red blood cells in circulation. In short, an improvement in circulatory endurance will be caused by (1) an increase in the size and power of the heart muscles which results in an increased stroke volume; (2) an increase in the number of capillaries in the skeletal and cardiac muscles, thereby making more blood available in those muscles during exercises; (3) an increase in the number of capillaries in the lungs, thereby making more area available for transfer of gases (oxygen and carbon dioxide); (4) an increase in the number of red blood cells in circulation, enabling more oxygen to be carried to the muscles. See CIRCULO-RESPIRATORY ENDURANCE.

Several types of training require maximum endurance. Laurence E. Morehouse, Ph.D., and Philip J. Rasch, Ph.D., in their book *Sports Medicine for Trainers* discussed the various principles and aspects of training.

Anaerobic Training (without oxygen)—Anaerobic training requires short bursts of maximum effort. It would involve running or swimming as fast and as far as you can. If you are not exhausted (unable to sustain effort) after 20 to 30 seconds of effort, you did not work to your maximum capacity. Consequently, the work is accomplished before oxygen intake becomes a limiting factor. In effect, you should be able to work at a maximum rate for 20 to 30 seconds while holding your breath. This type of training affects the ATP cycle. See ANAEROBIC EXERCISE.

Aerobic Training (with oxygen)—Aerobic training is designed to increase the oxygen transportation and utilization systems. Exhaustion should result after about two minutes of effort. Running an 880-yard race in approximately that time would be a good example of aerobic training. Quoting the author: "This type of effort taxes heavily the cardiorespiratory and biochemical systems involved in oxygen transport and utilization. It promotes alveolar hyperplasia (sport lung), hypertrophy of the diaphragm, an increase in erythrocytes, a growth of new capillaries, an increase in blood volume and chemical changes in the blood and other body fluids that increase their buffering." See AEROBIC EXERCISE. These changes are all indicators of improvement in circulo-respiratory endurance.

Heat Training—Heat training helps the temperature-regulating systems of the body adapt to the increase in temperature which occurs as a result of exercise. Exhaustion should occur after eight minutes of sustained activity. If exhaustion occurs after ten minutes of exercising, or if exhaustion occurs before eight minutes, the workout was too light or too heavy to produce a maximum body temperature. The temperature inside the large muscle can rise 8 to 10 degrees Fahrenheit during heavy exercise.

Rhythm Training—Rhythm training involves practicing the endurance event at the desired speed. For example, if an athlete wants to run a mile in four minutes, he should practice the mile at that speed or run continuous 60-second quarter miles. Rhythm training enables the athlete to coordinate the movements that will be necessary for that effort, and establish the arm, leg and breathing patterns. It also conditions him to endure pain and to gain confidence in his ability to sustain the desired pace.

There are three other possible types of training for endurance. Unlike those previously mentioned which are basically physiological, the following types are related to the psychological aspects of the person.

Relaxation Training—Relaxation is an attempt to reduce tension in the muscles. The tension increases the effort that is required for movement and, therefore, reduces the speed of movement. You can voluntarily relax before, during and after a workout.

Psychological Training—In endurance training, it is necessary to endure pain, fatigue and a desire to quit. Each person has a different tolerance level to those phenomena, but everyone experiences them. To improve endurance, however, requires that you are exposed to those discomforts, and repeated exposure will increase your tolerance level.

Pace Training—Proper pace is a prime objective in training. Since you cannot go all out all the time, except in events of short duration, you must learn to conserve your energy to prolong the effort. A steady pace provides the most desirable and efficient performance, not repeated acceleration and deceleration.

Training Programs

There are several general training programs you can follow to develop maximum endurance. All have one common factor—hard work. Below is a resume of some of the programs. Most of the programs are more applicable to running and swimming training, although they may be modified somewhat for other sports and can be used by the person who wants to develop his circulo-respiratory endurance. Little equipment is needed, except a place to run or swim.

Over and under training involves work at over-distance (slower) and under-distance (faster) than the intended performance to develop endurance and speed respectively. Fartlek, or "speed play" training varies your speed according to pleasure. It is an excellent program to help an athlete get through a period of staleness or to help him avoid staleness. Interval training is a rigidly scheduled program that involves a fast lap followed by a slower lap, and so on. It is particularly good for pace of rhythm training. Repetition training requires you to run a given distance, a given number of times, at a given speed. The obstacle-course type of program that helps you develop general fitness is circuit training. It is particularly good in the off season.

Flexibility Training

Good flexibility at a joint indicates that you are able to move freely and easily through the full range of motion at that joint. Flexibility is specific to a joint, not to the entire body in general. You may have good arm and shoulder flexibility but poor hamstring flexibility (inability to touch the floor).

Good flexibility is desirable for at least four specific reasons. 1. A proper degree of flexibility is a possible safeguard against low-back pain and back and neck tension. 2. Flexibility acts as a precautionary measure against damage to muscle fibers. 3. An increase in the flexibility of the joints tends to decrease the possibility of injuries to those joints. 4. A greater range of motion of the joints results in better sports performance and efficient bodily movement.

In order for the body levers to move, the muscles opposite the contracting muscles (antagonist) must lengthen sufficiently so that full range of motion is established. Ligaments and other connective tissues also restrict movement, as will lack of activity.

An increase in flexibility can be obtained by stretching the muscles, ligaments and connective tissues that are limiting movement. The range of motion can be increased by slow, gentle and long-term stretching exercises performed several times daily. Continue the exercises to the point of discomfort and then slightly beyond.

There are three points of caution, however, in performing flexibility exercises. One, if pain is noted the next day, in all probability overstretching has occurred and you must use more discretion in performing the exercises. Two, "bounce and stretch" exercises are not recommended because muscle tears may result. Three, with an increase in flexibility, there should also be a development of muscular strength so that support can be given to the joints with increased flexibility. Earl L. Wallis, Ed.D. and Gene A. Logan, Ph.D., in their book, *Figure Improvement and Body Conditioning Through Exercise* indicate the necessity of strength and coordination in developing flexibility. They cite the example of developing increased flexibility in the ankle joint and the resultant ability to exert more force in some movements. Without proper strength and coordination, however, the foot may be placed in a weak position to bear the weight of the body.

See FLEXIBILITY and TESTS for specific exercise.

Skill Training—Regardless of the activity in which you are involved, there is a certain element of skill. Some activities require a greater amount of skill than others. During training much of the improvement in performance, even in running, is the result of an increase in your skill level. At first you may attribute your becoming more skilled to better conditioning. Although that is true, there is also the possibility that you are getting better because you are able to run more efficiently.

Skill training is largely the result of coordinating the various major muscle groups. A high level of skill is characterized by an ease of effort, while a lack of skill is typified by awkward movements.

Skillful movement is the result of a properly integrated neuromuscular system. The system perceives the stimulus, interprets it properly, and sends the proper impulses back to the muscles for the correct response. If the neuromuscular system is not properly integrated for a certain activity, somewhere along the line there will be a breakdown or delay, thereby causing an inefficient movement.

Laurence E. Morehouse and Augustus T. Miller, Jr. in their book *Physiology of Exercise* present an excellent review of some of the factors that influence skill training. If maximum skill in an activity is to develop, all the factors, with the exception of body height, must be improved or adjusted.

Body Weight—Excess fat will put a limitation on your physical skill. The added fat increases the effort that is required to perform a movement or skill and may also inhibit movement.

Body Height—The tall person has a higher center of gravity than the short person, and, therefore, he must move his center of gravity through a greater distance to perform a similar movement.

That applies to all directions except those movements in a horizontal plane. The shorter person, therefore, has the advantage in many skill activities, especially in diving and gymnastics. Errors in form appear to be magnified for the taller person. However, he has a distinct advantage in such skills as baseball pitching, basketball and tennis.

Timing—In skill activities, there is a fine coordination in the time of muscle contractions. There must be a proper contraction and relaxation of the various muscles involved. As learning progresses in a skill, the time of the muscular contractions and relaxations becomes more precise. The limiting factor in time, however, is the central nervous system. That system controls the relaxation and contractions of the various muscles. A person with an impaired or abnormal central nervous system can progress only to that level dictated by his nervous system, regardless of his degree of muscular development.

Eye-muscle coordination—Eye-muscle coordination is the most important factor in *learning* a skill. Later on, as the skill is better learned, the factor becomes less and less dominant. When the skill is finally perfected, it can often be done with the eyes closed. The coordination of eyes and muscles enables you to establish a relationship between your body and the target object so that there will be proper movement and successful execution of the activity.

Kinesthesis—Nerve endings stimulated by stretching or compression are located in the muscles, tendons and joints. Those endings respond to this stimulus of stretching or compression by presenting a *kinesthetic impression.* The impression is an awareness of a change in the position of the body or some part of the body. Through kinesthetic impressions, you are able to ride a bicycle without having to constantly check to see if your leg and arm positions are correct, if you adjusted the wheel properly to avoid falling and if your eyes are on the road. You will recall, however, that while you were learning to ride a bicycle, you had a great deal of trouble coordinating everything for the proper riding action. That was because you did not have the necessary experience to give your muscles the proper "feeling" for performing the complicated task. Practice, for that reason, is extremely important so that the body can become aware of the various positions it will assume during the activity. See KINESTHESIA.

Balance—Balance is important in any activity, for without it, coordinated movements would be impossible. Balance depends upon the nerve impulses which originate in the inner ear. You have experienced a lack of balance by turning your body very rapidly in a circle or after performing several somersaults. A feeling of dizziness or even nausea may have accompanied the poor balance. That dizziness or feeling of nausea must be reduced, for it limits skill and accuracy of movement, especially in such activities as dancing, figure skating, diving, tumbling and gymnastics. You can help reduce dizziness, when turning rapidly, by keeping your eye on a fixed point as long as possible. Then, when you are unable to hold your head in that position any longer, turn your head in the direction of the spin and look at another distant fixed point. Practice will develop the ability to concentrate on a fixed point, and skill and accuracy will be improved. See BALANCE.

Visual Aim—The eye is an amazing organ. Most people are able to see the finest hair at arm's length, and yet the eye is able to adjust to see objects miles away. The lens of the normal eye is flattened when viewing objects at least 20 feet away and must bulge for clear vision of objects closer than 20 feet. That change in the lens is called the *accommodation reflex.* Also associated with that reflex is the *convergence reflex.* That refers to the ability of the eyes to turn inward toward the nose to view closer objects. The convergence reflex enables you to estimate the distance through kinesthetic impressions. Objects within 20 feet of you can be estimated with regard to length, width and thickness, an ability called spatial discrimination. The discrimination is diminished, however, when an object is viewed from more than 20 feet, and lost when one eye is closed.

You are more accurate in your attempt to direct an object toward a distant target if a closer object is used as a reference point. That principle is utilized in many sport activities. In bowling, for example, many people use the spot system of bowling. In applying that principle, they do not look at the pins but rather at a point 16 feet down the lane. Archers also use the technique in point of aim sighting.

Muscular Tension—The amount of muscular tension evident during the performance of an activity affects the energy requirement (calories used), the rate of movement of the various body parts and the onset of fatigue.

The level of muscular tension exhibited by a person during physical performance is extremely critical. Too much tension produces jerky, uncoordinated movement. Too little tension makes the movement weak and unsteady.

The degree of muscular tension is dependent upon the central nervous system. A feel of depression or sadness can cause low muscle tension; a feeling of happiness and moderate excitement will cause a desirable level of muscular tension, while a fear or excessive excitement may cause an inhibiting degree of muscular tension.

Thinking about a muscular performance may increase the tension of the muscles that will be involved in the movement. That's why a person may improve his golf swing during the winter, or off season, simply by reading about the proper form and concentrating specifically on the technique employed. See SKILL.

Precision—Manual tasks in which movement is away from your body are made more accurately than those in which the movement is toward your body.

Most people under stress are less accurate in their movements and,

therefore, produce more efforts. The additional stress is largely the result of muscle tension. There are some people, however, who maintain efficiency under stress.

Movements with the right hand are made more quickly and accurately if the movement is counter-clockwise while the left hand is better at clockwise movements.

TRAMPING

"Tramping" is travel on foot across hilly or mountainous country, often in bush or forest, by self-contained parties who usually back-pack all necessary goods and equipment. It is often associated with deerstalking and mountaineering.

Travel may be along ridges either in or above the bush or in valleys which contain steep, fast-flowing rivers, often in gorges. Trips are mainly organized on weekends (i.e., 2-3 days), but longer trips lasting up to three weeks are often made during vacations. Pack weights vary from 20-40 pounds for weekend trips to 60-80 pounds for longer trips.

Tramping clubs construct shelter huts and maintain access tracks in some areas, but many parties traveling in hutless country carry lightweight tents.

The contribution to physical fitness is high. The moving and often lifting several thousand feet in vertical height of a weight equivalent to the tramper's own body plus pack and other equipment over a period of 8 to 14 hours a day, in many cases for several consecutive days, requires great cardiorespiratory endurance. Physiological adjustments are promoted which have lasting effects on the cardiorespiratory efficiency, particularly in respect to endurance.

The effect on muscle endurance is high. The benefit to strength and flexibility varies, tending to be lower where formed tracks reduce whole body movements, which are constantly required in dense bush or on rock faces. Trunk and leg muscles are chiefly affected, but associated activities frequently involve arms and shoulder girdle also. See HIKING, MOUNTAIN CLIMBING and ORIENTEERING.—*J. L. Anderson*

TWELVE MINUTE RUN

See TESTS.

ULCERS

Although heredity can predispose a person to getting an ulcer, the main cause is environmental stress. Such stresses are those encountered on the job or in the family are typical. A person who worries too much causes secretions of excess acid in the stomach. That overacid condition may promote ulcers. If the extra acid eats away at the lining of the stomach or the duodenum and is not reduced, blood vessels may be exposed and the result is a bleeding ulcer.

Once you have an ulcer, you must learn to calm down by either removing the stresses or learning to face them without apprehension. Your diet should be altered so that the food will be bland and will not aggrevate an acid condition. You may also be required to take medication to neutralize the excess acid. If the condition is very serious, surgery may be necessary.

Exercise and Ulcers

If it is regular, enjoyable, and fatiguing, exercise can go a long way in helping to neutralize or reduce the stomach acid and, therefore, can be a major factor in preventing or relieving ulcers for those people who are ulcer prone. Suitable exercise has a relaxing effect and affords a means of reducing tension and stress. See STRESS. Besides aiding the body physically, exercise provides an emotional outlet, relieves the acid condition of the digestive tract, works off aggression and releases hostility. See HYPOKINETIC DISEASE.

Note that the exercise must be enjoyable. If you select an activity that causes additional stress, you may be only adding to the unwanted condition. Likewise, if you select an activity that is highly competitive, you may also find that instead of getting away from the stress of the competitive world you are adding another stress.

USE AND DISUSE

The terms use and disuse refer to one of the physiological principles of training. If you require a part of your body to perform a certain task, the efficiency of that part will remain the same or improve (use). Conversely, if you do not require a part of the body to perform a certain task, or other tasks similar to it, the efficiency of that part will deteriorate (disuse). Muscles grow larger and stronger when exercised, while muscles that are unexercised decrease. Furthermore, the efficiency of the circulatory and respiratory systems deteriorates when endurance exercises are not performed regularly. But when these exercises are performed, the sluggishness of the circulatory and respiratory systems are reduced, and the efficiency is improved. In short, use promotes function while disuse may reduce the ability to function. See TRAINING.

VALSALVA PHENOMENON

Named after an 18th century Italian scientist, the Valsalva phenomenon is associated with the lifting of heavy weights. It occurs when you hold your breath during an intense effort. If the glottis is kept closed during a heavy lift, the pressure in the chest (intrathoracic cavity) increases and prevents the blood from returning to the heart.

Initially, the arterial blood pressure increases; but if the exertion is extended, the intrathoracic pressure also increases, and the blood pressure will fall very quickly and considerably because of the decreased blood flow to the heart. During that period of exertion the veins of the neck become distended. When the exertion is over, the heart is filled with blood, and the blood pressure again rises to levels above normal.

Cautions

The phenomenon has significant implications for older persons or for those who have circulatory and/or respiratory weaknesses. They should use extreme caution in weight training, for undue stress may be placed on the circulatory and respiratory systems. For the average individual, however, there is no real problem since most of the weight-training programs fall short of requirements necessary to produce the Valsalva phenomenon.

VARICOSE VEINS

The veins are vessels that collect the blood from the various tissues and send it back to the heart. The veins near the capillaries are very small but become larger as they join together. As the veins enlarge, they make the flow of blood easier or harder depending upon whether the blood flows downward (those vessels above the heart) or upward (those vessels below the heart). The veins in the legs must carry blood a considerable distance against gravity. The heart pumps the blood not only around the body, but moves it with such a force as to send it all the way back to the heart. When the heart does not pump—called the rest phase—the valves of the veins and the muscles that surround the veins prevent the blood from flowing backward.

Causes

Varicose veins develop when the valves or the walls of the veins become weakened. Some people may be born with varicose veins, or an injury or disease may cause damage. When the valves or veins are weak, after a period of time they give way under pressure and sag outward at the valves. As a result, the valves do not close tightly to regulate the flow of blood; and because of the lack of regulation, the pressure increases against the vein walls. That condition of the blood is called pooling in the veins, when you may suffer from that effect. Even if the veins are healthy, prolonged standing may cause the blood to pool in the legs, thereby preventing proper flow elsewhere in the body, particularly to the brain. As a result you may feel faint or actually faint. That happens in many military demonstrations when recruits are standing at attention for a long period of time. If this pooling continues over a period of years, even people with apparently healthy veins can develop varicose veins.

Varicose veins are usually a condition associated with aging. The veins lose their tone, they can no longer maintain their elasticity, and they begin to sag.

Treatment

Treatment of varicose veins traditionally has involved medical or surgical procedures. Medical treatment recommends that the person wear elastic stockings or bandages, the elastic stockings for a mild condition and the bandages for more serious cases. In both instances the patient is told to elevate his legs during the day and avoid excessive standing. Surgical treatment may be indicated if the varicose veins are very large and lie just underneath the skin. The enlarged veins are removed, and the blood is rerouted to the deep veins, where it is then carried to the heart.

There are other recommendations that have been made by doctors for people suffering from varicose veins.

If you take a long trip by train or plane, get up and walk around every ½ hour. If you are traveling in the car, stop every two hours and walk for a time. When you are watching TV, elevate your feet; the executive who always has his legs on his desk has the right idea. If your doctor approves, elevate your feet while sleeping.

Exercise and Varicose Veins

Another recommendation made by many doctors is that exercise is important for varicose veins, because it helps general circulation. The movements of the leg muscles when walking, jogging, running, cycling or swimming all aid to push the blood upwards.

Doctors suggest that people who suffer from varicose veins should:

1. Avoid wearing round garters that cut off circulation.

2. Not wear elastic girdles continuously, especially if sitting for long periods of time, for they may bunch up and inhibit the flow of blood.

3. Wear elastic stockings continuously throughout the day, but not to bed. They should be put on in the morning, however, before arising.

4. Not sit or stand for long periods of time to prevent pooling in the legs, especially the ankles. If you must stand for any length of time, move about. If that is impossible, make it a habit to contract your leg muscles while standing, a sort of isometric contraction. Or bend the knees slightly, straighten them and then rise upon your toes.

People who develop varicose veins are usually either obese and inactive or have had to carry a heavy weight for long periods of times, such as a pregnant woman. Exercise, naturally, can help the overweight person by reducing his obesity and getting him active again. Exercise also helps to keep the veins elastic by massaging them so that the blood can get back to the heart more readily. Exercise is one of the best preventive measures for varicose veins. See CIRCULATORY SYSTEM.

VOLLEYBALL

Origin and Popularity

In 1895 a student at Springfield College and a part-time Physical Director at the Holyoke, Massachusetts, YMCA put up a tennis net across the gym and used a basketball bladder for a game he called minonette. This game became volleyball, inasmuch as the ball was volleyed back and forth across the net. YMCA Physical Directors took both games to the far corners, and they became world-wide sports.

Volleyball today should be called "smash ball" when played at the top level of competition. It has been estimated it is played by more people as a team sport than any game in the world except soccer football.

Its past popularity may be due to many factors: it can be played on all levels of competition from back-yard fun to olympic tournaments; it is adaptable to all ages for both men and women, boys and girls; it requires a minimum of equipment; the rules have remained relatively simple; and it remains the only truly amateur sport in the world today.

Contribution to Physical Fitness

The value of volleyball for physical fitness ranges from near 0 to 100. The degree of fitness obtained is dependent upon the training program and the level of volleyball played.

The back-yard and noon-time military type produces little physical fitness. The training program and game as played at the level of the U.S. national championships rates very high. The training program of the Japanese Olympic team and the Russian and Czech teams contains as rich a physical fitness routine as contained in any other sports of world-wide prominence.

Cardio-Respiratory Endurance

In this area the back-yard type of fun game, even though having many desirable attributes, produces a very low degree of cardio-respiratory endurance.

It must be admitted, regretfully, that athletic directors in the U.S. have so "down-played" volleyball that we have, in comparison with the rest of the world, relatively little volleyball of the type that produces physical fitness.

Flexibility

In the upper levels of volleyball competition, great flexibility of the body is developed. In the pass and set up, there must be agility, flexibility and a high degree of body control involving the foot, ankle, knee and particularly the spine and pelvic regions. In making the pass, great flexibility of wrist and fingers is essential, especially when the players become set-up players.

Spiking entails even more flexibility in the foot movements for the take-off jump, the back, shoulder girdle and wrist snap. Tremendous speed and flexibility are now needed for defensive play in the modern game.

Muscle Endurance

Most volleyball tournaments are conducted on a double-elimination basis, and teams that are not easily eliminated are called upon to play many games in one day. The legal two time outs per game, with a 30-second limit each, allow very little time for recuperation. A player may be in action as many as 6 or 7 times a day, and this requires great muscle endurance of the whole lower extremities.

The other demands for muscular endurance come from the fact that a great deal of jumping is necessary for all players, not only for the attack man but also the blocking team. The net is 8 feet high, and players are called upon to jump with hands above that net as many as 1,200 times a day.

Muscle Strength

Muscle strength or power varies again as to the level of the game being played. For all blockers and spikers there needs to be a great amount of strength in order to propel the body weight off the floor.

The spiker needs a good deal of back, shoulder and arm strength with the hitting arm. The modern volleyball spiker hits a ball that travels faster than Boody Feller's fastest pitch.

Conditioning Programs for Volleyball

1. *Isometric*

Tension exercises of this type are not the most desirable training routine for volleyball. It is true that players need some degree of static strength; but the big emphasis must be upon endurance, speed, mobility, flexibility, explosive power. Isometrics furnishes none of these. See ISO-METRICS.

2. *Weight Training*

Specific types of weight training are used by the leading volleyball teachers and coaches. But, it must be carefully planned to produce the results needed for volleyball players. See WEIGHT TRAINING.

3. *General Training Programs*

Hundreds of drills and training programs have been and are being used by the coaches of the country who are connected with top-level play: those who have attended national championships and those who have traveled abroad and observed the high-gear training programs in other countries.— *Marshall L. Walters*

Association:

United States Volleyball Association (USVBA), 301 East Martin Street, San Antonio, Texas 78205.

Since volleyball is a high-energy-cost activity it may be used to help improve your fitness level, especially your circulo-respiratory and muscle

*VOLLEYBALL PROGRAM
(Vigorous)**

Chart 1	Chart 2
1. 10 minutes	1. 38 minutes
2. 15 minutes	2. 40 minutes
3. 18 minutes	3. 43 minutes
4. 20 minutes	4. 45 minutes
5. 23 minutes	5. 50 minutes
6. 25 minutes	6. 53 minutes
7. 30 minutes	7. 55 minutes
8. 33 minutes	8. 58 minutes
9. 35 minutes	9. 60 minutes

* See ENDURANCE and ENERGY COST OF ACTIVITIES for an explanation of these charts.
**Doesn't include rest periods, time outs, etc.

Fitness 1

If you achieved a score of poor or low average on the *Harvard Step Test* or a score of very poor or poor on the *12 Minute Run,* start on Chart 1-Level 1 and spend 1 week at each level until Chart 2-Level 9 is reached. It is recommended that you participate 4 to 5 days a week. When Chart 2-Level 9 is reached, 4 days a week is sufficient.

Fitness 2

If you achieved a score of high-average on the *Harvard Step Test* or fair on the *12 Minute Run,* start on Chart 1-Level 4. Spend 1 week on Chart 1-Levels 2, 4, 6, 7, and 9 and when Chart 2-Level 9 is reached, 4 days a week is sufficient.

Fitness 3

If you achieved a score of good or excellent on either the *Harvard Step Test* or *12 Minute Run,* continue your current program or select Chart 2-Level 9 as your level of participation. Four days a week is sufficient.

endurance. Below is a volleyball program which takes into account the important principles of training.

WAIST

Your natural girdle—the muscular network of the abdominal region—can do everything an elastic girdle can do. Just consider the way your body is constructed and how your natural girdle fits into that structure. The bones of your skeletal system are so arranged that the several groups of bones each perform some vital function. For example, the legs are used for locomotion; the pelvis or pelvic girdle for support, and the rib cage for protection. Draped on the bony framework, skeletal muscles provide the basic form of the body. On top of and within some areas of muscle are located fat deposits that may vary in thickness from a fraction of an inch to several inches. A typical example is the abdominal fat depository. Much of the effectiveness of your external girdle in shaping the figure depends on how easy it is to restrict, restrain and control the fat depositories of the abdomen, the thighs and the buttocks.

All four sets of muscles of your abdominal girdle acting in combinations can perform the following finds of functions: give shape to the waist, hold in the organs of the abdominal cavity, squeeze the contents of the abdomen, protect the internal organs from blows and keep the pelvis in its proper position. Although helping only slightly in turning and bending movements when standing, they play a major role in turning and bending movements when lying on the back because now the weight of the trunk acts as a resistance to movement. Almost everyone appreciates the sight of a well-proportioned female figure. To be considered well-proportioned implies shoulder, chest and hip measurements that are somewhat similar and waist measurements that are a few inches less. Abdominal musculature that has sufficient muscular endurance can maintain that position and contribute to a well-proportioned figure with athletic appeal. How then can you insure that each of those muscles behave as they are intended to behave? Simply by using them in the intended manner so they become accustomed to this new function and are able to perform easily and automatically.

Try These Exercises

A few simple exercises practiced daily will help to orient the muscles to their new role. Try the abdominal compression exercise first. Simply pull in the abdominal wall toward the backbone. It may be done in almost any body position, while lying, sitting or standing. Don't hold your breath, but just try to pull in the muscles to your new waistline for several seconds.

Start by practicing that exercise a few times each day and then gradually build up to ten to fifteen times. The more times you exercise during the day, the sooner you will develop the strength and the habit necessary to maintain the desired position. But remember start out easy and increase just a bit each day. That will help you avoid muscle soreness, which is quite discouraging and really unnecessary. You didn't get in your present condition in a day, so don't try to make the entire gain on the first day either.

Or try the abdominal curl. Lie flat on your back and, keeping your lower back in contact with the floor, curl your head and the upper part of your body forward and upward. Return slowly to the starting position by lowering your upper trunk and body to the floor. Try this several times, but be sure to work up to a specific number (5-10) rather than going all out the first time.

The lean back is a rather simple exercise that may provide ample measures of reward for the tummy area. Start by sitting on the floor with your hands interlocked behind the head and your legs fully extended. Lean back until your legs are slightly off the floor and you are balanced on your buttocks. That should put you into a perfect V position. Hold it for three counts before returning to the original sitting position.

Here's another. Interlace your fingers behind your head while lying on your back. Put your heels close to your buttocks with your knees together. Now ask your husband or wife (or anyone handy) to hold down your feet. In that position, attempt to sit up and touch your right shoulder with your left knee. Return to the starting position and repeat the exercise to the other side. Start with 10 sets and work up to 25.

The rowing curl is perhaps a bit more advanced, but if you can do several of these every day, you'll notice the benefits quickly. Lie on your back with your arms extended overhead. Curl your head and upper body forward just as in the abdominal curl. At the same time, bring your arms forward and raise your knees toward your shoulders. When the exercise is completed, you should be sitting with your knees next to your shoulders and your arms extended past the outside of your knees. When you return to the starting position, you have completed the "rowing" maneuver.

If you make these exercises a regular part of your daily schedule, you'll find that the muscles in your abdominal area will firm up quite nicely. As a result, your posture will improve, your measurements will trim into line, and you'll be able to think twice about using a girdle—a device that paradoxically contributes to the weakening of the very muscles that it is supposed to support.

A girdle is nothing more than a complex interworking of elastic bands. You already have all the physical requirements to produce a firm, interwoven network of tough, yet flexible, muscular links.—*Donald F. Mapes*

WALKING

Walking is one of the best exercises for people of all ages. It is a natural movement of man and requires no special equipment other than properly fitted clothing. The pace at which you walk depends upon your physical characteristics and physical condition. It is classified as a mild- to high-energy-cost activity depending upon the vigor. Walking is an excellent exercise provided that the pace is not leisurely. Although the usual pace of man is around 2.5 miles per hour, a pace of about 4 miles per hour is the minimum for worthwhile fitness benefits. That's about a mile in 15 minutes. You can walk anywhere—in the city or in the country. It is an exercise that can be performed without anyone really knowing that you are exercising.

Allow extra time to get to the train, to the store, to meetings, other places you have to go so you can go, at least now and then, by foot-power.

Whenever you feel tense and nervous, try a walk—the brisker and longer, the better; but even a brief one will help discharge tension. Use a before-bed walk as an aid to sleep; it can be a big help in overcoming insomnia.

On an occasional weekend, plan walking as a family enterprise. Set a goal; take a walking tour to a park, other scenic spot or some place of historical interest.

Walking is an excellent way to get you exercising again, but it is not to be a leisurely stroll around the block. A good brisk walk of 30 minutes should be a minimum; and if you can extend that to an hour a day, so much the better. Get off the bus or train 10 blocks from work and walk the rest of the way. With today's traffic problems, you'll probably get there before or just about the time the bus does. *Time* magazine recently noted that traffic up Broadway in New York City moves at a pace of 3 to 4 miles per hour. You can walk that fast. Try it yourself some time; you'll find that the time differential, if there is any, is not very significant. And its a small price to pay for improved physical condition.

Benefits of Walking

Second Heart

Doctors have been recommending for years that people take up walking. It improves your physiological as well as your psychological condition. In a recent survey sponsored by "Patterns of Disease," a publication for doctors, the advice of 3,753 physicians, nationwide, was recorded. All supported brisk walking as the most effective way to battle short breath, excessive weight and the general "run-down" feeling.

A little more attention to what some researchers call "the second heart" would take a lot of people off pills and keep them out of hospitals. Nature has provided our busy hearts with an auxiliary system to ease the load of pushing some 72,000 quarts of blood through the system every 24 hours, over almost 100,000 miles of circulatory "roads." The help comes from the muscles in the feet, calves, thighs, buttocks and abdomen. As they work, they rhythmically contract and release, squeezing the veins, forcing the blood along. It's nature's way of moving the blood to the heart and brain in spite of gravity.

The key to the efficiency of this system is walking. Walking makes the muscles below the abdomen do their part in helping the heart. Without the push from the muscles, the blood tends to pool in the belly and the feet. The heart has to pitch in with more and bigger beats to move that blood, delivering essential nutrition to the tissues and flushing dangerous wastes.

Man is unique in his need for a "second heart." In four-legged animals, the circulation doesn't have much of a struggle against gravity because all the vital organs are on the same level; the heart, the brain, the lungs and even the reproductive glands have an easy time getting all the blood they need. But man stands up! Nature had to devise a way to pump the blood straight up, and the muscles around the veins were pressed into service. They work best when we walk.

Researchers have also noted that a regular regimen of walking helps bring down high blood pressure and pulse rates. Doctors have also noted that man was made to walk. Your

muscles, limbs, toes, organs and lungs were adapted to locomotion. When you walk, virtually all parts of the body are called upon to perform. All of that explains a lot about why walking has become so important in the treatment of heart patients. Doctors know now that it's the best way to make the muscles take over their share of the work and relieve a damaged heart. Even a little walk improves circulation, and it costs the heart nothing. In truth, say authors Aaron Sussman and Ruth Goode, in *The Magic of Walking*, people whose heart rate and blood pressure are high will find that a regimen of regular walking —not necessarily far or fast—brings the heart rate and blood pressure down to normal levels.

The "second heart" system worked

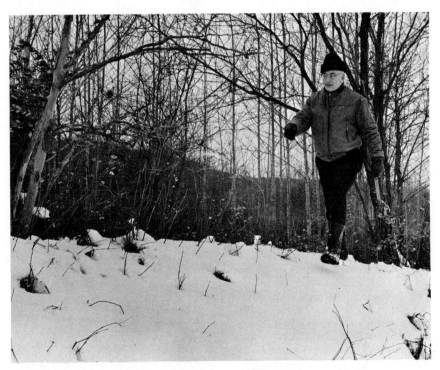

Despite the season, a brisk walk is an excellent activity for all ages. Many people have found it the only practical way they can achieve a big exercise goal.

like a charm for half a million years, then a lot of us stopped walking. No need anymore for walking to hunt or for walking to farm. Now we no longer even walk to our jobs. If people are getting more heart disease, more digestive and elimination problems and more flabby muscles than ever before, a good share of the blame is surely due to physical inactivity.

Surgeons prescribe walking a few steps within hours after an operation. That hospital procedure, which began originally as a measure against blood clots forming in patients kept inactive too long, showed its value in other unexpected ways—more rapid circulation, faster healing, improved muscle tone, better digestion and elimination. Patients forced to get out of bed and on their feet, no matter how painful it seems, feel a boost in morale. How sick can you be if you can stand up and move around on your own?

Weight Control

If people would walk more, they would probably weigh less. Not that walking is the quickest way to chop off a fast 20 pounds. It isn't. But regular walking can keep your weight at the proper level. If you put yourself on an easy, daily walking schedule at the first sign of an unwanted pound, you have an excellent chance of holding your own in the eternal battle of the beltline.

A walk can skim the fat off the top of your calorie day. An hour's worth of walking uses up about 300 calories, and those are the few extra calories that pack themselves into wide waistlines, unflattering hips and multiple chins. As Sussman and Goode point out, nobody gains weight suddenly. It's just the discovery that's sudden—and painful. If you gain a fifth of a pound a week you may not notice it until the end of a year when the fifths have piled up into ten pounds.

So many of us gain weight after 35, because our activities lessen and we don't realize it. As a man gets older, he becomes more successful. He moves from the old two-story to a ranch house or even a fashionable apartment. And there go the stairs. He can afford a second car so walking to the bus stop is out. His executive job no longer calls for trotting around the plant; he sits behind a desk. Economic progress is costing him a healthy heart.

Back home after a tension-filled day, he heads for a snack and a drink (both heavy on calories) to help him relax. A brisk walk would do it better. More than that, the walk eliminates drinking time and takes off some of the excess calories accumulated during the day.

Overweight people hate to work at losing. They come up with this one: walking makes you hungry, makes you eat more, eventually makes you heavier than ever. To quote Dr. Jean Mayer, Harvard nutritionist, "If you don't walk at all, you may well become a little less hungry if you start walking for an hour a day. If you are already active, increase your activity; your appetite will go up, but not so much that you won't profit from the activity."

If you're overweight, take a chance. Walking can't hurt you. On the whole, habitual walkers tend to be moderate eaters; they rarely need a reducing diet; they run lean, not pudgy.

Mental Relaxant

Walking is also an excellent means for mental relaxation. In the American society, everything is go-go-go. People do not take time to enjoy the works of nature. You jump in your car and speed to the local drug store or supermarket. When you do so, you are completely oblivious to the wonders of nature. If you just take the additional time to walk and enjoy the beauty around you, you'll find a great means of unwinding and getting your mind off the problems of society. It is one of the best tranquilizers known to man.

How to Walk

There is a special way to walk, and it is very important that it be done correctly. Be sure to keep your knees and ankles limber, and point the toes straight ahead. Holding your head and chest high, swing your legs directly forward from the hip joints. Don't shuffle your feet. Push them directly off the ground. Shoulders and arms should swing freely and easily.

The position of the hips is one reliable indicator of posture. They should rest squarely upon the legs without tilting forward or backward.

Flabby abdominal muscles and excess weight—particularly in the abdominal region—are frequent causes of poor posture and improper walking. Weak abdominal muscles permit the internal organs to drop. The results: the abdomen protrudes, the pelvis tilts forward and the curve of the lower back is accentuated. Lower back pains may occur.

The obese person's "paunch" upsets his center of gravity. As it pulls him forward, he compensates by leaning backward, bending his knees slightly and increasing the curve of his back. That produces the characteristic "old man's stance."

Excessive use of high heeled shoes can produce the same effect in women —even young women. Additionally, the muscles in the calves and the backs of the thighs are shortened, so that it may be uncomfortable to go barefoot or wear low heels.

Adequate dress for walking requires loose fitting, comfortable clothing and good shoes. Comfortable clothing normally offers no problem to most walkers. It's their footwear that most often causes concern. Pointed toes, thin soles, and spiked heels all make for some upleasant walks, causing many people to complain about burning or aching feet.

The walk to work, to lunch, or even around the block is a chore for those men who wear pointed-toed shoes and elevated (cuban) heels. And women who are subject to the whims of fickle fashion are even less fortunate. The style-conscious distaff set is forced to wear pointed-toed shoes, high heels and thin soles, all of which are not conducive to good walking.

In recent years, however, many women have achieved a compromise between style and comfort by wearing square toes and lower heels. But the problem of the thin sole still remains.

Ask several walkers what type of shoe is best and you will get a variety of answers. Actually the shoe should be firm, solid, thick-soled and arch supported. Walkers differ on their feelings about the weight of the shoe —some prefer it light and flexible, while others like it rather heavy and sturdy.

Manufacturers have tried to combine these points of view by making shoes both sturdy and light. They also have added non-skid soles, fleece linings, sweat absorbent insole and water proofing—all with a minimum of weight allowance.

Walkers normally recognize several basic elements as essential to a good walking shoe.

They are:

(1) A wide flat heel

(2) A broad rounded toe

(3) A straight line from inner toe to inner heel

(4) Ample room for toes

(5) A heel gripped firmly so that blisters are kept at a minimum

(6) A tongue to keep out dirt, etc.

(7) A firm heel and toe for protection

(8) A non-skid heel and sole. (Essential for city walking, but not as critical for walks in the country.)

(9) If shoes have laces, they should not cut. In long distance walking, hooks on the outside of the shoe are desirable.

°WALKING PROGRAM

Chart 1	Chart 2
1. Walk 1 mile in 15 minutes	1. Walk 3 miles in 43 minutes
2. Walk 1 mile in 14 minutes	2. Walk 3½ miles in 51 minutes
3. Walk 1¼ miles in 22 minutes	3. Walk 3½ miles in 50 minutes
4. Walk 1¼ miles in 21 minutes	4. Walk 3¾ miles in 54 minutes
5. Walk 2 miles in 30 minutes	5. Walk 3¾ miles in 53 minutes
6. Walk 2 miles in 28 minutes	6. Walk 4 miles in 57 minutes
7. Walk 2¼ miles in 37 minutes	7. Walk 4 miles in 56 minutes
8. Walk 2¼ miles in 36 minutes	8. Walk 4 miles in 55 minutes
9. Walk 3 miles in 44 minutes	9. Walk 4 miles in 54 minutes

° See ENDURANCE and ENERGY COST OF ACTIVITIES for an explanation of the charts.

Fitness 1

If you achieved a score of poor or low average on the *Harvard Step Test* or a score of very poor or poor on the *12 Minute Run*, start on Chart 1-Level 1 and spend 1 week at each level until Chart 2-Level 9 is reached. It is recommended that you participate 4 to 5 days a week. When Chart 2-Level 9 is reached, 4 days a week is sufficient.

Fitness 2

If you achieved a score of high average on the *Harvard Step Test* or fair on the *12 Minute Run*, start on Chart 1-Level 4. Spend 1 week on Chart 1-Levels 1, 3, 5, 7, 9, and Chart 2-Levels 1, 3, 5, 6, 9. It is recommended that you participate 4 to 5 days a week. When Chart 2-Level 9 is reached, 4 days a week is sufficient.

Fitness 3

If you achieved a score of good or excellent on either the *Harvard Step Test* or *12 Minute Run,* continue your current program or select Chart 2-Level 9 as your level of participation. Four days a week is sufficient.

---

(10) A waterproofed space between the sole and upper part of the shoe

(11) A shoe that's flexible and not too heavy

Since walking is a mild- to high-energy-cost activity, it may be used to help improve your fitness level, especially your circulo-respiratory and muscle endurance.

Below is a walking program that takes into account the important principles of training. See HIKING for a related program.

WARM-UP

The value of warm-ups, or working into an activity gradually, has been investigated frequently in the past twenty years. The results have been conflicting. Because of that disunity, it has been difficult to establish general principles or guidelines regarding warm-up.

All investigators agree that there are two types of warm-up. The general (informal) and the formal. The general warm-up involves exercising the large muscles of the body. Calisthenics, such as the daily dozen, are an excellent example of the general type. Showers, whirlpool baths, diathermy and massage are also considered to be a general warm-up. The formal warm-up, on the other hand, involves practicing the skills to be used in the forthcoming competition or activity. Shooting clay pigeons for the skeet shooter, serving a tennis ball for the tennis player, and swinging a baseball bat for a baseball player are excellent examples of the formal warm-up. Although all the experimental evidence regarding the value of the warm-up on performance, prevention of injuries, and the like is incomplete, most of the investigators agree on the following statements.

1. The formal warm-up affects the nervous and muscular systems and is beneficial in affecting performance. In effect, the person practices the skill with the formal warm-up just prior to the actual event. That procedure, of formal warm-up, therefore, should be continued in activities which require skillful controlled movements.

2. The value of the warm-up to improve performance in enduring events, which have low elements of skill, speed or strength, is questionable.

3. Showers, diathermy and massage generally are not found to improve performance.

4. The formal warm-up is superior to the general warm-up in improving performance.

5. The mental attitude or psychological ramifications play a critical role in the effect of warm-up on performance.

6. If the temperature is so low that the limbs are numb, there is a need for a general warm-up.

There are several points, however, on which the investigators do not agree due to conflicting evidence.

1. Failure to warm up before vigorous activity may lead to an actual tearing of muscle fibers from their tendinous attachments.

2. A general warm-up is unnecessary unless the external temperature is so low that the limbs are numb.

3. Investigators agree that logically the rise in body temperature due to exercise stimulates biochemical reactions to supply energy for muscular contraction; and an increased body temperature (therefore, muscle temperatures) shortens the period of muscle contraction. The same investigators, however, have not been able to demonstrate that those two phenomenon will affect performance.

Oldsters and Warm-Up

What effect will exercise have on an older person if he does not warm up properly? Dr. Thomas K. Cureton at the University of Illinois feels that a warm-up is necessary to prepare the circulatory system for demanding exercise. He states that it is unwise for an older person to go right out and start working at a very hard rate without first warming up. Their circulatory system is not as flexible as it was in younger days. Hence, an overexertion may cause serious consequences to the human organism. It is very important that the older person work very gradually into the exercise routine, slowly increasing the intensity of exercise. That will allow the circulatory system to adjust to the increased work gradually.

Dr. V. Wright, Consultant Physician in Rheumatology, at the University of Leeds, has reported that a lack of movement increases the stiffness of joints while movement lessens the stiffness of joints. He has conducted experiments at the rheumatism research laboratory which have demonstrated that exercise will reduce physical stiffness. That reduction is due to the interesting plasticity which tissues around the joints possess. The studies have also indicated that there is an improvement in grip strength and a reduction in stiffness if there is an increase in body temperature. He notes that those findings have strong implications for warming up. Other investigators agree that deep body temperature must be raised sufficiently.

Furthermore, the majority of research findings tend to indicate that a warm-up is unnecessary in preventing injury. Many people who have been actively engaged in prescribing exercise programs, training athletes, and coaching teams, however, feel that a sufficient warm-up lessens the chance of injury. Since empirical evidence seems to indicate that a warm-up may be beneficial, it is wise that the practice be continued until research becomes conclusive.

As a general rule, people who are involved in sport should warm up with activities closely related to their particular event. Other individuals, following more general exercise programs, such as walking, running and jogging, will find it to their benefit to start the exercises slowly, gradually increasing the intensity of exercise. At least 10 to 15 minutes should be spent by the older person in preparing his body for more demanding activities. See TAPERING OFF.

WATER CONSUMPTION AND RETENTION

Should athletes or fitness seekers drink water during a workout in warm weather?

Physiological evidence, and some unfortunate experiences, have reversed the trend of restraining water intake during workouts. During physical exertion, particularly in warm weather, a considerable amount of water and salt may be lost through the skin in the cooling process of sweating. Since the body is made up of approximately 60 per cent water, such a water loss can adversely affect body chemistry. Salt plays an important regulating role in body functions, and the replacing of water without replacing salt at the same time serves only to dilute the salt reserves of the body, thereby decreasing its effectivenes as a regulator. Therefore, it has become common practice to administer salt tablets with water during a workout.

Water consumption and retention depend upon a number of factors: the amount of liquid intake, the weather, physical exertion and other chemical considerations. The water control mechanisms are the lungs, the skin and the kidneys. During increased respiratory activity, more moisture is lost via the lungs in the exhalation phase of the breathing cycle. Increased physical exertion tends to increase the amount of urine since more wastes are forming in the muscles and must be removed. A greater amount of water is needed to sufficiently dilute the wastes and carry them out of the body. On a hot day, the kidneys return more water to the blood stream so that it can be used to cool the body by evaporation through the skin.

The control of the amount of water filtered by the kidneys comes from the pituitary gland. A hormone secreted by the cortex of the adrenal gland controls the amount of salt affected. See SALT TABLETS.

WATER SKIING

Water skiing is an American sport by origin and, simply defined, consists of a participant on one or two skis being towed behind a motor boat. The necessary equipment includes a maneuverable boat with adequate horsepower, a light towline with handle, appropriate skis and suitable flotation gear. The remaining essentials are a competent driver and a qualified observer for the boat.

The various skills and stunts of the sport are: skiing on two skis, single or slalom skiing, trick riding, jumping, competitive skiing and novelty acts such as barefooting and kite-flying. Water skiing can afford you as much challenge as you want or simply the opportunity to enjoy the exhilarating effect of skimming across the water.

Contrary to oft-expressed opinion, water skiing is easily learned and relatively safe. Over 10 million participants attest to its popularity, and the number continues to increase.

Contribution to Physical Fitness

Water skiing can make an important contribution to physical fitness, primarily in the areas of muscular strength and endurance. The potential contribution to cardio-respiratory endurance falls somewhere between low and medium, since the boat provides the prime source of propulsion. The activity does foster ankle, knee and hip flexibility, particularly in assuming a deep crouch position to take off or start skiing.

The potential contribution of water skiing to physical fitness is a function of the workload involved relative to the existing fitness level of the participant. The workload is determined by: (1) the length of the period spent in continuous skiing, and the total time involved on a given occasion; (2) the amount of activity entailed; and (3) the type of skiing done. For instance, 10 minutes of continuous skiing requires more energy expenditure than does comparable skiing for a 3-minute period. And crossing the wake (waves left behind) of a boat 30 times compared to 10 in the same time interval entails more work done. It is more strenuous to jump the wake each time

rather than simply riding over it. Finally, slalom skiing is more vigorous than skiing on two skis.

While the contribution of water skiing to cardio-respiratory endurance appears limited, your level of cardio-respiratory endurance will determine the overall vigor with which you can water ski. Do not anticipate the development of increased cardio-respiratory endurance to any great extent through water skiing.

The prime and significant contribution of water skiing to physical fitness is in muscular strength and endurance. Through the variables determining workload, you can noticeably enhance the development of muscular strength and endurance, particularly the muscles of the arms and shoulder girdle. However, since the activity entails resisting the pull of the boat and the force of the water and also initiating bodily movement apart from those two forces, virtually

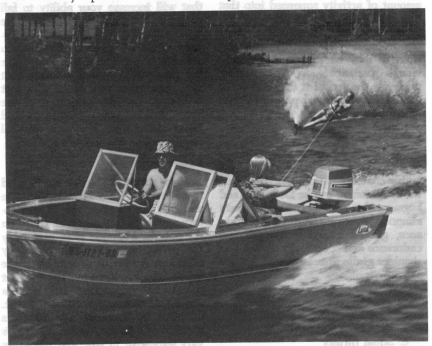

Successful water skiers combine strength and flexibility into plenty of exercise fun.

all muscle groups of the body have a part to play. The abdominal, back and buttock muscles undergo considerable stress in maintaining and changing body positions. Obviously, the hip and leg muscles are active in absorbing the pounding of waves, jumping and executing turning movements. Certain takeoffs and changes in direction demand considerable muscular strength to maintain a grip on the handle of the towrope. As you persist for prolonged periods in performing those aspects of skiing that require considerable strength, you will naturally develop the endurance of the active muscles.

Water skiing affords everyone the opportunity to develop muscular strength and endurance while literally "having a ball." You will progress easily in skill, and by gradually increasing the amount of time spent skiing (for which the inherent fun will provide the motivation), the amount of activity squeezed into that time and the energy demands of the type of activity, you will noticeably improve your overall muscular strength and endurance. Most individuals participate in water skiing solely for the fun of it and derive the concomitant improved physical fitness as a dividend.

Conditioning Programs

Graduated, progressive participation in water skiing itself affords a pleasurable conditioning process. However, the conditioning can be facilitated and augmented by programs that direct attention to cardio-respiratory endurance, general muscular strength and endurance and specifically to arm and shoulder girdle muscle groups that are active in pulling.

General Exercise
  a. Running
  b. Bent knee sit-ups
  c. Squat thrusts
  d. Squat jumps
  e. Treadmill
  f. Standing broad jump
  g. Vertical jump
  h. Chinning
  i. Rope or pole climbing
  j. Hanging and walking by hands on horizontal ladder
  k. Repetitive squeezing of soft rubber ball in each hand

See ISOMETRICS and WEIGHT TRAINING for additional exercises.

The prospective water skier should be physically sound and in reasonably good health. Age is of no consequence; skiers range from preschoolers to senior citizens who are well into their retirement years. It is imperative that you be at ease in the water and be able to swim well enough to move about for several minutes, with or without flotation gear. That quality is not only a safety precaution but also eliminates the fear of being "dumped." You should be able to jump and dive into the water with relative ease, for that will increase your ability to fall properly. It is also desirable to have some muscular strength and endurance, which will prolong the time you are able to spend on skis and minimize the resultant muscular soreness that may accompany your initial efforts. It is best to be fully cognizant of the hand signals, voice commands and safety skiing tips. They are essential for the safety and enjoyment of all.

Equipment

Make sure that the skis are in good repair and suitable in style and size and that the flotation gear is satisfactory and worn properly with straps on the outside. Flotation gear, preferably the jacket type, should be worn by all skiers—novice to expert. Even the expert who has the wind knocked out due to an unexpected fall is in a serious predicament without a jacket. Children up to about age 10 years should use a junior size ski. Adult skis vary somewhat in size, and the larger size is preferable behind smaller horsepower boats and for heavier individuals. Finally, the towline should be 75 feet long with a single handle —and preferably made of a buoyant synthetic material, such as polypropylene.

Most Common Injuries

Water skiing is a relatively safe sport. Despite the fact that about ¾ of a million more Americans learn to ski each year, accidents and injuries are amazingly few. Water skiing mishaps are classified as pleasure-boating accidents and occur less frequently than those attributable to all other causes such as falling overboard, capsizing and collisions. Accidents that do occur usually are attributable to an uninformed amateur or reckless practices.

Injuries that appear most often are:

1. Low back strain, largely attributable to skiing for too long a period, assumption of poor and rigid body positions and unexpected falls or sudden changes in position.

2. Bruises about limbs and body, particularly the lower legs, resulting from bumping against the skis in falls, takeoffs and landings.

In *Today's Health,* Earl Hilligan and E. E. Maxwell delineated six precautions for skiers to heed, which seem very pertinent in promoting safe skiing:

Do not ski in shallow water. (Usually five feet is the minimum depth considered safe for adults.)

Do not wrap the towrope around any part of the body or put any part of the body through any so-called bridle or loop.

Do not attempt fast landing directly toward shore. Good practice is to run parallel with the shore and come in slowly when landing.

Quit before you become overly tired.

Do not ski in front of another boat.

Do not ski at night.—*Carlton R. Meyers*

Association:

American Water Ski Association (AWSA), Seventh Street and G Ave-

* WATER SKIING PROGRAM

Chart 1	Chart 2
1. 25 minutes	1. 75 minutes
2. 35 minutes	2. 85 minutes
3. 40 minutes	3. 90 minutes
4. 45 minutes	4. 95 minutes
5. 50 minutes	5. 100 minutes
6. 55 minutes	6. 105 minutes
7. 60 minutes	7. 110 minutes
8. 65 minutes	8. 115 minutes
9. 70 minutes	9. 120 minutes

* See ENDURANCE and ENERGY COST OF ACTIVITIES for an explanation of these charts.

Fitness 1

If you achieved a score of poor or low average on the *Harvard Step Test* or a score of very poor or poor on the *12 Minute Run,* start on Chart 1-Level 1 and spend 1 week at each level until Chart 2-Level 9 is reached. It is recommended that you participate 4 to 5 days a week. When Chart 2-Level 9 is reached, 4 days a week is sufficient.

Fitness 2

If you achieved a score of high average on the *Harvard Step Test* or fair on the *12 Minute Run,* start on Chart 1-Level 1. Spend 1 week on Chart 1-Levels 1, 3, 5, 7 and 9 and Chart 2-Levels 1, 2, 4, 6, 8 and 9. It is recommended that you participate 4 to 5 days a week. When Chart 2-Level 9 is reached, 4 days a week is sufficient.

Fitness 3

If you achieved a score of good or excellent on either the *Harvard Step Test* or *12 Minute Run,* continue your current program or select Chart 2-Level 9 as your level of participation. Four days a week is sufficient.

nue, S.W., Winter Haven, Florida 33880.

Since water skiing is a moderate-high-energy-cost activity, it may be used to help improve your fitness level, especially your circulo-respiratory and muscle endurance. Below is a water skiing program that takes into account the important principles of training.

Does not include putting skis on, swimming and so on. If those are included, water skiing is more demanding and need not take as long. If a single ski is used water skiing is a much more strenuous activity.

WEIGHT CONTROL

In today's society going on a diet is somewhat of a status symbol—a mark of the "In-Crowd." People seem to talk incessantly about such things as calories, dietary specialties, midriff bulge, overweight, non-sweetened sodas, the drinking man's diet, low calorie foods, obesity and heart disease.

Their concern often advances with an increase in years because usually there is a gradual increase in weight after the age of 25. In an effort to combat "creeping overweight," people turn to all forms of weight reducing techniques. The end result for most of those people is unsatisfactory. In fact, some may actually increase in weight.

There are others who claim that the increase in weight is just a sign of aging and that little can be done about it. While that may be typical, it is not necessary or desirable. Life insurance companies have published statistics indicating that people who are overweight have a greater possibility of dying prematurely than those of normal weight. The death rate for an individual 15 to 24 per cent overweight is about 20 per cent greater than those of people who are not overweight, yet of a comparable age. The statistics are even more frightening for men who are 35 per cent over-

weight. For with them, there is a 50 per cent greater death rate than the average. Why that is true has not been firmly established. However, indications are that there is a strong relationship between being overweight and many cardiovascular disorders. The extra strain placed on the heart, the high blood pressure, and the incidence of atherosclerosis are a few examples. Not to be discounted are the aesthetic qualities of a slim and trim figure. Many aspects of social, cultural and business life depend a great deal upon an attractive figure. Your physique plays an important role in the impression (especially the first) others have about you.

Being overweight can also restrict body movements, thereby making you less graceful and efficient. That aspect is critical for those who need certain physical skills for recreational and vocational purposes.

Height-Weight Tables

Perhaps you need to consider how much you should really weigh. Are you under- or overweight? Should you diet? In an effort to find the answers, people turn to height-weight tables, many of which have been published by various life insurance companies. But those charts may provide a rough guide at best. Use caution in interpreting them. Even though they provide for various builds (small, medium and large), many people don't know what size frame they have, or fail to consider their muscle structure (muscle weighs more than fat).

Calorie Charts

A calorie is the heat necessary to raise approximately one quart of water two degrees Fahrenheit. It is a term used by nutritionists for measuring the energy needs and expenditures of man and the energy value of various foods.

There are charts indicating the calories in different foods, charts that indicate the approximate calories con-

DESIRABLE WEIGHTS FOR MEN AND WOMEN
According to Height and Frame, Ages 25 and Over

WEIGHTS FOR WOMEN

Height (with shoes on) 2-inch heels	Small Frame	Medium Frame	Large Frame
4'10"	92- 98	96-107	104-119
11"	94-101	98-110	106-122
5' 0"	96-104	101-113	109-125
1"	99-107	104-116	112-128
2"	102-110	107-119	115-131
3"	105-113	110-122	118-134
4"	108-116	113-126	121-138
5"	111-119	116-130	125-142
6"	114-123	120-135	129-146
7"	118-127	124-139	133-150
8"	122-131	128-143	137-154
9"	126-135	132-147	141-158
10"	130-140	136-151	145-163
11"	134-144	140-155	149-168
6' 0"	138-148	144-159	153-173

WEIGHTS FOR MEN

Height (with shoes on) 1-inch heels	Small Frame	Medium Frame	Large Frame
5' 2"	112-120	118-129	126-141
3"	115-123	121-133	129-144
4"	118-126	124-136	132-148
5"	121-129	127-139	135-152
6"	124-133	130-143	138-156
7"	128-137	134-147	142-161
8"	132-141	138-152	147-166
9"	136-145	142-156	151-170
10"	140-150	146-160	155-174
11"	144-154	150-165	159-179
6' 0"	148-158	154-170	164-184
1"	152-162	158-175	168-189
2"	156-167	162-180	173-194
3"	160-171	167-185	178-199
4"	164-176	172-190	182-204

Weight in Pounds According to Frame (In Indoor Clothing)

sumed during various activities and charts that are a combination of the two. See CALORIES.

Counting calories at each meal can become quite a chore. The charts serve merely as a guide so that you have a general idea of the calorie requirements of various foods and the number of calories burned with different activities. Then logical judg-

ments can be made regarding the selection of activities and foods.

Calorie charts do not consider individual differences. Body weight, body build, skill level in the activity and present physical condition are all neglected.

For that reason, further information is necessary to evaluate truly the total calories burned during normal activity or exercise. Such information would include the energy cost of the activity and the total body surface area. (See charts.)

Don't rely solely on the charts. They are presented as a reference to help you establish guidelines for your exercise program. The charts also stress that you should be careful in attempting to balance your calorie intake (food eaten) and calorie expenditure (energy required for daily living).

There are several misunderstandings concerning exercise and the effect on body weight. Jean Mayer, Ph.D. and Frederick J. Stare, M.D. state that there are three general misconceptions about muscular exercise and weight control. The misconceptions are:

a. Exercise requires relatively little calorie expenditure, and, therefore, increased physical activity is of little use in weight reduction.

b. An increase in physical activity will be accompanied by an increase in appetite and food intake, thereby negating weight reduction.

c. Body weight is always a reliable measure of degree of obesity regardless of muscular development.

The authors systematically refute the misconceptions and conclude that exercise is the most practical way to increase energy expenditure. A person who is gaining weight or who is already overweight will require more energy to perform a given amount of work than one who is underweight or at normal weight, simply because of the extra weight that has to be moved during exercise. Research indicates that energy cost of exercise is approximately proportional to body weight.

Furthermore, a decrease in physical activity is not necessarily followed by a decrease in appetite, nor is an increase in physical activity followed by an increase in appetite, thereby discarding the second misconception.

Finally, the authors refute the third

misconception by using as an illustration, college football players. Many linemen average 5 feet 10 inches and weigh 200 pounds. According to desirable height and weight tables, those boys could be overweight and some even obese. Yet much of the body weight is muscle and not fat.

Mayer and Stare conclude with the caution that vigorous exercise occasionally or even weekly is of little value in weight reduction and may be hard on the cardiovascular system. Moderate, frequent and consistent exercise is the best route to weight control.

Heredity also plays an important role in weight control. If you are the child of stout or lean parents, you too may have a tendency toward stoutness or leanness, respectively. That tendency may be a result of heredity or it may be a similarity in eating habits. However, heredity can affect the rate at which your body uses its fuel (burns up the calories).

Your basal metabolism rate (BMR) —the rate at which your body uses energy to maintain itself while at complete rest—differs from that of your neighbor. You may know of someone who can eat a great deal but never seems to put on any excess weight. He is called a "fast burner," or one who has a high BMR.

Another heredity factor is body build. Some body types tend to put weight on more easily than others, see BODY TYPE. The key factors, however, in the majority of people are exercise and diet.

Basically, there are two distinct problems in weight control. One is the problem of reducing, while the second is the equally important problem of maintaining desirable weight.

If you are trying to take off just a few pounds, you may begin by regulating your calorie intake and outgo with an emphasis on increased activity without fear of harmful effects. If, however, you find yourself consider-

A Comparison of Energy Costs in Some Usual Activities vs. Sports

Normal Activity	*Cal./Min./Sq.M.**
Sitting, normal	0.70
Sitting, reading	0.70
Sitting, eating	0.80
Sitting, playing cards	0.83
Resting in bed	0.68
Standing, normal	0.81
Standing, light activity	1.41
Personal toilet	1.09
Shower	1.84
Dressing	1.84
Making bed	2.64
Shining shoes	2.11
Mopping floor	2.67
Walking indoors	1.68
Walking outdoors	3.07
Walking upstairs	10.00
Walking downstairs	3.80
Kneeling	0.68
Squatting	1.12
Washing clothes	1.46
Sport	
Football	5.04
Basketball	4.31
Ping-pong	2.42
Bowling	4.07
Swimming	6.06
Golfing	2.76
Tennis	3.50
Squash	5.00
Table tennis	2.00
Badminton	1.91
Rowing	4.00
Sailing	1.30
Snooker pool	1.50
Dancing	2.00
Riding	1.50
Boxing, sparring	5.00

* Based on basal metabolic rate of 0.59 calories per minute per square meter of body surface area. Cal./Min./Sq.M. = calories per minute per square meter of body surface area.

ably overweight, you should consult your physician before attempting any program of weight loss.

To maintain normal weight, you must attempt to balance your calorie intake and outgo so that your present weight remains constant.

The concern about weight control has stimulated much commercial interest. Companies and individuals have "sold" the public on machines and ideas that will supposedly help them lose weight or relocate their fat.

There are gimmicks such as vibrators, machines used to increase fitness, lose weight and promote relaxation. They range from small machines that are to be used to spot reduce (that is, concentrate on specific parts of the body such as the abdomen, bust, and so on) to vibrating chairs and beds.

Dr. Steinhaus in his article entitled

How to Determine Body Surface Area from Height and Weight (after Du Bois)

A given individual may determine his body surface area from his height and weight. Multiplication of body surface area by any one of the factors in the table gives caloric expenditure in calories per minute for that individual engaging in that particular activity.

Height in Feet	Weight in Pounds																
	55	66	77	88	99	110	121	132	143	154	165	176	187	198	209	220	231
6' 8"							1.84	1.91	1.97	2.03	2.09	2.15	2.21	2.26	2.31	2.36	2.41
6' 6"							1.80	1.87	1.93	1.99	2.05	2.11	2.17	2.22	2.27	2.32	2.37
6' 4"				1.56	1.63	1.73	1.77	1.84	1.90	1.96	2.02	2.08	2.13	2.18	2.23	2.28	2.33
6' 2"				1.53	1.60	1.70	1.74	1.80	1.86	1.92	1.98	2.04	2.09	2.14	2.19	2.24	2.29
6' 0"				1.49	1.57	1.67	1.71	1.77	1.83	1.89	1.95	2.00	2.05	2.10	2.15	2.20	2.25
5' 10"	1.19	1.28	1.36	1.46	1.53	1.64	1.67	1.73	1.79	1.85	1.91	1.96	2.01	2.06	2.11	2.16	2.21
5' 8"	1.17	1.26	1.34	1.43	1.50	1.57	1.63	1.69	1.75	1.81	1.86	1.91	1.96	2.01	2.06	2.11	
5' 6"	1.14	1.23	1.31	1.40	1.47	1.54	1.60	1.66	1.72	1.78	1.83	1.88	1.93	1.98	2.03	2.07	
5' 4"	1.12	1.21	1.29	1.37	1.44	1.50	1.56	1.62	1.68	1.73	1.78	1.83	1.88	1.93	1.98		
5' 2"	1.09	1.18	1.26	1.33	1.40	1.46	1.52	1.58	1.64	1.69	1.74	1.79	1.84	1.89			
5' 0"	1.06	1.15	1.23	1.30	1.36	1.42	1.48	1.54	1.60	1.65	1.70	1.75	1.80				
4' 10"	1.03	1.12	1.20	1.27	1.33	1.39	1.45	1.51	1.56	1.61	1.66	1.71					
4' 8"	1.00	1.09	1.17	1.24	1.30	1.36	1.42	1.47	1.52	1.57							
4' 6"	0.97	1.06	1.14	1.20	1.26	1.32	1.38	1.43	1.48								
4' 4"	0.95	1.04	1.11	1.17	1.23	1.29	1.35	1.40									
4' 2"	0.93	1.01	1.08	1.14	1.20	1.26	1.31	1.36									
4' 0"	0.91	0.98	1.04	1.10	1.16	1.22	1.27										

"Do Mechanical Vibrators Take Off or Redistribute Fat?" concluded that the vibrator used in the study (a fifteen-minute period of continuous vibrating of a most vigorous type with the belt placed around the abdomen) is not to be taken seriously as a device for reducing or redistributing fat. To lose one pound of fat would require approximately one fifteen-minute period per day for a year. See MECHANICAL DEVICES and MYTHS OF EXERCISE.

WEIGHT GAINING

A small segment of the population has a unique problem—they want to gain weight, usually to improve their appearance or to gain greater body mass for contact sports, such as football.

The easiest way to gain weight is to increase the intake of food and to conserve activity—the opposite of the technique employed for weight control. Eat high energy foods, use dietary supplements, eat regular meals, and take a few extra bits more than you feel you want. Snacking between meals will also help you increase caloric intake. Avoid eating too many sweets. Get adequate sleep, at least eight hours, daily.

For some people, however, that procedure may be unsuccessful because of their nervous temperament. They may seem to burn up more calories than they can consume. Furthermore, the weight-gaining program outlined above results in excessive fat tissue.

To avoid the depositing of unwanted fat tissue, select an exercise program that is designed to provide muscular hypertrophy (increase in size) with a minimum of energy expenditure. One of the best exercise programs, therefore, is weight training. See WEIGHT TRAINING for the various techniques. Weight training may be used successfully by men or women. Many times, however, women reject the idea of weight training for fear of developing unsightly muscles. Unless you carry the exercises to an extreme, sex differences prevent such an occurrence. The development of unsightly muscles in women is often called *masculinizing*. The masculinizing effects, however, are controlled by the endocrine glands and by body type and not by participation in sports. See BODY TYPE.

WEIGHT LOSS IN SPORTS

The practice of losing weight through dieting, dehydration, laxatives and diuretics in sports such as wrestling and boxing has been a concern of athletes and coaches for many years.

Many athletes engage in the practice of weight reducing, thinking that if they lose the weight, they will be able to participate at a lower weight class, thereby being relatively stronger than their opponent.

Research

Studies Indicating Deleterious Effect

K. Ahlman and M. J. Karvonen, in a 1962 issue of *Journal of Sports Medicine and Physical Fitness*, investigated the effects of sweating as a means of weight reduction and found that those individuals who lost 5 to 7 pounds had a less efficient cardiovascular system. An unpublished study conducted by Jennings B. Edward, supported Ahlman and Karvonen's investigation. He found that although semi-starvation and dehydration did not materially affect the strength of the subjects, their endurance was reduced. Other researchers have reported similar findings.

Studies Indicating Non-Deleterious Effect

About 25 years ago, W. W. Tuttle, in the *Research Quarterly* examined the neuromuscular, cardiovascular and respiratory responses of subjects who had been subjected to dehydration and semi-starvation. He found that except for a slight increase in heart rate and lung capacity the resulting weight loss did not affect the various physiological responses. He concluded that five per cent of an athlete's body weight may be lost without affecting his physical performance. A study by Nathan Doscher in the *Research Quarterly* a year later, supported Tuttle's work.

Howard M. Byram in an unpublished Master's Thesis from the State University of Iowa in 1953, conducted an experiment in which athletes lost up to 18.7 per cent of their body weight. The weight loss had no detrimental effect on strength, muscular endurance or cardiorespiratory endurance.

Harold Nichols, in his unpublished Doctoral Dissertation, studied the effect of weight loss (1.67 per cent to 11.11 per cent of the total body weight, with an average loss of 6.78 per cent) on various performance measures. The weight loss did not affect the performance of the wrestlers on their tests. In fact, in each of the tests, the results favored the wrestlers who lost the weight.

C. Kuntzleman's study of the effects of a limited diet on cardiovascular and neuromuscular performance revealed similar results. A person may lose five per cent of his body weight without adversely affecting his physical performance.

Limitations of Cited Research

All of those investigators, however, fail to evaluate what effect the starvation and dehydration have on the internal organs of the body, such as the kidneys. That consideration is an extremely important area of investigation that has been neglected. Extended periods of weight loss should also be investigated. Furthermore, the majority of the research has been conducted on college-age or older subjects, thereby neglecting what effect starvation and dehydration has on the development of a younger athlete.

Because of those unknown areas, coaches and physical educators must exercise caution in permitting a person to lose a sizable percentage of weight. Even though physical performance and the ability to do well on fitness tests are not affected by weight loss, there is no indication from research that nothing is seriously wrong internally. There are several clinical reports of Olympic athletes at the peak of training and condition who are stricken with various physical disorders, i.e., tuberculosis, cutaneous infections, infantile paralysis and the like.

Philip Rasch and Walter Kroll summarize very nicely the most recent thinking on the problem of making weight. They state:

"Making weight is an undesirable practice for the adolescent. The older individual in good training may take off up to approximately 10 per cent of his normal weight for brief periods without adversely affecting his strength endurance, reaction time, fatigue rate or blood pressure. Reducing weight by restriction of caloric intake over long periods of time involves the risk of vitamin and mineral deficiency. Reducing by restricting water intake may result in fatigue. The physiological effects of dehydration are apparently more severe than those of semi-starvation."

Moreover, the withholding of food and water may cause psychological problems. In the experiment conducted by C. Kuntzleman, some of the subjects complained about their inability to sleep because of the desire for food and water. Others complained about dreaming of being on a desert without water. Still others felt they were unable to concentrate while studying. All the subjects felt they became fatigued more rapidly. At the time of the test, however, they prepared themselves mentally to do their very best.

The psychological aspects, therefore,

cannot be discounted; for a young man in the heat of competition may extend himself to a maximum performance despite the severe weight loss, thereby possibly jeopardizing his physical health.

WEIGHT TRAINING AND WEIGHT LIFTING

Man's interest in his strength and its development has been of concern, probably, from the beginning of his existence. In no phase of his sporting endeavor has that interest been more noticeably present than in weight lifting. Although the terms weight training and weight lifting are frequently interchanged, they are really quite distinctly different.

Weight lifting, as we know it today, is a competitive sport, the object of which is to lift a greater total poundage than your competitors with three basic lifts. The lifts, usually referred to as the Olympic lifts because of their inclusion in the Olympic Games, are the press, snatch, clean and jerk. Each of the lifts is governed by a strict performance code, enforced by the presence of judges. Most weight lifting competition in the United States is sponsored by the Amateur Athletic Union.

Weight training, on the other hand, refers to the process of developing muscular strength and/or endurance by exercising with weights or resistive devices. Weight training is based upon the principle that the body is capable of adapting to stresses placed upon it, called overload, and in doing such will generally bring about an overcompensation. By progressively increasing the intensity of the effort, you can effect a series of compensatory readjustments and, thereby, gain in strength and/or endurance. For that reason, weight training is technically referred to as progressive resistance exercise. As a conditioning method, weight training is, therefore, applicable to any

sport including weight lifting. The training methods may be adapted toward the development of strength, endurance, flexibility or other physical characteristics depending upon the objectives of the training program.

Body building is another possible objective of weight training in which primary emphasis is placed upon the aesthetic aspects of the body. Body building contests (Mr. America, Mr. Universe, etc.) are sponsored by various organizations on a regular basis. Many people train with weights merely as a method of developing and/or maintaining physical fitness.

Contribution of the Activity to Physical Fitness

Weight training is unsurpassed as a method of developing and maintaining muscular strength. Because of that, the use of weights in the conditioning program has been so widely adopted by coaches and athletes in a great variety of sports. Although the main value of weight training lies in the efficacy with which it can develop strength, you can modify procedures to place more emphasis upon endurance. Flexibility may also be promoted by emphasizing that the movements be carried out through the full range of motion about the joint. Failure to adhere to that principle may bring about quite the opposite, a loss of flexibility. It is probably due to a failure to train throughout the full range of motion that the misleading term *muscle-bound* has sprung into existence. The term is misleading because an extremely muscular person can still possess superior flexibility if, in his training program, he has emphasized development of all muscle groups. Without adequate emphasis being placed upon the development of the antagonistic muscle or muscles he would tend to facilitate asymmetrical development and reduce flexibility. Remember that the effects of training are highly specific and the qualities of strength, endurance and flexibility will be developed only to the degree that they are emphasized in the training program and will be specific to those areas of the body that are focused upon for the training program. See MUSCLE-BOUNDNESS.

In order to develop cardio-respiratory endurance, the cardio-respiratory stress must be reflected not only in an increased pulse rate but also in the maintenance of such an increased rate for a sustained period of time. Relatively short bursts of activity as generally practiced in weight training are usually effective in elevating the pulse rate; but since the activity is of relatively short duration, that is not conducive to development of cardio-respiratory endurance. By increasing

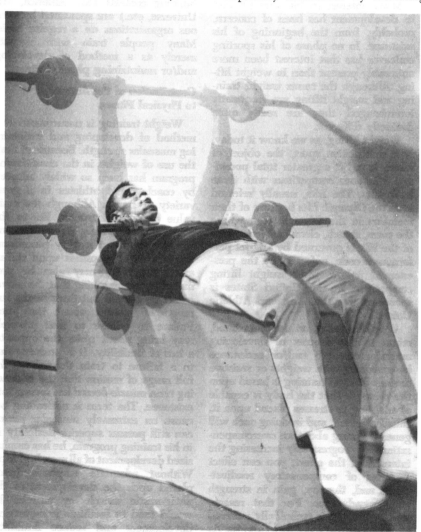

Weight training doesn't have to be an exercise in extremism. Here a weight trainer uses a bench press as an effective method of increasing upper torso strength.

the intensity of the work (work done per unit of time), you can increase the cardio-respiratory stress and, therefore, increase cardio-respiratory endurance. Circuit training, when practiced with weights, will lead to the development of good cardio-respiratory endurance. Participation in weight lifting alone, without regard to the weight training procedures employed in conditioning, would have little effect on the cardio-respiratory system.

Conditioning Programs for the Activity

Since the effects of training are highly specific, the best conditioning program for competitive weight lifting involves performance of the actual lifts for competition. Preparation for actual lifting of limit weight is best done by practicing the lift in sets of few repetitions with a progressive increase in poundage. Practice on a three day a week schedule, alternating days of rest. Maximum limit lifting should be done no more than one day each week and perhaps even less frequently depending upon the competitive schedule and stage of training. There are many different methods of training for the development of strength, however, only three of the better known systems will be discussed here. Regardless of the system you follow, begin with a relatively light weight and progress to increasingly greater resistance.

The DeLorme Method—Prior to World War II, there was little emphasis placed upon physical conditioning with the use of weights. Athletic coaches were skeptical of the results of training with weights, and fear of becoming "muscle-bound" led them to discourage their athletes' interest in that type of activity. The attitude was probably due to their observation of the "strongmen" of that era who were large, corpulent men capable of tremendous feats of strength. The results

of physical rehabilitation of combat-dehabilitated veterans directed by Dr. Thomas DeLorme was one of the factors that led to a change of attitude toward the use of weights in physical conditioning. The DeLorme method is based on the performance of 3 sets of 10 repetitions* as follows: first set-10 repetitions using a weight equal to one-half of that which could be lifted a total of 10 repetitions maximum (RM); second set = full ten RM.

The Oxford Technique—The Oxford technique, sometimes referred to as the Zinovieff method, involves the performance of a greater total number of repetitions and a greater range of proportionate resistance than the DeLorme method. Ten sets are performed, each set consisting of 10 repetitions. The first set consists of a full 10 RM, and the resistance for each successive set is reduced so that 10 repetitions may be completed. The basic principle is to keep the muscle working against maximal resistance even though performance capacity is being reduced by fatigue. All present systems are variations of those two classical approaches.

Set System—The set system is based on the performance of a number of sets (three is usually thought to be optimal) during which the resistance remains constant, thereby reducing the repetitions of each succeeding set. The optimal number of repetitions per set are between 4 and 8, with 6 the most commonly practiced number. That system, or other mild variations of it, appears to be the most widely practiced one among present day weight trainers.

---

* A repetition is a complete performance of the exercise, frequently referred to as an execution. If the exercise were to be repeated ten times, it would be described as ten repetitions. Although that is, in reality, only *nine repetitions but ten executions,* the term repetitions seems to be inextricably lodged in the weight training nomenclature. A set is a given number of repetitions. Repetitions maximum (RM) refers to the maximum number of repetitions that can be performed with a given weight.

Physical Qualities Needed for Participation

Before participation in weight lifting or weight training, as in the case of any strenuous activity, you should be declared medically fit by a physician. Weight training is widely employed in rehabilitative work and, therefore, can be adapted to the physical condition of most people. However, limitations should be realistically appraised. The beginning participant must realize that there are individual rates of response to that type of training and should not expect to progress at any preconceived rate. Your limits are set by a combination of heredity and intensity of training. The psychological characteristics of determination, perseverance and ability to tolerate discomfort are essential. Since competitive lifting is based upon weight classification, a smaller person enjoys the same degree of potential success as a much larger individual; in fact, a shorter man has several advantages over the taller man, e.g., better leverage, less distance to lift the weight, and greater relative strength.

Most Common Injuries

Contrary to popular opinion, weight training and weight lifting are among the safest of all types of physical activity. Sprains and strains, the most common injuries, are neither overly frequent nor exceptionally severe when compared with other sports. Practice proper lifting techniques in order to avoid back injuries resulting from placing the spinal column in an unfavorable position. Keep the back as straight as possible with the large muscles of the legs being responsible for initiating the lift from the floor. Hernia does not seem to be a serious problem among weight lifters. However, individuals suffering from such an ailment should not participate in the activity unless medically prescribed.

The greatest source of potential danger in weight training or lifting is being struck by a weight. That would be most likely to occur from failure to observe proper safety procedures. Many inexperienced lifters, when attempting to lift maximal weights, have a tendency to seriously disrupt breathing by straining against the resistance which results in an increased intrathoracic pressure and tends to interfere with the return of blood to the heart. If sustained long enough, that could result in a temporary loss of consciousness (cerebral anoxia). Since, following that exertion, there is a compensatory high elevation of the blood pressure, perform such exercises with caution if you have dysfunction of the cardio-respiratory system. If you adhere to proper safety procedures by working with spotters when lifting heavy weights overhead, little danger of injury exists. See VALSALVA PHENOMENON.—*Gere B. Fulton*

Progressive Resistance Exercises

People lift weights for one of three purposes: weight training, weight lifting or body building. Weight training is the development of increased physical capacity—namely increased muscle endurance, strength, speed of movements and power. Weight lifting is the sport of raising heavy amounts of weight overhead, using a certain type of lift. Body building is concerned with the size of the muscles and developing a well-proportioned body. Here are some exercises used primarily for weight training and body building.

Neck

1. *Neck Curl*—Assume a supine position on the floor with a weight (plate) held in place on the forehead with both hands. The legs are straight or bent. Curl your head forward until your chin touches the throat. Return slowly. The curl develops the muscles that draw the head forward.

2. *Side Neck Lift*—Assume a side-

lying position with a weight (plate) held in place on the side of the head. Lift your head upward and (sideward) as far as possible. Return slowly. This lift develops muscles that draw the head to the side. Repeat on other side.

3. *Neck Extension*—Assume a prone position on the floor, with a weight (plate) held in place on back of the head. The legs and toes touching the floor. Lift your head backward and upward as high as possible. Return slowly. The extension develops the muscles that draw the head backward.

Shoulder

4. *Arm Press*—Assume a standing position with a barbell in front of the chest, palms forward. Extend the barbell over the head with your arms straight; return. The press develops shoulder, upper back, upper chest and back of upper arm muscles.

5. *Bench Press*—Lie on a bench with the knees bent and feet on the floor (flat). The barbell is across the chest with the palms forward. Press the barbell upward until the arms are fully extended. Then return to the chest. The press develops the muscles of the chest, front shoulders and back of the upper arms.

6. *Shoulder Shrug*—Stand with the arms extended forward. The barbell is held with palms facing body grip; and the barbell is resting against the thighs. Elevate the shoulders and attempt to touch the top of your shoulders to the ears. Return slowly. The muscles of the upper shoulders and side of the neck are affected.

7. *Lateral Raise*—Stand with the palms facing the body and the dumbbells at the sides of the body. Lift the dumbbells sideways to a horizontal level or beyond to an overhead position. The muscles of the outer shoulders are developed (deltoid, trapezius and serratus anterior).

8. *Rowing*—Stand with the feet spread apart. Your trunk is flexed at a 90° angle. The knees and back are straight. Grasp the bar at a little more than shoulder width with the palms on top and the arms straight. Lift the bar to the chest, by bending the elbows and bringing the bar to the chest. Rowing develops the muscles of the back, back of the shoulders and the front of the upper arms.

9. *Prone Arm Lift* (on stomach)— Assume a prone position with the arms extended at right angles to the body. The dumbbells are grasped with the palms toward the floor. Raise the arms as high as possible, toward the ceiling. Lower slowly. The lift develops muscles of the upper back and the back of the shoulder.

Chest

10. *Supine Pull-Over* (on back)— Assume a supine position; your arms are extended above the head. The palms are facing forward. Raise the arms to a 90° angle, and then return to the original position. The arms must be kept straight through the entire movement. The pull-over develops muscles of the front of the chest, back of the upper arms and sides of the chest.

11. *Forward Raise*—Stand with the dumbbells at the sides of the body, palms facing the body. Elevate the dumbbells forward to the horizontal position, lower to original position. The raise develops muscles of the upper chest and front shoulders.

Upper Arms

12. *Barbell Curls*—Stand with the arms extended downward, the barbell against the thighs and the palms forward. Flex your forearms so that the bar is brought to the shoulders. Return until the arms are fully extended. The muscles of the front of the upper arms and forearms are developed.

13. *Reverse Curl*—Assume a standing position with palms facing the thighs as the barbell is held directly in front of the thighs. The bar is brought to the shoulders, as in the

arm curl, except that the palms are facing in the opposite direction. The curl develops the front of the upper arm and back of the forearm muscles.

14. *Triceps Press*—Assume a standing position with the dumbbell held overhead. The arms are completely extended with the palms facing inward. Lower the weight slowly behind the neck, bending the elbows. Then return. The press develops the muscles of the upper arm.

Forearms

15. *Wrist Curl*—Sit on a bench with the forearms resting on the thighs, and the wrists extended beyond the knees. The barbell is held with the palms facing forward. Extend the hands at the wrists, lowering the bar as far as possible. Then flex the wrists bringing the bar upward as far as possible. The curl develops the flexor muscle of the forearm and hand.

16. *Wrist Extensor*—Sit on a bench with the forearm resting on the thigh and the wrists extended beyond the knees. The barbell is held with the palms facing downward. Lift the weight by extending the wrist upward, through its maximum range of movement. The extensor develops the extensor muscles of the forearm and hand.

17. *Supinator-Pronator*—Sit on a bench with the forearm on the table and only the wrist and hand extended over the support. Grasp a dumbbell bar with a weight on only one end in an upright position. Lower the weight to the one side so that the palm is facing upward, then return to an upright position, and lower it to the other side so that the palm is facing downward. The exercise develops the supinator and pronators of the forearms.

18. *Wrist Abduction*—After loading a dumbbell at one end only, grasp the other end. Allow the dumbbell to drop slowly in an arc until it points to the

floor and then return it to its original position.

19. *Wrist Adduction*—Load the dumbbell as in the previous exercise but reverse the loaded end so that it points to the rear. Allow the dumbbell to drop slowly in the arc until it points to the floor and then return in the same arc to the original position.

20. *Wrist Roller*—Take a cylindrical handle about 12 inches long and fasten a rope or window sash cord to its center. Tie a weight to the opposite end of the rope. Roll all the rope onto the handle and then reverse the movement, allowing the weight to return to the starting position.

Abdomen

21. *Sit-Ups*—Assume a supine position with the knees bent and the feet held by a barbell or assistant. A weight (plate) is held behind the head. Sit up, touching the left elbow to the right knee and then the right elbow to the left knee and return. Sit-ups develop the abdominal muscles.

22. *Side Bend*—Assume a standing position with a barbell resting on the shoulders. Bend the body to the right side as far as possible. Return carefully to the erect position. Then repeat to the other side. The side bend develops the muscles on the side of the abdomen.

23. *Leg Press Out*—Assume a sitting position with the hands located directly behind the buttocks. Draw the legs up in a tuck position and have all the weight resting on the buttocks and hands. Slowly extend the legs together until they are fully extended and approximately 8-12 inches from the floor. Weighted or heavy shoes should be used. The press out develops the muscles of the abdomen and upper legs and hips.

Lower Back

24. *Dead Lift*—Assume a position so that the body is bent at the waist and the upper body is horizontal to

the floor; the legs are straight. The arms are straight and the barbell is held by the hands with the palms facing the body. Lift with the back and come to a standing position, then return to original position. The lift develops the muscles of the lower back. (The exercise may also be performed with the knees bent.) Most adults should use light weight as a warm-up until they are well conditioned.

25. *Leg Extensor Lift*—Assume a prone position with the arms extended above the head. With a weighted or heavy shoe, lift one leg upward (straight) as far as possible, return slowly. Then repeat on the other side. The lift develops muscles of the lower back, hips, back of upper leg.

26. *Trunk Extension*—Assume a prone position with the hips supported by a small bench. A weight (plate) is held behind the head, the feet are held by an assistant. Start with the head on the floor, then raise the upper body as high as possible.

Hip and Pelvis

27. *Hip Flexor*—Assume a sitting position on a table with the edge of the table touching the back of the knee and grasping the edges of the table with the hands. With a weighted boot or very heavy shoe, raise the knee toward the chest, as far as possible. Lower slowly and repeat. Do not bend your body forward or backward. The muscles of the front of the hip and upper leg are developed.

28. *Hip Abductor*—Assume a side lying position with the under arm extended above the head. The top arm is across the front of the body for support. With a weighted boot or very heavy shoe, raise the top leg as far as possible, working toward 45° or more. Lower slowly. Repeat. Keep the knee extended at all times. The abductor develops muscles on the side of the hip area.

Thigh

29. *One-half Squat*—Assume a standing position with a barbell on the shoulders behind the neck and the feet comfortably spread. Bend the knees so that a one-half squat (90°) is performed. Then return to a starting position. The squat develops muscles of the front thigh and lower leg.

30. *Straddle Lift*—Crouch with the legs straddling the barbell. One foot is slightly in front of the other. Grasp the bar with the hands, one in front of the body, the other behind. The thumbs are facing forward. Keep the head up and the back straight. Extend the knees and trunk coming to an erect position. Return to the crouch. The lift develops muscles of upper and lower leg and the lower back. Anyone who has had a hernia should avoid this exercise.

31. *Walking Squat*—Stand with a barbell resting on the shoulders behind the neck. One foot is 12-18 inches in front of the other. Take one step forward and execute a one-half knee bend, return to an upright position. Take one step forward—repeat. The squat develops muscles of the upper and lower leg.

32. *Knee Curl*—Assume a prone position with hands extended above the head. With a weighted boot or very heavy shoe on the foot, curl the leg inward until the boot nearly or actually touches the buttocks, slowly return. The curl develops the muscles of the back of the leg.

33. *Sitting Knee Curl*—Sit on the edge of a table with your legs hanging over the edge. With a weighted boot raise your lower leg to a horizontal position, return slowly. Develops the extensors of the leg.

34. *Toe Raise*—Assume a standing position with a barbell resting on the shoulders behind the neck. The balls of the feet are resting on a 1-2 inch block of wood, and the feet are on the floor. Raise up on the toes as far as

EXERCISE	All Around	Archery	Australian Rules Football	Badminton	Baseball	Basketball	Bicycling	Bowling	Boxing	Canoeing
Neck:										
Neck Curl	X		X	X						
Side Neck Lift	X									
Neck Extension	X	X	X	X						
Shoulder:										
Arm Press	X		X	X		X	X			X
Bench Press	X	X		X	X					X
Shoulder Shrug	X	X	X	X	X	X		X		
Lateral Raise		X		X	X	X			BE SURE ALL MUSCLE GROUPS ARE INCLUDED	
Rowing	X	X	X	X						X
Prone Arm Lift		X								
Chest:										
Supine Pull-Over	X			X	X					
Forward Raise	X	X		X		X				
Upper Arm:										
Barbell Curls	X	X	X	X	X			X		X
Reverse Curl		X						X		X
Triceps Press	X									X
Forearms:										
Wrist Curl	X	X	X	X	X	X		X		X
Wrist Extensor	X	X	X	X	X	X		X		X
Supinator-Pronator				X	X			X		
Wrist Abduction				X	X			X		
Wrist Roller					X			X		
Abdomen:										
Sit-Ups	X	X	X	X	X	X	X	X		X
Side Bend	X									
Leg Press Out	X				X		X			
Lower Back:										
Dead Lift										
Leg Extensor Lift	X									
Trunk Extension	X	X	X	X	X		X			
Hip & Pelvis										
Hip Flexor	X						X			
Hip Abductor	X								ALL MAY BE USED	
Thigh:										
One-half Squat	X		X	X	X	X	X			X
Straddle Lift								X		
Walking Squat			X	X		X	X	X		
Knee Curl										
Sitting Leg Raise					X		X			
Lower Leg:										
Toe Raise	X		X		X	X	X			
Ankle Turn			X		X	X				

Diving	Equestrian Act	Fencing	Field Hockey	Football	Gaelic Football & Hurling	Golf	Gymnastics	Handball	Hunting	Ice Boating	Ice Hockey	Jai Alai	Lacrosse	Motor Sports
X				X			X						X	
				X										
X				X			X						X	
	X	X	X	X	X	X	X	X	X		X	X	X	X
X				X	X	X	X	X				X		X
	X		X	X	X	X	X	X			X	X	X	X
							X	X	X		X	X	X	X
X				X	X		X	X				X		X
			X			X	X	X				X		
	X	X	X	X				X				X		
X	X	X	X	X	X		X	X	X		X	X	X	X
		X	X						X		X	X	X	X
					X						X	X	X	
X		X		X	X	X	X	X			X	X	X	X
X		X		X	X	X	X				X	X	X	X
	X	X				X	X	X		SEE SAILING	X	X	X	
		X				X	X	X			X	X	X	
		X					X				X			
X	X	X	X	X	X	X	X	X	X		X	X	X	X
				X										
X			X						X		X	X		
			X								X		X	
	X				X									
X		X		X		X	X	X	X					
	X			X					X					
	X			X					X					
	X	X	X	X	X		X	X	X		X	X	X	
		X	X		X	X	X	X	X					
		X		X							X	X	X	
X			X											
X	X			X	X	X			X		X	X	X	
		X		X	X				X		X		X	

SEE SAILING (Ice Boating)

SPORT

EXERCISE	Rodeo	Rowing	Sailing	Shooting	Skating	Skiing Snow & Water	Skin & Scuba Diving	Softball	Soccer	Swimming
Neck:										
Neck Curl	X								X	
Side Neck Lift	X								X	
Neck Extension	X						X		X	X
Shoulder:										
Arm Press	X						X			X
Bench Press		X		X						
Shoulder Shrug	X	X	X			X	X		X	X
Lateral Raise					X		X			X
Rowing	X	X	X				X		X	X
Prone Arm Lift										
Chest:										
Supine Pull-Over	X				X		X		X	X
Forward Raise	X				X					
Upper Arm:										
Barbell Curls	X	X	X	X	X	X	X			X
Reverse Curl		X	X	X		X				
Triceps Press									X	
Forearms:										
Wrist Curl	X		X				X	SEE BASEBALL		X
Wrist Extensor	X		X				X			X
Supinator-Pronator										
Wrist Abduction										
Wrist Roller										
Abdomen:										
Sit-Ups	X	X	X	X	X	X	X		X	X
Side Bend	X									
Leg Press Out				X	X	X	X			X
Lower Back:										
Dead Lift	X	X				X	X			
Leg Extensor Lift	X		X							
Trunk Extension	X		X			X	X		X	X
Hip & Pelvis:										
Hip Flexor		X				X				
Hip Abductor						X	X		X	X
Thigh:										
One-half Squat	X	X	X	X	X	X	X		X	X
Straddle Lift				X						
Walking Squat	X						X			X
Knee Curl						X	X		X	X
Sitting Leg Raise	X						X		X	X
Lower Leg:										
Toe Raise	X	X				X	X		X	
Ankle Turn	X					X	X		X	

	Tennis	Track & Field	Sprints	Middle Distance	Long Distance	Hurdles	Discus Throw	Hammer Throw	High Jump	Javelin Throw	Long Jump	Pole Vault	Shot Put	Triple Jump	Volleyball
										X			X		
								X	X	X		X			
		X	X	X			X	X		X	X		X	X	X
		X	X	X			X		X		X	X		X	
		X	X	X			X	X	X	X		X	X	X	
SEE BADMINTON			X	X	X			X	X			X	X		X
						X	X		X			X	X	X	X
										X		X	X		X
									X			X			
										X		X	X		X
										X		X	X		X
												X			
												X			
												X			
												X			
		X	X	X	X	X	X	X	X	X	X	X		X	X
		X	X	X			X		X						
								X						X	
						X									
									X	X		X		X	X
						X			X		X	X		X	X
		X	X	X	X	X	X	X	X	X	X	X	X	X	X
		X	X	X	X			X	X			X		X	X
		X	X	X					X					X	X
		X	X	X		X	X								
		X	X	X	X		X	X	X		X		X		X

SEE BADMINTON

possible, then return to original position. The raise develops muscles of the back of the lower leg.

35. *Ankle Turn*—Sit on a table with the leg hanging over the end of the table. With a weight or a weighted shoe, turn the entire foot inward and outward as far as possible. Return. The turn develops muscles of the ankle joint and front of the lower leg.

WOMEN

The phrase, physical fitness for women, evokes numerous reactions and images from the general public. There are those who feel that little emphasis should be placed on physical fitness for women. So long as the woman is able to push the dishwasher and vacuum cleaner buttons, care for the children and get the groceries home, she is fit enough. After all, the woman is not required to fight a war, nor is she plagued with heart disease to the same extent as men. To others, physical fitness in women is a picture of a lady Amazon with bulging muscles and a masculine character. In contrast to the Amazon image, there are the women figure skaters, tennis players, fencers, some track and field participants and gymnasts, whose high degree of physical fitness is combined

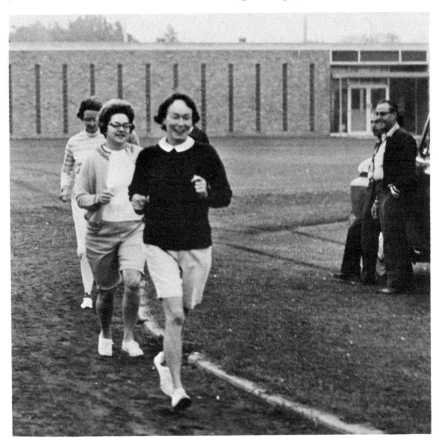

Many women mistakenly feel that inactivity is feminine. Others, like these Detroit joggers, realize that vigorous and compatible women must have high energy reserves.

with graceful movements. Those women bring stand-up ovations from men and women alike.

If the mode of life requires that a woman perform the duties of a wife and mother, the criteria for fitness is that she be able to do the daily household tasks and still have enough reserve of energy, vim and vigor to be a compatible and cheerful wife to the man she promised "for better or for worse." If a woman aspires to play tennis, then the criteria for physical fitness is that she be able to play tennis at her particular skill level without collapsing from fatigue at the end of the match. When "overtime" (loss of sleep to care for a sick child, a night out with her husband or an extra set of tennis) incapacitates the woman or causes her to operate at less than optimum the next day or for several days, then she is not physically fit.

Biological Need

Fortunately, the recent emphasis on physical fitness at the national level is permeated with a concern for all people; the young and the old, males *and* females. That concern for all is undoubtedly based on the fact that the biological needs of the human organism are basically the same regardless of age or sex. Examination of the gross anatomy and physiological systems of the male and of the female reveals striking similarity except for the reproductive system. Both sexes have the same number of bones and muscles. Those bones and muscles are structured so that the same patterns of movement are possible for both the male and the female. The cardiorespiratory, endocrine, excretory and nervous systems are basically the same. Malfunction of any aspect of the systems affects the body of the female in the same way that it affects the male. The bodies of the male and female respond in a very similar manner to nourishment, exercise, nurturing, deprivation or other stimuli.

There are, of course, individual differences, but the differences are as prevalent within a particular sex as between the sexes. So far as the physical health of the human is concerned, exercise that is good for the male body is also good for the female body. That statement, however, must be tempered with an understanding of the system that truly differentiates the male and the female; the reproductive system and the associated hormone differences. The male has a larger proportion of the body weight in the chest and shoulder area, additional height and weight and greater muscle mass than his female counterpart, each of which gives the male an advantage over the female in physical performances that require strength, endurance and speed. From a biological standpoint, physical activity is a requisite to physical fitness. The difference between the development of physical fitness through physical activity for the male and for the female is not a matter of what kind of physical activity, but rather, how much is desirable.

Prototypes

Some women, even in the United States, lift tubs of wash water, plow the fields, harvest the crops or perform other types of physical activity that may be considered manual labor. Certain of those women may represent a malnourished and medically neglected segment of society, but such is not always the case. In the presence of good nutrition and medical attention for the ill, women who labor manually are probably more physically fit than less active women.

Other women aspire to be champions in sport. They may spend long, even grueling hours in physical training and practice. They have learned that training which develops men champions also develops women champions. They may even lift weights and use progressive resistance exercises. The epitome of desirable physical activity for some women is a friendly game of golf or tennis, ordinary calisthenic exercises or light gardening. Participation in such activities may occur on a regular or sporadic basis. The reactions of the regular participator may run something like this: the activity period is a time of diversion from the routine of daily living; the physical activity is mentally refreshing; to be physically tired is a good feeling; sleeping habits are better; skillful performance in an activity is a satisfying experience.

On the other hand, the experiences of the sporadically active woman may be quite a different story: fatigue to the point of having to sit down to rest; muscle soreness to the point of sheer misery for days; actual physical injury such as blisters, tendonitis or bursitis; frustrations that come with lack of skill or realization that the "old grey mare ain't what she used to be." Those latter reactions may be physical health hazards. There will always be the exceptions: the physically active woman who appears to be a physical and mental wreck and the almost inert woman who is in apparent perfect health.

The last prototype includes the largest number of women, and most women will fit into that category at one time or another during a lifetime. Those are the women who have *no time* for planned physical activity. They are the mothers who are caught up in the syndrome of daily living; get the children off to school; stack the dishes; make the beds; make telephone calls; shop; deliver, wait for or pick up the children from scout meetings, music lessons, swimming lessons; prepare dinner; get the family off to night meetings or to bed. In fact, those women hardly sit down during the entire day except to drive the car. In the way of physical activity, they have walked, stooped, lifted, reached and twisted, all of which is good physical activity, provided the *quantity* is adequate. The problem arises when there

is no longer a need to rush through the day. Those are the women who, then, may devote most of the time and energy to service and social organizations. Or they may fall into the group of women who haunt the medical doctor's office with nonspecific aches and pains; or they may join the ranks of the career women who, aside from the demand of gainful employment, are tending the duties associated with family and household.

Underlying Causes for Inactivity

At a very early age, the little girl learns that dolls are for girls and that balls and bats are for boys. Later she learns that throwing and batting abilities are of little importance for her since there are few softball teams for girls. Throughout life, a society clearly differentiates feminine and masculine activities. She conforms to what is expected of her. The unfortunate aspect of her conformity is that she may fail to develop some of the basic movement skills, such as throwing and running. Many women truly would like to play golf or tennis, but they meet defeat in learning the necessary skills. The woman who uses poor mechanics in ordinary running probably will have difficulty moving to the tennis ball on the tennis court. The woman who cannot throw a ball with speed and accuracy also will have problems hitting the tennis ball or golf ball with speed and accuracy. Although the fine points of the skills involved in various sports may differ, the movement patterns of the body necessary to produce the force to apply to the ball are very similar. It is certainly possible to learn new physical skills as an adult, but it takes a great deal of practice to develop timing and coordination necessary for most skills. Children practice throwing, running, jumping or any activity for hours on end. Unfortunately, adults are often so impatient or embarrassed that they quit when they do not quickly meet success.

Related to the problem of skill is that of strength. Many women have never developed adequate strength in chest, arm and hand muscles to handle sports implements. Muscular strength in the chest and arms is required to swing the implement with speed, and wrist strength is required to hold the implement firm at impact. Lack of sufficient strength is a real handicap in successful skill development.

Women also lack the experience of having trained for physical fitness. Even if they played sports in high school, physical conditioning probably was not emphasized. Frequently, a man may be heard to make a statement to the effect that he never felt better than when he was in condition for the varsity or collegiate team. Most women, however, have no conception of the meaning of such a statement, since they have never experienced the feeling of well-being that accompanies physical conditioning. Consequently "to feel better" is not motivation to them.

Last, but certainly not least, the fashions of a culture often dictate the type of physical activity that is desirable or possible. Today, hair styles probably present the greatest problem to women. Wind and perspiration play havoc with most female hair styles, not to mention the steamy shower room or the water in the swimming pool. A few minutes of vigorous physical activity can negate several hours (and several dollars) spent on a hair style. Some cosmetics and apparel commonly used by women may also discourage participation in physical activity either because the particular item cannot be worn or because its effect will be spoiled. Aside from specific annoyances related to grooming, many women dislike the feeling of perspiration-soaked clothing that almost certainly accompanies vigorous physical activity. Underlying that aversion may be their dislike for showering without the privacy and convenience afforded at home.

Positive Action

In setting a course of positive action, consider first, kinds of activities that are best for overall body conditioning and, consequently, for physical fitness. Running, swimming and bicycling are among the best activities. Fortunately, those activities are adaptable to all ages, to both sexes, and to most levels of fitness. Although swimming may involve some expense and may be seasonal, running and cycling entail minimal expense and are not limited greatly in most climates. Many sport and dance activities can also be good body conditioners *provided you develop a high skill level.* A game of pitter-pat badminton in which you are not required to take a step is not highly skilled badminton playing. In general, an activity that requires movement of the total body and that is vigorous enough to cause a definite increase in breathing rate is an activity that is probably a definite asset to physical fitness. However, any type of physical activity is better than no activity.

Consider next the factors which will encourage you to participate in physical activity, as well as factors which will prevent you from participating.

1. *Choose an activity that you enjoy.* From a psychological standpoint, you do the things that you want to do and that you enjoy doing. Many well-intentioned exercisers give up calisthenic exercises after one week or one month out of sheer boredom.

2. *Select an activity in which you will experience success.* Few individuals relish the idea of doing anything that cannot be done with a fair degree of proficiency. When success is doubtful, rent or borrow equipment and make an honest effort to learn the skills involved. Remember that skill development as well as skill maintenance requires constant practice. The

typist, pianist, or the sportsman who practices only once a month will probably give a poor performance, compared to his capability.

3. *Make a definite commitment to regular exercise.* Include exercise in the regular schedule in such a manner that you will feel obligated to follow through with the plan. For some people, it is sufficient to promise that on Monday, Wednesday and Friday at 2:00 there shall be one hour set aside for physical activity. Joining a team or a club may be motivating and enjoyable. Still others may participate only if they buy expensive memberships or pay for instruction. Whatever the plan, it should be one which does not encourage indefinite postponements.

4. *Develop an attitude of self-testing and self-appraisal.* Keep records of times, scores, number of repetitions per unit of time or pulse rates in the case of endurance activities such as running.

5. *Vary the activity.* Seasonal changes sometimes dictate a change in activities. When such is not the case, it is probably wise to alternate between several activities to prevent boredom and staleness.

6. *Choose an activity that is compatible with grooming requirements.* Hair is the greatest problem for most women. There are numerous inexpensive accessories such as hair bands or kerchiefs which aid in maintaining the hair style during most activities. You can also schedule the activities immediately prior to the hair styling appointment.

7. *Select an activity that is within financial reason.*

8. *Select an activity that is reasonable in terms of time requirement.* Competent female golfers often forego the sport when home responsibilities will no longer permit them to have a minimum of two to three hours to play nine holes of golf. Consider all aspects of the time element: travel time to and from the activity; time spent in waiting for the facility; and the time it takes to play the game or to engage in the activity for a satisfactory period.

All women should participate regularly in some type of vigorous physical activity, preferably an activity from which she can derive social and psychological benefits as well as physical benefits. Fortunate is she who is not plagued by social stigmas and personal biases that deter such participation. Even more fortunate is she who has the initiative, ingenuity and wisdom to make some type of vigorous physical activity a regular part of her habitual living pattern.—*Louise E. Kindig*

WORK

The human body is a dynamic machine. As it moves to perform its many functions, it expends energy. The components of the machine, the body segments and organs, cannot distinguish between movements made while performing occupational tasks from those made conducting leisure time pursuits. Energy is expended on the basis of the demands made on the machine (rate of movement, load moved, number of movement repetitions and rest pauses between movements). Likewise, the intake of energy is accomplished without regard to the name of the activity causing energy depletion but upon the depletion itself.

The accompanying table illustrates broad categories in which human movements might be placed. The categories and, therefore, the placement of movements are based on energy values. Both intake and expenditure of energy are usually expressed in calories. The categories have been developed by investigators who have determined the calories expended in a variety of activities and by evaluation of the effects of continuous participation in those activities. It should be emphasized that the categorization of human effort is subject to wide variation both within and between activities.

Classification of human effort, according to energy expenditure, includes both occupational and leisure efforts. The average energy expenditure of bricklaying falls into the same category (light effort) as playing baseball (pitcher excluded). If the energy expenditure is the same, what is the difference between work and exercise?

"Going to work" is a common phrase which conveys an action that is universally understood. That is to say, you are going to the place where you carry out the tasks of a chosen occupation. However, the stress resulting from work can be much different, depending on the occupation and between different job classifications within the same occupation. From the standpoint of energy expenditure, "going to work" at the mill is probably much different from "going to work" at the office. Mill work is usually thought of as being more physically demanding than working in a more sedentary office environment. On the other hand, some jobs in a mill, such as a foreman, are relatively sedentary at least when compared to a laborer.

Historically, man could be described by his occupation, his work. A man's trade or profession occupies the great majority of his waking hours. Little time, energy and few facilities were available for leisure time pursuits. Therefore, job titles, such as carpenter, fireman and farmer, which described the type of work performed, also defined the major component of a man's life. That is no longer true since shorter work weeks have resulted in a greater proportion of total time available for leisure. Modern man, therefore, is not only a creature of work but a creature of leisure.

"Going to exercise" may not result in such universal understanding as "going to work." The word "exercise" is not generally used when describing occupational work, even though occupational work may evoke the same type of physical responses; that is, profuse sweating, shortness of breath and pounding of the chest. However, when participating in very heavy exercise, for example running, you may hear the activity referred to as "work." "Work" is often used extra-occupationally as a general term to mean hard exertion.

Exercise, as presently defined, must be accomplished during the leisure hours primarily (until such time as employers become convinced of the utility of including exercise breaks within the working day). Whereas man formerly had no time for exercise, the reduction of work time provides the opportunity for exercise to occur. The technological revolution which stimulated the reduction in work time is also responsible for the more sedentary behavior of man and, therefore, a greater need and opportunity to exercise during the leisure hours.

Overload of muscles can be accomplished during work as well as exercise activities. Therefore, health benefits derivable from the application of the overload principle are not limited to exercise. The occupation may also offer a positive benefit to health. Several studies have attempted to relate the presence of good health and physical fitness to the amount of habitual physical activity involved in certain occupations. Those studies are complicated by many factors not the least of which is the inability, or failure, to account for leisure time exercise which would also have an effect on the health of men. Even though unintentional health benefits may be derivable from some occupational activities, it is questionable whether most modern occupations, with many automated and semi-automated jobs, provide a suitable exercise overload.

The dictionary definition of "exercise" indicates that "use of the limbs

EFFORT - ENERGY CONTINUUM

	Light Effort	Moderate Effort	Heavy Effort	Very Heavy Effort
Cal./Min.	2.5	5.0	7.5	10.0
Cal./Hr.	150	300	450	600
Occupations:	Housekeeping Bricklaying House Painting Carpentry	Pick and Shovel Work Coal Mining Agriculture	Chopping Wood Iron & Steel Work	Lumber Work
Leisure:	Calisthenics Walking (2 mph) Dancing (Moderate) Baseball	Bicycle Riding (Rapid) Swimming (1 mph)	Skating (9 mph) Skiing (3 mph)	Mt. Climbing Fencing Running (5.7 mph) Wrestling Rowing (11 mph) Football

for health" is the preferential meaning. Generally, exercise is *not* motivated by the same goals as occupational tasks. It is health related. The work goal is usually economically related and is placed in a more primary position on the priority scale of most people.

The fact that you *must* work in order to survive while exercise is usually initiated voluntarily, represents a major difference between the two activities. Voluntary participation results in a much different psychological reaction than does forced participation. "Exercise" automatically denotes willingness while "work" may indicate indifference or reluctance. There is no reason to believe that work cannot be performed for reasons other than monetary gain and at an energy level which is of benefit to the general health. Although good health ultimately may result in financial gains, exercise is never undertaken for monetary reward.—*Bruce J. Noble*

Work-Exercise Ideas

Walking to and from your office or factory is wonderful exercise, if you live within reasonable distance of where you work. It is a productive form of work-oriented exercise. You save money on gasoline and auto depreciation. Perhaps that is a small incentive to exercise, but it shouldn't be ignored. If you want to walk an hour or two a day, you will find it much easier to maintain that schedule by walking to and from work than just by going out for a stroll. If you live too far from your office or factory, consider parking your car within 2 or 3 miles of your destination. Or get off the bus before it gets to your usual stop.

Another idea is to return to the habit of using muscle to do some of the household and garden tasks that have been taken over by machines in most homes. Cut some grass with a hand mower, for example. You wouldn't have to give up your power mower for the big stretches of grass, but consider using a hand mower for some of the smaller sections. Rake up the grass clippings by hand. Stretch your hamstring muscles by bending down to pick up pine cones, acorns, or anything else littering your lawn. Spade part of your flower beds by hand. Take it as a project to dig out a stump that has been bothering you, or level off that hump of ground you have been looking at for years.

There are also plenty of indoor opportunities to increase the work-exercise quotient of the average home. Do you really need that power can opener or an electric shoe-shine kit? Shining your shoes by hand every morning is a good wake-up exercise. Electric food mixers are very convenient, but sometimes you can do the job by hand and enjoy the change. How about your extension telephones? Can you do with one less? Check all the electric motors in your home and see if they are all necessary. An electric drill makes you feel like a professional craftsman, but maybe you would also like some of the exercise you could get by drilling holes by hand. Scraping and sanding of furniture is wonderful exercise. Do you remember how people used to beat carpets before they had vacuum cleaners? Are you doing anything now that gives you that kind of exercise? Throw away the remote control for your television set and return to the habit of stretching your legs when you want to change channels.

Make-Work Builds Strength

Training with weights is a way of substituting formal exercise for the professional type of body-building achieved by laborers. Barbells are a relatively new invention, but rocks and heavy loads of all kinds have been lifted by human muscles for millions of years. Most young men would rather work out with barbells than lift rocks, but that doesn't mean that the right kind of actual work wouldn't produce the same results.

There is nothing crazy about setting up a work situation in or around your home that creates fitness as a primary product. Many people I know have not really needed the garden improvements in which they have invested long hours—but they tackled those tasks just to get exercise that they craved for. Stone and brick walls have been built with that primary motivation. Garden steps have been built for

exercise, and wood lots thinned out. Cutting up trees for firewood is an excellent physical conditioner, as many young people of the past have found out. There is no reason why people today can't take the same route to fitness, even if they do have less need for the wood.

In these days when "labor-saving" has robbed us of activity which is extremely important to our health, it may even pay to set up work-type situations which are completely with-

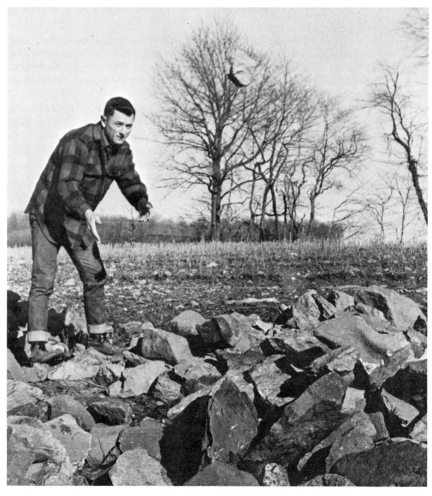

It's easy to set up work situations that satisfy the urge to be constructive and are productive of fitness. Often a physical chore can have built-in fitness benefits.

out any useful purpose except exercise. A friend of mine would certainly benefit by chopping wood or digging in his garden every day of the year, even if that work wasn't really needed. Why then shouldn't he go through the motions if he enjoys that route to fitness? Perhaps there are many more people like him—who enjoy vigorous movement most when it is cloaked in the disguise of some useful task. I know that some of the most enjoyable workouts I have ever had were gained during some youthful experience as a quarry worker. My father was building some stone walls, and sent me to pick up the rock. Picking up heavy stones from the ground and throwing them up into the bed of a 5-ton dump truck built strength the like of which I did not have before or since. I thoroughly enjoyed that change of routine from school chores, and often thought it would be fun and beneficial to do work like that again once in a while. Using smaller rocks, of course.

Although I have not yet had the courage to call the quarry, I have given some serious thought to ordering a load of stone delivered to my back yard, for the sole purpose of allowing me to do some outdoor weight training. I am sure that it would be more fun to move those stones around than to do sit-ups and push-ups indoors on a bright, spring-like day. Aside from getting the satisfaction of going through the motions of work, a setup like that would also lend itself to measurement of performance. I could check the time it takes to move the stones from place to place, thereby keeping a record of improvements in strength. A wheelbarrow could be used instead of our old dump truck, providing even more exercise.

There are plenty of other opportunities for work-exercise, limited only by the space you have available and your imagination. Of course, there is also the matter of enthusiasm. Perhaps you are like the English humorist Jerome Jerome, who said back in the 1800's: "I like work. It fascinates me.

*DIGGING AND SHOVELING

Chart 1	Chart 2
1. 50 minutes	1. 80 minutes
2. 55 minutes	2. 85 minutes
3. 58 minutes	3. 90 minutes
4. 60 minutes	4. 95 minutes
5. 65 minutes	5. 100 minutes
6. 70 minutes	6. 105 minutes
7. 73 minutes	7. 108 minutes
8. 75 minutes	8. 110 minutes
9. 78 minutes	9. 115 minutes

* See ENDURANCE and ENERGY COST OF ACTIVITIES for an explanation of the charts.
**Doesn't include rest periods, times out, etc.

Fitness 1

If you achieved a score of poor or low average on the *Harvard Step Test* or a score of very poor or poor on the *12 Minute Run*, start on Chart 1-Level 1 and spend 1 week at each level until Chart 2-Level 9 is reached. It is recommended that you participate 4 to 5 days a week. When Chart 2-Level 9 is reached, 4 days a week is sufficient.

Fitness 2

If you achieved a score of high average on the *Harvard Step Test* or fair on the *12 Minute Run*, start on Chart 1-Level 1. Spend 1 week on Chart 1-Levels 1, 2, 4, 6, and 8 and Chart 2-Levels 1, 3, 5, 8, and 9. It is recommended that you participate 4 to 5 days a week. When Chart 2-Level 9 is reached, 4 days a week is sufficient.

Fitness 3

If you achieved a score of good or excellent on either the *Harvard Step Test* or *12 Minute Run*, continue your current program or select Chart 2-Level 9 as your level of participation. Four days a week is sufficient.

I can sit and look at it for hours." If so, then you will have to look elsewhere for your exercise.

But I think that there may be more people who agree with Voltaire's thoughts on the subject of work. "Not to be occupied and not to exist amount to the same thing," he said.—*Robert Rodale*

Since work is a mild to high energy cost activity, it may be used to help

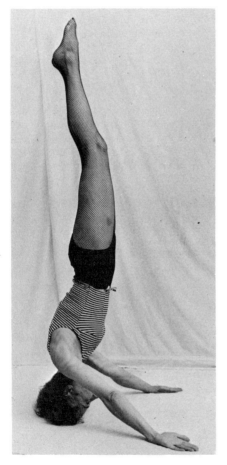

Yoga fuses mental and physical development. The head stand position is one of many inversion positions that stretch muscles and ligaments while concentrating on relaxation.

improve your fitness level, especially your circulo-respiratory and muscle endurance. Below are work programs that take into account the important principles of training.

For a closely allied discussion and program, see GARDENING.

YOGA

Originating in India as one of its classic philosophical systems, Yoga literally means a union of mind and body to achieve a state of unexcelled physical health and mental well-being. Although many people, especially those in Eastern countries, practice Yoga to gain both physical and mental development, the main emphasis in this country is on the Hatha or physical portion of the science of Yoga. And to many people, practicing Yoga means little more than standing on your head.

Contribution to Fitness

Take a look at what Yoga really is and what it has to offer. That head stand which most people identify with Yoga is actually only one of 84 main postures (asanas) or Yoga exercises. The exercises are classified as either stretching, inversion (head and shoulder stands), balancing, standing and sitting postures. Combined with simple breathing exercises, groups of those postures and the movements of getting into and out of them plus relaxation make up a typical Yoga workout. Actually the positions can be so grouped that specific body parts can be exercised.

Proper breathing helps to avoid the fatigue and strained feeling so common at the end of other exercises. And Yoga's prescription to "move as slowly in coming out of Yoga posture as in going into it" is another important deterrent to that tired feeling immediately after calisthenics and other traditional exercises. Edith Nobel Zarifis and her husband, Frank, co-directors of the Sivananda Yoga Vedanta Center in New Haven, Connecticut, state that "in general, exercises are done vigorously by the quick movement of the muscles. Yoga exercises involve slow and graceful movement, with proper breathing, followed by relaxation. They, therefore, cause practically no fatigue. They stretch the muscles and ligaments and are meant to increase circulation and the intake of oxygen. Yogic exercises have a lasting effect because they work scientifically on the entire body."

Furthermore, the exercises are simple and can be varied to correspond with the individual's limitations. For example, the athletic type of person will be able to exert more effort and spend more time in each position than the ordinary person who has just started on a physical fitness program. Yoga is for all ages and for all physical makeups. A full Yoga exercise schedule can be worked out to suit any mild exercise requirements.

Another aspect of Yoga that makes it so welcome and successful is that it works scientifically on a specific part of the body to do a required job. It is sometimes slow, but always sure. Yoga postures performed correctly will always bring positive results.

What actual physical benefits can you expect? In addition to restoring some of the original body flexibility which seems to be sapped out by sedentary living, the stretching, inversion and sitting postures of Yoga strengthen and recondition the entire body and actually help to remove excess weight. The stretching exercises are an especially good tonic for vibrant muscle tone and a trim, slim figure. The stretching exercises are also a fine way to remove tension and develop grace and poise.

Conditioning for Yoga

There's really nothing complicated about Yoga. At first you should hold a particular posture for only a few seconds—gradually working up to 10 seconds or more. As you progress with your program, however, you can lengthen the time of your daily workout. But again, that will depend on the time limitations of your daily schedule. It is generally recommended that you set aside a regular time each day (preferably before breakfast) and practice at least 20 minutes. (Although experts on Yoga agree that individuals of all ages can benefit from Yoga, they point out that the exercises are especially beneficial to individuals over the age of 30.)

Remember to get into each position in slow motion. You should take at least 10 seconds to move into and out of a certain position. Once in a position, remain motionless. Any fidgeting or other movement detracts from the physical effects that are taking place at the time. Never go too far in your stretching when getting into or holding a position. Stretch, but do not strain. If you get to the point where you are generally uncomfortable, then you know you are applying yourself too strenuously.

Recommended Yoga Regimen for Beginners

Here is a starter program similar to that practiced by intermediate students, but the asanas or positions are not as strenuous:

This exercise should precede all Yoga work. It limbers up muscles and makes it easier to carry out the other positions. 1. Fold hands, stand erect with legs together. 2. Inhale and raise the arms. Bend backwards. 3. Exhale and bend forward till the hands are touching the floor and in line with the feet. Touch the knees with your head. In the beginning, of course, the knees may be slightly bent so that the head can touch them. 4. Inhale and move the right leg away from the body in a big backward step. Keep the hands and left foot firmly on the floor and bend the head to the rear. 5. Inhale and hold the breath. Move the left leg along side the right; raise up on your hands, keeping the body in a straight line from head to foot. 6. Exhale and lower the body to the floor. In that position, known as Sastanga Namaskar or eight-curved prostration, only the feet, knees, hands, chest, and forehead touch the floor. 7. Inhale and bend backwards as much as possible. 8. Exhale and lift the body, keeping the feet and hands on the floor, hips high, heels flat and head down. 9. Inhale and assume position number four. 10. Exhale and take up position number three. 11. Raise the arms over head and bend backwards inhaling as in position number two. 12. Exhale, drop the arms, and relax.

Leg Lifts

After limbering up with the sun exercises, you're ready to try some of the basic positions of Yoga. One of the easiest and simplest for the beginner is the leg lift. That exercise will also get you ready for the head stand. Start by lying down on your back, arms to the sides and hands with palms down. Inhale and raise one leg high, keeping your back flat on the floor. Move the leg slowly, continuously stretching it. Don't lift the leg up automatically. Let the leg down slowly—do not drop it. That exercise should be done 5 to 10 times, alternating legs and breathing rhythmically. Then raise both legs 5 to 10 times.

Benefits:
1. Removes stiffness and tension and strengthens the back area.
2. Firms buttocks, thighs and legs.
3. Strengthens hamstring muscles.

Shoulder Stand

1. Lie flat on your back. Slowly raise the legs, trunk and hips to a vertical position. Rest elbows firmly on the floor and support the back with both hands. In that position, the back of the neck, the posterior part of the head and the shoulders should touch the floor. Breathe slowly and do not allow the body to shake to and fro. 2. Bring one leg down over the head until the toe touches the floor. Repeat with other leg, then with both together. The knees remain straight. 3. To come down, bend knees to forehead and place hands and arms on the floor in front of you. Arch the neck, raise the chin and lower the back to the floor. Slowly lower the legs to the floor and relax two or three moments.

Benefits:
1. Improves blood circulation in the legs.
2. Tones up abdominal muscles.
3. Strengthens back.

Plough

1. Lie flat on your back, heels and toes together and the hands—palms down—near the thighs. 2. Without bending the knees, slowly raise the legs straight up in the air until they are at a 90-degree angle to the rest of the body. Remember that this movement, like all other Yoga movements, should take at least 10 seconds. 3. Slowly raise the hips and the lumbar part of the back so that your legs come over your body toward your head. Continue that movement until the toes touch the floor. 4. Press the chin against the chest and breathe slowly through the nose. Remain in this position for 10 to 15 seconds. 5. Return to the original position. This exercise can be repeated three times.

Benefits:
1. Stretches and limbers the hips, legs and entire spine with a minimum of energy.
2. Strengthens the abdominal and neck muscles.
3. Helps reduce weight in the legs, thighs, hips and abdomen.
4. Improves circulation.

Basic Standing Positions

1. Stand with the feet three to four feet apart. Twist the body and look

back. Slowly bend the whole body sideways until you touch the right foot with the left hand. Keep the right hand straight, making a straight line from the left to the right. Alternate sides and repeat. 2. Keeping the legs apart, raise your arms until they are parallel to the floor. Now twist the body and look upward. Slowly bend and touch the right foot with the left hand. Perform the same movements with the right hand and left foot.

Benefits

1. Strengthens the ankles and helps develop the chest muscles.
2. Stretches the hamstring muscles and muscles of the back.
3. Firms those muscles around the waist and hips.
4. Firm leg muscles.

Limitations

1. Yoga does not place a stress on the circulo-respiratory system.
2. Some of the positions are potentially dangerous. See EXCESSIVE EXERCISE for a more complete discussion.
—*John Haberern*

Selected References

ABDUCTION
Rasch, P. J. and R. K. Burke, *Kinesiology and Applied Anatomy*, Lea and Febiger, 1967.

ADAPTATION
McCristal, K. J. and others, *Foundations of Physical Activity*, Stipes Publishing, 1965.

ADDUCTION
Rasch and Burke, *op. cit.*

AEROBIC EXERCISE
Cooper, K. H., *Aerobics*, M. Evans, 1968.

AGE AND ATHLETIC PERFORMANCE
Jokl, E., *Physiology of Exercise*, Charles C. Thomas, 1964.
Karpovich, P. V., *Physiology of Muscular Activity*, W. B. Saunders, 1965.
Lehman, H. C., *American Journal of Psychology*, 1951, p. 161.

AGILITY
Fleishman, E. A., *The Structure and Measurement of Physical Fitness*, Prentice-Hall, 1964.

AGING
Committee on Aging of the American Medical Association, *Health Aspects of Aging*, American Medical Association.
McCloy, C. H., *Journal of the American Association for Health, Physical Education and Recreation*, January 1945, p. 20.
Michigan State Medical Society, *Journal of the Michigan State Medical Society*, 1967, p. 589.
Shock, N., *Scientific American*, January, 1962, p. 100.

ALBUMINURIA
Steinhaus, A., *Toward an Understanding of Health and Physical Education*, Wm. C. Brown, 1963.
Wesson, L. G., In *Science and Medicine and Sports*, Harper and Row, 1960.

ALCOHOL
Cooper, *op. cit.*
Graham, M. F., *Prescription for Life*, David McKay, 1966.

ALL-OR-NONE LAW
Best, C. H. and N. B. Taylor, *The Human Body*, Holt, Rinehart and Winston, 1963.
Karpovich, *op. cit.*

ANAEROBIC EXERCISE
Cooper, *op. cit.*
Morehouse and Rasch, *Sports Medicine for Trainers*, W. B. Saunders, 1964.

ANGINA
American Heart Association, *Journal of the American Medical Association*, March 15, 1965, p. 31.
Dimond, E. G., *Medical World News*, January 15, 1965, p. 43.

ANTHROPOMETRY
Sills, F. D., *Science and Medicine of Exercise and Sports*, *op. cit.*

APPETITE
Mayer, J., *Science and Medicine of Exercise and Sports*, *op. cit.*
Mayer, J. and others, *American Journal of Clinical Nutrition*, 1956, p. 169.

ARCHERY
McKinney, W. C., *Archery*, Wm. C. Brown, 1966.

ARTERIOSCLEROSIS
American Heart Association, *Heart Disease Caused by Coronary Atherosclerosis*, American Heart Association.
Crosby, A. L., *Your Blood Pressure and Your Arteries*, Public Affair Committee.

ARTHRITIS
Arthritis Foundation, *Osteoarthritis*, The Arthritis Foundation, 1967.

ASTHMA

McElhenny, T. R., *Medical Tribune,* April 13, 1965.

Scherr, M. S. and L. Frankel, *Journal of the American Medical Association,* December 13, 1958, p. 1996.

ATHLETE'S HEART

Jokl, E. J., *op. cit.*

Karpovich, *op. cit.*

Time-Life, *The Healthy Life,* Time-Life, Inc., 1965.

ATHLETIC PARTICIPATION FOR YOUNGSTERS

Cureton, T. K. and A. Barry, *Improving the Physical Fitness of Youth,* Society for Research in Child Development, Inc., Vol. 29, No. 4, 1964.

Division of Men's Athletics, *Athletics in Education,* American Association of Health, Physical Education and Recreation, 1963.

Kral, J., "Sports Competitions During Youth," Atti dell VIII Congress o Intavazionale di Medicina Sportiva, Firenze, Montecantini 28-31, Maggio, 1950.

BACKYARD FITNESS

Ruffer, W. R., *Research Quarterly,* 1965, p. 183.

BADMINTON

Friedrich, J. A. and A. Rutledge, *Beginning Badminton,* Wadsworth Publishing, 1963.

BALANCE

Fleishman, *op. cit.*

BLOOD

Brumbach, W. B., *Research Quarterly,* 1961, p. 147.

Chapman, C. B. and J. H. Mitchell, *Scientific American,* 1965, p. 212.

McDonald, G. D. and H. W. Fullerton, *Lancet,* 1958, p. 600.

Montoye, H. J. and others, *American Journal of Clinical Nutrition,* 1959, p. 1959.

Steinhaus, *op. cit.*

BLOOD PRESSURE

Best and Taylor, *op. cit.*

Morehouse, L. E. and A. T. Miller, *Physiology of Exercise,* C. V. Mosby, 1963.

BODY COMPOSITION

Behnke, A. R. and others, *Journal of the American Medical Association,* 1942, p. 495.

Brozek, J., *Annals of the New York Academy of Sciences,* 1963, p. 1.

———, *American Journal of Physical Anthropology,* 1966, p. 239.

Brozek, J. and A. Henschel, *Techniques for Measuring Body Composition,* National Academy of Science—National Research Council, 1961.

Brozek, J. and A. Keys, *British Journal of Nutrition,* 1951, p. 194.

Dempsey, Y., *The Relationships between the Strength of the Elbow Flexors and Muscle Size of the Upper Arm in Children,* unpublished master's thesis, University of Wisconsin, 1955.

Forbes, G. B., *Pediatrics,* 1965, p. 825.

Ismail, A. H. and others, *Research Quarterly,* 1963, p. 463.

Leedy, H. E. and others, *Research Quarterly,* 1965, p. 158.

Johnston, F. E. and R. M. Malina, *Human Biology,* 1966, p. 1.

Malina, R. M. and F. E. Johnston, *Research Quarterly,* 1967, p. 216.

———, *Human Biology,* 1967, p. 211.

Novak, L. P., *Journal of the American Medical Association,* 1966, p. 891.

Parizkova, J., *Current Anthropology,* 1968, p. 273.

Pascale, L. R. and others, *Human Biology,* 1956, p. 165.

Rarick, L. and J. A. J. Thompson, *Research Quarterly,* 1956, p. 321.

Royce, J., *Research Quarterly,* 1958, p. 60.

Tanner, J. M., *American Journal of Physical Anthropology,* 1952, p. 427.

Young, C. M., *New York State Journal of Medicine,* 1961, p. 1928.

Body Composition Determination

Behnke, *op. cit.*

Best, W. R., *USAMRNL Report No. 113,* August 31, 1953.

Bischoff, E., *Zeitschr. f. ration, Med. III,* Reihe, 1863, p. 75.

Boyd, E., *Human Biology,* 1933, p. 646.

Brozek, J. and A. Keys, *op. cit.*

Forbes, R. M. and others, *Journal of Biological Chemistry,* 1953, pp. 203 and 359.

Insull, W. J., Jr. and others, *USAMRNL Report No. 129,* May 14, 1954.

Keys, A. and others, *Physiological Reviews,* 1953, p. 245.

Miller, A. T., Jr. and C. S. Blyth, *Journal of Applied Physiology,* 1955, p. 139.

Parizkova, J., In *International Research in Sport and Physical Education*, (E. Jokl, and E. Simon, Eds.) Charles C. Thomas, 1964.

Pascale, *op. cit.*

Rathbun, E. N. and N. Pace, *Journal of Biological Chemistry*, 1945, p. 667.

Siri, W. E., *Advances in Biological and Medical Physics*, 1956, p. 239.

Von Dobeln, W., *Acta Physiological Scandinavica, suppl.*, 1956, p. 1.

von Liebig, G., *Arch. f. Anat., Physiol. und wiss. Med.*, 1874, p. 96.

Welch, B. E. and C. E. Crisp, *USAMRNL Rept. No. 207*, July, 1957.

BODY TYPE

Cureton, *op. cit.*

——, *Physical Fitness of Champion Athletes*, University of Illinois Press, 1951.

Kin-Itsu, H., *The Journal of Sports Medicine and Physical Fitness*, 1966, p. 207.

Sheldon, W. H., *Varieties of Human Physique*, Harper and Brothers, 1940.

Sills, F. D. and P. W. Everett, *Research Quarterly*, May 1953, p. 228.

BOWLING

Day, N. and M. Raymer, *Bowling, Instructor's Guide*, The Athletic Institute, 1953.

McMahon, J. and M. Goodman, *Modern Bowling Techniques*, The Ronald Press, 1958.

Raymer, M., *The Teaching of Classroom Bowling*, Spencer-Walker Press, 1958.

BUSINESS

Johnson, H., *U. S. News and World Report*, August 22, 1960, p. 72.

CANOEING

American Red Cross, *Canoeing*, Doubleday, 1956.

CHILDHOOD FITNESS

Astrand, P. O., *International Research in Sport and Physical Education, op. cit.*

Keogh, J., *Motor Performance of Elementary School Children*, Department of Physical Education, University of California, Los Angeles, March, 1965.

Metheny, R. E., *Breathing Capacity and Grip Strength of Preschool Children*, Dissertation, State University of Iowa, 1940.

Robb, E., *The Energy Requirement of Normal Three- and Four-Year-Old Children Under Standard Basal Metabolism Conditions and During Periods of Quiet Play*, Bureau of Publications, Teachers College, Columbia University, Child Development Monograph No. 16.

Robinson, A. S., *Arbeit Physiologie*, 1938, p. 279.

CHOLESTEROL

Brown, C. E., and others, *Journal of Gerontology*, 1956, p. 296.

Brumbach, *op. cit.*

Chapman and Mitchell, *op. cit.*

Graham, *op. cit.*

McDonald and Fullerton, *op. cit.*

Montoye, *op. cit.*

Myasnikov, A. L., *Circulation*, 1958, p. 110.

CIRCUIT TRAINING

Morgan, R. E. and G. T. Adamson, *Circuit Training*, G. Bell and Sons, 1961.

Sorani, R., *Circuit Training*, Wm. C. Brown, 1966.

CIRCULATORY SYSTEM

Anthony, C. P., *Textbook of Anatomy and Physiology*, C. V. Mosby Company, 1959.

Guyton, A. C., *Function of the Human Body*, W. B. Saunders, 1964.

Rice, T. B. and F. V. Hein, *Living*, Scott, Foresman, 1954.

Turner, C. E., *Personal and Community Health*, C. V. Mosby Company, 1963.

CIRCULO-RESPIRATORY ENDURANCE

Balke, B. and R. T. Clarke, *In Health and Fitness in the Modern World*, Athletic Institute, 1961.

Cooper, *op. cit.*

deVries, H. A., *Physiology of Exercise*, Wm. C. Brown, 1966.

Graham, *op. cit.*

Johnson, P. B. and others, *Physical Education, A Problem Solving Approach to Health and Fitness*, Holt, Rinehart and Winston, 1966.

CLAUDICATION

Larsen, A. and N. A. Tassen, *Modern Medicine*, May 22, 1967, p. 64.

COLLATERAL CIRCULATION

Eckstein, R. W., *Circulation Research*, 1957, p. 230.

CONTINUOUS RHYTHMICAL EXERCISE

Cureton, T. K., *Physical Fitness and Dynamic Health*, Dial Press, 1965.

COORDINATION

Fleishman, *op. cit.*

DAILY ACTIVITIES

Steinhaus, A., *How to Keep Fit and*

Like It, The Dartnell Corporation, 1963.

DEGENERATIVE CARDIOVASCULAR DISEASE

Eckstein, *op. cit.*

Karvonen, M. and A. J. Barry, *Physical Activity and the Heart,* Charles C. Thomas, 1967.

Norris, J. N., *Lancet,* 1953, pp. 1053 and 1111.

Ochsner, A., *Medical Tribune,* March 17, 1965, p. 11.

Selye, H., *The Stress of Life,* McGraw-Hill, 1957.

Taylor, H. L., *Exercise and Fitness,* Athletic Institute, 1960.

Time-Life, *op. cit.*

DIET

Adlersbug, D., *Journal of the American Medical Association,* 1956, p. 619.

Anonymous, *Medical World News,* February 26, 1965, p. 50.

Bogert, J. L. and others, *Nutrition and Physical Fitness,* W. B. Saunders, 1966.

Keys, A., *Modern Medicine,* March 1, 1957, p. 78.

Keys, A. and M. Keys, *Eat Well and Stay Well,* Doubleday, 1965.

Moses, M., *Journal of the American Medical Association,* 1956, p. 492.

Russek, H. I., *Journal of the American Medical Association,* 1959, p. 503.

Stare, F. J., *Eating for Good Health,* Doubleday, 1964.

Yudkin, J., *American Heart Journal,* 1963, p. 835.

DIGESTIVE SYSTEM

Anthony, *op. cit.*

Barcroft, J. and H. Florey, *Journal of Psychology,* 1929, p. 181.

Basmajian, J. V., *Primary Anatomy,* Williams and Wilkins, 1964.

Carlson, A. J., *The Control of Hunger in Health and Disease,* University of Chicago Press, 1916.

Hamilton, W. J., *Textbook of Human Anatomy,* Macmillan, 1957.

Morehouse and Miller, *op. cit.*

Stickney, J. C. and E. J. VanLiere, *Science and Medicine of Exercise and Sports, op. cit.*

DRUGS

American College of Sports Medicine, Unpublished Report of the Committee to Study the Use of Drugs in Athletics, Philadelphia, April 29, 1958.

Karpovich, P. V., *Journal of the American Medical Association,* 1959, p. 558.

Lovingood, B. W., *The Effects of Dextro-Amphetamine and Caffeine on Selected Psychomotor, Strength, and Intellectual Performance Tasks and Physiological Parameters of Young White Men Exposed to a Restricted Environment (125.6°F.),* Unpublished Ph.D. Dissertation, The University of North Carolina, 1963.

Office of Naval Research, Department of the Navy, Washington, D.C., ONR-Report ACR-29, August, 1958.

Pierson, William R., *Journal of the American Medical Association,* 1961, p. 345.

Plotnikoff, N. and others, *Drug Enhancement of Performance,* Stanford Research Institute, SRI Project No. SU-3024, Office of the Navy, September 15, 1960.

Seashore, Robert H. and A. C. Ivy, *Psychological Monographs: General and Applied,* 67: No. 365, The American Psychological Association, Inc., 1953.

Smith, G. M. and H. K. Beecher, *Journal of the American Medical Association,* 1960, p. 1502.

Sommerville, W., *Canadian Medical Association Journal,* 1946, p. 470.

Tyler, David B., *The American Journal of Physiology,* 1947, p. 253.

EFFECTS OF EXERCISE

Steinhaus, A. H., *Physiological Reviews,* 1933, p. 103.

——, *Toward an Understanding of Health and Physical Education, op. cit.*

EMPHYSEMA

Ambrus, L., *Exercise in Emphysema,* Veterans Administration Hospital, 1965.

ENDOCRINE

Anthony, *op. cit.*

Asimov, I., *The Human Body, Its Structure and Operation,* Houghton Mifflin, 1963.

Otto, J. J. and others, *Modern Health,* Holt, Rinehart and Winston, 1967.

ENERGY COST OF EXERCISE

Asmussen, E., *Acta Physiologica Scandinavica,* 1946, p. 197.

Consolazio, E. F. and others, *Physiological Measurements of Metabolic Functions in Man,* McGraw-Hill, 1963.

Morehouse and Miller, *op. cit.*

Passmore, R. and J. V. G. A. Durnin, *Physiological Reviews,* 1955, p. 801.

Ricci, B., *Physiological Basis of Human Performance,* Lea and Febiger, 1967.

Wells, J. G. and others, *Journal of Applied Physiology,* 1967, p. 51.

ENVIRONMENT
Iampietro, P. F. and others, *Journal of Applied Physiology,* 1960, p. 632.
Karpovich, P. V., *Physiology of Muscular Activity, op. cit.*
Morehouse and Miller, *op. cit.*
Vernon, H. M., *Physiological Reviews,* 1928, p. 130.

Altitude

Balke, B., *Science and Medicine of Exercise and Sports, op. cit.*
Balke, B. and others, *Journal of the American Medical Association,* 1965, p. 646.
Cervantes, J. and P. N. Karpovich, *Research Quarterly,* 1964, p. 446.
Goddard, R. F., *The Effects of Altitude on Physical Performance,* Athletic Institute, 1967.
Shephard, R. J., *Research Quarterly,* 1967, p. 291.
EQUIPMENT
Rodhl, C. W., *Be Fit For Life,* Harper & Row, 1964.
ERGOGENIC AIDS
Cureton, T. K., *Scholastic Coach,* 1959, pp. 24, 26, 48.
Doherty, J. K., *Journal of Health, Physical Education and Recreation,* 1960, pp. 32-33.
Hurt, H. W., *Goals—The Life of Knute Rockne,* Murray Book, 1932.
Johnson, W., *Athletic Journal,* 1953, p. 14.
Karpovich, P. V., *Physiology of Muscular Activity, op. cit.*
——, *Exercise and Fitness,* Athletic Institute, 1960.
Mayer, J. and B. Bullen, *Exercise and Fitness, op. cit.*
Nelson, D. O., *Research Quarterly,* 1959, p. 312.
——, *Research Quarterly,* 1960, p. 627.
——, *Scholastic Coach,* 1961, p. 32.
Samko, W., *Scholastic Coach,* 1963, p. 40.
Upjohn, H. and others, *Journal of the American Medical Association,* 1953, p. 818.
Van Huss, W. D. and others, *Research Quarterly,* 1962, p. 120.
Van Itallie, T. B. and others, *Science and Medicine of Exercise and Sports, op. cit.*
——, *Journal of the American Medical Association,* 1956, p. 1120.

EXCESSIVE EXERCISE
Irwin, T., *Today's Health,* American Medical Association, July, 1966, p. 46.
EXCRETORY SYSTEM
Anthony, *op. cit.*
Asimov, *op. cit.*
Berger, A. J., *Elementary Human Anatomy,* John Wiley and Sons, 1964.
Dayton, O. W., *Athletic Training and Conditioning,* The Ronald Press, 1960.
Easton, D. M., *Mechanisms of Body Functions,* Prentice-Hall, 1963.
Grant, J. C., *An Atlas of Anatomy,* Williams and Wilkins, 1947.
Kahn, F., *Man in Structure and Function,* Alfred A. Knopf, 1960.
Kimber, D. C. and others, *Textbook of Anatomy and Physiology,* Macmillan, 1959.
Lockhart, R. D. and others, *Anatomy of the Human Body,* J. B. Lippincott, 1959.
Wesson, L. G., Jr., *op. cit.*
EXTENSION
Rasch and Burke, *op. cit.*
FATIGUE
Dill, D. B., *Physiological Reviews,* 1936, p. 263.
Karpovich, *Physiology of Muscular Activity, op. cit.*
National Safety Council, Inc., *Practical Methods for Reducing Fatigue,* Safe Practices Pamphlet No. 50, National Safety Council, 1940.
FLEXIBILITY
Colson, J., *Rehabilitation of the Injured,* Cassell, 1949.
Cureton, T. K., *Research Quarterly,* 1941, p. 381.
deVries, *op. cit.*
Fleishman, E., *op. cit.*
Hupperich, F. L. and P. O. Sigerseth, *Research Quarterly,* 1950, p. 25.
Leighton, J., *Archives of Physical Medicine,* 1957, pp. 24, 580.
Munrow, A. D., *Pure and Applied Gymnastics,* Arnold, India, 1963.
Steinhaus, *Toward an Understanding of Health and Physical Education, op. cit.*
Wells, K., *Kinesiology,* W. B. Saunders, 1966.
Wells, K. F. and E. K. Dillon, *Research Quarterly,* 1952, p. 115.
FLEXION
Rasch and Burke, *op. cit.*
FUTURE OF ATHLETIC RECORDS
Jokl, E. and P. Jokl, *The Physiological*

Basis of Athletic Records, Charles C. Thomas, 1968.

GOLF

Bruce, B. and E. Davies, *Beginning Golf,* Wadsworth Publishing, 1962.

Nance, V. L. and E. C. Davies, *Golf,* Wm. C. Brown, 1966.

GROWTH

Adams, E. H., *Research Quarterly,* 1938, p. 102.

Bready, C. F., Jr., *A Study of the Effects of Heavy Resistance upon the Pattern of Muscular Development as Indicated by Strength Endurance, and Girth of the Right Elbow Flexors,* unpublished master's thesis, University of Maryland.

Buskirk, E. R. and others, *Research Quarterly,* 1956, p. 127.

Donaldson, H. H., *American Journal of Anatomy,* 1933, p. 403.

Donaldson, H. H. and R. E. Meeser, *American Journal of Anatomy,* 1932, p. 559.

Evans, F. G., *Stress and Strain,* Charles C. Thomas, 1957.

Gillespie, J. A., *Journal of Bone and Joint Surgery,* 1954, p. 464.

Godin, P., *Growth during School Age* (translated by S. L. Eby), Gorham Press, 1920.

Hatai, S., *Anatomical Record,* 1915, p. 647.

Helander, E. A. S., *Biochemical Journal,* 1961, p. 478.

Montoye, H. J. and others, *Research Quarterly,* 1960, p. 474.

Rarick, G. L., *Science and Medicine of Exercise and Sports, op. cit.*

Rasch, P. J., *Archives of Physical Medicine and Rehabilitation,* 1963, p. 507.

Rasch, P. J. and W. R. Pierson, *Arbeitsphysiologie,* 1963, p. 1.

Simon, E., *Health and Fitness in the Modern World, op. cit.*

Steinhaus, A. H., *Physiological Reviews, op. cit.*

Stewart, D. M., *American Journal of Physiology,* 1962, p. 281.

Tanner, *op. cit.*

Weinmann, J. P. and H. Sicher, *Bones and Bone: Fundamentals of Bone Biology,* C. V. Mosby, 1955.

Wells, J. B. and others, *Journal of the Association for Physical and Mental Rehabilitation,* 1962, p. 69.

————, *Journal of the Association for Physical and Mental Rehabilitation,* 1963, pp. 37, 56.

GUERRILLA EXERCISES

Casady, D. R. and others, *Handbook of Physical Fitness Activities,* Macmillan, 1965.

HANDBALL

Phillips, B. E., *Handball—Its Play and Management,* Ronald Press, 1957.

Yessis, Michael, *Handball,* Wm. C. Brown, 1966.

HANDICAPPED

American Association of Health, Physical Education and Recreation, *Recreation and Physical Activity for the Mentally Retarded,* American Association of Health, Physical Education and Recreation, 1967.

Clarke, H. and D. Clark, *Developmental and Adapted Physical Education,* Harper & Row, 1965.

Daniels, A. S., *Adapted Physical Education,* Harper and Brothers, 1954.

Dolch, E., *Helping Handicapped Children in School,* Barrard Press, 1954.

Fait, H. F., *Adapted Physical Education,* W. B. Saunders, 1960.

Heck, A. O., *The Education of Exceptional Children,* McGraw-Hill, 1953.

Matthews, D. K. and others, *The Science of Physical Education for Handicapped Children,* Harper & Row, 1962.

Stafford, G., *Sports for the Handicapped,* Prentice-Hall, 1947.

Stafford, G. T., and E. D. Kelly, *Preventive and Corrective Physical Education,* Ronald Press, 1958.

HEART DISEASE

Enos, W. F. and others, *Journal of The American Medical Association,* 1955, p. 912.

Karvonen and Barry, *op. cit.*

Proceedings of the International Symposium on Physical Activity and Cardiovascular Health, *Journal of the Canadian Medical Association,* March 25, 1966.

HEART STRAIN

Jokl, E., *Physiology of Exercise, op. cit.*

HEREDITY

Gedda, L., *Health and Fitness in the Modern World, op. cit.*

HIKING AND CAMPING

Clarke, H. H., *Muscular Strength and Endurance in Man,* Prentice-Hall, 1965.

Cox, J., *Camping for All,* Ward, Lock, 1953.

Hunt, J., *Accident Prevention and Life Saving*, E. S. Livingstone, 1965.

Kjellstrom, B., *Be Expert With Map and Compass*, American Orienteering Service, 1955.

Melbourne University Mountaineering Club, *Equipment for Mountaineering*, Melbourne University Mountaineering Club, 1967.

Ministry of Education, *Camping and Education*, H. M. S. O., 1961.

Young, G., *National Heart News*, No. 10, National Heart Foundation of Australia, May, 1966.

HYPOKINETIC DISEASE

Kraus, H. and W. Raab, *Hypokinetic Disease*, Charles C. Thomas, 1960.

INDIVIDUAL RATES OF RESPONSE

Evaul, T. and others, *Basic Concepts of Physical Education*, Temple University Bookstore, 1966.

INFECTION

Jokl, *Physiology of Exercise, op. cit.*

Karpovich, *op. cit.*

INTELLIGENCE

DiGiovanna, V. G., *Research Quarterly*, 1937, p. 96.

Hart, M. and C. T. Shay, *Research Quarterly*, 1964, p. 443.

Ilsley, M. L., *Research Quarterly*, 1940, p. 115.

Johnson, G. B., *Research Quarterly*, 1942, p. 57.

Shaw, J. H. and H. J. Cordts, *Science and Medicine of Exercise and Sports, op. cit.*

INTENSITY OF EXERCISE

Cooper, *op. cit.*

Graham, *op. cit.*

Morehouse and Miller, *op. cit.*

Weiss, R. A. and P. V. Karpovich, *Archives of Physical Medicine*, 1947, p. 447.

ISCHEMIC HEART DISEASE

Graham, *op. cit.*

ISOMETRICS

Bender, J. A. and others, *Journal of Health, Physical Education and Recreation*, May, 1963, p.

JOGGING

Bowerman, W. J. and W. E. Harris, *Jogging*, Grosset and Dunlap, 1967.

KINESIOLOGY

Guyton, A. C., *Function of the Human Body*, W. B. Saunders, 1964.

Rasch and Burke, *op. cit.*

Steindler, A., *Kinesiology of the Human Body*, Charles C. Thomas, 1955.

Wells, K., *op. cit.*

KINESTHESIA

Botelho, S. Y., *Physical Therapy*, 1965, p. 667.

Christina, R. W., *Research Quarterly*, 1967, p. 177.

Divoli, E., *Relationship of Fatigue to Certain Measures of Hand Function and Kinesthesis*, unpublished Doctoral Dissertation, State University of Iowa, 1958.

Gardner, E., *Fundamentals of Neurology*, W. B. Saunders, 1963.

Hellebrandt, F. A., *Cerebral Palsy Review*, 1958, p. 9.

Meday, H. W., The Influence of Practice on Kinesthetic Discrimination, unpublished master's thesis, University of California, 1952.

Mountcastle, U. B. and T. P. S. Powell, Bull. Johns Hopkins Hospital, 1969, p. 201.

Scott, M. G., *Analysis of Human Motion*, Appleton-Century-Crofts, 1963.

Singer, R. N., *Motor Learning and Human Performance*, Macmillan, 1968.

KNEE

Klein, K., *The Knee*, AAHPER, 1965.

LIFETIME SPORTS

Lifetime Sports Offered in Secondary Schools, AAHPER,

Lifetime Sports Education Project, National Recreation and Park Association.

LOAFER'S HEART

Kraus and Raab, *op. cit.*

LONGEVITY

Buskirk, E. R. and J. E. Counsilman, *Science and Medicine of Exercise and Sports, op. cit.*

Chapman, A. L., *U.S. News and World Report*, June 8, 1959, p. 104.

Cureton, T. K., Jr., *Research Quarterly*, 1952, p. 149.

———, *American Journal of Physical Anthropology*, 1954, p. 273.

———, *The Journal of the Association for Physical and Mental Rehabilitation*, 1957, p. 145.

Currens, J. H. and P. D. White, *New England Journal of Medicine*, 1961, p. 988.

Davis, E. C. and others, *Biophysical Values of Muscular Activity*, Wm. C. Brown, 1965.

Hein, F. and A. J. Ryan, *Research Quarterly*, 1960, p. 263.

Jokl, E., *Report of the International Congress on the Essentials of Physical Education for Youth,* AAHPER, 1954.

Jones, H. B., *Handbook of Aging and the Individual,* University of Chicago Press, 1960.

Karvonen, M. J., *Health and Fitness in the Modern World, op. cit.*

Kennedy, J. F., *Sports Illustrated,* December 1960, p. 16.

Mateeff, D., *Health and Fitness in the Modern World, op. cit.*

——, *NAPLA Proceedings,* December, 1964.

Montoye, J. J., *Journal of Michigan State Medical Society,* 1957, p. 589.

——, *Science and Medicine of Exercise and Sports, op. cit.*

Parick, L. C., *Journal of the Michigan State Medical Society,* 1957, p. 589.

Wakefield, M. B., *Research Quarterly,* 1944, p. 2.

Walters, C. E., *Journal of the Michigan State Medical Society,* 1957, p. 589.

White, P. D., *Journal of the American Medical Association,* 1957, p. 70.

LOW BACK PAIN

Rules to Live By—From Now On, McNeal Laboratories.

LYDIARD TRAINING SYSTEM

Doherty, J. K., *Modern Training for Running,* Prentice-Hall, 1964.

MASSAGE

Dayton, *op. cit.*

MECHANICAL DEVICES

Steinhaus, A., *Toward an Understanding of Health and Physical Education, op. cit.*

MENSTRUATION

AAAU, *Effects of Athletic Competition in Girls and Women,* AAAU, 1953. Cited in *Practitioner,* 177:73, 1956.

Astrand, P. O. and others, *Acta Paediatrica,* 1963.

Harris, R. and C. Walters, *Research Quarterly,* May, 1955.

MENTAL HEALTH

Carter, Gerald C., *School Review,* 1940, p. 127.

Clarke, H. H. and D. J. Clark, *Research Quarterly,* 1961, p. 326.

Cowell, C. C. and A. H. Ismail, *Research Quarterly,* 1962, p. 40.

Layman, E. M., *Journal of Health, Physical Education and Recreation,* 1957, p. 22.

——, *Mental Health Through Physical*

Education and Recreation, Burgess Publishing, 1955.

Menninger, W. C., *Recreation,* 1948, p. 340.

Merriman, J., *Research Quarterly,* 1960, p. 163.

Michael, E. D., *Research Quarterly,* 1957, p. 50.

Mohr, D. R., *Fitness for the Individual,* Bureau of Correspondence Study State University of Iowa, 70, undated.

Schendel, J., *Research Quarterly,* 1965, p. 52.

Scott, M. G., *Research Quarterly,* 1960, p. 313.

Seymour, E., *Research Quarterly,* 1956, p. 338.

Slusher, H. S., *Research Quarterly,* 1964, p. 539.

Tillman, K., *Research Quarterly,* 1965, p. 483.

Ulrich, C., *Research Quarterly,* 1957, p. 160.

Zion, L. C., *Research Quarterly,* 1965, p. 490.

METABOLISM

Cooper, *op. cit.*

deVries, *op. cit.*

Karpovich, *Physiology of Muscular Activity, op. cit.*

Morehouse and Miller, *op. cit.*

Rice, B., *op. cit.*

MIDDLE AGE

Astrand, P. O., *Physiological Reviews,* 1956, p. 307.

Buskirk and Counsilman, *Science and Medicine in Exercise and Sports, op. cit.*

Shock, *op. cit.*

MOTIVATION

Olson, A. L., *Pennsylvania Journal of Health, Physical Education and Recreation,* June, 1967, p. 14.

MOTOR ABILITY

Cureton, T. K., *Journal of Health, Physical Education and Recreation,* March 1945, p. 11.

MOTOR EDUCABILITY

Cratty, B., *Movement Behavior and Motor Learning,* Lea and Febiger, 1964.

MOTOR FITNESS

Clarke, H. H., *Application of Measurement to Health and Physical Education,* Prentice-Hall, 1967.

Roper, R. B., *Movement and Thought,* Blackie and Son, 1938.

Muller, A., *Ergonomics,* 1965, p. 409.

MUSCLE CRAMPS
Karpovich, P., *Physiology of Muscular Activity, op. cit.*

MUSCLE ENDURANCE
Clarke, H., *Muscular Strength and Endurance in Man*, Prentice-Hall, 1966.

MUSCLE TONE
Basmajian, J. V., *Muscle Alive*, Williams and Wilkins, 1967.

MUSCLES, SKELETAL
Anthony, *op. cit.*
Gray, H., *Anatomy of the Human Body*, Lea and Febiger, 1959.
Morehouse and Miller, *op. cit.*

NUTRITION
Diehl, H. S., *Healthful Living*, Mc-Graw-Hill, 1964.
Morehouse, and Miller, *op. cit.*
National Research Council, *The Role of Nutrition in International Programs*, National Academy of Sciences, July, 1961.
Van Itallie and others, *Science and Medicine in Exercise and Sports, op. cit.*

OBESITY
Barney, V. S. and others, *Conditioning Exercises*, C. V. Mosby, 1965.
Bauer, W. W., *Today's Health Guide*, American Medical Association, 1965.
Browe, J. H., *Preventive Medicine*, W. B. Saunders, 1965.
Bullen, B. A. and others, *American Journal of Clinical Nutrition*, 1964, p. 211.
Corbin, C. B., *Abstracts of Research Papers*, AAHPER, 1967.
Dempsey, J. A., *Research Quarterly*, 1964, p. 275.
Goodhart, R. S. and M. G. Wohl, *Manual of Clinical Nutrition*, Lea and Febiger, 1964.
Guthrie, H. A., *Introductory Nutrition*, C. V. Mosby, 1967.
Jalliffee, N., *Reduce and Stay Reduced*, Simon and Shuster, 1963.
Johnson, M. L. and others, *American Journal of Clinical Nutrition*, 1956, p. 231.
——, *American Journal of Clinical Nutrition*, 1956, p. 37.
Marks, H. H., *Bulletin of New York Academy of Medicine*, 1960, p. 15.
Mayer, J., *The New England Journal of Medicine*, 1966, pp. 24, 31.
——, *Science and Medicine of Exercise and Sports, op. cit.*
U. S. Department of Health, Education and Welfare, *Obesity and Health*, U. S. Government Printing Office.
Wohl, M. B. and R. S. Goodhart, *Modern Nutrition in Health and Disease*, Lea and Febiger, 1960.

ORIENTEERING
Disley, J., *Orienteering*, Stackpole Books, 1967.

OVERTRAINING
Wolf, W., *Health and Fitness in the Modern World*, Athletic Institute, 1961.

OXYGEN DEBT AND OXYGEN INTAKE
deVries, *op. cit.*
Henry, F. M., *Physiology of Work*, University of California Associated Students Store, 1950.
Karpovich, *Physiology of Muscular Activity, op. cit.*

OXYGEN REQUIREMENTS
Hill, A. V. and H. N. Lupton, *Quarterly Journal of Medicine*, 1923, p. 135.
Hill, A. V. and others, *Muscular Exercise, Lactic Acid and the Supply and Utilisation of Oxygen*, Proc. Roy. Soc., 1924-1925, p. 438, 455, 155.

PERSONALITY
Behrman, R. M., *Research Quarterly*, 1967, p. 163.
Bendien, J. and J. Groen, *Journal of Psychosomatic Research*, 1963, p. 11.
Booth, E. G., *Research Quarterly*, 1958, p. 127.
Brozek, J. and others, Paper presented at the Conference on the Biology of Human Variation, February 11-13, 1965.
Cathey, C. and others, *The American Journal of Medical Sciences*, 1962, p. 421.
Cattell, R. B., *Exercise and Fitness, op. cit.*
Flanagan, L., *Research Quarterly*, 1951, p. 312.
Harlow, R. G., *Journal of Personality*, 1951, p. 312.
Havel, R. C., Proceedings of the 62nd Annual Meeting of the College Physical Education Association, 1959.
Hellerstein, H. K. and A. B. Ford, *Circulation*, 1960, p. 1166.
Henry, F. M., *Psychological Bulletin*, 1941, p. 745.
Johnson, W. R. and others, *Research Quarterly*, 1954, p. 484.
Kemple, C., *Psychosomatic Medicine*, 1945, p. 85.
Kroll, W., *Research Quarterly*, 1967, p. 49.

Lakie, W. L., *Research Quarterly*, 1962, p. 566.

LaPlace, J. P., *Research Quarterly*, 1954, p. 313.

McPherson, B., *The Psychological Effects of an Exercise Program for Post-Cardiac and Normal Adult Men*, unpublished master's thesis, London, Ontario, University of Western Ontario, 1965.

———, *Journal of Sports Medicine and Physical Fitness*, 1967, p. 95.

New, H. N., *Geriatrics*, 1958, p. 640.

Schendel, J., *Research Quarterly*, 1965, p. 52.

Slusher, H. S., *Research Quarterly*, 1964, p. 539.

Sperling, A., *Research Quarterly*, 1942, p. 351.

Thune, J. B., *Research Quarterly*, 1949, p. 296.

Tillman, K., *Research Quarterly*, 1965, p. 483.

Whiting, H. T. and D. E. Stembridge, *Research Quarterly*, 1965, p. 348.

Wilder, R. M., *General Practitioner*, 1964, p. 115.

PHYSICAL FITNESS

Cureton, T. K. and others, *Physical Fitness Appraisal and Guidance*, C. V. Mosby, 1947.

PREGNANCY

Erdelji, G. J., *Journal of Sports Medicine*, 1962, p. 174.

Pfeifer, W. A., *Practitioner*, 1956, p. 73.

PROGRAMS

Cooper, *op. cit.*

Mathews, D. K., *Beginning Conditioning*, Wadsworth Publishing, 1965.

President's Council on Physical Fitness and Sports, *Adult Physical Fitness*, Superintendent of Documents, U. S. Government Printing Office.

Royal Canadian Air Force, *5BX Plan for Physical Fitness*, Queen's Printer and Controller of Stationery, 1963.

———, *XBX Plan for Physical Fitness*, Queen's Printer and Controller of Stationery, 1963.

PULSE RATE

Brouha, L. and E. T. Radford, Jr., *Science and Medicine of Exercise and Sports*, *op. cit.*

Bruce, R. A. and others, Rodale's *Health Bulletin*, January-February, 1965.

Graham, *op. cit.*

RACES

Baker, P. T. and R. W. Newman, *American Journal of Physical Anthropologists*, 1957, p. 601.

Bayley, N., *Child Development*, 1965, p. 379.

Broman, G. E. and others, *American Journal of Physical Anthropologists*, 1958, p. 197.

Cobb, W. M., *Journal of Negro Education*, 1934, p. 340.

Codwell, J. E., *Journal of Negro Education*, 1949, p. 452.

Connolly, J. A., *A Comparison of the Buoyancy of Negro and White High School Girls as It Affects Swimming Power*, unpublished master's thesis, State University of Iowa, Iowa City, 1965.

Damon, A., *Human Biology*, 1966, p. 380.

Damon, A. and others, *American Journal of Physical Anthropologists*, 1962, p. 461.

Espenschade, A., *Child Development*, 1946, p. 245.

———, *Research Quarterly*, 1958, p. 274.

Fraley, L. M., *Comparison of the General Athletic Ability of White and Negro Men of College Age*, unpublished doctoral dissertation, George Peabody College for Teachers, Nashville, Tenn., 1939.

Glass, B., *American Journal of Human Genetics*, 1955, p. 368.

Hampton, M. C. and others, *American Journal of Clinical Nutrition*, 1966, p. 422.

Herzstein, J. N., *A Comparison of the Jumping Ability of American Negro Male College Students with American White Male College Students as Measured by the Sargent Vertical Jump Test*, unpublished master's thesis, University of Maryland, 1961.

Hrdlicka, A., *Anthropological Investigations on One Thousand White and Colored Children of Both Sexes, the Inmates of the New York Juvenile Asylum, with Additional Notes on One Hundred Colored Children of the New York Colored Orphan Asylum*, Anthropological Report on New York Juvenile Asylum, 1900.

———, *American Journal of Physical Anthropologists*, 1928, p. 15.

Hutinger, P. W., *Research Quarterly*, 1959, p. 366.

Johnston, F. E., *Annals of New York Academy of Science*, 1966, p. 507.

Karpinos, B. D., *Human Biology*, 1961, p. 335.

Knobloch, H. and B. Pasamanick, *Journal of Genetic Psychology*, 1953, p. 137.

Krogman, W. M., *Height, Weight and Bodily Growth of American White and American Negro Boys of Philadelphia, Age 6-14 Years*, Growth Center, Philadelphia, 1959.

——, *Height, Weight and Bodily Growth of American White and American Negro Girls of Philadelphia, Age 6-14 Years*, Growth Center, Philadelphia, 1959.

Laeding, L., *Assessment of the Difference in Power, Agility, Strength and Reaction Time of Negro and White Male Subjects at the Tenth Grade Level*, unpublished master's thesis, Michigan State University, 1964.

Lane, E. C., *Research Quarterly*, 1964, p. 21.

Malina, R. M., *Human Biology*, 1966, p. 89.

——, *New Perspectives of Man in Action*, Prentice-Hall in press.

Malina, R. M. and F. E. Johnston, *Research Quarterly*, 1967, p. 219.

Marino, A., *Anthropometric Measurements in the Lower Leg of White and Negro High School Boys in Relation to Vertical Jumping Ability*, unpublished master's thesis, University of Oklahoma, Norman, Oklahoma, 1966.

Meredith, H. V., *Human Biology*, 1952, p. 290.

Metheny, E., *Research Quarterly*, 1939, p. 41.

Montpetit, R. R. and others, *Research Quarterly*, 1967, p. 231.

Newman, R. W., *Human Biology*, 1956, p. 154.

Ohlson, M. A. and others, *Body Measurements and Human Nutrition*, Wayne University Press, 1956, pp. 79-92.

Piscopo, J., *Research Quarterly*, 1962, p. 255.

Ponthieux, N. A. and D. G. Barker, *Research Quarterly*, 1965, p. 468.

Rhodes, A., *Child Development*, 1937, p. 369.

Roberts, D. F., *American Journal of Human Genetics*, 1955, p. 361.

Sessoms, J. E., *Common Motor Abilities of Negro Preschool Children*, unpublished master's thesis, State University of Iowa, 1942.

Smith, M., *Life*, October 23, 1964, p. 81.

Steggerda, M. and C. E. Petty, *Research Quarterly*, 1940, p. 110.

——, *Research Quarterly*, 1942, p. 275.

Steinkamp, R. C., *California Health*, 1965, p. 113.

Stern, C., *Scientific American*, October, 1954, p. 80.

Tanner, J. M., *The Physique of the Olympic Athlete*, George Allen and Unwin, 1964.

Todd, T. W., *Human Biology*, 1929, p. 57.

Trotter, M. and others, *The Leech*, 1958, p. 139.

——, *American Journal of Physical Anthropologists*, 1959, p. 19.

——, *Journal of Bone and Joint Surgery*, 1960, p. 50.

Williams, J. R. and R. B. Scott, *Child Development*, 1953, p. 103.

REHABILITATION

Clark, H. and D. H. Clarke, *op. cit.*

Delagi, E. F. and others, *Physical Therapy Review*, January, 1955, p. 1.

Howorth, M. B., *Journal of Bone and Joint Surgery*, October, 1963, p. 7.

Jokl, E., *The Clinical Physiology of Physical Fitness and Rehabilitation*, Charles C. Thomas, 1958.

Kottke, F. J., *Journal of the American Medical Association*, 1966, p. 825.

Krusen, F. H. and others, *Handbook of Physical Medicine and Rehabilitation*, W. B. Saunders, 1965.

Wessel, V. A. and W. Van Huss, *Science and Medicine of Exercise and Sports, op. cit.*

RELAXATION

Jacobson, E., *Progressive Relaxation*, Lippincott, 1964.

——, *Anxiety and Tension Control*, University of Chicago Press, 1938.

——, *Tension Control for Businessmen*, McGraw Hill, 1963.

RESPIRATION

Morehouse and Miller, *op. cit.*

ROPE SKIPPING

Baker, J. A., *Research Quarterly*, 1968, p. 240.

Jones, D. M. and others, *Research Quarterly*, 1962, p. 236.

ROWING

International Rules of Rowing, Fédération Internationale des Sociétés d'Aviron, Switzerland.

Scott, A. C. and J. G. P. Williams (ed.), *Rowing—A Scientific Approach,* Kaye and Ward, Ltd., 1967.

SAILING

American National Red Cross, *Basic Sailing,* The American National Red Cross, 1966.

McDermott, T. J., *Manual of Sailboat Racing,* Macmillan, 1964.

SAUNA

Fornoza, A. and C. G. Salgada, *Health and Fitness in the Modern World,* The Athletic Institute, 1961.

Huikko, M. and others, *Acta Physiologica Scandanavia,* 1966, p. 316.

SCUBA DIVING

Ciampi, E., *The Skin Diver,* Ronald Press, 1960.

Conference for National Cooperation in Aquatics, *The New Science of Skin and Scuba Diving,* Association Press, 1962.

Superintendent of Documents, *United States Navy Diving Manual,* NAVSHIPS 250-538, United States Government Printing Office, 1958.

SECOND WIND

Karpovich, *Physiology of Muscular Activity, op. cit.*

Morehouse and Miller, *op. cit.*

SKIING

Editors of Ski Life Magazine, *Ski Pointers by the Experts,* Harper & Row, 1961.

Editors of Ski Magazine, *The Skiers Handbook,* Harper & Row, 1965.

SKILL

Lundervold, A., *Health and Fitness in the Modern World,* Athletic Institute, 1961.

Nettleton, B. and E. Sandstrom, *Australian Journal of Physical Education,* November, 1963, p. 17.

Steinhaus, A., *Journal of Health and Physical Education,* 1931, p. 217.

——, *Physiological Reviews, op. cit.*

Welford, F., *Discovery,* July, 1962, p. 27.

SKIN DIVING

Conference for National Cooperation in Aquatics, *The New Science of Skin and Scuba Diving,* Association Press, 1962.

Tailliez, P. and others, *The Complete Manual of Free Diving,* G. P. Putnams, 1957.

Tillman, A., *Skin and Scuba Diving in*

Underwater Education, Wm. C. Brown, 1962.

SMOKING

Cooper, K. H., *op. cit.*

Cooper, K. H. and others, *Journal of the American Medical Association,* January 15, 1968, p. 123.

Mathews, D. K. and others, *Physiology of Muscular Activity and Exercise,* Ronald Press, 1965.

Morehouse and Miller, *op. cit.*

Royal College of Physicians Report, *Smoking and Health,* Royal College of Physicians, 1962.

SOCIAL CONTEXT

Broom, L. R. and P. Selunick, *Sociology, A Text With Adapted Readings,* Harper & Row, 1963.

Caillois, R., *Man, Play and Games,* Free Press, 1961.

Cartwright, D. and A. Zander, *Group Dynamics: Research and Theory,* Row, Peterson, 1960.

Coleman, J. S., *The Adolescent Society,* Free Press of Glencoe, 1961.

Mills, C. W., *Power, Politics, and People,* Ballantine Books, 1963.

Rosen, B. C., *American Sociological Review,* 1959, p. 47.

Sears, R. R. and others, *Patterns of Child Rearing,* Row, Peterson, 1957.

SPEED

Deford, F., *Sports Illustrated,* May 22, 1967, p. 34.

deVries, *op. cit.*

SQUASH

Hawkey, R. B., *Improving Your Squash,* Faber & Faber, 1967.

Mattick, W., *Squash—An Introduction,* Turner and Henderson Pty., Ltd., 1963.

McCausland, A., *The Step to Squash Success,* W. and K. Purhrieh, 1962.

STRENGTH

Hettinger, T., *Physiology of Strength,* Charles C. Thomas, 1961.

Obeck, V., *How to Exercise Without Moving a Muscle,* Pocket Books, 1964.

Steinhaus, A., *How to Keep Fit and Like It, op. cit.*

STRESS AND PHYSICAL FITNESS

Selye, H., *The Stress of Life,* McGraw-Hill, 1956.

Ulrich, C., *Science and Medicine of Exercise and Sports, op. cit.*

TARGET TRAINING

Lewis, A. S., *The Journal of Physical*

Education of Great Britain and Northern Ireland, Vol. 53, No. 158, 1959.

——, New Zealand Journal of Physical Education, No. 18, 1959.

TENNIS

Jaeger, Eloise M. and Harry "Cap" Leighton, Teaching of Tennis, Burgess Publishing, 1960.

TESTS

Carlson, H. C., Research Quarterly, October, 1945, p. 169.

Cooper, Aerobics, op. cit.

Karpovich, Physiology of Muscular Activity, op. cit.

TRAINING

Klafs, C. and D. Arnheim, Modern Principles of Athletic Training, C. V. Mosby, 1963.

Morehouse and Miller, op. cit.

Morehouse and Rasch, Sports Medicine for Trainers, op. cit.

Wallis, E. L. and G. A. Logan, Figure Improvement and Body Conditioning Through Exercise, Prentice-Hall, 1964.

WALKING

Sussman, A. and R. Goode, The Magic of Walking, Simon and Schuster, 1968.

WATER SKIING

Hardman, T. C. and W. D. Clifford, Let's Go Water Skiing, Hawthorn Books, 1965.

Hilligan, E. and G. E. Maxwell, Today's Health, August, 1966, p. 40.

WEIGHT CONTROL

Mayer, J. and F. J. Stare, The Journal of the American Dietetic Association, 1953, p. 340.

Pollack, H. and others, Journal of the American Medical Association, 1958, p. 216.

Steinhaus, A., Toward an Understanding of Health and Physical Education, op. cit.

WEIGHT LOSS IN SPORTS

Ahlman, K. and M. J. Karvonen, Journal of Sports Medicine and Physical Fitness, 1962, p. 58.

Byram, H. M., Effect of Weight Reduction on Strength and on Muscular Endurance, unpublished master's thesis, State University of Iowa, 1953.

Doscher, N., Research Quarterly, 1944, p. 317.

Edward, J. B., A Study of the Effect of Semi-Starvation and Dehydration on Strength and Endurance with Reference to College Wrestlers, unpublished master's thesis, University of North Carolina, 1951.

Kuntzleman, C. T., The Effects of 1200 Calorie Diets and Partial Dehydration on Selected Neuromuscular and Cardiovascular Performances of Well-Conditioned College Men, unpublished master's thesis, Temple University, 1965.

Nichols, H., The Effect of Rapid Weight Loss on Selected Physiologic Responses of Wrestlers, unpublished doctoral dissertation, University of Michigan, 1957.

Rasch, P. and W. Kroll, What Research Tells the Coach About Wrestling, American Association of Health, Physical Education and Recreation, 1965.

Tuttle, W. W., Research Quarterly, 1943, p. 158.

WEIGHT TRAINING AND WEIGHT LIFTING

Amateur Athletic Union, Weight Lifting, AAU, Annual.

Massey, B. H., The Kinesiology of Weight Lifting, Wm. C. Brown, 1959.

Rasch, P. J., Weight Training, Wm. C. Brown, 1966.

INDEX